Third Edition

Rehabilitation
of the
Coronary
Patient

Edited by

Nanette Kass Wenger, M.D.
Professor
Division of Cardiology
Department of Medicine
Emory University School of Medicine
Director
Cardiac Clinics
Grady Memorial Hospital
Atlanta, Georgia

Herman K. Hellerstein, M.D.
Professor
Division of Cardiology
Department of Medicine
Case Western Reserve University School of Medicine
Attending Physician
University Hospitals of Cleveland
Cleveland, Ohio

Churchill Livingstone
New York, Edinburgh, London, Melbourne, Tokyo

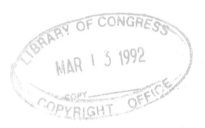

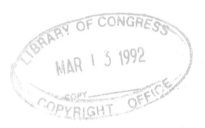

Library of Congress Cataloging-in-Publication Data

Rehabilitation of the coronary patient / edited by Nanette Kass
Wenger, Herman K. Hellerstein. — 3rd ed.
        p. cm.
    Includes bibliographical references and index.
    ISBN 0-443-08765-2
    1. Coronary heart disease—Patients—Rehabilitation. I. Wenger,
Nanette Kass. II. Hellerstein, Herman K., date.
    [DNLM: 1. Myocardial Infarction—rehabilitation. WG 300 R3455]
RC 685.C6R44 1992
616.1'23'03—dc20
DNLM/DLC
For Library of Congress   91-34216
                                                        CIP

Third Edition © Churchill Livingstone Inc. 1992
Second Edition © Churchill Livingstone Inc. 1984
First Edition © John Wiley & Sons Inc. 1978

Distributed in the United Kingdom by Churchill Livingstone, Robert Stevenson
House, 1–3 Baxter's Place, Leith Walk, Edinburgh EH1 3AF, and by associated
companies, branches, and representatives throughout the world.

Accurate indications, adverse reactions, and dosage schedules for drugs are provided in this book, but it is possible that they may change. The reader is urged to
review the package information data of the manufacturers of the medications
mentioned.

The Publishers have made every effort to trace the copyright holders for borrowed material. If they have inadvertently overlooked any, they will be pleased
to make the necessary arrangements at the first opportunity.

Acquisitions Editor: *Avé McCracken*
Copy Editor: *Elizabeth Bowman-Schulman*
Production Designer: *Angela Cirnigliaro*
Production Supervisor: *Christina Hippeli*

Printed in the United States of America

To Julius Wenger, M.D.
and
Mary Hellerstein, M.D.

Contributors

Thomas G. Allison, Ph.D., M.P.H.
Assistant Professor, Division of Cardiovascular Diseases, Department of Internal Medicine, Mayo Medical School; Consultant, Division of Cardiovascular Diseases, Department of Internal Medicine, Mayo Clinic, Rochester, Minnesota

William F. Armstrong, M.D.
Associate Professor, Department of Internal Medicine, University of Michigan Medical School; Director, Echocardiography Laboratory, University of Michigan Hospital, Ann Arbor, Michigan

Gary J. Balady, M.D.
Associate Professor, Department of Medicine, Boston University School of Medicine; Director, Cardiovascular Exercise Center and Cardiac Rehabilitation, The University Hospital, Boston, Massachusetts

George A. Beller, M.D.
Head, Division of Cardiology; Professor, Department of Medicine, University of Virginia School of Medicine, Charlottesville, Virginia

Kathy Berra, B.S.N.
Director, YMCA Cardiac and Pulmonary Rehabilitation, Palo Alto, California

Richard A. Carleton, M.D.
Professor, Department of Medicine, Brown University Program in Medicine, Providence, Rhode Island; Physician-in-Chief, Memorial Hospital of Rhode Island, Pawtucket, Rhode Island

Patricia McCall Comoss, R.N., B.S.
Nurse Consultant for Cardiac Rehabilitation, Nursing Enrichment Consultants, Inc., Harrisburg, Pennsylvania

Mark W. Connolly, M.D.
Assistant Professor, Division of Cardiothoracic Surgery, Department of Surgery, Emory University School of Medicine; Cardiothoracic Surgeon, Division of Cardiothoracic Surgery, Department of Surgery, Emory University Affiliated Hospitals, Atlanta, Georgia

Michael J. Cowley, M.D.
Professor, Division of Cardiology, Department of Internal Medicine, Virginia Commonwealth University Medical College of Virginia School of Medicine, Richmond, Virginia

Anthony N. DeMaria, M.D.
Professor and Chief, Division of Cardiology, University of Kentucky College of Medicine, Lexington, Kentucky

Gordon A. Ewy, M.D.
Professor and Associate Head, Department of Internal Medicine, Director, University Heart Center, and Chief, Section of Cardiology, University of Arizona College of Medicine, Tucson, Arizona

Barry A. Franklin, Ph.D.
Associate Professor, Department of Physiology, Wayne State University School of Medicine, Detroit, Michigan; Director, Cardiac Rehabilitation and Exercise Laboratories, Division of Cardiology, William Beaumont Hospital, Royal Oak, Michigan

Seymour Gordon, M.D.
Clinical Professor, School of Health Sciences, Oakland University, Rochester, Michigan; Medical Director, Cardiac Rehabilitation and Exercise Laboratories, Division of Cardiology, William Beaumont Hospital, Royal Oak, Michigan

Robert A. Guyton, M.D.
Professor and Chief, Division of Cardiothoracic Surgery, Department of Surgery, Emory University School of Medicine; Chief, Division of Cardiothoracic Surgery, Department of Surgery, Emory University Affiliated Hospitals, Atlanta, Georgia

Larry F. Hamm, Ph.D.
Lecturer, Division of Kinesiology, School of Kinesiology and Leisure Studies, University of Minnesota; Exercise Physiologist, Cardiovascular Consultants, Ltd., Minneapolis, Minnesota

William L. Haskell, Ph.D.
Professor, Division of Cardiovascular Medicine, Department of Medicine, Stanford University School of Medicine, Stanford, California

Herman K. Hellerstein, M.D.
Professor, Division of Cardiology, Department of Medicine, Case Western Reserve University School of Medicine; Attending Physician, University Hospitals of Cleveland, Cleveland, Ohio

David L. Herbert, J.D.
Senior Partner, Herbert, Benson and Scott, Attorneys and Counselors–at–Law, The Belpar Law Center, Canton, Ohio

William G. Herbert, Ph.D.
Director, Cardiac Therapy and Intervention Center; Professor, Division of Health and Physical Education, Virginia Polytechnic Institute and State University, Blacksburg, Virginia

J. Willis Hurst, M.D.
Professor, Division of Cardiology, and former Chairman, Department of Medicine, Emory University School of Medicine, Atlanta, Georgia

Thomas E. Kottke, M.D.
Associate Professor, Division of Cardiovascular Diseases, Department of Internal Medicine, Mayo Medical School; Consultant, Department of Cardiology and Health Sciences Research, Mayo Clinic, Rochester, Minnesota

Jules Lam, M.D.
Assistant Professor, Department of Medicine, University of Montreal Faculty of Medicine; Cardiologist, Montreal Heart Institute, Montreal, Quebec, Canada

Richard W. Lee, M.D.
Assistant Professor, Division of Cardiovascular Diseases, Department of Internal Medicine, Mayo Medical School, Rochester, Minnesota; Consultant, Division of Cardiovascular Diseases, Department of Internal Medicine, Mayo Clinic Scottsdale, Scottsdale, Arizona

Stephen Lenhoff, M.B. Ch. B.
Assistant Professor, Division of Cardiology, University of Kentucky College of Medicine, Lexington, Kentucky

Arthur S. Leon, M.D.
Henry L. Taylor Professor of Exercise Science and Health Enhancement, Division of Kinesiology, School of Kinesiology and Leisure Studies, College of Education, and Division of Epidemiology, School of Public Health, University of Minnesota; Chief Cardiologist, Heart Prevention Clinic, Department of Medicine, University of Minnesota Medical School—Minneapolis, Minneapolis, Minnesota

Nancy Houston Miller, R.N., B.S.
Program Nurse Director, Stanford Cardiac Rehabilitation Program, Stanford University School of Medicine, Stanford, California

Barbara Packard, M.D., Ph.D.
Associate Director for Scientific Program Operation, National Heart, Lung, and Blood Institute, National Institutes of Health, Bethesda, Maryland

Chris Papadopoulos, M.D.
Clinical Associate Professor, Department of Medicine, University of Maryland School of Medicine; Chief of Cardiology, Department of Medicine, Harbor Hospital Center, Baltimore, Maryland

Fredric J. Pashkow, M.D.
Medical Director of Cardiac Health Improvement and Rehabilitation, Department of Cardiology, The Cleveland Clinic Foundation, Cleveland, Ohio

Charles E. Rackley, M.D.
Professor, Division of Cardiology, Department of Medicine, Georgetown University Medical Center, Washington, D.C.

William C. Roberts, M.D.
Chief, Pathology Branch, National Heart, Lung, and Blood Institute, National Institutes of Health, Bethesda, Maryland

M. Nagui Sabri, M.D.
Assistant Professor, Division of Cardiology, Department of Medicine, Virginia Commonwealth University Medical College of Virginia School of Medicine, Richmond, Virginia

John L. Shuster, M.D.
Assistant Professor, Department of Psychiatry and Behavioral Neurobiology, University of Alabama at Birmingham School of Medicine, Birmingham, Alabama

Hugh C. Smith, M.D.
Professor, Division of Cardiovascular Diseases, Department of Internal Medicine, Mayo Medical School; Consultant and Chair, Division of Cardiovascular Diseases, Department of Internal Medicine, Mayo Clinic, Rochester, Minnesota

Ray W. Squires, Ph.D.
Assistant Professor, Division of Cardiovascular Diseases, Department of Internal Medicine, Mayo Medical School; Consultant, Division of Cardiovascular Diseases, Department of Internal Medicine, and Director, Cardiovascular Health Clinic, Mayo Clinic, Rochester, Minnesota

Theodore A. Stern, M.D.
Associate Professor, Department of Psychiatry, Harvard Medical School; Psychiatrist and Director, Resident Psychiatric Consultation Service, Massachusetts General Hospital, Boston, Massachusetts

Mario Talajic, M.D.
Assistant Professor, Department of Medicine, University of Montreal Faculty of Medicine, Montreal, Quebec, Canada

C. Barr Taylor, M.D.
Professor, Department of Psychiatry and Behavioral Sciences, Stanford University School of Medicine, Stanford, California

George E. Tesar, M.D.
Assistant Professor, Department of Psychiatry, Harvard Medical School; Associate Psychiatrist and Director, Acute Psychiatry Service, Department of Psychiatry, Massachusetts General Hospital, Boston, Massachusetts

Gerald C. Timmis, M.D.
Clinical Professor of Health Sciences (Medical Physics), Oakland University, Rochester, Michigan; Medical Director of Clinical Research, Division of Cardiology, William Beaumont Hospital, Royal Oak, Michigan

David Waters, M.D.
Associate Professor, Department of Medicine, University of Montreal Faculty of Medicine; Cardiologist, Montreal Heart Institute, Montreal, Quebec, Canada

Donald A. Weiner, M.D.
Associate Professor, Department of Medicine, Boston University School of Medicine; Director, Exercise Laboratory, The University Hospital, Boston, Massachusetts

Nanette Kass Wenger, M.D.
Professor, Division of Cardiology, Department of Medicine, Emory University School of Medicine; Director, Cardiac Clinics, Grady Memorial Hospital, Atlanta, Georgia

Byron R. Williams, Jr., M.D.
Clinical Assistant Professor, Department of Medicine, Emory University School of Medicine; Director, Cardiac Services; Director, Department of Nuclear Cardiology, St. Joseph's Hospital of Atlanta, Atlanta, Georgia

Preface to the Third Edition

During the seven years since the publication of the Second Edition of Rehabilitation of the Coronary Patient in 1984, the management of patients with coronary heart disease, with and without myocardial infarction, has changed dramatically. These changes have been designed to reduce mortality; decrease emotional, physical, sexual, and vocational morbidity and disability; and to improve the patients' quality of life. Contributing to these changes have been better understanding of and insight into factors influencing the pathogenesis, progression, regression, and manifestations of coronary artery atherosclerotic disease; earlier recognition of myocardial ischemia and dysfunction; earlier use of coronary angiography; and improvement of coronary blood flow and revascularization to conserve myocardium by coronary thrombolysis, coronary angioplasty, coronary atherectomy and laser techniques, and by coronary artery bypass surgery. Also of importance have been the applications of multifaceted evaluative studies at rest and with exercise (echocardiography; imaging of myocardial dynamics, perfusion, and metabolism by positron emission tomography, magnetic resonance imaging, computed tomography, etc.); shortened periods of bed rest and hospitalization; and implementation of exercise training to enhance the functional capacity and prognosis of coronary patients, including both low- and high-risk subgroups, the elderly, and even patients after heart transplantation.

The extraordinary growth of our knowledge and advances in the care of coronary patients since the Second Edition of this book has necessitated extensive rewriting and rearrangement of almost every chapter in the Third Edition. However, the basic objectives of delineating the components of comprehensive care and rehabilitation of the patient with coronary heart disease (i.e, presenting the multi-disciplinary nature of optimal rehabilitation as addressed in the First and Second Editions) have been preserved.

Throughout the Third Edition, emphasis has been placed on the importance of individualization of the process of coronary rehabilitation, on the increased scope of patients eligible for rehabilitative care (e.g., elderly patients, patients with congestive heart failure, those with implanted pacemakers and/or cardioverter defibrillators, and following heart transplantation); and on the changing characteristics of exercise rehabilitation (i.e., earlier time of onset, lesser intensity, variable sites of exercise training and amounts of professional supervision) and the dependency of these aspects on risk classification or stratification of coronary patients.

Several chapters have been devoted to pharmacologic therapy, including coronary thrombolysis; newer imaging techniques (radionuclide testing, positron emission tomography, magnetic resonance imaging), to clinical aspects and rehabilitation of coronary heart disease in women and in the elderly, reflecting major demographic changes in the U.S. population; and to associated psychological, personality, and sexual problems.

Sections have been expanded that address myocardial revascularization: coronary angioplasty, coronary atherectomy, coronary bypass surgery, and other surgical procedures for coronary heart disease and its complications, including implantation of pacemakers and cardiac defibrillators and heart transplantation.

Several chapters of this edition have been devoted to risk characterizations. Risk factors have been identified and quantitated that determine the progression and regression of coronary artery atherosclerotic disease, which in turn influence the need for specific therapies and suggest the likelihood of efficacy of coronary risk factor changes. Risk attributes have been delineated that contribute to the discrepancy between functional capacity as determined at work evaluation and the successful return to work. High-risk characteristics have been established (low functional capacity, impaired ventricular function, decreased ejection fraction, exercise-induced myocardial ischemia and dysfunction, and complex arrhythmias) that influence prognosis and therefore many aspects of clinical decision-making. Evidence is presented that conventional coronary risk reduction and behavioral approaches, often utilizing new technology, for the education and counseling of coronary patients can result in improved survival, lesser morbidity, and retardation and even reversal (regression) of the underlying process of coronary atherosclerosis.

We acknowledge with gratitude the enthusiastic acceptance and application of the concepts and recommendations of the First and Second Editions by national and international colleagues and students; and the adoption and incorporation of guidelines for rehabilitative care by several national professional societies. The authors of the chapters for this edition, selected both for their acknowledged expertise and their excellence in communication, have more than fulfilled our expectations in forging the gateway to the rehabilitation of the coronary patient in the twenty-first century. We express our appreciation to them and their respective secretaries. Our sincere appreciation goes to Avé McCracken and the staff at Churchill Livingstone, who facilitated the timely completion of a multi-authored book and served as liaison among the editors, authors, and publisher.

A special acknowledgment is due Vera M. Husselman of Dr. Hellerstein's office.

To Julia Wright and Jeanette Zahler in the "Atlanta Office," our admiration and appreciation for their skills in organization and coordination, their meticulous attention to detail and accuracy, their precision in verification of references and citations, their tireless proofreading and correction of galleys, and their provision of encouragement and emotional support to authors attempting to meet deadlines or respond to last-minute queries for additional information or clarification. Their caring has likely contributed to improved patient care.

Nanette Kass Wenger, M.D.
Herman K. Hellerstein, M.D.

Preface to the Second Edition

As emphasized in a recent United Nations report, "the more a society recognizes that disability will create a cost, regardless of whether or not rehabilitation services exist, and the more it attempts to ameliorate the social effects of disability, whether on the basis of humanitarian concern or socioeconomic planning, the greater is the overall economic return to society."

In recent years, the rehabilitative approach to the coronary patient has become increasingly incorporated into routine clinical care in the United States. This is attested to in the results of a recent physician survey.[1] During the past decade, general practitioners, internists, and cardiologists have altered their management of patients with myocardial infarction in a manner designed to limit disability and improve functional status. Among these changes in the pattern of care are earlier ambulation during the hospitalization and earlier discharge when appropriate, early angiography leading to coronary artery bypass surgery for appropriately selected patients, increased use of exericse testing to assess function, application of pharmacotherapy and exercise training (as well as coronary surgery) to enhance both prognosis and functional capacity, and increased education of the patient and family about preventive and therapeutic aspects of coronary disease.

The national professional societies have reemphasized the importance of the rehabilitative approach in the management of patients with symptomatic coronary disease and have provided guidance both to the practicing physician and to the health care community in the form of specific standards and guidelines for rehabilitative services.[2-6] These data and recommendations, with methods for their implementation, are incorporated in the second edition of this text.

The scope of the rehabilitative approach to the coronary patient has undergone a remarkable expansion since the first edition of this book was published. This is due in large part to the development and application of a variety of diagnostic and therapeutic procedures and techniques relating to coronary disease. Morphologic aspects of atherosclerotic coronary artery disease have been defined that may influence the potential role of thrombolytic therapy. There is increasing emphasis on stratification of risk, that is, identification of patients excessively susceptible to recurrent events, in an attempt to improve their outlook by pharmacologic, exercise, and surgical treatments.

Many of these advances in the care of patients are included in the expanded second edition. There is an update of the traditional medical management of the patient with myocardial infarction. Considerable insight and experience have developed regarding early ambulation and patient education. The noninvasive evaluation of coronary patients by echocardiography, ambulatory electrocardiography, and radionuclide myocardial imaging is discussed. Much has been learned about the varied roles of exercise testing, and the procedure is an accepted standard of care. The concept of prescribed exercise is also a validated approach, and advances have been made in the design of safe, effective, and practical exercise programs. Considerable attention is directed to coronary artery bypass surgery, which has fulfilled its promise as a beneficial rehabilitative procedure; guidelines are available for selection of patients, preoperative management, and physical, psychologic, and pharmacologic components of care.

New problems and opportunities that have occurred since publication of the first edition have mandated attention to such diverse areas as the rehabilitation of aged coronary patients, patients with congestive heart failure, patients with implanted pacemakers, and those after cardiac transplantation. It is expected that these areas will become increasingly important in the near future. Included are the delineation of the research data that form the basis for contemporary medical decision making and suggested plans for the application of this new information in the care of coronary patients.

Several exciting developments are not addressed in this volume because of their limited clinical application to date: positron emission tomography in delineating information about myocardial metabolism; nuclear magnetic resonance imaging in measuring blood flow velocities and in identifying cardiac structures and studying myocardial metabolism and energy transfer; reduction of coronary artery obstruction by thrombolysis, angioplasty or laser techniques; ambulatory blood pressure monitoring; newer medications, including modifications of current beta-adrenergic blocking and calcium-entry blocking preparations; behavior modification, biofeedback or operant conditioning, and so forth.

We may reasonably expect current research to provide, within the next several years, considerable new information regarding myocardial metabolism and contractility, the genesis and potential reversal of atherosclerosis, the noninvasive quantification of coronary atherosclerosis, the role of the nervous system and personality in atherogenesis, and the value of alternate choices of behavior in influencing the development of coronary disease, arrhythmias, and sudden cardiac death. These may be topics for a third edition.

We have attempted to maintain the multidisciplinary appeal of the text, because optimal rehabilitative care of the coronary patient requires an interdisciplinary effort. We acknowledge with gratitude the enthusiastic acceptance of the first edition by our colleagues and students, which encouraged our preparation of this updated version. The authors of the chapters, selected both for their acknowledged expertise and their skills in communication, have more than fulfilled our expectations; we would also like to thank their respective secretaries. A special acknowledgment is due Vera Husselman of Dr. Hellerstein's office. Our appreciation goes to John de Carville, formerly of John Wiley & Sons, who launched the second edition, and Ray Moloney, who shepherded it to completion with the able assistance of Clara Perez and Audrey Pavey.

To Julia Wright and Jeanette Zahler in the "Atlanta office" our sincerest appreciation and admiration for their skills in organization, their attention to detail and accuracy in typing, verification of references, and proofreading; and their patience with us. The authors and their manuscripts, as well as the publisher's deadlines, have been a part of their lives for over two years.

Nanette Kass Wenger, M.D.
Herman K. Hellerstein, M.D.

References

1. Wenger NK, Hellerstein HK, Blackburn H, and Castranova SJ: Physician practice in the management of patients with uncomplicated myocardial infarction—Changes in the past decade. Circulation 65:421, 1982.

2. Subcommittee on Rehabilitation. Target Activity Group: The Exercise Standards Book. American Heart Association, 70-041-A, 1979

3. Subcommittee on Exercise/Rehabilitation. Target Activity Group: Standards for supervised cardiovascular exercise maintenance programs. Circulation 62:669A, 1980

4. Council on Scientific Affairs: Physician-supervised exercise programs in rehabilitation of patients with coronary heart disease. JAMA 245:1463, 1981

5. American College of Sports Medicine. Guidelines for Graded Exercise Testing and Exercise Prescription. Lea & Febiger, Philadelphia, 1980

6. Coronary Heart Disease Study Group: Optimal resources for the care of patients with acute myocardial infarction and chronic coronary heart disease. Circulation 65:654B, 1982

Preface to the First Edition

One of the most exciting features of the rehabilitative approach to the cardiac patient during the past decade has been the establishment of its validity and its acceptance and progressive incorporation into the mainstream of traditional medical care.

We have witnessed the increasing use of exercise testing to evaluate objectively function and responses to various types of therapy and the subsequent institution of exercise training programs to improve the patient's functional capacity. Equally significant attention is currently being focused on the psychosocial factors affecting the patient after myocardial infarction, since these factors often contribute more to disability than physiologic impairment. Patient, public, and professional educational efforts have begun, appropriately, to emphasize that most patients after myocardial infarction and after aortocoronary bypass surgery can and should return to their customary normal or near-normal lifestyle. Aortocoronary bypass surgery has also received increasing acceptance as a sound method of rehabilitation.

The rehabilitative approach should begin at the onset of illness and remain as a continuing feature in the long-term care of the patient; however, the initiation and coordination of rehabilitation efforts must be the responsibility of the patient's primary physician, although he may utilize the knowledge, skills, techniques, and services of a variety of medical consultants and health care professionals to implement the actual rehabilitative processes.

The important components of myocardial infarction rehabilitative programs include physical activity, functional evaluation, prescriptive training, patient and family education, and psychosocial and vocational counseling.

This book is designed to provide background information about the physiologic, medical, and social problems associated with myocardial infarction, to present insight into the scientific bases for rehabilitation programming, and to furnish a detailed description of a realistic rehabilitative approach to the patient after myocardial infarction. It is hoped that the primary care physician and other members of the health team will find the presentations helpful in improving the care of their patients who have sustained a myocardial infarction or who have undergone aortocoronary bypass surgery. The clinical advent of coronary atherosclerotic heart disease is overwhelming because of the residual functional impairment, both physiologic and psychologic. Appropriate attention is directed to the recognition, assessment, prevention, and management of this impairment.

Several currently developing methods are not included in this book because their practical application to rehabilitation, although promising, is not yet established. These methods include isotopic myocardial imaging scanning, radionuclide cineangiography, ventricular systolic intervals, psychologic (quiz) stress testing, etc.

In the text, the terms *heart attack* and *myocardial infarction* are used synonymously, and the terms *heart patient* and *cardiac patient* are used interchangeably. The individual identified as a *myocardial infarction patient* or a *coronary patient* is considered to have *coronary atherosclerotic heart disease*. Finally, *primary care physician* designates the individual responsible for the continuing care of the patient; this individual may be an internist, cardiologist, family physician, etc.

It is our hope that the readers will share our view that the health sciences are entering the dawn of the scientific era of rehabilitation, which encompasses basic and clinical sciences and humanism.

We would like to express our gratitude to Betty Martin for the administrative coordination of the text; she served as liaison among editors, authors, and publisher, shepherding the myriad of details required for the coordination of a multiauthored book. Special appreciation goes to Julia Wright for verifying references, typing manuscripts, responding to authors' concerns, and working with Betty Martin in the proofreading and correction of galleys. Special thanks also go to Vera Husselman, Charline Hutton, and Elaine Shaw for typing chapters. And we give sincerest appreciation to John Wiley & Sons, particularly John de Carville, Ruth Wreschner, and Margery Carazzone for their ongoing encouragement, help, and expertise.

We would like to thank the specialists who contributed to this text. They are leaders in their respective fields of endeavor and have painstakingly summarized the newest knowledge in each area, emphasizing scientific background information and application to patient care.

Nanette Kass Wenger, M.D.
Herman K. Hellerstein, M.D.

Contents

Background Information

1

Coronary Heart Disease: The Overview of a Clinician

J. Willis Hurst, M.D.

The clinician's approach to the recognition of coronary atherosclerotic heart disease was rather passive until the era of modern technology. Prior to the development of coronary angiography in the late 1950s, a diagnostic problem was solved by edict; when a history of chest discomfort was confusing, it was settled by asking an "authority" to render the final opinion. Master's two-step exercise test was sometimes used. Now the problem is usually settled by coronary angiography and nuclear scanning.

The ability to delineate the coronary anatomy and, in turn, to identify many different clinical syndromes (subsets) has converted clinicians into aggressive warriors who fight the disease rather than passive observers of the natural history of a very serious condition. Accordingly, new methods of treatment have been devised including drugs, coronary bypass surgery and percutaneous transluminal coronary angioplasty (PTCA).

The new aggressiveness of clinicians has not been limited to the diagnosis and treatment of the disease, but has been extended to the prevention of the condition itself. Although the concept of prevention was emphasized as far back as the late 1940s, it is now being taught to every man, woman, and child in the United States.

So, we clinicians have become more aggressive warriors against coronary atherosclerotic heart disease. Our ammunition is powerful, and, as with any powerful ammunition, we must be careful how we use it.

The items discussed above dominate the current medical scene. Because of this, I have selected five of my favorite subjects for more detailed discussion.

DEFINITIONS OF WORDS AND TERMS

There was a time when the definitions of medical words and terms were relatively unimportant. This is not true today, because, as clinical syndromes are clarified and divided into subsets, it is important to know the precise definitions of the words and terms used to identify and discuss them. A subset becomes important when it can be defined, linked to specific pathophysiology, and, in turn, linked to specific treatment. For example, the conditions known as stable and unstable angina pectoris are different, yet both of them are subsets of coronary atherosclerotic heart disease.

This is not the place for a lengthy discussion of all the subsets of coronary atherosclerotic heart disease. The interested reader is referred to a

3

more detailed discussion of this point.[1] The point is that we must not be flippant in our use of the words and terms used to describe the subsets of clinical syndromes caused by coronary atherosclerotic heart disease.

The poor understanding of the meaning of words can cause other types of mischief. In the early 1950s, the medical world heralded the first chemical test for myocardial necrosis.[2] The physicians who described the serum glutamic-oxaloacetic transaminase (SGOT) test for myocardial necrosis were disturbed when members of the profession used the test improperly. Some physicians would state that the patient had no coronary artery disease when the SGOT test result was normal, even though the patient had retrosternal discomfort that lasted 20 minutes and had a history of angina pectoris. The physicians who made this serious error did not perceive the difference in the terms *coronary artery atherosclerosis* and *coronary atherosclerotic heart disease*.

Coronary atherosclerosis may be present for years before it becomes sufficiently severe to produce myocardial ischemia. Such patients have atherosclerosis of the *coronary arteries* but do not have coronary atherosclerotic heart disease. The patient with evidence of myocardial ischemia due to coronary atherosclerosis is said to have coronary atherosclerotic *heart disease*. This occurs when the internal diameter of a coronary artery is narrowed to about 50%. It may also be said to be present when there is a high-grade (90% diameter) narrowing of a coronary artery but overt myocardial ischemia is avoided because of abundant collateral circulation or marked limitation of physical activity. In this situation, however, it should be remembered that ischemia of the myocardium is present, even if not identified as a syndrome, because collateral vessels are present; collateral vessels will not develop or persist without the stimulus of chronic ischemia.

Readers may say that we have come a long way and that mistakes related to the misuse of such words are not made today. Bear with me as I relate an example of the modern counterpart of the misinterpretation of the same words. This favorite story of mine is retold here with the permission of the Emory University Journal of Medicine.[3] Suppose a coronary angiogram is performed in a patient with chest discomfort in an effort to determine whether the discomfort is due to myocardial ischemia caused by coronary atherosclerosis. The angiographer reports only "luminal irregularity" of one coronary artery. The jargon is understood by other angiographers, cardiologists, and cardiac surgeons, but may not be understood by physicians who do not use such language daily. These physicians may not understand that "luminal irregularity" implies that there is angiographic evidence of a small amount of coronary artery atherosclerosis but does not imply that there is coronary atherosclerotic heart disease. The patient must not be labeled, from this information alone, as having coronary heart disease. Such an error can ruin a patient's life.

This example serves to illustrate that we must not use words, as Humpty Dumpty did, to mean anything we wish them to mean.[4] Words must be used with care, and terms must be carefully defined.

CLASSIFICATION OF HEART DISEASE

Paul Dudley White deserves the credit for insisting that it is necessary for the physician to classify a patient's heart disease in a specified manner in order to be certain that a *complete cardiac diagnosis* is made. A complete diagnosis is needed to understand the cardiovascular problem, its treatment, and its impact on the patient's life. Paul White considered his publication on this subject, written with Werrell Myers in 1921, to be one of his most important contributions to cardiology.[5] He originally required that the physician identify the etiology, the anticipated pathology of the disorder, and the functional status of the patient in order to create the complete diagnosis. The New York Heart Association (NYHA) recognized the importance of the views of White and others and published its first book, *Criteria for the Classification and Diagnosis of Heart Disease*, in 1928.[6] The Criteria and Nomenclature Committee of the NYHA prepared eight editions of the book. For many years the complete cardiac diagnosis was defined as having

Table 1-1. New York Heart Association Classification of a Complete Diagnosis of Cardiovascular Disease (Prior to 1973)

Etiology	
Anatomy	Functional capacity[a]
Physiology	Therapeutic

[a] The old "functional capacity" was abandoned in 1973[7] and has been replaced by "cardiac status and prognosis" (see Table 1-2).

Table 1-2. New York Heart Association Classification of a Complete Diagnosis of Cardiovascular Disease (After 1973)

Etiology	
Anatomy	Cardiac status and prognosis[a]
Physiology	Specific recommendations

[a] The old "functional capacity" category was abandoned in 1973.[7] The new category, "cardiac status and prognosis," is created by utilizing all of the clinical data that are available, rather than symptoms alone.

four parts: etiology, anatomy, physiology, and function. Function was determined by the symptoms of a patient. The symptoms being assessed were *angina* due to myocardial ischemia and *dyspnea* due to heart failure. The functional classification that was used until 1973 is shown in Table 1-1.[7]

By 1973 the Nomenclature Criteria Committee of the NYHA recognized that new technology had produced new insights into the understanding of cardiovascular disease.[7] The members recognized several things: (1) that symptoms alone could not always be used to indicate the seriousness of heart disease; (2) that heart failure due to serious heart disease could occur and that a patient might have little dyspnea; (3) that "mild" angina did not always indicate "mild" coronary atherosclerotic heart disease; and (4) that the result of exercise electrocardiogram (ECG) testing, the use of radionuclear technology, the determination of the ejection fraction, and the location and extent of the atherosclerotic lesions determined angiographically determined the seriousness of coronary disease; and that an estimate of seriousness should not be based on symptoms alone. Accordingly, the separate functional status of the classification was abandoned in 1973 and replaced by *cardiac status*.[7] The difference in the two terms is that the old *functional status* was determined by symptoms only, whereas the new *cardiac status* is determined by integrating *all* of the data into the final appraisal of the patient (Table 1-2).

Does this imply that a functional assessment is not needed? Of course not! The Canadian Cardiovascular Society Classification (CCSC) of angina pectoris is used almost universally now.[8] The CCSC classification of angina pectoris is

shown in Table 1-3.[8] It should be listed under the *physiologic* portion of the complete cardiac diagnosis. Should dyspnea due to heart failure be a problem, it can be graded as mild, moderate, or severe or the old classification of the NYHA can be used. The class designation of heart failure should be listed in the physiologic portion of the complete cardiac diagnosis; it is not listed as a separate category.

We are all influenced by carefully conducted clinical trials. The patients entering a clinical trial must be carefully chosen to fit the well-thought-out guidelines. The physician who ap-

Table 1-3. The Canadian Cardiovascular Society's Classification of Angina Pectoris[a]

1. Ordinary physical activity does not cause . . . angina, such as walking and climbing stairs. Angina with strenuous or rapid or prolonged exertion at work or recreation.
2. Slight limitations of ordinary activity. Walking or climbing stairs rapidly, walking uphill, walking or stair climbing after meals, or in cold, or in wind, or under emotional stress, or only during the few hours after awakening. Walking more than two blocks on the level and climbing more than one flight of ordinary stairs at a normal pace and in normal conditions.
3. Marked limitation of ordinary physical activity. Walking one to two blocks on the level and climbing one flight of stairs in normal conditions and at normal pace.
4. Inability to carry on any physical activity without discomfort—anginal syndrome may be present at rest.

[a] This classification of angina pectoris has replaced the New York Heart Association's classification.
(From Campeau,[8] with permission.)

plies the results of a clinical trial to his or her patients must select patients who are similar to those who participated in the trial. Patients who are entered into most clinical trials must have a specified etiology for their disorder, a specified cardiac anatomy, and specified altered physiology. Accordingly, we must be skilled in identifying these attributes in patients with heart disease, including those with coronary atherosclerotic heart disease. Obviously, the skills of examination must be maintained in order to create complete diagnoses, otherwise clinical trials cannot yield accurate information.

Therefore, it is important that we learn to classify patients with heart disease, including those with coronary atherosclerotic heart disease, with reproducible precision. The NYHA method of doing so stimulates the physician to think deeply about his or her patients. It is important, however, to appreciate the change in the NYHA classification that was published in 1973.[7] It is also necessary to maintain the skills required to accurately classify patients, both for use in practice and in order that clinical trials may be implemented with precision.

EVOLVING CONCEPTS

Etiology of Atherosclerosis

The etiology of coronary atherosclerosis is not known. It is clear, however, that many factors are involved in the creation of obstructive coronary artery lesions. Some of the factors may incite the process while other factors may simply accelerate it. The field of molecular biology is churning with activity and excitement. For example, we now realize that endothelial cells are busy creatures. They do far more than form the inside limit of the coronary arteries; they generate a substance that can dilate the coronary arteries and another substance that stimulates myocardial contractility.

The work of Ross forms the basis for the following scenerio.[9] The atherosclerotic lesion may begin when the endothelium becomes injured. The cause of the injury is not known, but it is undoubtedly multifactorial. Low-density lipro-

tein (LDL) from the blood enters the subendothelial area, where it becomes oxidized. Just how the oxidation takes place is now the subject of much research. However it happens, the oxidized LDL is more toxic than native LDL. Monocytes in the blood dive through the cracks in endothelial cells and enter the subendothelial portion of the arteries. They seem to be attracted there by the oxidized LDL and other substances. The monocytes become macrophages and begin their cleanup duties; they engulf the LDL. The macrophages become foam cells. All of this activity creates a bulge into the lumen of the artery known as a fatty streak; it is the earliest sign of atherosclerosis. The more advanced atherosclerotic lesions are produced by additional mechanisms. The macrophages deteriorate, leaving the oxidized LDL, which produces further damage to the endothelium. Platelets clump together like a platoon of soldiers in an effort to protect the injured endothelium. The endothelial cells and monocytes, in addition to the platelets, produce growth factors that become involved in the process that is designed to repair the injury to the inner surface of coronary artery. The growth factors also stimulate the smooth muscle cells to increase in number and pass outside of the natural wall of the artery into the developing plaque. Platelets, as well as the endothelial cells, produce substances that constrict and dilate the coronary arteries. Although the repair process itself is needed, it seems to run amok, and when this occurs the artery becomes obstructed. Finally, when a coronary artery becomes sufficiently narrow and when other factors such as coronary spasm occur, a thrombus may develop to produce the final blockade to coronary blood flow. It is now accepted that a thrombus usually occus in an obstructed artery to produce myocardial infarction. It is also highly likely that a thrombus contributes to the syndrome of unstable angina, especially when the angina is recent in onset.

The players in this dramatic scene are more precisely identified than formerly, but the monologue of each character and the dialogue between them is still not perfectly understood by those who observe the play. Despite this, the overall plot is understood. Still missing are the identity of the playwright who called the players together in the first place (inciting cause and causes) and the way to stop the play when it gets out of hand. For example, enthusiastic extras may be in the wings ready to run on stage and produce havoc. This is why the hypothesis of Steinberg et al, Beyond Cholesterol, is so important.[10]

So, as we clinicians struggle to understand coronary atherosclerotic heart disease, we should divide our study into four parts. They are lipoprotein metabolism, the molecular biology of the intima, the clotting mechanism, and the multiple causes of coronary artery spasm.

In summary, it is necessary to watch the players involved in atherosclerosis carefully because the exact culprit is not yet known. New characters are about to enter the play, and, when they do, they may provide the missing link to the mystery regarding the etiology of atherosclerosis. In the meantime, a conglomerate approach to the prevention of the disease is prudent. This includes not smoking, maintaining normal blood pressure, achieving desirable levels of serum cholesterol and LDL, and performing the appropriate amounts of exercise.

Active and Inactive Stages of the Atherosclerotic Process

There is an active and an inactive stage of the atherosclerotic process. Some high-grade obstructive lesions may not progress. Of the patients with high-grade lesions in the left main coronary artery or high-grade triple vessel lesions, 10 to 20% are alive 10 years or longer after the discovery of the lesions. On the other hand, a 50% diameter obstruction of a single artery may become a 90% obstructive lesion within 6 months to 1 year. A patient may have a 90% diameter obstruction in one coronary artery and a 40% obstruction in another artery, and with the passage of time the 90% diameter obstruction may remain unchanged and the lesion that formerly produced a 40% diameter obstruction of a coronary artery may progress so that the artery becomes totally occluded. There is evolving recognition that some lesions may even regress. Additionally, patients may have angina pectoris for several years

and may then be free of angina pectoris for years, only to have it return later.

The controlling factors that determine the onset of the active and inactive phases of the disease are not known. The practical value of this perception is obvious. Unstable angina is a signal that an active phase of the disease is in progress. This is why balloon dilatation during the early stage of unstable angina may produce total occlusion of the artery more often than it will in patients with stable angina. The growth factors described earlier are already active in patients with unstable angina. Accordingly, when the endothelial and subendothelial area is damaged by balloon dilatation, even more rapid repair appears to be stimulated, and so the overgrowth of the repair process, as well as other factors, closes the artery. It is therefore important to understand that the activity of the atherosclerotic process seems to wax and wane in the same individual. The factors controlling this activity are not known.

The Supply-Demand Concept

Stable angina pectoris occurs when the atherosclerotic obstructive process is either inactive or progressing so slowly that collateral circulation is able to keep pace with the obliterative process. Angina pectoris is produced when the heart muscle needs more blood (oxygen) as a result of an increase in myocyte work but the obstructed artery cannot deliver the amount of blood (oxygen) that is needed. In effect, there is a mismatch between the amount of blood (oxygen) needed by the myocardium and the amount delivered by the coronary arteries. Stable angina pectoris is said to be present when the angina has not changed in 60 days.

Unstable angina pectoris occurs when, during an active phase of the atherosclerotic process, there is rapid narrowing of a coronary artery. The development of collateral circulation is too slow to compensate for the impaired coronary artery blood flow caused by the rapid obstruction of the coronary arteries. Angina pectoris may occur at rest or after less effort than when the atherosclerotic process is inactive. Unstable angina is said to be present when angina occurs for the first time, when it has developed during the last 60 days, or when stable angina is increasing in frequency or occurs after less effort.

When the obstruction occurs suddenly in a major coronary artery and persists for a sufficient period, *myocardial necrosis (myocardial infarction)* may occur.

In summary, it has long been accepted that certain clinical syndromes are created when the myocardium has an increased need for oxygen and that other syndromes are due to a decrease in coronary arterial supply of oxygen to the myocardium. At times, the latter syndromes are related to a rapid growth phase of obstructing atherosclerotic lesions (including thrombosis). Therapy is determined by the physician's perception of the presence of these mechanisms.

The Ischemic Cascade

Nesto and Kowalchuk[11] emphasized the abnormalities that occur when the left ventricle becomes ischemic and remains so for a time. The initial abnormality produced by ischemia is diastolic dysfunction of the left ventricle. The ventricle becomes less compliant; i.e., it becomes stiff. The next abnormality to develop is systolic dysfunction, which is followed by a rise in diastolic pressure in the left ventricle. The ECG may then show ST segment displacement, and finally the patient may have angina pectoris.

Although this exact sequence of abnormalities may not be evident in every example of myocardial ischemia, it is an excellent model to illustrate why certain clinical abnormalities occur. For example, the patient with *silent ischemia* has either an abnormal exercise ECG or thallium scan, and the patient who has *anginal equivalents* may experience dyspnea on effort, acute pulmonary edema due to a rise in the left ventricular diastolic pressure, or exhaustion due to a decrease in cardiac output. Silent ischemia may also occur at rest or with the ordinary activities of daily living. These conditions may occur during the early stages of ischemia before angina pectoris occurs.

Obviously, if the ischemia of the ventricular myocardium continues for a sufficient period, the myocytes die; i.e., a myocardial infarction develops. So, when the chest discomfort that is characteristic of myocardial ischemia is present for 20 minutes or more, it is highly likely that a certain number of myocytes have died, even when the ECG or serum creatine kinase (CK) determinations do not reveal signs of myocardial infarction. We must remember that a finite number of myocytes must die before the ECG becomes abnormal or the serum cardiac enzymes become elevated. Stable angina pectoris usually lasts one to several minutes. It subsides when the effort that produced it ceases and the ischemic heart muscle returns to normal. Prolonged chest discomfort that lasts 20 minutes or more should not be labeled angina pectoris but should be called *prolonged myocardial ischemia with or without ECG or laboratory (CK elevation) signs of infarction.*

It can also be stated that *dead myocytes don't hurt.* This realization has considerable clinical value because, when the chest discomfort that is consistent with myocardial ischemia recurs in the setting of myocardial infarction, it is a signal that more myocytes are in danger of dying and, at times, that specific therapeutic measures are needed to save the ischemic, but not yet dead, myocytes.

Therefore, knowledge of the effect of the ischemic cascade on the working myocytes enables one to understand the development of silent ischemia, anginal equivalents, certain ECG abnormalities, angina pectoris, and myocardial infarction.

Coronary Artery Spasm

In 1957 Prinzmetal et al.[12] described the clinical syndrome of variant angina pectoris due to coronary artery spasm. In 1948, Frank Wilson and Franklin Johnston[13] described a patient who developed angina pectoris and ST segment displacement whenever he smoked a cigarette; they attributed the condition to coronary artery spasm.

It appears that *Prinzmetal's angina,* a syndrome of coronary artery spasm, occurs most often in patients with obstructive coronary atherosclerosis. As a rule, the angina occurs at rest and tends to recur at the same time each day. The ST segment elevation occurs during the episode and resolves as the angina subsides. This observation is the best clue that coronary artery spasm has occurred. Some patients may have ST segment elevation at some time and ST segment depression at others. Atrioventricular block may occur. Transient abnormal Q waves may also occur; this clue to a "stunned" myocardium was first observed many decades ago. When the chest discomfort is prolonged, it is difficult to separate the syndrome from an ordinary acute myocardial infarction when thrombolytic therapy has been given, because the ST segment abnormality may subside spontaneously in Prinzmetal's angina and may subside when thrombolytic therapy is successful in patients with infarction.

Coronary artery spasm without coronary atherosclerosis should be suspected in young people with angina pectoris or infarction who smoke. Coronary spasm may also occur as a result of using cocaine.

An internal mammary artery graft and a venous graft used in bypass surgery may undergo spasm during and perhaps after the postoperative period.

Although typical Prinzmetal's syndrome is characterized by recurrent angina pectoris, I suspect, but cannot prove, that an isolated episode of intense coronary artery spasm may cause sudden death or myocardial infarction in rare patients in whom the coronary angiogram is normal.

In summary, coronary artery spasm can play a role whether or not coronary atherosclerosis is present.

Isoembolism

When a thrombus forms in a diseased coronary artery, it may be the source of an embolus that travels to a more distal portion of the same artery. This may be more likely to occur when there is moderate dilatation of the coronary artery above or below the obstructed area. It is especially likely to occur when there is a saccular aneurysm of the coronary artery.

Isoembolism may be responsible for ischemic cardiomyopathy due to coronary atherosclerosis in some patients. It may also explain why some patients with obstruction of the left anterior descending coronary artery have ECG signs of inferior myocardial infarction rather than of an anterior infarction. The left anterior descending coronary artery of such patients "wraps around" the left ventricle and supplies coronary blood flow to the inferior surface of the left ventricle.[14] So, when an embolus obstructs the distal part of the artery, it produces an inferior infarction. Finally, isoembolism may occur following balloon dilatation of an atheromatous obstruction of a coronary artery.

The above discussion shows that isoembolism of a coronary artery is not rare; it may be the cause of ischemic cardiomyopathy, unusual infarctions, and infarction after PTCA.

DETERMINATION OF THE PRETEST PROBABILITY THAT CHEST DISCOMFORT IS DUE TO CORONARY ATHEROSCLEROTIC HEART DISEASE

Heberden described angina pectoris in 1766.[15] This antedated Jenner's identification that angina could be caused by coronary atherosclerosis.[16] It also preceded Burns' physiologic explanation for the syndrome.[17] Only one autopsy was performed in Heberden's patients, and, even through the pathologist did not know what to look for, he reported that the arteries were normal. It is highly likely that some of Heberden's patients did not have coronary atherosclerosis. Some of the patients probably had aortic valve stenosis or cardiomyopathy (including hypertrophic cardiomyopathy), and some of the patients who did not die probably had noncardiac causes of chest discomfort. It has been clear for at least a century that some patients with characteristic Heberden's angina do not have coronary atherosclerotic heart disease and that some patients with chest discomfort that was not characteristic of Heberden's angina did, in fact, have coronary atherosclerotic heart disease. This is why the term *atypical angina pectoris* is confusing and it should not be used (see the discussion of predictive value).

Coronary angiography will undoubtedly be accepted as one of the greatest technologic advances of this century, and Mason Sones[18] deserves credit for its development. This new tool permitted physicians to measure their ability to determine the presence or absence of coronary atherosclerotic heart disease after analyzing the chest discomfort of patients. When all patients with chest discomfort were considered, the ability of the physician to correctly determine that the discomfort was due to coronary atherosclerotic heart disease was about 75%.[19,20] In other words, 25% of patients with chest discomfort who were thought to have angina pectoris due to coronary atherosclerotic heart disease in fact did not have it. The accuracy varied according to the characteristics of the symptoms and the age and sex of the patients studied. This finding led to the concept that it is important to establish the pretest probability that a patient's chest discomfort is caused by coronary atherosclerotic heart disease. It was soon learned that no symptoms had a predictive value of 100%. It was also learned that the pretest probability that angina pectoris was present could be estimated and that the estimate could be used to determine the technology that should be used to clarify the problem.

The problem was studied by workers at the Cleveland Clinic[19] and by our group at Emory University.[20] The following discussion is based on these studies.

Classification of Patients with Chest Discomfort

It is possible to divide patients with chest discomfort into five groups according to the characteristics of the chest discomfort, their age, and their gender.

Group 1. This group is typified by a *man* who is *45 years old* (or older) who has at least a 2-month history of recurrent retrosternal chest discomfort lasting 1 to 3 minutes, produced by effort and relieved by rest. The history is easy to obtain, and the relationship of the discomfort to effort is definite. The chances are 90% or greater that the patient is having episodes of *stable angina pectoris*. The same is true when the discomfort is felt in the throat, lower jaw, left arm, left elbow, wrist, or precordial area. It is the relationship to effort that is the diagnostic feature of the clinical syndrome. Two additional points should be made about the patient who has a history of recurrent retrosternal discomfort for more than 2 months. The patient has had ample time to study the reproducibility of the discomfort; he can confirm that the discomfort is produced by effort. In addition, he has usually noted that he experiences the discomfort when he walks up a slight incline but not when he walks on level ground.

Group 2. This group is typified by a *man* who is *45 years old* (or older) who has had retrosternal chest discomfort for more than 2 months. He does not know the exact duration of the discomfort, nor is he certain what precipitates the discomfort. He is vague regarding the reproducibility of the discomfort. He does not know whether walking up a small incline produces the discomfort but walking on level ground does not. The predictive value of this type of history indicating *stable angina pectoris* due to coronary atherosclerotic heart disease is about 75%. The same would be true for a woman older than 55 years. When the discomfort has been present for a short period, say 1 to 7 days, and the history is vague, the predictive value of the complaint indicating coronary atherosclerotic heart disease is about 75%. This clinical syndrome must be managed carefully because, if it is *unstable angina pectoris*, it is far more serious and demands more intense treatment than stable angina pectoris.

Group 3. This group is typified by a woman who is younger than 45 years and who has chest discomfort produced by effort and relieved by rest. She may also have discomfort at rest. There is no history in women this age that has a predictive value in indicating coronary atherosclerotic heart disease that is greater than 50%.

Group 4. The middle-aged patient who has persistent retrosternal discomfort for the first time must be considered to be having myocardial infarction until proven otherwise.[21] A normal ECG does not exclude a myocardial infarction and the subsidence of the discomfort after administration of a gastric antacid does not prove that the discomfort is due to esophageal reflux (heartburn). About 80% of patients with acute myocardial infarction will exhibit abnormal ECG signs of infarction and will be candidates for immediate thrombolytic therapy. Also, we must never forget that myocardial infarction may be present but the ECG may not reveal it.

Group 5. A man or woman of any age may have "sticks and stabs" of chest discomfort that last no longer than the time it takes to snap the fingers.[22] Such discomfort is not due to coronary atherosclerotic heart disease. Even if the patient has coronary atherosclerotic heart disease, such symptoms are not related to it. A man or woman of any age may have precordial discomfort that lasts for hours.[23] They experience the discomfort day after day. This type of discomfort is not due to coronary atherosclerotic heart disease.

The proper selection of high technology is determined by the physician's ability to judge the pretest probability that a certain clinical syndrome is present.

Group 1 Patients

Patients in group 1 should, unless there are noncardiac contraindications to the test, have a coronary angiogram performed as the initial procedure.[23] The test is not done to determine the presence of coronary atherosclerosis because the predictive value of the history indicating the presence of the disease is more than 90%. It is done in an effort to judge the seriousness of the disease, establish a prognosis, and determine whether PTCA, coronary bypass surgery, or medical treatment should be implemented. An exercise ECG or exercise thallium scan is not indicated because it will not answer the question the physician is asking and, in addition, there is some small danger associated with exercising some patients.

Group 2 Patients

The patients in group 2 may be tested in several different ways, but certain exceptions must be known. A man with a history that has a predictive value of 75% may, if the discomfort has been present for more than 2 months, have an exercise ECG or an exercise thallium scan.[24] The latter yields results that are more sensitive and more specific, but the test may not always be available. If the exercise test is abnormal, a coronary angiogram is indicated. If, in a local setting, coronary angiography is more reliable than exercise testing, it is proper to have a coronary angiogram performed as the initial procedure.

Whenever the discomfort has been present for only a few days, it is proper to have a coronary angiogram performed rather than have one of the exercise tests. This is because, even though the predictive value of the patient's history is only 75%, the chest discomfort must be regarded as being unstable angina until proven otherwise. It is not wise to exercise a patient who might have unstable angina pectoris.

Group 3 Patients

The women who compose group 3 have special problems. An exercise ECG is useful only if it is negative, because, for unexplained reasons, a positive response will be a false-positive response about 50% of the time.[25] A thallium exercise test can give a false-positive result in women with large breasts. Because of these problems, it is usually wise to use coronary angiography to answer the diagnostic question.

Group 4 Patients

The patients in group 4 are believed to be having a myocardial infarction.[26] There are several different approaches to such patients; at present, the preferred approach has not been determined. Two major determinants of treatment are the length of time that has passed since the onset of chest pain and the immediate availability of a cardiac catheterization laboratory. When the patient is seen within a few minutes after the onset of chest pain, and a cardiac catheterization laboratory is immediately available, coronary angiography may be performed. A decision is then made regarding the need for PTCA or surgery. When a cardiac catheterization laboratory is not immediately available, thrombolytic therapy may be used when the *diagnosis is definite* and a coronary angiogram and possible angioplasty may be performed 2 or 3 days later. When myocardial infarction is strongly suspected but cannot be confirmed (left bundle branch block or permanent pacemaker), coronary angiography may permit a definitive diagnosis and appropriate therapy. When the patient is seen 6 hours or more after the onset of chest pain, he or she is placed in a coronary care unit for a few days. Should any complications arise, such as recurrent angina, coronary angiography should be performed. PTCA or bypass surgery is then performed, depending on the results of the test. When no complications of infarction occur, risk stratification is implemented before the patient is dismissed from the hospital; a modified exercise ECG or thallium test may be used, but many physicians prefer coronary angiography.

Group 5 Patients

The patients in group 5 require no additional study. The characteristics of the symptoms alone indicate that they are not caused by coronary atherosclerotic heart disease. At times, additional testing may be needed in an effort to reassure the patient but, when possible, should be avoided.

In summary, data are now available that enable the physician to determine the pretest probability that chest discomfort is due to coronary atherosclerotic heart disease. The predictive value that is calculated should be used to determine which technology is used to clarify the problem.

THERAPEUTIC ADVANCES, PREVENTION, AND REHABILITATION

Therapeutic Advances

Modern technology, including exercise ECG, nuclear cardiology, echocardiography, and coronary angiography have made it possible to delineate the clinical syndromes that make up the subsets of coronary atherosclerotic heart disease.[27] In addition to these important advances, modern technology has made it possible to link the clinical syndrome to the pathophysiology that causes it and then, in turn, to link both to a specific therapeutic approach to the problem. In other words,

data can be obtained that permit the physician to choose between medical therapy, PTCA, or coronary bypass surgery.

Medical Treatment

Stable Angina Pectoris.   The medical treatment for stable angina pectoris includes[28]: the use of sublingual nitroglycerin, nitroglycerin skin patches, dinitroisosorbide, beta-blocking drugs such as propranolol and atenolol, calcium-blocking drugs, aspirin, a weight reduction diet that is low in saturated fat and cholesterol, abstinence from smoking, and an appropriately prescribed exercise program. Almost all patients, except the elderly and patients with serious concomitant disease(s) should have a coronary angiogram to determine the need for PTCA or bypass surgery.

Unstable Angina Pectoris.   Unstable angina pectoris is treated with the same drugs listed above.[28] Calcium-blocking drugs should be emphasized more than beta-blocking drugs because coronary artery spasm is a more important factor in patients with unstable angina than it is in patients with stable angina. When angina pectoris is crescendic, it may be necessary to use intravenous nitroglycerin to prevent the episodes; intravenous heparin should also be used in such patients together with aspirin. Patients should be placed at bed and chair rest. Smoking must be discontinued, and a weight reduction diet low in saturated fat and cholesterol should be started. Almost all patients should have coronary angiography to determine the need for PTCA or bypass surgery.

Prinzmetal's Angina.   Nitrate drugs and calcium-blocking drugs are used to treat Prinzmetal's angina. Coronary angiography should be performed because most patients with this syndrome have coronary atherosclerotic heart disease as well as coronary artery spasm. Coronary bypass surgery or PTCA may be indicated. Such patients must not smoke tobacco and should eat a low-fat, low-cholesterol diet.

Patients with proven sole coronary spasm are treated with nitrate drugs, calcium-blocking drugs and aspirin. These patients must not smoke tobacco.

Myocardial Infarction. Patients with myocardial infarction who are seen within a few minutes after the onset of chest discomfort may have coronary angiography performed immediately if a catheterization laboratory is available. The result of the study can be used to determine whether PTCA or bypass surgery is needed. Patients who are not seen immediately, but are seen within 4 hours after the onset of chest discomfort, should have intravenous thrombolytic therapy unless there is a contraindication to its use or evidence of cardiogenic shock necessitating a more aggressive approach.[29] The issue has not been settled regarding the use of heparin and aspirin and when coronary angiography should be performed following thrombolytic therapy. The precise role of PTCA and bypass surgery has not yet been delineated. Today, there is a tendency to wait 2 or 3 days after successful thrombolytic therapy before coronary angiography and possibly PTCA or bypass surgery are performed. However, should ischemic episodes continue after thrombolytic therapy, coronary angiography and possible PTCA or bypass surgery are performed without delay.

Patients with myocardial infarction who are seen more than 4 to 6 hours after the onset of chest discomfort are treated by admission to the coronary care unit, administration of oxygen, relief of chest pain with opiates, intravenous nitroglycerin, calcium-blocking drugs, beta-blocking drugs (if the blood pressure is sustained and tachycardia is present), aspirin, and heparin. Thrombolytic therapy, or immediate coronary angiography followed by possible PTCA, may be considered in patients whose chest pain has waxed and waned, suggesting intermittent reperfusion. Thrombolytic therapy, or immediate coronary angiography followed by possible PTCA, may also be considered in patients with clear-cut persistence of severe ischemic pain for more than 4 hours because these phenomena suggest that some viable myocardium remains. Coumadin should be used for anterior infarctions and large inferior infarctions in an effort to decrease the incidence of mural thrombi. The patient usually remains in the hospital for 10 to 14 days. A submaximal exercise ECG, thallium scan, or coronary angiogram should be performed on the un-

complicated patient before the patient is discharged from the hospital. If the submaximal exercise ECG or thallium scan is abnormal, a coronary angiogram should be performed. Many physicians, and I am among them, recommend a coronary angiogram rather than an exercise ECG or thallium scan. A judgment is then made as to the need for PTCA or bypass surgery.

Cardiac arrhythmias following myocardial infarction are treated promptly, but prophylactic antiarrhythmic drugs are generally not used. Coronary angiography is performed without delay in patients with recurrent angina after acute myocardial infarction.

A carefully planned rehabilitation program should be organized for the patient who is recovering from myocardial infarction. Almost all patients who were working prior to the infarction should return to work. One of Paul White's great contributions to medicine was his insistence that most patients who survive a myocardial infarction can lead active lives and should return to work.

Coronary Bypass Surgery

Coronary bypass surgery has stood the test of time.[30] Variables used to determine the need and feasibility for surgery are the physiologic age of the patient, subjective and/or objective signs of myocardial ischemia, the ejection fraction of the left ventricle, and location and extent of the atherosclerotic lesions in the coronary arteries, the presence of noncardiac disease that would increase the risk of surgery or shorten the patient's life, and the surgical expertise at the facility where the surgery will be performed.

In general, few symptoms should be required for surgical intervention in patients under the age of 65 years who have appropriate coronary anatomy. Disabling angina should be required for surgical intervention in patients who are over 75 years of age. The reason for this difference in management is clear: the operative mortality and likelihood of stroke related to surgery in older patients is about double the likelihood of these events in younger patients, being at least 4 and 6%, respectively, in the older patients.

Patients with class 1 to 4 angina pectoris, or

objective signs of myocardial ischemia, who have left main coronary artery obstruction should have coronary bypass surgery. Patients with triple-vessel disease who have class 1 to 4 angina (or objective signs of myocardial ischemia) should have coronary bypass surgery. Patients with double-vessel disease in which one of the obstructive lesions is located in the proximal portion of the left anterior descending artery who have class 1 to 4 angina, or objective signs of myocardial ischemia, should have coronary bypass surgery. Patients with single-vessel disease who have class 3 to 4 stable angina, or objective signs of myocardial ischemia, should have coronary bypass surgery when the lesion is not suitable for PTCA.

In general, patients with unstable angina are more urgent candidates for coronary bypass surgery than are patients with stable angina. Patients with coronary spasm and no atherosclerosis are not candidates for bypass surgery, whereas patients with coronary spasm and obstructive coronary atherosclerotic heart disease are candidates for surgery.

The operative risk of coronary bypass surgery varies from 1 to 10% depending on the ejection factor, age, gender, presence of noncardiac disease, and expertise of the surgical team and support system. The occurrence of stroke is 1 to 6%, depending on the age of the patient, presence of atrial fibrillation, and aortic and carotid artery disease.

Surgery can also be used for the treatment of a ruptured papillary muscle, ruptured septum, ventricular aneurysm, and certain categories of arrhythmias.

PTCA

PTCA was first used by Gruentzig in 1979.[31] Although the procedure is common, the research studies that were designed to determine the indications for its use and value have not been completed.

The current indication for PTCA is stable or unstable angina caused by single-vessel coronary artery disease due to atherosclerosis when the obstructed area is less than 2 cm in length and is not located at a bend in the artery and when there are no side branches exiting from the area of obstruction.[32]

Workers at numerous institutions are now performing PTCA on patients with multivessel coronary atherosclerotic heart disease, and our institution is no exception. We are engaged in a prospective, randomized, clinical trial designed to compare certain aspects of PTCA with coronary bypass surgery. Several other trials are under way in the United States and abroad. In the meantime, one must rely on common sense and the local expertise of the operators.

PTCA should not be used for dilatation of left main coronary artery disease. Balloon dilatation has been used to dilate saphenous vein graft stenosis with reasonable success.

The problems with PTCA are as follows: *Acute closure* of the coronary artery immediately after the procedure occurs in 4 to 6% of the patients; 3% or more of those who have emergency coronary bypass surgery die; and *restenosis* occurs in 25 to 30% of the patients within 6 months.

Prevention of Coronary Atherosclerosis

The *prevention of coronary atherosclerosis* should be a major goal for all of us.[33] We cannot and should not guarantee a patient that he or she will not have coronary atherosclerotic heart disease if the rules are followed. We should, however, indicate that it is prudent to observe the guidelines laid down by the American Heart Association; these include discontinuing smoking, maintaining a normal blood pressure, attaining a normal body weight, eating less saturated fat and cholesterol, maintaining a serum cholesterol under 200 mg/dL, and participating in an active exercise program. There is increasing evidence that this approach may not only decelerate the atherosclerotic process but also occasionally reverse the process.

THE NEGATIVE SIDE OF MEDICAL AND SURGICAL ADVANCES IN CARDIOLOGY

It is far better to have cardiac disease in 1990 than it was 20 years ago because the advances in technology have been enormous. There is, however, a "down-side" to the progress that has been made, and these "negatives" should be addressed.

Effect on Initial Screening

As new diagnostic techniques have been developed, there may well have been deterioration in the training of young physicians in history taking, physical examination, ECG, and the interpretation of chest x-rays.[34] These skills remain the essential first step in diagnostic work because the results are used by the physician to establish his or her first view of the patient's cardiac problem. This initial perception should be considered carefully, and the physician should determine whether there are sufficient data to make a complete cardiac diagnosis. If there are sufficient data to make a complete diagnosis, then additional diagnostic procedures cannot be justified unless the results of the studies will produce additional information that is needed for treatment or follow-up of the cardiac problem. When the initial examination does not permit the formulation of a complete cardiac diagnosis, it is necessary for the physician to define the question with precision. Having done so, the physician must ask whether he or she *should* order the studies that answer the question; this judgment is made by considering the patient's noncardiac diseases and determining, from the data available, whether answering the remaining questions about the patient might or might not alter the medical approach. If it is concluded that an answer to the questions will assist in the care of the patient, the physician should order the procedure that will answer the question with a predictive value that can be defended as useful in his or her decision-making process.

When the initial screening examination is performed poorly, it may influence the results of clinical trials. The selection of patients who are entered into certain clinical trials is determined by the results of the initial examination; if the patients are not selected properly, the results of the trial will not be reliable.

Public Perception of Treatment Modalities

The hyperbole associated with certain procedures has become uncontrollable. When there is a smell of commercialism to the "pitch," the claims are less believable, but, despite the odor, the claims have an impact on the public at large and physicians in particular.

At times the public has been misled because newspapers, magazines, radio, and television "news" has transmitted a new medical "breakthrough" as if the truth has been found. The articles in medical journals should be there to encourage scientific debate within the medical community; they rarely indicate a "breakthrough" that should be presented as "news." It is still generally true that a procedure or treatment must be tried in the field for several years before it can be accepted as useful. This caveat is often ignored today.

The educational programs for the public may be so simple that they injure some patients. In other words, when we insist that everyone should have a serum cholesterol level under 200 mg/dL, we simplify the objective to the point that we create harm. When the message comes through that the approach will prevent "heart attacks," the individual members of the public believe it will prevent their own personal heart attack. We must try to teach the public that the approach may help decrease the chances of "heart attacks" but that it does not guarantee that every individual who follows the rules will not have a "heart attack."

Should an individual who is 80 years old, with no evidence of coronary disease and a serum cholesterol of 230 mg/dL be placed on a low-fat, low-cholesterol diet and a lipid-lowering drug? Should a 70-year-old patient with ischemic cardiomyopathy due to coronary disease, whose level of serum cholesterol is 220 mg/dL, be placed on a low-fat, low-cholesterol diet plus a lipid-lowering drug? Should a patient with early Alzheimer's disease be placed on a low-cholesterol, low-fat diet? Despite the recent arguments that such individuals will benefit from the regimen, this approach is probably not useful.[35]

Each new antiarrhythmic drug is parlayed as the panacea for the treatment of arrhythmias. As time passes, many of the new antiarrhythmic drugs are found to be proarrhythmic. This leads physicians and members of the public to be wary of other new drugs. The physician's phone begins to ring soon after the "news flash" reporting that "it has just been determined that drug so-and-so is dangerous."

Consensus Reports and Preliminary Findings

We now live and prescribe according to consensus reports. Consensus reports are issued when there are conflicting data about a subject. Regrettably, the report is often viewed as a statement of truth, whereas the statement is merely a guideline indicating how to function while searching for the truth. The report, of necessity, represents the negotiating ability of the chair of the committee who must lead the members of the committee to acceptable and agreed-upon conclusions.

We must also be cautious in accepting the results of research that is reported in "abstracts" that are presented at national meetings. The word "abstract" implies that a summary of a final manuscript has been prepared. When an abstract is presented, there may or may not be a completed manuscript, and it is not uncommon for the data in an oral presentation to be different from the data in the written abstract. This is understandable because the work has continued and the data may change after the abstract has been submitted for inclusion at a presentation. Finally, a completed manuscript may not evolve from the work that generated the abstract, and when it does, the data and conclusions may be different from those written in the abstract. Members of the press may report data found in the written abstract, not realizing that the forum where the abstract is presented is (or should be) a "debate society" where *work in progress* is discussed with knowledgeable colleagues. A scientific meeting is an arena where truth is sought—not a place where all that is uttered is true.

Risks Associated with Treatment

PTCA is a medical miracle. Despite this, we must not ignore the problems associated with it[36] (see earlier discussion). Coronary bypass surgery has stood the test of time. We must, however, recognize that the operative risk and risk of stroke related to the procedure are increased after the age of 65. Accordingly, the need for the procedure in the elderly (beyond 65 years of age) must take into account the increase in risk that is associated with the procedure in such patients.

SUMMARY

A personal overview of coronary atherosclerotic heart disease has been presented. It is not all-inclusive, because entire books can be written on the subject. In fact, the remainder of this book addresses many other issues related to this disease and covers in more detail some of the items discussed here.

Great progress has been made and will continue to be made during the next few decades. There is always a "down-side" to progress, so a few "negatives" have been mentioned. We must also address the negative aspects with vigor, and, when possible, they must be eliminated. Stated another way, aggressive warriors must not use their new weapons inappropriately.

REFERENCES

1. Hurst JW: Atherosclerotic coronary heart disease: Historical benchmarks, methods of study and clinical features, differential diagnosis, and clinical spectrum. p. 994. In Hurst JW (ed): The Heart. 7th Ed. McGraw-Hill, New York, 1990
2. LaDue JS, Wroblewski F, Karmen A: Serum glutamic oxaloacetic transaminase in human acute myocardial infarction. Science 120:497, 1954
3. Hurst JW: A cardiovascular crotchet. Emory Univ J Med 4:143, 1990
4. Carroll L: Through the Looking Glass. 1872
5. White PD, Myers MM: The classification of cardiac diagnosis. JAMA 77:1414, 1921

6. The Criteria Committee of the New York Heart Association: Criteria for the Classification and Diagnosis of Heart Disease. 1st Ed. New York Heart Association, New York, 1928

7. The Criteria Committee of the New York Heart Association: Nomenclature and Criteria for Diagnosis of Diseases of the Heart and Great Vessels. 7th Ed. New York Heart Association/Little, Brown and Company, Boston, 1973

8. Campeau L: Letter to the editor. Circulation 54:522, 1976

9. Ross R: The pathogenesis of atherosclerosis—an update. N Engl J Med 314:488, 1986

10. Steinberg D, Parthasarathy S, Carew TE et al: Beyond cholesterol. Modifications of low-density lipoprotein that increase its atherogenicity. N Engl J Med 320:915, 1989

11. Nesto RW, Kowalchuk GJ: The ischemic cascade: Temporal sequence of hemodynamic, electrocardiographic and symptomatic expressions of ischemia. Am J Cardiol 57:23C, 1987

12. Prinzmetal R, Kennamer R, Merliss R et al: Angina pectoris. I. A variant form of angina pectoris: preliminary report. Am J Med 27:377, 1959

13. Wilson FN, Johnston FD: The occurrence in angina pectoris of electrocardiographic changes similar in magnitude and in kind to those produced by myocardial infarction. Am Heart J 22:64, 1941

14. Hurst JW, Pollak SJ, Brown CL, Lutz JF: Electrocardiographic signs suggesting inferior infarction associated with angiographic evidence of obstruction of the left anterior descending coronary artery of its branches. Emory Univ J Med 2:170, 1988

15. Heberden W: Some account of a disorder of the breast. Med Trans (published by the College of Physicians, London) 2:59, 1772

16. Baron J: The Life of Edward Jenner, M.D. p.39. Henry Coburn, London, 1838. (Letter to Dr. William Heberden, dated 1786)

17. Burns A: Observations on Some of the Most Frequent and Important Diseases of the Heart. Thomas Bryce, Edinburgh, 1809

18. Sones FM, Jr, Shirey EK, Proudfit WL, Westcott RN: Cine coronary arteriography. Circulation 20:773, 1959 (abstract)

19. Proudfit WL, Shirey EK, Sones FM, Jr: Selective cine coronary arteriography: correlation with clinical findings in 1000 patients. Circulation 33:901, 1966

20. Douglas JS, Jr, Hurst JW: Limitations of symptoms in the recognition of coronary atherosclerotic heart disease. p. 3. In Hurst JW (ed): Update I. The Heart. McGraw-Hill, New York, 1979

21. Morris DC, Walter PF, Hurst JW: The recognition and treatment of myocardial infarction and its complications. p. 1055. In Hurst JW (ed): The Heart. 7th Ed. McGraw-Hill, New York, 1990

22. Hurst JW: Atherosclerotic coronary heart disease: historical benchmarks, methods of study and clinical features, differential diagnosis, and clinical spectrum. p. 983. In Hurst JW (ed): The Heart. 7th Ed. McGraw-Hill, New York, 1990

23. Franch RH, King SB III, Douglas JS, Jr: Techniques of cardiac catheterization including coronary arteriography. p. 1881. In Hurst JW (ed): The Heart. 7th Ed. McGraw-Hill, New York, 1990

24. Steingart RM, Scheuer J: Assessment of myocardial ischemia. p. 354. In Hurst JW (ed): The Heart. 7th Ed. McGraw-Hill, New York, 1990

25. Hurst JW: Atherosclerotic coronary heart disease: Historical benchmarks, methods of study and clinical features, differential diagnosis, and clinical spectrum. p. 972. In Hurst JW (ed): The Heart. 7th Ed. McGraw-Hill, New York, 1990

26. Morris DC, Walter PF, Hurst JW: The recognition and treatment of myocardial infarction and its complications. p. 1055. In Hurst JW (ed): The Heart. 7th Ed. McGraw-Hill, New York, 1990

27. Hurst JW: Methods of treating atherosclerotic coronary heart disease. p. 994. In Hurst JW (ed): The Heart. 7th Ed. McGraw-Hill, New York, 1990

28. Pratt CM, Roberts R: Pharmacologic therapy of atherosclerotic coronary heart disease. p. 1019. In Hurst JW (ed): The Heart. 7th Ed. McGraw-Hill, New York, 1990

29. Morris DC, Walter PF, Hurst JW: The recognition and treatment of myocardial infarction and its complications. p. 1054. In Hurst JW (ed): The Heart. 7th Ed. McGraw-Hill, New York, 1990

30. Whalen RE, Hurst JW: The surgical treatment of atherosclerotic coronary heart disease. p. 1029. In Hurst JW (ed): The Heart. 7th Ed. McGraw-Hill, New York, 1990

31. Hurst JW: The first coronary angiography as described by Andreas Gruentzig. Am J Cardiol 57:185, 1986

32. King SB III, Douglas JS, Jr: Percutaneous transluminal coronary angioplasty. p. 1041. In Hurst JW (ed): The Heart. 7th Ed. McGraw-Hill, New York, 1990

33. Wenger NK, Schlant RC: Prevention of coronary atherosclerosis. p. 893. In Hurst JW (ed): The Heart. 7th Ed. McGraw-Hill, New York, 1990

34. Hurst JW: The examination of the heart: The importance of initial screening. Masters in Medicine. p. 251. In Bone RC (ed): Disease-A-Month. Vol. 36. No. 5. Mosby-Year Book, Chicago, 1990

35. Commissioned by the Task Force on Cholesterol Issues, American Heart Association: Special Report. The cholesterol facts: A summary of the evidence relating dietary fats, serum cholesterol, and coronary heart disease—A Joint Statement by the American Heart Association and the National Heart, Lung, and Blood Institute. Circulation 81:1721, 1990

36. Douglas JS, Jr, King SB III, Roubin GS: Technique of percutaneous transluminal angioplasty of the coronary, renal, mesenteric, and peripheral arteries. p. 2146. In Hurst JW (ed): The Heart. 7th Ed. McGraw-Hill, New York, 1990

2

Morphologic Aspects of Coronary Heart Disease and Its Complications

William C. Roberts, M.D.

Atherosclerotic coronary heart disease (CHD) is the most common cause of death in the western world. One person dies every minute of CHD in the United States and about 6 million persons have symptomatic myocardial ischemia because of CHD. About 250,000 coronary artery bypass grafting operations and 300,000 percutaneous transluminal coronary angioplasty (PTCA) procedures were performed in 1990 in the United States. The major cause of the atherosclerosis is now clear; the evidence is overwhelming that atherosclerosis is a cholesterol problem. The higher the blood total cholesterol level (specifically the low-density lipoprotein level), the greater the chance of developing symptomatic CHD, the greater the chance of having fatal CHD, and the greater the extent of the atherosclerotic plaques. Furthermore, lowering the blood total cholesterol level decreases the chances of having symptomatic or fatal CHD and increases the chance that some atherosclerotic plaques will actually regress. Although the coronary arteries have been examined visually at necropsy for over 100 years, only in recent years has the extent of the atherosclerotic process in the coronary arteries in patients with symptomatic or fatal CHD become appreciated. This chapter initially reviews the status of the major epicardial coronary arteries in various subsets of patients with fatal CHD. It then describes the effects of PTCA on these arteries, presents some observations in patients having thrombolytic therapy and coronary bypass surgery, and delineates various complications of myocardial ischemia.

NUMBER OF MAJOR EPICARDIAL CORONARY ARTERIES SEVERELY NARROWED IN THE VARIOUS "CORONARY EVENTS"

The most common method for describing the severity of coronary artery disease (CAD) in patients with clinical evidence of myocardial ischemia is by the number of major epicardial coronary arteries narrowed by more than 50% in luminal diameter by coronary angiogram. Thus, patients are divided into groups of one-vessel, two-vessel, three-vessel, and "left main" CAD. Because a 50% diameter reduction, in general, is equivalent to a 75% cross-sectional area narrowing, the cutoff point of "significant" as opposed to "insignificant" luminal narrowing at necropsy is the 75% cross-sectional area point. Physiologically, there is no significant obstruction to arterial flow until the lumen is narrowed by more than 75% in cross-sectional area.

Table 2-1 summarizes the number of major

Table 2-1. Number of Major Coronary Arteries Narrowed by More than 75% in Cross-Sectional Area by Atherosclerotic Plaque in Fatal CHD

Coronary Event	No. of Patients	Mean Age (yrs)	No. of Patients with Following No. of Arteries Narrowed > 75% CSA				
			4	3	2	1	Mean
Sudden coronary death	31	47	3	20	6	2	2.8
Acute myocardial infarction	27	59	3	14	10	0	2.7
Healed myocardial infarction							
Asymptomatic	18	66	0	7	7	4	2.2
Chronic CHF without aneurysm	9	63	0	3	5	1	2.2
Left ventricular aneurysm	22	61	1	12	6	3	2.5
Angina pectoris/unstable	22	48	10	8	3	1	3.2
Total (%)	129	56	17 (13)	64 (50)	37 (29)	11 (8)	2.7
Controls (%)	40	52	0 (0)	5 (5)	12 (13)	21 (23)	0.7

Abbreviations: CHF, congestive heart failure; CSA, cross-sectional area. (Courtesy of National Institutes of Health.)

(right, left main, left anterior descending, and left circumflex) epicardial coronary arteries narrowed by more than 75% in cross-sectional area by atherosclerotic plaque alone in patients with fatal CHD.[1] Among the 129 patients with fatal CHD studied at necropsy, 516 major epicardial coronary arteries were examined and 345 (67%) of them were narrowed at some point by 76 to 100% in cross-sectional area by atherosclerotic plaque. By contrast, of 40 control subjects, mainly victims of acute leukemia and without clinical evidence of myocardial ischemia during life, 160 major epicardial coronary arteries were examined and 60 (37%) of them were narrowed at some point by more than 75% in cross-sectional area by plaque. Among the 129 coronary patients, only 11 (8%) had a single coronary artery severely narrowed (23% in the controls); 37 (29%) had two arteries severely narrowed (13% in the controls); 64 (50%) had three arteries severely narrowed (5% in the controls); and 17 (13%) had all four major arteries severely narrowed (0% in the controls). Thus, of the four major coronary arteries in the coronary patients, an average of 2.7 were narrowed >75% in cross-sectional area by plaque; the equivalent number among the control subjects was 0.7 of 4.

The number of major coronary arteries severely narrowed by atherosclerotic plaque among the various subsets of coronary patients was relatively similar, except for being higher in the un-

stable angina patients (Table 2-1). Among the 31 *sudden coronary death* patients,[2] all of whom died outside the hospital, usually within a few minutes of onset of symptoms of myocardial ischemia, an average of 2.8 of the 4 major arteries were severely narrowed, a number virtually identical to that of the 27 patients with *transmural acute myocardial infarction*,[3] all of whom died in a coronary care unit. Only 2 of the 31 sudden-death victims and none of the 27 acute myocardial infarction patients had only a single coronary artery (one-vessel disease) severely narrowed.

The *healed myocardial infarction* group was divided into three subgroups. One consisted of patients who had had an acute myocardial infarction in the past; the infarcts had healed, and thereafter there was never evidence of myocardial ischemia clinically; these patients died of a noncardiac cause, usually cancer.[4] Nevertheless, the average number of major coronary arteries severely narrowed at necropsy was 2.2 of 4. Another subgroup consisted of patients who had chronic congestive heart failure after healing of an acute myocardial infarct, but in the absence of a left ventricular aneurysm.[5] This subgroup might be called the ischemic cardiomyopathy subgroup. The average number of major coronary arteries severely narrowed in it was also 2.2 of 4. The final subgroup of healed myocardial infarction patients had a true left ventricular aneurysm[6]; the average number of severely narrowed major coronary arteries was 2.5 of 4.

The final group consisted of 22 patients with *unstable angina pectoris*, all of whom had had coronary artery bypass grafting procedures within 7 days of death.[7] Preoperatively, all had normal left ventricular function and none had had a clinically apparent acute myocardial infarction or congestive heart failure at any time. The average number of major coronary arteries severely narrowed by plaque was 3.2 of 4, and 10 of the 22 patients had severe narrowing of the left main coronary artery, as well as severe narrowing of the other three major coronary arteries (four-vessel disease). Another study[8] has indicated that severe narrowing of the left main coronary artery usually is an indicator that the other three major arteries also are severely narrowed. The *unstable angina* group thus had the largest average number of major coronary arteries severely narrowed of any of the groups, but this group of patients, nevertheless, had excellent left ventricular function.

QUANTITATIVE APPROACH TO CAD: AMOUNTS OF NARROWING IN EACH 5-mm SEGMENT OF EACH OF THE FOUR MAJOR CORONARY ARTERIES

Although the one-, two-, three-, and four-vessel disease approach has been useful clinically, this type of severity analysis might be thought of as a *qualitative* approach, and differences in degrees of coronary narrowing in the various subsets of coronary patients are usually not discernible by this approach. To obtain a better appreciation of the extent of the atherosclerotic process in patients with fatal CHD, several years ago my colleagues and I began examining each 5-mm segment of each of the four major coronary arteries.[1] In adults, the average length of the right coronary artery is 10 cm; the left main, 1 cm; the left anterior descending, 10 cm; and the left circumflex, 6 cm. Thus, 27 cm of major epicardial coronary artery is available for examination in each adult. Because each 1 cm is divided into 2 five-mm seg-

ments, an average of 54 five-mm segments is available to examine in each heart. This approach not only allows one to ask how many of the 5-mm segments are narrowed 76 to 100% in cross-sectional area, but also how many are narrowed 51 to 75%, 26 to 50%, and 0 to 25%. This approach, in contrast to the one-, two-, three-, and four-vessel disease approach, might be considered a *quantitative* one.

The same patients previously described by the qualitative approach also were evaluated at necropsy by the quantitative approach; the findings are summarized in Table 2-2. A total of 6,461 five-mm segments were sectioned and later examined histologically. The sections were stained by the Movat method to delineate the internal elastic membrane. The findings in the 129 coronary patients were compared with those in 1,849 five-mm segments in 40 control subjects. In each coronary subgroup, the 5-mm segments from each of the four major coronary arteries were pooled, so, by this approach, the amount of narrowing in an individual patient was not discernible. The percentage of 5-mm segments narrowed 76 to 100% in cross-sectional area by atherosclerotic plaque was 35% for the coronary patients and 3% for the control subjects; the percentage narrowed 51 to 75% was 36% for the coronary patients and 22% for the control subjects. Thus, 71% of the 5-mm segments in the coronary patients were narrowed by more than 50% in cross-sectional area by atherosclerotic plaque and 25% were narrowed by this amount in the control subjects. In contrast, only 29% of the 5-mm segments in the coronary patients were narrowed <50% and only 8% even approached normal, i.e., narrowed 25% or less in cross-sectional area. In contrast, 75% of the 5-mm segments in the control subjects were narrowed by less than 50% and 31% of them were normal or nearly normal. Thus, in the coronary patients 92% of the 6,461 five-mm segments of the four major epicardial coronary arteries were narrowed by more than 25% in cross-sectional area by atherosclerotic plaque. Accordingly, the coronary atherosclerotic process is a diffuse one in patients with fatal CHD. To believe that the atherosclerotic process is a *focal* one in patients with fatal CHD is to believe a *myth*.

Among the various subsets of coronary patients,

Table 2-2.   Amounts of Cross-Sectional Area Narrowing of Each 5-mm Segment of the Four Major Epicardial Coronary Arteries by Atherosclerotic Plaque in Subjects with Fatal CHD

Subgroup	No. of Patients	Mean Age (yrs)	No. of 5-mm Segments	No. of Patients with Following Percentage of Segments Narrowed				Mean Score	Mean % Narrowing/ 5-mm Segment
				0–25%	26–50%	51–75%	76–100%		
Sudden coronary death	31	47	1,564	7	23	34	36	2.98	67
Acute myocardial infarction	27	59	1,403	5	23	38	34	3.01	68
Healed myocardial infarction									
Asymptomatic	18	66	924	11	23	35	31	2.87	64
Chronic CHF without aneurysm	9	63	529	11	23	37	29	2.78	61
LV aneurysm	22	61	992	4	21	42	33	3.03	68
Angina pectoris/ unstable	22	48	1,049	11	12	29	48	3.12	70
Total	129	56	6,461	8	21	36	35	2.98	67
Controls	40	52	1,849	31	44	22	3	1.97	32

(Healed myocardial infarction group: 31%)

Abbreviations: CHF, congestive heart failure; LV, left ventricular. (Courtesy of National Institutes of Health.)

those with sudden coronary death[2] and acute myocardial infarction[3] had similar percentages of 5-mm segments narrowed 76 to 100% in cross-sectional area by plaque (36 and 34%, respectively); patients with healed myocardial infarcts[4–6] as a group had the least severe narrowing (31% of segments narrowed by more than 75%), and the patients with unstable angina pectoris[7] had the most severe narrowing of all (48% of the 5-mm segments were narrowed by more than 75%).

In an attempt to provide a single number for the amount of coronary arterial narrowing in each patient, a score system was used. A segment narrowed 0 to 25% was assigned a score of 1; a segment narrowed 26 to 50%, 2; a segment narrowed 51 to 75%, 3; and one narrowed 76 to 100%, 4. The mean score for all 129 coronary patients or for each of the 6,461 five-mm coronary segments was 3.0, and that for the 40 control subjects or their 1,849 five-mm segments was 2.0. Again, the *unstable angina* patients had the most extensive coronary narrowing by this approach.

A possible criticism of the 5-mm segment approach to quantifying coronary artery narrowing is that the epicardial coronary arteries were fixed in an unphysiologic pressure state, namely a zero-pressure state, rather than at a systemic arterial diastolic pressure. In an attempt to take into account the unphysiologic fixation state, the degrees of narrowing were conservatively judged; that is, if a segment was more or less between two quadrants (e.g., between 51 to 75% and 76 to 100%), the lesser degree of narrowing always was chosen. Second, for any segment in which a portion of wall was collapsed by the fixation process, the degree of narrowing was determined as if the segment was expanded. Finally, and most important, the segments narrowed the most, i.e., more than 75% in cross-sectional area, were affected the least by the fixation process. Irrespective of whether the histologic technique used in this study is perfect or imperfect, the same technique was used in all subsets of coronary patients and all control subjects; therefore, the comparison data are highly reliable. Irrespective of whether the degrees of luminal narrowing should be slightly greater or slightly less than that determined by this technique, it is clear that the atherosclerotic process is a diffuse one in nearly all patients with fatal CHD. The accuracy of the technique of determining degrees of cross-sectional area narrowing by estimation from stained histologic sections magnified about 40 times is similar (less than or equal to 5%) to that determined by planimetry.[9]

Another possible concern of the aforementioned quantitative data is its applicability to living patients with symptomatic or other clinical evidence (positive exercise test, for example) of myocardial ischemia. It is my view that the major difference in coronary arterial narrowing occurs at the stage of conversion from the asymptomatic to the symptomatic myocardial ischemic state and that there is relatively little difference in degrees of coronary narrowing between the symptomatic and the fatal states. This view is supported by the presence of severe and extensive coronary narrowing (as shown in a coronary angiogram) during life and by a study of the coronary tree at necropsy in patients who, during life, had a coronary event and who died later from a noncardiac cause. Although data from the latter situation are minimal, the degrees of coronary narrowing at necropsy are similar to those in other patients with fatal symptomatic myocardial ischemia. Finally, among the subsets of coronary patients described here, those with unstable angina pectoris had by far the worst degrees of coronary narrowing; the subjects in this group were the only ones in whom their natural course was interrupted by an iatrogenic event, namely coronary artery bypass grafting (within 7 days of death).

DISTRIBUTION OF SEVERE NARROWING IN EACH OF THE THREE LONGEST EPICARDIAL CORONARY ARTERIES IN FATAL CHD

In all the quantitative coronary arterial studies just reviewed, the amount of cross-sectional area luminal narrowing by atherosclerotic plaque in the right, left anterior descending, and left circumflex coronary arteries was similar if results for the 5-mm segments in each of the three longest coronary arteries were pooled for a number of patients. This statement is best understood by examining a single subset of coronary patients with fatal CHD. Among the 27 patients with fatal transmural acute myocardial infarction, a total of 1,358 five-mm segments was analyzed from the right, left anterior descending, and left circumflex cor-

onary arteries, and the percentage of segments narrowed 0 to 25%, 26 to 50%, 51 to 75%, and 76 to 100% was similar for each of these four categories of cross-sectional area narrowing in each of these three major epicardial coronary arteries. The same findings were observed in the patients with sudden coronary death, healed myocardial infarction, and unstable angina pectoris.[1]

In a single patient, however, the percentage of 5-mm coronary segments severely (more than 75% in cross-sectional area) narrowed by atherosclerotic plaque in one major epicardial coronary artery may be greater or smaller than that for another major coronary artery. If the results for segments from one coronary artery (right, for example), however, were pooled for several patients with fatal CHD and compared with pooled 5-mm segments from another coronary artery (left anterior descending, for example) for several patients with fatal CHD, the percentage of segments narrowed at each of the four categories of cross-sectional area narrowing in each artery are similar. The definition of "several" has not yet been established, but, with few exceptions, this principle may apply to as few as three patients with pooled 5-mm segments from each of the three major coronary arteries. Thus, the quantity of atherosclerotic plaque is similar for similar lengths of the right, left anterior descending, and left circumflex coronary arteries, and, because the amount of atherosclerotic plaque is similar, the amount of resulting luminal narrowing also is similar. The cholesterol thesis might not be tenable if the amount of atherosclerotic plaque was very different in the different major epicardial coronary arteries, because the same serum cholesterol level presumably is present in each major coronary artery.

CLINICAL USEFULNESS OF THE QUANTITATIVE APPROACH TO CAD

The information derived at necropsy quantitating the severity and extent of atherosclerosis in the four major epicardial coronary arteries in fatal CHD is potentially useful clinically in two

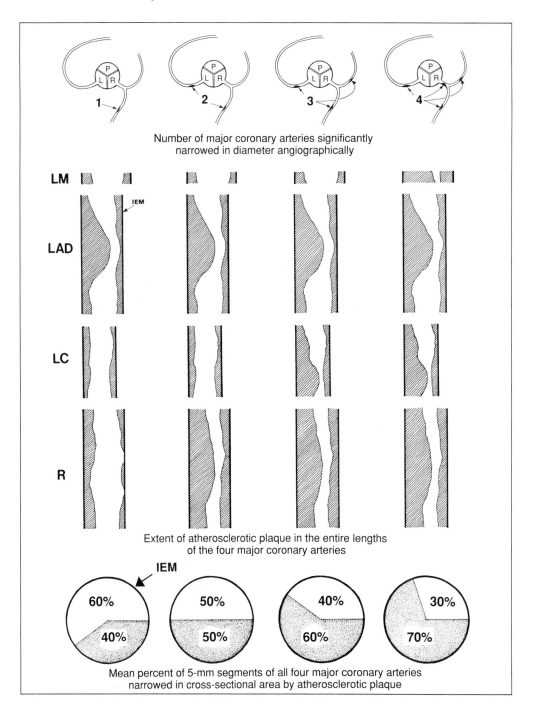

Number of major coronary arteries significantly
narrowed in diameter angiographically

LM

LAD

IEM

LC

R

Extent of atherosclerotic plaque in the entire lengths
of the four major coronary arteries

IEM

60%

40%

50%

50%

40%

60%

30%

70%

Mean percent of 5-mm segments of all four major coronary arteries
narrowed in cross-sectional area by atherosclerotic plaque

Fig. 2-1. Diagram showing numbers of coronary arteries significantly narrowed by angiogram (top), the amounts of plaque in the entire lengths of the four major (left main [LM], left anterior descending [LAD], left circumflex [LC], and right [R]) epicardial coronary arteries (middle), and a cross-sectional area view (bottom) of the average amount of plaque in each 5-mm segment of the entire lengths of the four major coronary arteries according to the numbers of major arteries significantly narrowed by angiogram. (From Roberts,[51] with permission.)

areas: (1) in interpreting degrees of coronary narrowing by coronary angiography during life, and (2) in deciding which of the major coronary arteries needs a conduit at the time of coronary artery bypass grafting.

Without coronary angiography, neither coronary bypass surgery nor PTCA would be done. The only way, during life, to obtain information on the status of the epicardial coronary arteries is coronary angiography; therefore, this procedure revolutionized the diagnosis of CHD just as

aortocoronary bypass grafting revolutionized therapy of CHD. But coronary angiography—as good as it is—has certain deficiencies. The angiogram is a luminogram, and a narrowed segment is compared to a less narrowed segment, which is assumed to be normal. The angiogram does not delineate the internal elastic membrane of the artery, and, therefore, the artery's true lumen remains uncertain (Figs. 2-1 and 2-2).

The quantitative coronary studies discussed above demonstrated that, in fatal CHD, 93% of

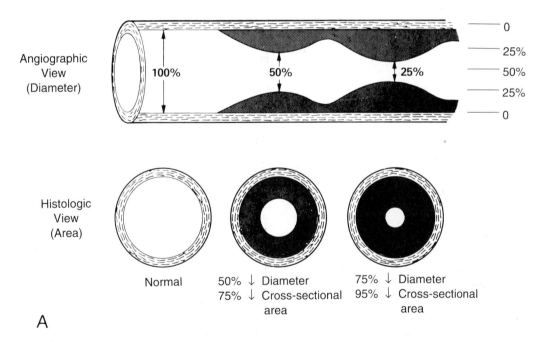

Fig. 2-2. Diagram showing differences in units used for designating degrees of narrowing by angiography (diameter reduction) and that used for histologic examination (cross-sectional area narrowing) of coronary arteries. In general, a 50% diameter reduction (by angiography) is equivalent to a 75% cross-sectional area narrowing. (**A**) A segment of a coronary artery which is entirely normal. This situation rarely exists in persons with symptomatic myocardial ischemia. (*Figure continues.*)

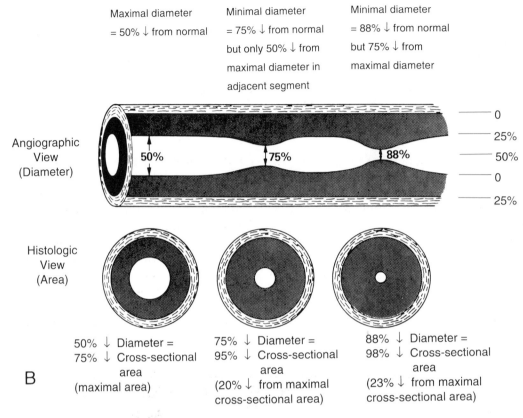

Maximal diameter = 50% ↓ from normal

Minimal diameter = 75% ↓ from normal but only 50% ↓ from maximal diameter in adjacent segment

Minimal diameter = 88% ↓ from normal but 75% ↓ from maximal diameter

Angiographic View (Diameter)

50%   75%   88%

0
25%
50%
0
25%

Histologic View (Area)

50% ↓ Diameter = 75% ↓ Cross-sectional area (maximal area)

75% ↓ Diameter = 95% ↓ Cross-sectional area (20% ↓ from maximal cross-sectional area)

88% ↓ Diameter = 98% ↓ Cross-sectional area (23% ↓ from maximal cross-sectional area)

B

Fig. 2-2. (*Continued*). (**B**) The usual situation is depicted, which indicates that the severest narrowing is compared with an adjacent area which by angiography may be considered to be normal but in actuality is simply less narrowed. (From Arnett et al.[10] with permission.)

the 5-mm segments of the four major epicardial coronary arteries were narrowed by more than 25% in cross-sectional area by atherosclerotic plaque. Thus, only 7% of the 5-mm segments even approached normal and virtually none was normal. Therefore, at least in fatal CHD, and probably also in living patients with symptomatic myocardial ischemia, an angiographically severely narrowed segment of a coronary artery can infrequently be compared with a segment of coronary artery that is actually normal. In other words, in patients with symptomatic myocardial ischemia, the coronary angiogram measures degrees of narrowing by comparing severely narrowed segments with segments which are simply less narrowed and by no means normal (Fig. 2-1). Accordingly, coronary angiograms in patients with symptomatic myocardial ischemia usually *underestimate* the degrees of luminal narrowing.[10,11]

The unit of measuring degrees of narrowing by coronary angiography is different from the unit of measurement at necropsy. In the anatomic quantitative studies discussed above, the unit was *cross-sectional area* narrowing. The unit of coronary angiography is *diameter* narrowing. In general, a 75% cross-sectional area narrowing is equivalent to a 50% diameter reduction, and, therefore, a 50% or more diameter reduction during life has generally been considered the cutoff point between clinically significant and clinically insignificant coronary narrowing.

The second potential usefulness of the information derived from the quantitative CAD studies at necropsy is the appreciation that the atherosclerotic process in patients with symptomatic myocardial ischemia is usually diffuse and severe and, therefore, that more rather than fewer aortocoronary conduits provide a higher frequency of relief of or improvement in symptoms of myocardial ischemia, an improvement in results of exercise testing, and an improvement in prolonging life. Among patients surviving less than 30 days or longer after aortocoronary bypass operations, the amount of severe narrowing in the *nonbypassed native* coronary arteries is usually similar to that in the *bypassed native* coronary arteries.[12,13] From study at necropsy of 102 patients dying either early (up to 60 days) or late (2.5 to 108 months [mean, 35 months]) after coronary bypass operations, Waller and Roberts[12] found that the bypassed and nonbypassed native coronary arteries had similar degrees of severe luminal narrowing by atherosclerotic plaque. Specifically, in 213 (94%) of the 226 bypassed native arteries and in 73 (91%) of 80 nonbypassed native arteries, the lumens were narrowed by more than 75% in cross-sectional area by atherosclerotic plaque. The reason the native arteries were not bypassed was not that they were too small or severely narrowed distally, but because by coronary angiogram the lumens were judged not to be sufficiently narrowed to warrant the insertion of a conduit. Thus, if a coronary angiogram shows that two of the major coronary arteries are severely narrowed and the third major artery is "insignificantly" narrowed, and if a coronary bypass operation is to be done, the insertion of a conduit in all three major coronary arteries could be reasonably argued. There is, of course, potential danger to inserting a conduit in an artery that is insignificantly narrowed, but, nevertheless, it may be more advantageous to err on the side of too many conduits than too few. At necropsy, three-vessel disease is far more frequent than two-vessel disease and even when only two of the three major coronary arteries at necropsy are narrowed by more than 75% in cross-sectional area, the third one is usually narrowed by 51 to 75% in cross-sectional area. Thus, an appreciation of the diffuse nature of coronary atherosclerosis in fatal CHD and probably also in symptomatic myocardial ischemia encourages the tilt toward more, rather than fewer, conduits at coronary bypass operations.

SIGNIFICANCE OF CORONARY ARTERIAL THROMBUS IN TRANSMURAL ACUTE MYOCARDIAL INFARCTION

Thrombi in the coronary arteries of patients with transmural acute myocardial infarction have been observed at necropsy in numerous studies.[14–16] Herrick[17] found them in four patients with fatal acute myocardial infarction, and for many decades thrombi were believed to have precipitated acute myocardial infarction. They were considered so important in causing this acute event that the term "coronary thrombosis" was used for years to describe the event that more physicians now call "acute myocardial infarction." To evaluate the significance of coronary thrombus in acute myocardial infarction, Brosius and Roberts[18] examined in detail the coronary arteries containing thrombi in 54 autopsied patients with transmural acute myocardial infarction.

A coronary arterial thrombus was defined as a collection of fibrin (with or without engulfed erythrocytes) or platelets or both within the residual lumen, with attachment of the fibrin/platelets to the luminal surface of the artery. In the 54 patients with fatal acute myocardial infarction, the luminal surface was always the surface of an underlying atherosclerotic plaque. The thrombus was always attached to the intimal surface in its distal portion, but in a few patients it was not attached in its most proximal portion. The thrombus was considered occlusive when it totally occupied the residual lumen of the artery, that is, the portion not occupied by atherosclerotic plaque. The thrombus was considered nonocclusive when it filled the residual lumen incompletely. The area of the occlusive thrombus was the difference between the area of the original lumen and the area of the atherosclerotic plaque. In the nonocclusive thrombus, the residual lumen was the difference between the artery's original lumen and the sum of the area occupied by atherosclerotic plaque plus the area occupied by the nonocclusive thrombus. In the sections of coronary artery proximal and distal to the thrombus, the residual lumen was the difference between the artery's original lumen and the area occupied by atherosclerotic plaque. The percentage of cross-sectional area narrowed by atherosclerotic plaque and by thrombi (in the case of nonocclusive thrombi) was calculated. The area of each artery enclosed by the internal elastic membrane (original lumen), the area of the atherosclerotic plaque, and that of the nonocclusive thrombus provided by videoplanimetry were converted into actual areas. At the site of attachment of thrombi, the underlying atherosclerotic plaques contained extravasated erythrocytes in 21 (39%) of the 54 patients. In none of the 21, however, did the hemorrhage into the pultaceous debris of the plaque appear to compromise the lumen.

The Brosius–Roberts[18] study raises questions regarding the importance of coronary thrombi in patients with fatal transmural acute myocardial infarction. The major finding at autopsy is that in patients with fatal acute myocardial infarction, thrombi are found in major coronary arteries that already are severely narrowed by old atherosclerotic plaques at, immediately proximal to, and/or immediately distal to the site of thrombosis. The lumen of the coronary artery containing the thrombus was already narrowed an average of 79% (range, 26 to 98%) in cross-sectional area by atherosclerotic plaque alone at and within 2 cm proximal to and distal to the thrombus; that is, an "average" coronary artery with a thrombus was severely narrowed (75% in cross-sectional area) at three sites (at, proximal to, and distal to the thrombus). The average coronary arterial narrowing at the site of thrombus, however, actually underestimates the true severity of the narrowing in the vicinity of the thrombus. The site of most severe narrowing was within the 2 cm proximal to the thrombus in 16 of 54 (30%) coronary arteries, at the site of the thrombus in 25 (46%), and within the 2-cm segment distal to the thrombus in 13 (24%). At the site of most severe narrowing, 96% of the coronary arteries were narrowed by 76 to 98% in cross-sectional area by atherosclerotic plaque and half were narrowed by 91 to 98%. In contrast, the percentage of coronary lumen narrowed by thrombus alone averaged 19% of the original cross-sectional area of the artery (range, 2 to 67%) in the 47 patients with occlusive thrombi and 7% (range, 2 to 24%) in the 7 patients

with nonocclusive thrombi. Thus, if thrombus were the only luminal material, the amount of thrombus within the coronary artery, with a few exceptions, probably would not by itself diminish or slow blood flow. Thus, the frequent need for coronary bypass surgery or PTCA after successful thrombolysis is readily understandable. A corollary is that, among necropsy patients with fatal acute myocardial infarction, the coronary thrombus, when present, is always superimposed on an atherosclerotic plaque. The exception is coronary embolism, when clot may be present without underlying atherosclerotic plaque.[19]

The coronary thrombi found at necropsy in patients with fatal acute myocardial infarction are usually short. Among the 54 patients studied by Brosius and Roberts,[18] the average coronary thrombus was 1.6 cm long (range, 0.5 to 10 cm); the occlusive thrombi were longer than the nonocclusive thrombi (1.8 versus 0.7 cm). Also, occlusive thrombi in the right coronary arteries tended to be longer than those in the left anterior and circumflex coronary arteries (2.4 versus 1.4 and 1.1 cm). Because the right and left anterior descending coronary arteries in adults are more than 10 cm long and the left circumflex artery is usually about 6 cm long, the actual length of a coronary artery occupied by thrombus is small, and in no patient was the entire length of a coronary artery occupied by a thrombus. In the right coronary artery, there was a weak, but significant, positive correlation between the length of an occlusive thrombus and the duration of survival of a patient between the time of onset of acute myocardial infarction and death. This relation suggests that thrombi may lengthen or "grow" with time.

CARDIAC MORPHOLOGIC FINDINGS IN ACUTE MYOCARDIAL INFARCTION TREATED WITH THROMBOLYTIC THERAPY

Until thrombolytic and revascularization therapy of acute myocardial infarction was introduced, virtually all acute myocardial infarcts observed at necropsy were nonhemorrhagic. Treatment with thrombolytic agents has been shown to restore the patency of occluded coronary arteries, but this has been associated with an apparently marked, although heretofore undetermined, increase in the frequency of hemorrhagic infarcts. It has been suggested that myocardial hemorrhage after coronary reperfusion is confined to zones of the myocardium that were already necrotic and that the hemorrhage is probably a consequence of severe microvascular injury and not its cause. Gertz et al.[20] studied at necropsy the hearts of 52 patients who had received recombinant tissue plasminogen activator (rt-PA) during acute myocardial infarction and compared clinical and cardiac morphologic findings in patients with hemorrhagic infarcts to those with nonhemorrhagic infarcts. The acute infarcts were hemorrhagic by gross inspection (with histologic confirmation) in 23, nonhemorrhagic in 20, and not visible grossly in 2; in 7, there was no acute necrosis by either gross or histologic examination of multiple sections of the myocardium. In 4 of these 7 patients without acute infarcts, the interval from chest pain to death was less than 10 hours, which is often too early to detect the presence of necrosis by gross examination.

No significant differences were found between patients with hemorrhagic and nonhemorrhagic infarcts with respect to mean age, heart mass, interval from chest pain to rt-PA infusion, interval from chest pain to peak creatine kinase level, interval from chest pain to death, location of the myocardial necrosis, frequency of left ventricular dilatation, frequency of myocardial rupture (left ventricular free wall or ventricular septum), or frequency of cardiogenic shock, fatal arrhythmias, or fatal bleeding. Furthermore, the frequencies of thrombi and plaque rupture in coronary arteries and the sizes of the infarcts were similar in patients with hemorrhagic and nonhemorrhagic infarcts. Thus, although the frequency of hemorrhagic infarct increases after thrombolytic therapy, the hemorrhage does not appear to extend the infarct or to increase the frequency of complications of infarction.

In a separate study, Gertz et al.[21] compared cardiac findings at necropsy in 23 patients who had received thrombolytic therapy during acute myocardial infarction with those in 38 patients with acute myocardial infarction who had not received thrombolytic therapy. Although each group of patients had similar baseline characteristics, the patients receiving thrombolytic therapy (rt-PA) had a greater frequency of platelet-rich (fibrin-poor) thrombi in the infarct-related coronary arteries, more nonocclusive than occlusive thrombi, and a lower frequency of myocardial rupture.

COMPOSITION OF ATHEROSCLEROTIC PLAQUES IN FATAL CHD

Kragel et al.[22,23] studied atherosclerotic plaque composition in the four major (right, left main, left anterior descending, and left circumflex) coronary arteries at necropsy in 15 patients who died of consequences of acute myocardial infarction, 12 patients with sudden coronary death without associated myocardial infarction, and 10 patients with isolated unstable angina pectoris with pain at rest. The coronary arteries were sectioned at 5-mm intervals, and a Movat-stained section of each segment of artery was prepared and analyzed by using a computerized morphometry system. Among the three subsets of coronary patients, there were no differences in plaque composition between any of the four major epicardial coronary arteries. Within all three groups, the major component of plaque was a combination of dense acellular and cellular fibrous tissue with much smaller portions of plaque being composed of pultaceous debris (amorphous debris containing cholesterol clefts, presumably rich in extracellular lipid), calcium, foam cells with and without inflammatory cells, and foam cells alone (Fig. 2-3). Within all three groups, plaque morphology varied as a function of cross-sectional area narrowing of the segments. In all three groups, the amount of dense, relatively acellular fibrous tissue, calcified tissue, and pultaceous debris increased in a linear fashion with increasing degrees of cross-sectional area narrowing of the segments and the amount of cellular fibrous tis-

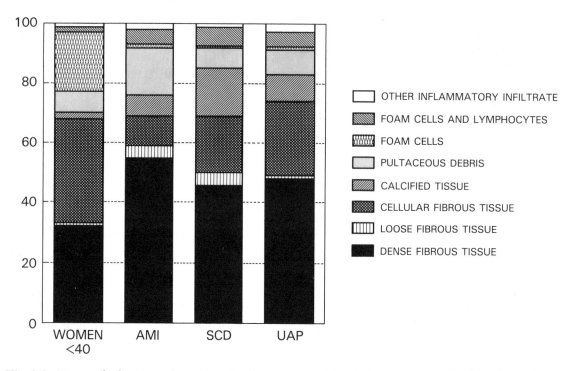

Fig. 2-3. Bar graph showing atherosclerotic plaque composition (mean percentage) in histologic 5-mm sections of the four major epicardial coronary arteries narrowed by more than 75% in cross-sectional area. The patients included 8 women aged 31 to 39 years (mean, 34 years) with fatal coronary artery disease and 35 patients over 40 years of age (mean, 59 years) with fatal acute myocardial infarction (AMI), sudden coronary death (SCD), and unstable angina pectoris (UAP). The dominant component of the atherosclerotic plaques in all groups was fibrous tissue. (From Dollar et al,[52] with permission.)

sue decreased linearly. The percentage of plaque consisting of pultaceous debris was highest in the subgroup with acute myocardial infarction. Multiluminal channels were most frequent in the subgroup with unstable angina pectoris. The studies by Kragel et al.[23,23] are the first to analyze quantitatively the composition of coronary arterial plaques in the various subsets of coronary patients.

EFFECTS OF PTCA ON ATHEROSCLEROTIC PLAQUES AND RELATION OF PLAQUE COMPOSITION AND ARTERIAL SIZE TO OUTCOME

To delineate their relation to outcome of PTCA, the atherosclerotic plaque composition and coronary artery size in 82 five-mm segments of 28

PTCA sites in 26 patients were determined by Potkin and Roberts.[24] The 26 patients were subdivided into three groups according to the degree of angiographic patency at the end of the PTCA procedure and to the duration of survival after PTCA (up to and including 30 days or more than 30 days): *early success* (13 patients, 16 PTCA sites, and 49 five-mm segments); *early failure* (4 patients, 4 PTCA sites, and 16 five-mm segments) and *late success* (9 patients, 8 PTCA sites, and 17 five-mm segments). The mean percentage of plaque made up of fibrous tissue among the three groups was $80 \pm 18\%$, $71 \pm 23\%$, and $82 \pm 16\%$, respectively; the mean percentage of plaque made up of lipid was $17 \pm 16\%$, $21 \pm 24\%$, and $16 \pm 15\%$; and the mean percentage of plaque made up of calcium was $3 \pm 4\%$, $8 \pm 10\%$, and $2 \pm 3\%$, respectively. The mean coronary arterial internal diameter was 3.3 ± 0.6, 3.9 ± 1.2, and 3.2 ± 0.7 mm, respectively. Plaque tear was present in one or more histologic sections in 25 of the 26 patients, and the single patient without it had the longest interval (nearly 3 years) between PTCA and death. Plaque tear extending from intima into media with dissection was observed only in the early and late success groups. Hemorrhage into plaque was present in 16 (80%) of 20 PTCA sites in the two early groups and in three of eight sites in the late group. Occlusive thrombus (5 of 16, 1 of 4, and 1 of 8) and plaque debris (7 of 16, 1 of 4, and 2 of 8) in residual lumens were insignificantly different among the three groups and their 82 five-mm segments. Plaques that had more than 25% lipid content had an increased frequency of hemorrhage into plaque, occlusive thrombus, and plaque debris in residual lumens. These findings suggest that the coronary arterial size and plaque composition are strong determinants of PTCA outcome. The ideal coronary arterial atherosclerotic narrowing for both technically and clinically successful PTCA appears to be a small artery (less than 3.3 mm in internal diameter) in which the plaque contains relatively little calcium and lipid. This study[24] was the first to quantify the composition of atherosclerotic plaque at the site of successful and unsuccessful PTCA and also the first to measure the coronary arterial internal diameter at sites of PTCA.

MORPHOLOGIC FINDINGS IN SAPHENOUS VEINS USED AS CORONARY ARTERIAL BYPASS CONDUITS

Studies of Changes in Saphenous Veins Used as Conduits

Saphenous veins, when used as aortocoronary conduits, undergo changes in their intimal, medial, and adventitial layers. The predominant late intimal change is a proliferation of fibrous tissue, a finding observed within 2 months after coronary artery bypass grafting. Other late changes in saphenous vein grafts include deposits of lipid, thrombus, and, rarely, aneurysm formation. Most published studies describing changes in saphenous veins used as coronary bypass conduits have

involved few necropsy patients, only operatively excised specimens, or cases with relatively short intervals from coronary bypass surgery to death or reoperation. Kalan and Roberts[13] studied at necropsy the hearts and grafts of 53 patients who lived longer than 1 year after coronary bypass surgery. They examined 123 saphenous vein grafts and 1,865 five-mm segments of the grafts in these 53 patients, some of whom died of consequences of myocardial ischemia and some of whom died of noncardiac conditions.

The 53 patients died from 13 to 185 months (mean, 58) after a single aortocoronary bypass operation. Of the 53 patients, 32 (60%) died of a cardiac cause and 36 of their 72 saphenous vein aortocoronary conduits (49%) were narrowed at some point by more than 75% in cross-sectional area by atherosclerotic plaque; the remaining 21 patients (40%) died of a noncardiac cause, and 10 of their 50 saphenous vein conduits (20%) were narrowed at some point by more than 75% in cross-sectional area by plaque. Thus, the noncardiac mode of death in a large percentage of the patients suggests that the coronary bypass operation prolonged life to a degree sufficient for another condition to develop. The 123 saphenous vein conduits were divided into 5-mm segments, and a histologic section was prepared from each. Of the 1,104 five-mm segments in the 32 patients who died as a consequence of myocardial ischemia, 291 (26%) were narrowed by more than 75% in cross-sectional area by plaque; in contrast, of the 761 five-mm segments of veins in the 21 patients with a noncardiac mode of death, 86 (11%) were narrowed by more than 75% by plaque. Of the total 1,865 five-mm segments of vein, only 395 (21%) were narrowed by 25% or less in cross-sectional area by plaque. Thus, in patients who die late after coronary bypass surgery, the atherosclerotic process continues in all segments of the saphenous veins used as aortocoronary conduits. Therapy after the operation must be directed toward prevention of progression of the atherosclerosis in the "new" coronary "arteries."

In the study by Kalan and Roberts,[13] the amount of luminal narrowing in the saphenous veins used as aortocoronary conduits was significantly greater in patients who died of a cardiac cause than in those who died of a noncardiac cause. Additionally, the percentage of vein conduits and the percentage of 5-mm segments of the vein conduits totally occluded or nearly so (>95% in cross-sectional area) were significantly greater in the patients who died of a cardiac cause than in those who died of a noncardiac cause (22 [30%] of 73 veins versus 7 [14%] of 50 veins, and 152 [14%] of 1,104 segments versus 57 [27%] of 213 segments).

Surprisingly, the interval from coronary bypass surgery to death did not correlate with either the percentage of vein conduits or the percentage of 5-mm segments of vein conduit narrowed more than 75% in cross-sectional area by plaque. The percentage of venous conduits that were narrowed severely (more than 75%) was similar in the 18 conduits (seven patients) in place from 13 to 24 months and in the 9 conduits (five patients) in place for longer than 10 years. Moreover, the percentage of 5-mm segments of saphenous vein conduit that were severely narrowed was similar in the 35 patients surviving up to 5 years to that in the 18 patients surviving more than 5 years (268 [19%] of 1,387 segments versus 113 [24%] of 478 segments).

Why some saphenous vein conduits became severely narrowed or occluded or nearly so and others did not may be related more to the status of the native coronary artery containing the graft than to the graft itself. Of the 123 native coronary arteries containing a saphenous vein conduit, 49 (40%) of the arteries distal to the anastomotic site were narrowed more than 75% in cross-sectional area by plaque, and the anastomosed saphenous vein was severely narrowed in 33 (67%) of them. In contrast, of the 74 native coronary arteries narrowed less than 75% distal to the anastomotic site, the attached saphenous vein was severely narrowed in only 14 (19%). Thus, the amount of narrowing in the native coronary artery distal to the anastomotic site plays a major determining role in the fate of the attached saphenous vein.

Composition of Plaque in Saphenous Vein Conduits

The composition of the plaques in the saphenous venous conduits is similar to that in the native coronary arteries. Fibrous tissue or fibro-

muscular tissue was the dominant component of the plaques in the saphenous vein conduits, just as it was the dominant component of plaques in the native coronary arteries in patients with fatal CHD without coronary bypass surgery. Lipid was present in plaques in saphenous veins in much smaller amounts than was fibrous tissue. Intracellular lipid was found in a saphenous vein as early as 14 months after coronary bypass surgery, and it did not increase in either frequency or amount as the interval from coronary bypass surgery to death increased. Extracellular lipid was first seen at 26 months after coronary bypass surgery, and it did not appear to increase thereafter as the interval from the coronary bypass operation increased. Hemorrhage into plaque, which occurred almost entirely into extracellular lipid deposits (containing cholesterol clefts within pultaceous debris), was first seen at 32 months after coronary bypass surgery. Intraluminal thrombus was found in saphenous veins in 14 patients (26%) and was first observed at 32 months. Thrombus was always superimposed on underlying lipid in the plaque. Calcific deposits were found in saphenous vein conduits in 11 patients (21%); they were first noted at 34 months after coronary bypass operation, and they did increase in frequency with time.

Cause of Death in Patients With and Without Coronary Bypass

The frequency of the various modes of death among the patients who died late after coronary bypass surgery is a bit different from that of patients with symptomatic myocardial ischemia without coronary bypass surgery. Of the 53 coronary bypass surgery patients studied, only 32 (60%) died of a cardiac cause, and therefore 21 (40%) died of a noncardiac cause. Among patients with symptomatic myocardial ischemia who do not have coronary bypass operations, approximately 95% die of a cardiac cause, and therefore only about 5% die of a noncardiac cause. The fact that 40% of the coronary bypass surgery patients studied died of a noncardiac cause supports the view that the coronary bypass operation in many patients prolongs life long enough for various fatal noncardiac conditions to develop. Of the 53 coronary bypass surgery patients studied by Kalan and Roberts,[13] 10 (19%) died of cancer, a percentage far higher than in patients with symptomatic myocardial ischemia who did not have coronary bypass surgery.

The Kalan-Roberts study[13] reemphasizes that coronary bypass surgery is useful but that it does not, per se, deter progression of the underlying atherosclerotic process. In a slight way, the coronary bypass operation might even cause acceleration of the atherosclerotic process because in about 25% of persons having coronary bypass surgery, the serum total cholesterol level increases and the body weight increases substantially during the first year after the operation. Because lowering the serum (or plasma) total cholesterol level (and specifically the low-density lipoprotein cholesterol level) may cause some portion of atherosclerotic plaques to regress and the chances of a fatal or nonfatal subsequent atherosclerotic event to decrease, a strong case can be advanced for combined simultaneous initiation of both low-fat, low-cholesterol diet therapy and lipid-lowering drug therapy as soon as is reasonably feasible after a coronary bypass operation.[25]

MORPHOLOGIC FEATURES OF COMPLICATIONS OF TRANSMURAL ACUTE MYOCARDIAL INFARCTION

Cardiogenic Shock

Cardiogenic shock is the leading cause of death in patients hospitalized for acute myocardial infarction. Since the advent of coronary care units, the frequency of cardiogenic shock in patients with fatal acute myocardial infarction has at least doubled (40% to about 80%). Necropsy studies have shown important differences in the hearts of patients with acute myocardial infarction and cardiogenic shock compared with patients with acute myocardial infarction who died of other complications, such as arrhythmias or emboli. The major differences are the amount of myocardium damaged and the frequency of coronary arterial thrombi. The location of myocardial necrosis bears no relation to the occurrence of cardiogenic shock. Shock occurs with approximately equal frequency in patients with anterior and inferior wall infarcts. The size of the infarct, in contrast, does correlate with the occurrence of shock. Shock is more frequent in patients with larger than smaller acute infarcts, and myocardial scars are more frequent in patients with cardiogenic shock than in those without. Thus, the total amount of damaged myocardium appears to be more important than the size or location of the acute infarct in determining the occurrence of cardiogenic shock (see also Ch. 3).

To determine the extent of myocardial necrosis and fibrosis, Page et al.[26] studied 20 patients with fatal acute myocardial infarction and shock and 14 others with fatal acute myocardial infarction without shock. Of the 20 with acute infarction and shock, 19 had lost 40 to 70% of the left ventricular myocardium and one had lost 35%; 13 had combined acute and healed infarcts, and 7 had recent infarcts only. Of the 14 patients with acute myocardial infarction without shock, 12 had lost 30% or less of left ventricular myocardium, 1 had lost 35%, and 1 had lost 40%; 6 had combined acute and healed infarcts, and 8 had recent infarcts only. The patients with cardiogenic shock, in contrast to those with infarction without shock, had microscopic foci of necrotic myocardial cells at the edges of the infarcts and at other sites in both left and right ventricles. Similar widespread microscopic foci of necrosis also were observed in the hearts of the 20 patients who had died of shock not due to acute myocardial infarction. Thus, cardiogenic shock in acute myocardial infarction is associated with extensive left ventricular myocardial damage due to recent or to both acute and healed infarcts, and additional widespread acute myocardial damage appears to occur secondary to the shock.

A second important feature of cardiogenic shock in acute myocardial infarction is its association with a high frequency of recent coronary thrombosis. Of 37 patients with fatal acute myocardial infarction studied by Walston et al.,[28] 24 (65%) had cardiogenic shock. No differences between the two groups of patients were observed in the extent of coronary atherosclerosis, which was extensive and severe in all but two patients. The frequency of coronary arterial thrombi in the two groups differed greatly: thrombi were found in 17 (71%) of 24 patients with, and in only 2 (15%) of 13 patients without the "power failure syndrome" (cardiogenic shock). Of the 37 patients, 19 had coronary arterial thrombi and 17 (90%) had the "power failure syndrome;" of the 18 patients without thrombi, 7 (39%) had the "power failure syndrome." Of their 20 patients with cardiogenic shock, 5 had coronary occlusions from hemorrhage into old atherosclerotic plaques, whereas occlusion due to this mechanism occurred in only 1 of the 13 patients without shock. Thus, 22 (88%) of the 24 patients with cardiogenic shock had coronary occlusions due to thrombus or intramural hemorrhage, whereas only 3 of 13 patients without shock had an acute occlusion. Kurland et al.[28] also studied the association of acute coronary occlusion and cardiogenic shock in patients with fatal acute myocardial infarction. Of 46 patients with cardiogenic shock 31 (67%) had acute coronary occlusions; of 81 patients without shock, 39 (48%) had acute coronary occlusions. In the study by Page et al.[26], a high (18 of 20 patients [90%]) frequency of coronary thrombosis occurred in patients with cardiogenic shock and fatal infarction, but a high frequency (11 of 14 patients [78%]) also was found in their patients with fatal myocardial infarction without shock.

In other studies of fatal acute myocardial infarction, the frequency of coronary arterial thrombosis has varied from 21 to 100%.[15] Several factors probably contributed to this variation: (1) the inclusion of cases of subendocardial infarction and sudden death ("acute cardiovascular collapse in the absence of myocardial necrosis") with cases of transmural necrosis; (2) the varying frequency of cardiogenic shock in the different studies; and (3) the differing techniques used in studying the coronary arteries.

On the basis of the thrombolytic-infusion studies during acute myocardial infarction, it would appear that the clinical frequency of coronary thrombosis during the infarction is higher than might be discerned from the necropsy studies. Coronary thrombus is diagnosed clinically by injection of contrast material into a coronary artery, finding the lumen to be totally occluded, and, after infusing a thrombolytic agent and injecting contrast material again, finding that the lumen is patent. This sequence clearly suggests that thrombus was present and that is was dissolved by thrombolysis. Diagnosing thrombus by using contrast material, however, is a presumption, and the coronary lumen has become patent during myocardial infarction in several patients when saline rather than a thrombolytic agent was infused into the occluded coronary artery. Exactly what a 2- or 3-hour old thrombus looks like is unclear. At this stage, it probably consists mainly or entirely of platelets, and it may or may not be adherent to the intimal lining of the artery. The absence of fibrin and the possible lack of adherence of the thrombus to the intimal lining clearly make the early thrombus quite different from the later thrombus. Possibly these early thrombi are missed at necropsy or are dissolved after death.

Papillary Muscle Dysfunction

A significant advance in cardiology during the 1960s was appreciation of the importance of the left ventricular papillary muscles for closure of the mitral orifice during ventricular systole. Hypoxemia, necrosis, or fibrosis of the left ventricular papillary muscles may be associated with various degrees of mitral regurgitation. Although coronary atherosclerosis is the most common cause of papillary muscle dysfunction, scarred or necrotic papillary muscles have been observed in a number of conditions in which the coronary arteries were normal. Despite increased awareness of disorders of the papillary muscles, a number of discrepancies indicate that knowledge about these structures is incomplete. For example, some patients without precordial murmurs during life have been observed at necropsy to have severe necrosis or fibrosis or both of one or both left ventricular papillary muscles; severe mitral regurgitation by clinical examination during or after acute myocardial infarction has been found at necropsy to be associated with normal papillary muscles, normal mitral leaflets and chordae tendineae, and normal-sized mitral annuli. Some necropsy observations on the cardiac papillary muscles are described below.[29]

Anatomically Normal Left Ventricular Papillary Muscles but "Papillary Muscle Dysfunction"

Transient ischemia of the papillary muscles is believed to be extremely common and probably results in various degrees of mitral regurgitation. A murmur of mitral regurgitation can occur during an episode of angina pectoris at rest and frequently during effort and be absent during pain-free periods. Transient systolic murmurs during and after myocardial infarction probably result from papillary muscle ischemia. Arterial perfusion of the left ventricular papillary muscles also may be influenced by body position, emotional stress, or cigarette smoking.

Left ventricular dilatation of any origin is a frequent cause of papillary muscle dysfunction. Under such circumstances, the papillary muscles may contract normally, but the spatial relations between the papillary muscles, the chordae tendineae, and the mitral orifice are altered by the caudal and lateral migration of the left ventricular wall away from the mitral annulus. The valve leaflets are thus pulled downward into the left ventricle, and, consequently, the mitral orifice becomes incompetent. Also, the axes of the papillary muscles become more oblique with respect to the mitral annulus.

Although it can accompany left ventricular dilatation, mitral annular dilatation is probably a rare cause of mitral regurgitation. Most patients with mitral regurgitation, attributed in the past to mitral annular dilatation, probably had papillary muscle dysfunction instead.[30] Mitral annular dilatation to a degree capable of causing mitral regurgitation occurs, in my experience, only in association with mitral valve prolapse, and annular dilatation is a major contributor to mitral regurgitation in patients with mitral valve prolapse.[31,32] In patients with dilated left ventricles not associated with mitral valve prolapse, the widest diameter occurs not at the left ventricular base, the area that includes the mitral annulus, but in the midportion of the chamber between the apex and the base. Indeed, the base of the left ventricle is prevented from dilating freely be-

cause the "fibrous skeleton" is attached to it, whereas the midportion of the left ventricle is not so inhibited. Severe left ventricular dilatation can occur without any dilatation of the mitral annulus, and, in patients with mitral valve prolapse, considerable mitral annular dilatation can occur in the absence of significant left ventricular dilatation.

Although it is now appreciated that mitral regurgitation can occur in patients with dilated left ventricles from any cause, without associated left ventricular necrosis or fibrosis, it is less well recognized that necrosis or fibrosis of the left ventricular free wall unassociated with left ventricular dilatation or papillary muscle or mitral valve lesions may also be associated with mitral regurgitation. Generally, the scarred or necrotic myocardium adjacent to the papillary muscles fails to move or moves paradoxically during ventricular systole, and the abnormal ventricular contraction may lead to abnormal papillary muscle anchoring, with resulting mitral regurgitation. Anatomic left ventricular aneurysms unassociated with papillary muscle necrosis or fibrosis can cause mitral regurgitation by the same mechanism. Abnormal traction on the papillary muscles, unassociated with left ventricular necrosis or fibrosis or with cavity dilatation, can occur in patients with hypertrophic cardiomyopathy, and this mechanism may account for the mitral regurgitation in these instances.

Necrosis or Fibrosis of Papillary Muscles Without Rupture

Necrosis and fibrosis of one or both left ventricular papillary muscles is extremely common. The necrosis or fibrosis may be either focal or diffuse, involving either one or both papillary muscles, and auscultatory mitral regurgitation may or may not be present. When they are focal, the papillary muscle lesions generally are of two types: (1) those that involve nearly all the distal or apical portion of the papillary muscle, and (2) those that involve many areas throughout the entire papillary muscle. The latter lesions usually are small and spare areas adjacent to intramural coronary arteries. When only one papillary muscle contains foci of necrosis or fibrosis, it is virtually always the posteromedial one, since this one has the poorer blood supply.

It is now clear from experimental studies that mitral regurgitation is not a consequence of fibrosis involving only the papillary muscles themselves. If one or both left ventricular papillary muscles were made fibrotic in the dog, either by injection of formalin or by ligation of the base of the muscle, no regurgitation of contrast material from the left ventricle to the left atrium occurred on later angiographic studies. If, however, the free wall beneath the papillary muscle was made fibrotic at the same time, so that ventricular contraction was impaired, mitral regurgitation did result. Excessive fibrosis or necrosis of one or both left ventricular papillary muscles has been observed at necropsy in many patients in whom no precordial murmur had been audible during life. Fibrosis or necrosis of the left ventricular papillary muscles and of the free walls beneath them does not necessarily ensure the appearance of a precordial murmur of mitral regurgitation during life. Several patients with "silent" auscultatory mitral regurgitation have been shown to have mitral regurgitation after left ventricular injection of contrast material.[33] "Silent" mitral regurgitation during acute myocardial infarction has been attributed to a diminished flow velocity across the mitral valve secondary to diminished myocardial contractility.

The most common cause of papillary muscle necrosis or fibrosis is narrowing of the coronary arterial lumen by atherosclerosis. The posteromedial papillary muscle is more commonly involved, and therefore papillary muscle dysfunction is far more likely after inferior than after anterior wall acute myocardial infarction. In anterior wall infarction the anterolateral papillary muscle may be spared, presumably because its blood supply is better than that of the posteromedial muscle. Since infarction limited to the ventricular septum or to the lateral portion of the left ventricular free wall (i.e., the portions of the left ventricular wall unattached to papillary muscle) is rare, the papillary muscles are frequently involved when myocardial infarction occurs. It is therefore surprising that papillary muscle dysfunction is not more frequently observed during or after acute myocardial infarction.

Necrosis or fibrosis of one or both left ventricular papillary muscles is frequent in a number of conditions unassociated with luminal narrowing of the extramural coronary arteries. Inadequate oxygenation of the papillary muscles can result if the amount of oxygen in the blood is small (i.e., anemia) or if the cardiac output is inadequate for any reason. The left ventricular papillary muscles are the last portions of the heart to be perfused with coronary arterial blood. To perfuse the apices of the papillary muscles, the coronary artery must extend through the entire thickness of the myocardial free wall, turn "uphill," and ascend a distance equivalent to at least one, and often two, thicknesses of the free wall. Consequently, it is little wonder that these structures often show evidence of inadequate oxygenation. Furthermore, the papillary muscles serve as the most sensitive markers of inadequate myocardial oxygenation. Since the posteromedial papillary muscle is less well perfused than the anterolateral one, if only one papillary muscle shows foci of necrosis or fibrosis, it will nearly always be the posteromedial muscle.

Necrosis or Fibrosis of Papillary Muscle with Rupture

In contrast to necrosis of a papillary muscle, which occurs in more than 50% of patients with fatal acute myocardial infarction, rupture of a papillary muscle is rare, occurring in less than 1% of patients with fatal acute myocardial infarction. The rupture may be of two types. One involves the entire central muscle belly of the papillary muscle; this type of rupture is incompatible with survival, since half the support to each valve leaflet is destroyed and mitral regurgitation of overwhelming severity results. The second type of rupture involves only one or two apical heads of a papillary muscle. The resulting mitral regurgitation is less severe, and immediate survival is dependent upon the degree to which the function of the left ventricle has been impaired by the infarction. In patients who survive papillary muscle rupture, the functional capacity of the left ventricle also will govern the extent of clinical and hemodynamic improvement after mitral valve replacement.[34]

Although the entire papillary muscle is usually

necrotic, the mitral regurgitation resulting from rupture of an entire trunk of a papillary muscle may justifiably be attributed entirely to the rupture. In contrast, the mitral regurgitation following rupture of only one head of a left ventricular papillary muscle cannot necessarily be attributed entirely to the rupture, since the remainder of the papillary muscle is nearly always also necrotic. What percentage of the regurgitant volume is due to the rupture of a single head and what percentage to the associated papillary muscle necrosis is uncertain. Rupture of a single primary chorda tendinea in the dog, however, produces immediate severe mitral regurgitation; consequently, rupture of a head, which is equivalent to rupturing two primary chordae tendineae, must in itself be severe.

Barbour and Roberts[35] described certain clinical and necropsy findings in 22 patients, aged 45 to 80 years (mean, 64 years) including 15 men (68%), in whom rupture of a papillary muscle occurred during acute myocardial infarction. In most, the acute infarction associated with papillary muscle rupture was a first coronary event (only 18% had a myocardial scar consistent with prior infarction and 29% had angina pectoris). The posteromedial papillary muscle, presumably because of its more tenuous blood supply, ruptured almost three times more frequently than the anterolateral one (73 and 27%, respectively).

Quantitative examination of the amounts of narrowing by atherosclerotic plaque in each of the four major epicardial coronary arteries (right, left main, left anterior descending, and left circumflex) disclosed less narrowing in the patients with rupture than in the patients with fatal acute myocardial infarction unassociated with rupture. Of the 519 five-mm sections of coronary artery examined (11 patients), only 68 (13%) showed greater than 75% narrowing in cross-sectional area, compared with 34% of 1,403 sections from 27 patients with fatal myocardial infarction without rupture.

Rupture of the Left Ventricular Free Wall or Ventricular Septum

In the period before the introduction of coronary care units, the reported frequency of cardiac rupture (left ventricular free wall or ventricular septum) among necropsy cases of fatal acute myocardial infarction varied from 4 to 24% (mean, 8%).[36] Since the introduction of coronary care units, the reported frequency of rupture of the left ventricular free wall or ventricular septum among necropsy cases of fatal myocardial infarction has varied from 16 to 21% (mean, 17%). Reddy and Roberts[36] described the frequency of rupture of the left ventricular free wall or ventricular septum in 648 necropsy patients whom they studied from 1968 to 1988. Of 648 such patients, 204 (31%) had rupture of the left ventricular free wall or ventricular septum. Rupture occurred in 171 (40%) of 431 patients without healed myocardial infarcts (grossly visible left ventricular scars) and in 29 (13%) of 217 patients with healed myocardial infarcts. Thus, the frequency of rupture of the left ventricular free wall or ventricular septum during acute myocardial infarction appears to have increased substantially since the widespread use of coronary care units. Also, the frequency of rupture was nearly three times greater in those in whom rupture occurred during the first acute myocardial infarction than those with a previous infarction that healed. The reason why the frequency of cardiac rupture during acute myocardial infarction appears to have increased since the widespread use of coronary care units is unclear. The most plausible explanation is that the frequency of fatal arrhythmias during acute myocardial infarction has significantly decreased. If the frequency of one cause of death, namely arrhythmias, has decreased, that of another cause of death must increase, and that other cause appears to be cardiac rupture. A much less likely explanation is the increased use of nonsteroidal anti-inflammatory drugs in the last two decades. Anecdotal evidence has been presented by one center, but not by another, that patients with acute myocardial infarction receiving nonsteroidal anti-inflammatory agents for "pericarditis" have a higher frequency of cardiac rupture than do patients who do not receive these drugs during acute myocardial infarction. Corticosteroid therapy might also increase the frequency of cardiac rupture because these drugs delay the healing process.

It also has been suggested that thrombolytic therapy might increase the frequency of rupture of the left ventricular free wall or ventricular septum during acute myocardial infarction and that this increase accounts for the higher mortality during the first 24 hours after onset of acute myocardial infarction compared to patients not treated with thrombolytic agents. Among the 648 necropsy patients studied by Reddy and Roberts,[36] 56 (9%) had received either streptokinase or rt-PA during the first few hours after onset of infarction: 18 (32%) had rupture of the left ventricular free wall or ventricular septum, a percentage similar to that of patients who had not received thrombolytic therapy (186 of 592 [31%]).

Patients with rupture of a left ventricular papillary muscle during acute myocardial infarction presented a problem for inclusion in the study by Reddy and Roberts.[36] Among their 204 patients with rupture of the left ventricular free wall or ventricular septum, 5 (2%) also had rupture (partial or incomplete in all 5) of a left ventricular papillary muscle, and they were included among the rupture cases. Among their 444 patients with fatal acute myocardial infarction without rupture of the left ventricular free wall or ventricular septum, 18 patients had rupture (partial in 14) of a left ventricular papillary muscle. Reddy and Roberts considered it preferable to include these 18 papillary muscle rupture cases with the 444 who did not have rupture of the left ventricular free wall or ventricular septum because none of the 18 reports that included 7,905 necropsy cases reported from 1938 to 1968 mentioned rupture of a left ventricular papillary muscle.[36]

Finally, the question of biased case selection—accounting for the higher frequency of rupture in patients studied by Reddy and Roberts[36] compared with those reported before 1969—deserves comment. The frequency of rupture of either left ventricular free wall or ventricular septum varied considerably among the various submitting hospitals. Although case selection is a potential bias in any clinical study and probably was a factor in the study by Reddy and Roberts, it is unlikely that case selection by itself could have produced such a high frequency of cardiac rupture in their cases compared with those reported before 1969. The reported frequency of left ventricular free wall or ventricular septal rupture during acute myocardial infarction after widespread use of coronary care units is also much higher than that in the period before coronary care units.

Rupture of the Left Ventricular Free Wall

Mann and Roberts[37] compared clinical and necropsy findings in 138 patients (69 men and 69 women) with rupture of the left ventricular free wall during acute myocardial infarction with those in 50 patients who died during their first acute myocardial infarction without rupture. The frequency of systemic arterial hypertension (55 versus 52%), angina pectoris (13 versus 22%), and congestive heart failure (0 versus 0%) before the fatal acute myocardial infarction was similar for both groups. Mean heart masses for men (479 versus 526 g) and women (399 versus 432 g) with and without rupture also were similar. Left ventricular scar before the infarct that ruptured was present in 18 patients (13%); previous necropsy studies of patients with fatal acute myocardial infarction without rupture have indicated that 50% have left ventricular scars. The rupture group had significantly more frequent lateral wall location of the infarct (12 versus 2%). The number of three major (right, left anterior descending, and left circumflex) epicardial coronary arteries that were narrowed at some point by more than 75% in cross-sectional area by atherosclerotic plaque was significantly lower in the rupture group (39 versus 58%). The percentage of these three arteries that were totally occluded or nearly so (more than 95% in cross-sectional area) by plaque also was significantly less in the rupture group (24 of 198 arteries [12%]) than in the nonrupture group (38 of 144 arteries [26%]). Analysis of each 5-mm segment of these arteries in each group disclosed that the rupture group had significantly less narrowing than the nonrupture group. Of the 3,287 five-mm segments of artery examined in the rupture group (66 patients), 512 (15%) were narrowed >75% in cross-sectional area by plaque; in contrast, of the 1,848 five-mm segments in the nonrupture group (38 patients), 508 (28%) were narrowed to this degree by plaque. Thus, rupture of the left ventricular free wall is a complication primarily of the first acute myocardial infarction and is associated with considerably less coronary narrowing than is fatal acute myocardial infarction without rupture.

Rupture of the Ventricular Septum

Mann and Roberts[38] studied at necropsy 38 unoperated patients (24 men and 14 women) with an acquired ventricular septal defect during myocardial infarction (rupture group) and compared their clinical and necropsy findings with those in 50 patients who died during their first acute myocardial infarction without rupture (nonrupture group). The frequency of systemic arterial hypertension (54 versus 52%), angina pectoris (28 versus 22%) and congestive heart failure (5 versus 0%) before the fatal acute myocardial infarction was similar for both rupture and nonrupture groups. Mean heart masses for men (498 versus 526 g) and women (397 versus 432 g) with and without septal rupture also were insignificantly different. Although previous studies of fatal acute myocardial infarction cases have shown that 50% of patients with fatal acute myocardial infarction without rupture have left ventricular scars, only 4 (10%) of the patients with rupture had a left ventricular scar before the infarct that ruptured. The rupture group had a significantly more frequent inferior location of the infarct (74 versus 40%) and, hence a higher frequency of associated right ventricular infarcts (50 versus 18%). The number of three major (right, left anterior descending, and left circumflex) epicardial coronary arteries narrowed at some point by more than 75% in cross-sectional area by atherosclerotic plaque was the same in both groups. The percentage of these three arteries totally occluded or nearly so (more than 95% in cross-sectional area) by plaque was significantly less in the rupture group than in the nonrupture group (9 of 99 arteries [9%] versus 38 of 144 arteries [26%]). Analysis of each 5-mm segment of these arteries in each group disclosed that the rupture group had significantly less narrowing than the nonrupture group. Of the 825 five-mm segments of artery examined in the rupture group (18 patients), only 101 (13%) were narrowed more than 75% in cross-sectional area by plaque; in contrast, of the 1,848 five-mm segments in the nonrupture group (38 patients), 508 (28%) were narrowed to this degree by plaque. Thus, rupture of the ventricular septum primarily is a complication of the first acute myocardial infarction. It is associated with less severe coronary arterial narrowing than observed in fatal acute myocardial infarction without rupture, and it is a more frequent complication of inferior than anterior wall acute myocardial infarct.

Mann and Roberts[39] also described cardiac morphologic findings in 16 necropsy patients not surviving operative closure of an acquired ventricular septal defect during acute myocardial infarction. Of the 16 patients, 6 were women (mean age, 60 ± 7 years) and 10 were men (mean age, 60 ± 11 years). The acute myocardial infarction associated with the ventricular septal defect was the first coronary event in 13 patients (81%). At least six patients had a history of systemic arterial hypertension. Conduction disturbances were diagnosed by electrocardiogram in five patients (31%). The median interval from the onset of the acute myocardial infarction to death was 11 days, and the mean interval from the onset of the acute myocardial infarction to operative closure of the ventricular septal defect was 4 days. Eight patients died in the operating room or within 2 hours of operation. Coronary artery bypass grafting was performed simultaneously with the ventricular septal defect closure in seven patients. Death was attributed to unsuccessful ventricular septal defect closure in five patients, to inadequate left ventricular cavity size after resection of necrotic myocardium in five patients, and to inadequate viable left ventricular myocardium in four patients. Heart masses were increased in 14 patients (88%). The acute myocardial infarct associated with the ventricular septal defect was anterior in nine patients and inferior in seven. Healed myocardial infarcts were present in three patients. All 16 patients had severe (more than 75% in cross-sectional area) narrowing of one or more of the four major epicardial coronary arteries.

On rare occasion, both the ventricular septum and the left ventricular free wall may rupture (double rupture) during acute myocardial infarction. Such was the case in seven necropsy patients described by Mann and Roberts.[40]

True Left Ventricular Aneurysm

Some left ventricular wall motion abnormality—hypokinesia, akinesia, or dyskinesia—occurs at the time of transmural acute myocardial infarction. After healing of the infarct, a few patients are left with focal convex left ventricular protrusions, some during ventricular systole only (functional aneurysm) and some during both ventricular systole and ventricular diastole (anatomic aneurysm).[41] Cabin and Roberts[42] analyzed clinical and necropsy findings in 28 patients with true anatomic aneurysm at sites of healed left ventricular myocardial infarcts. Of the 28 patients, 24 were men, a greater sex difference than in other subsets of CAD patients. Also, in contrast to other subsets of coronary patients, chronic congestive cardiac failure was frequent (22 patients); angina pectoris was infrequent (4 patients) and, when present, was mild; recurrence of acute myocardial infarction (2 patients), sudden death (2 patients), and clinical events compatible with systemic emboli (1 patient) were infrequent; survival for longer than 5 years after healing of the infarction was limited (in 3 of 21 patients with clinically diagnosed infarction); and survival for longer than 12 months after aneurysmectomy was lacking (none of 7 patients). Additionally, most patients (23 of 28) had large hearts (>400 g [mean, 523 g]), 26 had dilated nonaneurysmal portions of the left ventricle, and all but 1 had large (more than 30% of left ventricular wall) myocardial infarcts.

Thus, from studies of necropsy patients with true anatomic left ventricular aneurysms and healed myocardial infarcts, the following conclusions appear justified: the myocardial infarcts are large; the heart weights are increased and nonscarred left ventricular walls are hypertrophied; the nonaneurysmal portions of the left ventricular cavities are dilated; the major epicardial coronary arteries are severely narrowed; chronic congestive heart failure is frequent and is the most common cause of death; angina pectoris is infrequent, as is recurrence of acute myocardial infarction; clinical events compatible with systemic emboli are infrequent despite frequent intra-aneurysmal thrombi; the long-term prognosis is poor; sudden death is infrequent; and the clinical diagnosis of the left ventricular aneurysm without left ventricular angiography or echocardiography is infrequent, despite the frequent (up to 20%) occurrence in cases with myocardial infarct at autopsy examination.

CAD, HEALED MYOCARDIAL INFARCT WITHOUT ANEURYSM, AND CHRONIC CONGESTIVE HEART FAILURE

Ross and Roberts[43] described clinical and necropsy findings in 81 patients (aged 29 to 91 years [mean, 62 years]; 77 [95%] men) with severe congestive heart failure of more than 3 months in duration, left ventricular transmural scar, and more than 75% cross-sectional area narrowing of one or more of the four major epicardial coronary arteries by atherosclerotic plaque. The duration of symptoms from initial onset of acute myocardial infarction (59 patients), congestive heart failure (18 patients), or angina pectoris (2 patients) to death ranged from 0.5 to 18 years (mean, 7.1 years) (two unknown). Angina pectoris occurred at some time, however, in 31 patients (38%). The cause of death was congestive heart failure in 48 patients (59%), sudden (arrhythmia) in 16 (20%), acute myocardial infarction in 11 (14%), and emboli in 6 (7%). The heart masses ranged from 410 to 800 g (mean, 585 g). Left or right ventricular thrombi or both occurred in 37 patients (46%), only 4 (10%) of whom had systemic emboli; of the 44 patients without intracardiac thrombi, none had any form of emboli. The severity of coronary narrowing was variable. In 24 patients (30%), only one artery was narrowed by more than 75% in cross-sectional area; in 22 patients (27%), two arteries were so narrowed; in 32 patients (39%), three arteries; and in 3 patients (4%), four arteries. The size of the left ventricular scar also varied. Of the 81 patients, 58 (72%) had large scars (involving more than 40% of the left ventricular wall); 10 (12%) had moderate-sized scars (6 to 40% of the left ventricular wall); and 13 (16%) had small scars (up to and including 5% of the left ventricular wall). The size of the left ventricular scar correlated inversely with a history of habitual alcoholism: of the 16 habitual alcoholics, 6 (38%) had small and 8 (50%) had large left ventricular scars; of the 65 nonalcoholics, 7 (11%) had small and 50 (77%) had large left ventricular scars. Chronic congestive heart failure in the 68 patients with either moderate-sized or large left ventricular scars is readily attributed to the left ventricular damage; in the 13 patients with small left ventricular scars, however, chronic congestive heart failure more reasonably may be attributed to another factor, e.g., alcoholism, despite coronary artery narrowing similar in severity to that in the patients with large left ventricular scars.

CAD, CHRONIC CONGESTIVE HEART FAILURE, BUT NO MYOCARDIAL INFARCT

Ross and Roberts[44] described clinical and necropsy findings in 18 patients (aged 38 to 73 years [mean, 58 years]; 16 [89%] men) studied at necropsy who had had chronic congestive heart failure for more than 3 months, more than 75% cross-sectional area narrowing of one or more of the four major epicardial coronary arteries, and no left ventricular fibrosis or necrosis. The duration of symptoms from onset of congestive heart failure to death ranged from 0.3 to 13 years (mean, 5.7 years). Angina pectoris occurred in two patients (11%). The mode of death was congestive heart failure in 12 (67%), sudden (arrhythmia) in 5 (28%), and emboli in 1 (5%). Heart masses ranged from 410 to 890 g (mean, 632 g). Of 72 major epicardial coronary arteries (right, left main, left anterior descending, and left circumflex) in the 18 patients, 30 (42%) were narrowed 76 to 100% in cross-sectional area by atherosclerotic plaque. A mean of 1.7 of 4 major epicardial coronary arteries per patient were narrowed 76 to 100% in cross-sectional area by atherosclerotic plaque. In 10 patients, each 5-mm segment of the four major coronary arteries was examined histologically (mean, 53 per patient): 23 segments (3%) were narrowed 96 to 100% in cross-sectional area by atherosclerotic plaque; 58 (11%), 76 to 95%; 93 (18%), 51 to 75%; 209 (40%), 26 to 50%;

and 146 (28%), 0 to 25%. Left and right ventricular thrombi were found in nine patients (50%); of the nine patients, one had a systemic embolus; of the nine patients without intraventricular thrombi, none had systemic emboli. Because grossly visible myocardial lesions were absent, the severe chronic congestive heart failure in these 18 patients cannot reasonably be attributed to CAD. It is most reasonable to believe that this group of patients had idiopathic dilated cardiomyopathy and that the CAD was coincidental.

RIGHT VENTRICULAR INFARCT

Relation to Left Ventricular Infarct

Acute myocardial infarction secondary to coronary arterial narrowing virtually always involves the left ventricular free wall and often also the ventricular septum. Involvement of the right ventricular free wall secondary to coronary luminal narrowing has, until recently, rarely been diagnosed clinically, and few morphologic studies have focused on its frequency or extent. One study, however, reported infarcts in the right ventricle in 14% of autopsied patients with myocardial infarction.[14] Isner and Roberts[45] examined the frequency of right ventricular infarcts in patients with associated transmural left ventricular infarct and determined its extent and relation to the accompanying location of the infarct of the left ventricular wall.

A total of 236 necropsy patients with transmural acute myocardial infarcts of the left ventricular wall were studied. The patients were divided into two groups: (1) those with transmural myocardial necrosis (acute infarct) and (2) those with transmural myocardial fibrosis (healed infarct). When both fibrosis and necrosis were visible grossly in the same heart (34 patients), the group in which the patient was placed was determined by which lesion was more extensive. The hearts were then further subdivided by location of the left ventricular infarct into two additional groups: (1) anterior wall and (2) inferior wall.

Of the 236 patients, 116 had acute and 120 had healed left ventricular myocardial infarcts. The myocardial infarcts involved the anterior wall in 97 patients and the inferior wall in the other 139. Of the 97 patients with anterior left ventricular infarcts (acute in 56 [40%] and healed in 83 [60%]), 33 (24%) had associated right ventricular infarcts. Of the total 236 patients, 133 had transmural infarcts of the ventricular septum, 68 had anterior left ventricular infarcts, and 65 had inferior left ventricular infarcts. All 33 patients with right ventricular infarcts were from the 65 with inferior left ventricular infarcts associated with transmural infarcts of the ventricular septum. Of the 74 patients with inferior ventricular infarcts without associated transmural infarcts of the ventricular septum, none had right ventricular infarcts. Of the patients with isolated anterior wall left ventricular infarcts, irrespective of whether the ventricular septum was involved, none had associated right ventricular infarct. In only 1 of the 33 patients was the right ventricular wall hypertrophied (more than 5 mm thick), whereas right ventricular dilatation was present in 12. Right ventricular thrombus occurred in three patients. The infarct of the right ventricle was limited to its posterior wall (types I or II) in 36 patients and to both posterior and anterolateral right ventricular free walls (types III and IV) in the other 7.

Comparison of the 33 patients who had inferior left ventricular wall infarcts with associated right ventricular wall infarcts with the 106 patients who had inferior left ventricular wall infarcts but without associated right ventricular wall infarcts disclosed no significant differences in the patients' age, sex, or length of survival after onset of symptoms of myocardial ischemia or the presence of right ventricular hypertrophy or thrombosis. Right ventricular dilatation, however, was significantly more frequent among the group with inferior left ventricular infarcts with associated right ventricular wall infarcts.

The three major (right, left anterior descending, and left circumflex) coronary arteries were examined in detail in 87 (63%) of the 139 patients with left ventricular inferior wall infarcts. Of these, 28 had associated right ventricular infarcts and 59 did not. No significant differences among the patients with inferior left ventricular infarcts were observed in the percentage of cross-sectional area luminal narrowing by more than 75% by old atherosclerotic plaque in each of the three major coronary arteries between those with and those without right ventricular infarcts. The degree of narrowing of the right coronary artery was similar in the patients with and without right ventricular infarct. The percentage of patients in whom the right coronary artery was narrowed 76 to 100% in cross-sectional area by old atherosclerotic plaque was significantly greater than the percentage of those in whom the left anterior descending coronary artery was narrowed to this degree, irrespective of whether infarct involved the right ventricular wall.

Among patients with fatal myocardial infarction secondary to severe coronary arterial luminal narrowing, right ventricular infarcts occurred only when the left ventricular infarct involved its inferior wall. Of the 139 patients with inferior left ventricular infarcts, 33 (24%) had associated right ventricular infarct. Even among the patients with inferiorly located left ventricular infarcts, however, transmural infarct of the ventricular septum was a prerequisite for development of right ventricular infarct. Of the 139 patients with inferior left ventricular infarcts, 74 did not have transmural infarcts of the ventricular septum and none had associated right ventricular infarct. Of the 65 with transmural infarcts of the ventricular septum, 33 (50%) had associated right ventricular infarcts. Thus, right ventricular infarct was a complication exclusively of transmural inferior left ventricular infarcts.

Extent of Right Ventricular Necrosis

The extent of the right ventricular necrosis or fibrosis varied from less than one-half of the posterior right ventricular free wall adjacent to the ventricular septum (nine patients) to involvement of nearly the entire right ventricular free wall (two patients). Of the 33 patients with right ventricular infarcts, the infarct was limited to the posterior right ventricular free wall in 26 (79%), and the remaining 7 (21%) had involvement of both posterior and anterolateral walls of the right ventricle.

Right Ventricular Hypertrophy and Right Ventricular Infarct

Right ventricular hypertrophy was not an important predisposing factor for the development of right ventricular myocardial infarct. Right ventricular hypertrophy was more frequent among the patients without associated right ventricular infarct. Right ventricular hypertrophy was observed at necropsy in only 1 (3%) of the 33 patients with right ventricular infarct and in 12 (6%) of the 203 patients with left ventricular myocardial infarct unassociated with right ventricular infarct. Furthermore, none had necropsy evidence of cor pulmonale. Although extensive right ventricular scarring has been described in various entities associated with right ventricular hypertrophy (including chronic pulmonary emboli and hypertrophic cardiomyopathy in the absence of significant coronary arterial luminal narrowing), such cases were excluded from the study by Isner and Roberts[45] unless they were associated with left ventricular scarring and significant coronary arterial luminal narrowing. Right ventricular dilatation was the single anatomic feature distinguishing the patients with from those without right ventricular myocardial infarct. Among the 139 patients with inferior wall left ventricular infarcts, the right ventricular cavities were dilated in 21 (36%) of the 33 patients with and 10 (9%) of the 106 patients without associated right ventricular infarcts. Right ventricular dilatation occurred in only 16 (16%) of the 97 patients with anterior wall left ventricular infarcts, a significantly lower percentage than in the patients with right ventricular infarcts.

Right Ventricular Mural Thrombus and Right Ventricular Infarct

Right ventricular mural thrombus is another necropsy finding reported to be more frequent among patients with associated right ventricular wall infarcts than in patients with isolated left ventricular wall infarcts. In the 237 patients with left ventricular wall infarcts, however, right ventricular thrombi occurred with similar frequency in those with and those without associated in-

farcts of the right ventricular wall. Among the 139 patients with inferior wall left ventricular infarcts, right ventricular thrombus occurred in 3 (9%) of the 33 patients with and 4 (4%) of the 106 patients without associated right ventricular infarcts; among the 97 patients with anterior wall left ventricular infarcts, right ventricular thrombus occurred in 8 (8%).

Among the patients with inferior wall left ventricular infarcts, the percentage with 76 to 100% cross-sectional area luminal narrowing of the right coronary artery by atherosclerotic plaque was similar (about 90%) in the patients with right ventricular infarcts and those without. All patients with right ventricular infarcts had severe (76 to 100% cross-sectional area) luminal narrowing of the dominant coronary artery, that is, either the right or the left circumflex, responsible for perfusing the inferior ventricular wall.

Diagnosis of Right Ventricular Infarction

Diagnosis during life of right ventricular infarction in patients with left ventricular infarction secondary to severe coronary arterial luminal narrowing is, at best, difficult. If the left ventricular infarct is isolated to the anterior wall, the chance of an associated right ventricular infarct is minimal. Thus, an inferior location of the left ventricular infarct is a prerequisite for right ventricular infarct. Nearly one-quarter of all patients with inferior wall infarct of the left ventricle had associated right ventricular infarcts. Thus, if the left ventricular infarct is inferior and transmural, there is a 1 in 4 chance of an associated right ventricular infarct. If, however, the ventricular septum is transmurally infarcted, the frequency of associated right ventricular infarct doubles, or becomes 50%. The electrocardiogram is not helpful in distinguishing infarct limited to the inferior left ventricular wall from that involving both the inferior and septal walls. The echocardiogram may show diminished motion of the ventricular septum in this circumstance, but the reliability of this technique in determining transmural septal infarct is unproved. One finding suggestive of right ventricular infarct is right ventricular dilatation, an occurrence nearly three times more frequent in patients with right ventricular infarct than in those without. Right ventricular hypertrophy is rare in patients with right ventricular infarct secondary to coronary narrowing and is therefore not helpful from a diagnostic standpoint.

Before the introduction of newer, noninvasive techniques, especially myocardial imaging, clinical validation of right ventricular myocardial infarct was limited to cardiac catheterization. The finding of elevated right atrial (or right ventricular end-diastolic) pressure has been suggested as the characteristic hemodynamic profile of right ventricular myocardial infarct. Three of the four patients studied by Isner and Roberts[45] with necropsy-confirmed right ventricular myocardial infarcts had hemodynamic profiles that were not suggestive of associated right ventricular infarct. The hemodynamic profile previously considered characteristic of right ventricular infarct is less diagnostically sensitive than previously believed, and right ventricular infarct may still be present in the presence of normal or near-normal intracardiac pressures. Conversely, in the absence of pericardial or valvular heart disease, the hemodynamic abnormalities described for right ventricular infarct appear to be relatively specific.

Cumulative clinical experience with right ventricular myocardial infarction complicating left ventricular myocardial infarction has clearly established the existence of a specific hemodynamic syndrome of right ventricular dysfunction characterized by underfilling of the left ventricle as a result of impaired right ventricular contractility. In such patients, right ventricular dilatation is the sole compensatory mechanism by which right ventricular contractility may be augmented. Under such circumstances, volume administration may be critical to maintain an optimal right ventricular filling pressure. Indeed, supplemental volume administration in patients with elevated right-sided pressures and a normal or near-normal left ventricular filling pressure (i.e., patients with right ventricular infarcts) has produced marked hemodynamic improvement. Therefore, it becomes important to recognize clues to the often occult syndrome of right ventricular dysfunction or right ventricular infarction. Evidence of an inferior myocardial infarct combined with the evidence of right ventricular dilatation should make one particularly suspicious of the presence of right ventricular infarct.

MODES OF DEATH IN FATAL CHD

Author's Study

Roberts et al.[46] described mode of death, frequency of a healed or an acute myocardial infarct (or both), number of major epicardial coronary arteries severely narrowed by atherosclerotic plaque, and heart mass at necropsy in 889 patients 30 years of age or older with fatal CHD. No patient had had a coronary bypass operation or PTCA. The 889 patients were classified into four major groups, and each major group was classified into two subgroups: (1) acute myocardial infarct without (306 patients) or with (119 patients) a healed myocardial infarct; (2) sudden out-of-hospital death without (121 patients) or with (118 patients) a healed myocardial infarct; (3) chronic congestive heart failure with a healed myocardial infarct without (137 patients) or with (33 patients) a left ventricular aneurysm; and (4) sudden in-hospital death without (20 patients) or with (35 patients) unstable angina pectoris.

The mean age of the 687 men (77%) was 60 ± 11 years, and that of the 202 women (23%) was 68 ± 13 years. Although men included 77% of all patients, they made up approximately 90% of the out-of-hospital (nonangina) sudden death group. The frequency of systemic arterial hypertension and angina pectoris was similar in each of the four major groups. The frequency of diabetes mellitus was lowest in the sudden out-of-hospital death group and similar in the other three major groups.

The mean heart mass and the percentage of patients with a heart of increased mass were highest in the chronic congestive heart failure group; values were lower and similar in the other three major groups. All patients in the chronic congestive heart failure group (by definition) had a healed left ventricular infarct which was similar in frequency in the other three major groups. The percentage of patients in whom three or four of the four major coronary arteries were severely narrowed (more than 75% in cross-sectional area) by atherosclerotic plaque was highest in the unstable angina subgroup and lower and similar in all other major groups.

Of the 437 patients (49%) with one or more grossly visible left ventricular scars, the fatal coronary event in 119 (27%) was an acute myocardial infarction; in 118 patients (27%) it was sudden out-of-hospital (or nearly so) cardiac arrest; in 170 patients (39%) it was chronic, intractable congestive heart failure; and in 30 patients (7%) it was sudden in-hospital death with or without preceding unstable angina pectoris. Of the 452 patients (51%) without a grossly visible left ventricular scar, the fatal coronary event in 306 (68%) was an acute myocardial infarction; in 121 patients (27%) it was sudden (or nearly so) out-of-hospital cardiac arrest; and in 25 patients (5%) it was sudden in-hospital cardiac arrest with or without preceding unstable angina pectoris. Thus, the patients without a previous acute myocardial infarction were more likely (nearly 70%) to die of an acute myocardial infarction, and the fatal events in the patients with a previous acute myocardial infarction were more or less equally divided among the subgroups with fatal acute myocardial infarction, sudden (or nearly so) out-of-hospital cardiac arrest, and chronic congestive heart failure.

One of the major tragedies of CHD is the relatively young age of its victims. Among the 687 men in this study, the average age at death was 60 years; among the 202 women, the average age at death was 68 years, roughly 10 years less than the average life expectancy for men and women in the United States.[47] Patients younger than 30 years at death were excluded from this study.

How representative of the modes of death from CHD are the patients in the present study? Most (73%) patients included in this study died in a hospital, and this fact almost surely increases the percentage of cases with a fatal acute myocardial infarction. Had more medical examiners' cases been included, the percentage of patients who died suddenly outside the hospital almost surely would have been higher. Had only hospital deaths been included in this study, the percentage of sudden deaths would have been consid-erably lower. Although the mode of death from CHD may or may not have been different from that in this study if all victims of CHD in a single community had been available for study at necropsy, this study nevertheless provides an opportunity to compare victims of one mode of death with victims of another mode of death when all cases were studied and classified by the same physician (W.C.R.).

Obstacles to Data Comparison among Studies

Although many reports have described findings at necropsy in patients with CHD, it is surprisingly difficult and probably relatively meaningless to compare contemporary data with those reported in earlier decades by others. There are several reasons why these comparisons are probably not useful, with one exception (to be described below).

Use of Obsolete and Ambiguous Terms in Older Studies

Terms that were used in older studies are sometimes meaningless today. For example, are the terms "coronary thrombosis, sudden or acute coronary occlusion, acute coronary, acute coronary obstruction and myocardial accident," as used in older reports, synonyms for "acute myocardial infarction" used today, or are some of these terms synonyms for "sudden coronary death"[48] as used today? Are "coronary insufficiency" and "coronary failure," as used in the past, synonyms for "unstable angina" or "sudden death," as used today? The term "unstable angina pectoris," introduced by Conti et al.,[49] has been used for less than two decades. Are "myocardial insufficiency" and "myocardial failure" old terms for "chronic congestive heart failure" or "ischemic cardiomyopathy" as used today? "Sudden death" and "gradual death" in older reports rarely were defined.

Use of Different Inclusion and Exclusion Criteria

Some past studies included only young individuals, others only older individuals; some studies intermixed cases in which CHD caused death and those in which death was not of coronary heart disease origin but CAD was present at necropsy or had produced symptoms of myocardial ischemia during life. Other studies included only patients who died in the hospital, whereas still others included only those who died outside the hospital; still other studies included only cases with a single coronary event—for example, acute myocardial infarction—and excluded those with sudden death, or vice versa.

Use of Relatively Few Cases in Older Studies

Obviously, meaningful data on the frequency of the various modes of death from CHD cannot be obtained by studying relatively small numbers of patients, irrespective of how detailed those studies might be.

Use of Data Collected by Many Nonspecialist Physicians in Older Studies

Nearly all publications focusing on the various modes of death from CHD or the cardiac findings in fatal CHD have been based on data recorded in autopsy protocols and collected by numerous physicians with little expertise in cardiovascular disease. In the Roberts et al. report,[46] all hearts were examined by a single physician who has specialized in cardiovascular diseases for three decades.

Advances in Treatment Over the Years

Coronary care units were not widely available until about 1970, and the mortality rate during acute myocardial infarction, and, therefore, subsequent mortality, probably has been affected by their use. Pharmacologic therapy for systemic arterial hypertension was not used until about 1950, and in 1972 only 15% of patients in the United States with systemic arterial hypertension had their blood pressure adequately controlled by therapy; by 1987, this percentage had climbed to nearly 60%. Thus, future studies of the heart at necropsy in fatal CHD may see a fall in the frequency of cardiomegaly and possibly other reflections of antihypertensive therapy on the heart. Future studies of modes of death from CHD may reflect the use or abuse of PTCA; coronary bypass grafting, and various thrombolytic therapies.

Rochester, Minn., Study

A superb study of the modes of death from CHD and cardiac findings at necropsy in its victims was reported by Spiekerman et al.[50] in 1962. Their study analyzed deaths of residents in a single community (Rochester, Minn.) during a 5-year period (1947 to 1952). During that period, 1,026 persons aged 20 years or older died (50% women and 50% men) and necropsy was performed in 691 (67%). Of the 1,026 patients, 563 (55%) died in the hospital and autopsy was done in 377 (67%), and 463 (45%) died outside the hospital and necropsy was done in 314 (68%). Of the 691 patients aged 20 years or over studied at necropsy, 221 (32%) died of CHD (40% of the men and 22% of the women). Of the patients aged 30 to 64 years, 54% died of CHD, and in the age group 65 years or older, 38% died of CHD.

In this Mayo Clinic study,[50] the modes of death in the 221 patients with fatal CHD were as follows: (1) "acute coronary failure" (sudden death), 94 patients (43%); (2) acute myocardial infarction, 87 patients (39%); (3) congestive heart failure, 32 patients (14%); and (4) "thromboembolism," 8 patients (4%). A healed myocardial infarct was seen at necropsy in 115 (52%) of the 221 patients, a percentage virtually identical to that of the Roberts et al. study.[46] In the Mayo Clinic study, nine patients included in their sudden death group actually had an acute myocardial infarct. If these nine patients were transferred from the sudden death to the acute myocardial infarction group, the frequency of acute myocardial infarction as the mode of death would climb to 43% and the frequency of sudden death would fall to 38%, percentages similar to those in the Roberts study (48 and 34%).

Association Between Heart Mass and CHD

Cardiomegaly (heart mass of greater than 400 g in men and greater than 350 g in women) occurred in 80% of our 889 patients.[46] The average heart mass was 505 g in the men and 427 g in the women. Of the 170 patients with congestive heart failure, 162 (95%) had a heart of increased mass; in contrast, of the 239 patients who died suddenly outside the hospital, 178 (74%) had a heart of increased mass. Of all 889 patients, only 20% had a heart of normal mass.

REFERENCES

1. Roberts WC: Qualitative and quantitative comparison of amounts of narrowing by atherosclerotic plaques in the major epicardial coronary arteries at necropsy in sudden coronary death, transmural acute myocardial infarction, transmural healed myocardial infarction and unstable angina pectoris. Am J Cardiol 64:324, 1989
2. Roberts WC, Jones AA: Quantitation of coronary arterial narrowing at necropsy in sudden coronary death. Analysis of 31 patients and comparison with 25 control subjects. Am J Cardiol 44:39, 1979
3. Roberts WC, Jones AA: Quantification of coronary arterial narrowing at necropsy in acute transmural myocardial infarction. Analysis and comparison of findings in 27 patients and 22 controls. Circulation 61:786, 1980
4. Virmani R, Roberts WC: Non-fatal healed transmural myocardial infarction and fatal non-cardiac disease. Qualification and quantification of coronary arterial narrowing and of left ventricular scarring in 18 necropsy patients. Br Heart J 45:434, 1981
5. Virmani R, Roberts WC: Quantification of coronary arterial narrowing and of left ventricular myocardial scarring in healed myocardial infarction with chronic eventually fatal congestive cardiac failure. Am J Med 68:831, 1980
6. Cabin HS, Roberts WC: True left ventricular aneurysm and healed myocardial infarction. Clinical and necropsy observations including quantification of degree of coronary arterial narrowing. Am J Cardiol 46:754, 1980
7. Roberts WC, Virmani R: Quantification of coronary arterial narrowing in clinically isolated unstable angina pectoris. An analysis of 22 necropsy patients. Am J Med 67:792, 1979
8. Bulkley BM, Roberts WC: Atherosclerotic narrowing of the left main coronary artery. A necropsy analysis of 152 patients with fatal coronary heart disease and varying degrees of left main narrowing. Circulation 53:823, 1976
9. Isner JM, Wu M, Virmani R, et al: Comparison of degrees of coronary arterial luminal narrowing determined by visual inspection of histologic sections under magnification among three independent observers and comparison to that obtained by video planimetry. An analysis of 559 five-mm segments of 61 coronary arteries from eleven patients. Lab Invest 42:566, 1980
10. Arnett EN, Isner JM, Redwood DR, et al: Coronary artery narrowing in coronary heart disease: Comparison of cineangiographic and necropsy findings. Ann Intern Med 91:350, 1979
11. Isner JM, Kishel J, Kent KM, et al: Accuracy of angiographic determination of left main coronary arterial narrowing. Angiographic-histologic correlative analysis in 28 patients. Circulation 63:1056, 1981
12. Waller BF, Roberts WC: Amount of narrowing by atherosclerotic plaque in 44 nonbypassed and 52 bypassed major epicardial coronary arteries in 32 necropsy patients who died within 1 month of aortocoronary bypass grafting. Am J Cardiol 46:956, 1980
13. Kalan JM, Roberts WC: Morphologic findings in saphenous veins used as coronary arterial bypass conduits for longer than one year: Necropsy analysis of 53 patients, 123 saphenous veins, and 1865 five-mm segments of veins. Am Heart J 119:1164; 1990
14. Wartman WB, Hellerstein HK: The incidence of heart disease in 2000 consecutive autopsies. Ann Intern Med 28:41, 1948
15. Roberts WC, Buja LM: The frequency and significance of coronary arterial thrombi and other observations in fatal acute myocardial infarction. A study of 107 necropsy patients. Am J Med 52:425, 1972
16. Kragel AH, Gertz SD, Roberts WC: Morphologic comparison of frequency and types of acute lesions in the major epicardial coronary arteries in unstable angina pectoris, sudden coronary death, and acute myocardial infarction. J Am Coll Cardiol 18:1991
17. Herrick JB: Thrombosis of the coronary arteries. JAMA 72:387, 1919
18. Brosius FC III, Roberts WC: Significance of coronary arterial thrombus in transmural acute myocardial infarction. A study of 54 necropsy patients. Circulation 63:810, 1981
19. Roberts WC: Coronary embolism. A review of causes, consequences, and diagnostic considerations. Cardiovasc Med 3:699, 1978

20. Gertz SD, Kalan JM, Kragel AH, et al: Cardiac morphologic findings in patients with acute myocardial infarction treated with recombinant tissue plasminogen activator. Am J Cardiol 65:953, 1990

21. Gertz SD, Kragel AH, Kalan JM, et al: Comparison of coronary and myocardial morphologic findings in patients with and without thrombolytic therapy during fatal first acute myocardial infarction. Am J Cardiol 66:904, 1990

22. Kragel AH, Reddy SG, Wittes JT, Roberts WC: Morphometric analysis of the composition of atherosclerotic plaques in the four major epicardial coronary arteries in acute myocardial infarction and in sudden coronary death. Circulation 80:1747, 1989

23. Kragel AH, Reddy SG, Wittes JT, Roberts WC: Morphometric analysis of the composition of coronary arterial plaques in isolated unstable angina pectoris with pain at rest. Am J Cardiol 66:562, 1990

24. Potkin BN, Roberts WC: Location of an acute myocardial infarct in patients with a healed myocardial infarct: Analysis of 129 patients studied at necropsy. Am J Cardiol 62:1017, 1988

25. Roberts WC: Lipid-lowering therapy after an atherosclerotic event. Am J Cardiol 65:16F, 1990

26. Page DL, Caufield JB, Kastor JA, et al: Myocardial changes associated with cardiogenic shock. N Engl J Med 285:133, 1971

27. Walston A, Hackel DB, Estes HE: Acute coronary occlusion and the "power failure" syndrome. Am Heart J 79:613, 1970

28. Kurland GS, Weingarten C, Pitt B: The relation between the location of coronary occlusions and the occurrence of shock in acute myocardial infarction. Circulation 31:646, 1965

29. Roberts WC, Cohen L: Left ventricular papillary muscles. Description of the normal and a survey of conditions causing them to be abnormal. Circulation 46:138, 1972

30. Bulkley BH, Roberts WC: Dilatation of the mitral annulus. A rare cause of mitral regurgitation. Am J Med 59:457, 1975

31. Roberts WC, McIntosh CL, Wallace RB: Mechanisms of severe mitral regurgitation in mitral valve prolapse determined from analysis of operatively excised valves. Am Heart J 113:1316, 1987

32. Dollar AL, Roberts WC: Morphologic comparison of patients with mitral valve prolapse who died suddenly with patients who died from severe valvular dysfunction or other conditions. J Am Coll Cardiol 17:921, 1991

33. Falcone MW, Ronan JA, Jr, Roberts WC: Silent mitral regurgitation complicating silent myocardial infarction. Hemodynamic and morphologic documentation. Chest 62:226, 1972

34. Morrow AG, Cohen LS, Roberts WC, et al: Severe mitral regurgitation following acute myocardial infarction and ruptured papillary muscle. Hemodynamic findings and results of operative treatment in four patients. Circulation 37–38 (suppl. II):II-124, 1968

35. Barbour DJ, Roberts WC: Rupture of a left ventricular papillary muscle during acute myocardial infarction: analysis of 22 necropsy patients. J Am Coll Cardiol 8:558, 1986

36. Reddy SG, Roberts WC: Frequency of rupture of the left ventricular free wall or ventricular septum among necropsy cases of fatal acute myocardial infarction since introduction of coronary care units. Am J Cardiol 63:906, 1989

37. Mann JM, Roberts WC: Rupture of the left ventricular free wall during acute myocardial infarction: Analysis of 138 necropsy patients and comparison with 50 necropsy patients with acute myocardial infarction without rupture. Am J Cardiol 62:847, 1988

38. Mann JM, Roberts WC: Acquired ventricular septal defect during acute myocardial infarction: Analysis of 38 unoperated necropsy patients and comparison with 50 unoperated necropsy patients without rupture. Am J Cardiol 62:8, 1988

39. Mann JM, Roberts WC: Cardiac morphologic observations after operative closure of acquired ventricular septal defect during acute myocardial infarction: Analysis of 16 necropsy patients. Am J Cardiol 60:981, 1987

40. Mann JM, Roberts WC: Fatal rupture of both left ventricular free wall and ventricular septum (double rupture) during acute myocardial infarction: Analysis of seven patients studied at necropsy. Am J Cardiol 60:722, 1987

41. Cabin HS, Roberts WC: Left ventricular aneurysm, intraaneurysmal thrombus and systemic embolus in coronary heart disease. Chest 77:586, 1980

42. Cabin HS, Roberts WC: True left ventricular aneurysm and healed myocardial infarction. Clinical and necropsy observations including quantification of degrees of coronary arterial narrowing. Am J Cardiol 46:754, 1980

43. Ross EM, Roberts WC: Severe atherosclerotic coronary artery disease, healed myocardial infarction and chronic congestive heart failure: Analysis of 81 patients studied at necropsy. Am J Cardiol 57:44, 1986

44. Ross EM, Roberts WC: Severe atherosclerotic coronary arterial narrowing and chronic congestive heart failure without myocardial infarction: Analysis of 18 patients studied at necropsy. Am J Cardiol 57:51, 1986

45. Isner JM, Roberts WC: Right ventricular infarction complicating left ventricular infarction secondary to coronary heart disease. Frequency, location, associated findings and significance from analysis of 236 necropsy patients with acute or healed myocardial infarction. Am J Cardiol 42:885, 1978

46. Roberts WC, Potkin BN, Solus DE, Reddy SG: Mode of death, frequency of healed and acute myocardial infarction, number of major epicardial coronary arteries severely narrowed by atherosclerotic plaque, and heart weight in fatal atherosclerotic coronary artery disease: Analysis of 889 patients studied at necropsy. Am J Cardiol 15:196, 1990

47. Roberts WC, Kragel AH, Potkin BN: Ages at death and sex distribution in age decade in fatal coronary artery disease. Am J Cardiol 66:1379, 1990

48. Roberts WC: Sudden cardiac death: A diversity of causes with focus on atherosclerotic coronary artery disease. Am J Cardiol 65:13B, 1990

49. Conti CR, Brawley RK, Griffith LSC, et al: Unstable angina pectoris: morbidity and mortality in 57 consecutive patients evaluated angiographically. Am J Cardiol 32:745, 1973

50. Spiekerman RE, Brandenburg JT, Anchor RWP, Edwards JE: The spectrum of coronary heart disease in a community of 30,000. A clinicopathologic study. Circulation 25:57, 1962

51. Roberts WC: Coronary "lesion," coronary "disease," "single-vessel disease," "two-vessel disease": Word and phrase misnomers providing false impressions of the extent of coronary atherosclerosis in symptomatic myocardial ischemia. Am J Cardiol 66:121, 1990

52. Dollar AL, Kragel AH, Fernicola DJ, et al: Composition of atherosclerotic plaques in coronary arteries in women <40 years of age with fatal coronary artery disease and implications for plaque reversibility. Am J Cardiol 67:1223, 1991

3

Pathophysiology of Coronary Heart Disease

Charles E. Rackley, M.D.

PATHOGENESIS OF ATHEROMA FORMATION

Current theories about the development of atherosclerosis include the contributions of lipids, circulating blood elements, abnormal cells within the vascular wall, and, finally, the influence of systemic disease conditions and external mechanical forces.[1] The lipid theory involves the attraction, deposition, and proliferation of lipid substances within the intimal surface of the blood vessel. Receptors are now recognized for both low-density lipoprotein (LDL) cholesterol and other lipid components, and excessive circulating LDL cholesterol is thought to be deposited within the endothelium and lining cells of the arteries. This lipid may then be accumulated in monocytes within the cell wall, which are subsequently converted to macrophages. Although the specific circulating lipid molecule responsible for excess fatty accumulation and proliferation within the lining of the vessel remains unrecognized, a current theory proposed by Steinberg is that oxidation of accumulated LDL cholesterol within the vascular wall serves as a stimulus for further accumulation and proliferation of lipid components within the macrophage.[2]

A second theory involves the role and contribution of circulating blood elements, in particular platelets. Although platelets and red blood cells are well recognized anatomically as leading to coronary occlusion when deposited on the surface of a severe atheromatous plaque, the initial steps may be merely adherence of platelets, monocytes and deposition of thrombin on the endothelial cells of arteries. This mechanism has support from animal models, which require some form of intimal injury and a high-cholesterol diet to produce the typical pathologic atheromatous lesions. In the course of platelet adhesion to the surface of an artery, vasoactive substances and growth factors such as thromboxane, serotonin, and platelet-derived growth factor can be released to produce further proliferation within the foam cell and the intima, leading to an enlarging atheroma and plaque.

Another theory of atheroma formation is the monoclonal hypothesis, which attributes atherosclerotic plaque development to proliferation of a single-cell precursor; such transforming agents influencing a single cell could include a virus, a chemical, a physical event, or a preexisting genetic defect.[2]

The components of all three theories involving lipids, thrombogenic substances, and the monoclonal origins may all be involved in the process of atheromatous development, and single theories are not necessarily mutually exclusive. Furthermore, the elaborated growth factors and vasoactive substances from circulating platelets, as well as the smooth muscle cells that have migrated into the intima, may further contribute to the overall plaque and atherosclerotic mechanisms. In addition to these theories about atherogenesis, other risk or contributing conditions include hypertension, diabetes mellitus, sedentary lifestyle, and cigarette smoking, all of which may initiate or augment the proliferative process in the atheromatous area within the wall.

The pathologic manifestations of atherosclerosis appear predominantly in arteries, but can be observed in veins implanted in the arterial system for use as a conduit in coronary bypass surgery. The initial lesion is a fatty streak, an intermediate lesion is a fibrous plaque, and the ultimate abnormality is a complicated plaque. The fatty streak is composed of lipid-laden myointimal cells, often observed at the bifurcation of arterial vessels. These streaks are shallow, small, and otherwise benign.

The more advanced lesions is the fibrous plaque, which represents the lipid-laden myointimal cells with additional fibrous tissue. The fiber and collagen can be either excreted or stimulated by the fat-laden monocytes, which are transformed into foam cells. In addition, these cells attract smooth muscle cells from the media. Invading smooth muscle cells are capable of excreting additional amounts of growth factor, similar to that released from platelets. In this manner, the fiber and collagen lipid-laden cells proliferate.

The most advanced atheromatous lesion is the complicated plaque, which is composed not only of the lipid-laden cells and fibrous and connective tissues, but also of calcium and sometimes necrotic debris. The necrotic material may be encapsulated and contained by a fibrous tissue cap. Furthermore, the size and intrusion of the complicated plaque into the lumen of the vessel may lead to further attraction of platelets, red blood cells, and fibrin. Thus, hemorrhage and necrosis can occur within the complicated plaque, as well as attracting additional circulating elements onto the surface of the plaque.

The metabolic and pathologic features of the atheromatous lesions can be further accentuated by progressive growth and intermittent reactions. Growth factors can be released from endothelial and smooth muscle cells within the plaque and by circulating platelets. Vasoactive substances such as thromboxane, serotonin, and acetylcholine contribute to spasm within and surrounding the plaque. Finally, the input into the central nervous system through various regulatory mechanisms can contribute to the development of the atheroma.

The circulating and neurohumoral mechanisms are activated in cigarette smoking, hypertension, and diabetes. Furthermore, genetic and hereditary tendencies contribute to mechanisms causing adherence of platelets and red blood cells to the surface of complicated plaques and to vasoconstriction around the plaques. These circumstances lead to the initial lipid deposition, to growth and proliferation of the plaque, and eventually to stenosis and vasoconstriction capable of severe narrowing or occlusion of vessels.

MECHANISMS OF MYOCARDIAL ISCHEMIA

Ischemia, by definition, indicates a reduction in blood flow to an organ. Ischemia can also be produced by an imbalance between flow and demand. In the heart, ischemia of the myocardium can be produced by increased myocardial oxygen demands with a fixed coronary blood flow or by stable oxygen demands with a temporary reduction in coronary blood flow. The determinants of myocardial oxygen consumption were initially identified in the isolated papillary muscle preparation as preload, afterload, contractile state, and frequency of stimulation (Table 3-1). Preload is the weight or force distending the relaxed papillary muscle. Afterload is the additional weight

Table 3-1.   Determinants of Myocardial Oxygen Consumption

Isolated Papillary Muscle	Intact Heart
Preload	End-diastolic pressure, volume, or wall stress
Afterload	Aortic pressure or wall stress
Contractile state	Ejection fraction, ventricular function curve
Stimulation frequency	Heart rate

(From Rackley et al,[3] with permission.)

or force added to the muscle preparation after the length of the muscle is fixed with the preload. The contractile state is defined by the force and velocity of the muscle contraction. The rate of stimulation influences the total oxygen demand of the muscle. In the intact left ventricle, preload represents theoretical stretch of the relaxed myocardial fiber and can be represented by either left ventricular end-diastolic pressure or, more precisely, left ventricular end-diastolic stress (which incorporates chamber pressure, chamber dimension, and thickness of the myocardial wall).[3] Afterload can be estimated from the systemic blood pressure and is the force generated in the myocardium to open the aortic valve. Systolic wall stress is a more precise measure of afterload and can be calculated from chamber pressure, volume, and wall thickness at the time of aortic valve opening. The contractile state is represented by measures of the ejection fraction or mechanical emptying, but can be derived more accurately from the rate of pressure development and the circumferential shortening rate of the left ventricle. The heart rate in patients with coronary artery disease can be measured as the frequency of myocardial stimulation. Additional considerations for myocardial oxygen consumption include the systemic metabolic state and areas of noncontracting myocardium. Normal myocardium utilizes predominantly fatty acids for the aerobic process of adenosine triphosphate (ATP) generation, whereas ischemic myocardium depends on utilization of glucose for anaerobic metabolism. Finally an area of acute myocardial infarction or myocardial akinesis can impose an additional burden on the viable myocardium for increased oxygen consumption.

In addition to the determinants of myocardial oxygen consumption, the balance between myocardial supply and demand of oxygen becomes important with regard to myocardial ischemia. A fixed reduction in the coronary luminal diameter can reduce coronary blood flow and produce ischemia when myocardial oxygen demands are increased by mechanical work of the heart. This is the most common mechanism for stable or predictable angina pectoris when there is a fixed stenosis in the coronary artery. When the myocardial oxygen demands are diminished, the reduced blood flow through the stenotic lesions may be adequate to meet the oxygen requirements of the heart. At other times, myocardial oxygen demands may remain constant, but further reductions in coronary blood flow and oxygen supply can occur when coronary vasoconstriction or spasm develops or when coronary perfusion pressure decreases as a result of the development of hypotension.

Normal coronary arteries dilate with exercise and the accompanying increase in myocardial oxygen demand. However, in atheromatous coronary arteries, coronary vasoreactivity is influenced by substances and mechanisms that constrict the vessels.[5] Normal coronary arteries dilate in response to exercise, as well as in response to infusion of acetylcholine. Diseased coronary arteries with atheromatous lesions and stenoses paradoxically constrict when exposed to acetylcholine. Substances such as serotonin and thromboxane can be released from platelets and induce vasoconstriction. Central nervous system mechanisms and the balance between the sympathetic and parasympathetic systems can also cause coronary vasoconstriction. This is observed clinically in patients with Prinzmetal's angina, a model of vasospastic angina during nocturnal hours. Furthermore, coronary vasoconstriction may occur upon awakening with the change from predominant parasympathetic to sympathetic influence on vascular tone. Similar circumstances occur in patients with stable and unstable angina, as well as in those with the early phases of acute myocardial infarction.

By definition, angina pectoris represents a sensation of discomfort within the chest initiated by effort or emotion and relieved by rest or nitroglycerin. These ischemic episodes are generally attended by abnormalities of the electrocardiogram (ECG) as well as abnormalities in ventricular wall motion, myocardial perfusion and substrate utilization. With ambulatory ECG recording, as well as with temporary occlusion of a coronary artery during coronary angioplasty, similar ischemic changes frequently have been observed in the left ventricle in the absence of chest discomfort. Monitoring of patients with known coronary heart disease and angina pectoris has confirmed that 70 to 80% of the episodes of ECG changes characteristic of myocardial ischemia are not accompanied by chest discomfort. Silent myocardial ischemia has become recognized in patients with known stable angina, as well as in individuals with unstable angina and those having sustained a recent myocardial infarction. Thus, alterations in the determinants of myocardial oxygen consumption, shifts in the supply-and-demand balance of coronary blood flow and oxygen, as well as mechanisms influencing vasoreactivity can produce critical reductions in myocardial oxygen availability, which may or may not be symptomatic in the patient with coronary heart disease.

MYOCARDIAL INFARCTION

Although coronary atherosclerosis is a consistent finding at autopsy in patients who died of myocardial infarction, several theories about the exact pathogenesis of the infarction have been proposed in the past. For several years, the thrombus on the atherosclerotic plaque was believed to be the result rather than the cause of myocardial infarction. In recent years, coronary angiographic studies of patients presenting with acute myocardial infarction have confirmed the presence of a thrombus in over 85% of patients studied within a few hours of acute myocardial infarction. The current prevailing theory is that platelets accumulate on the surface of a stenotic atherosclerotic plaque whose contents have appeared by rupture of a plaque or by dissection of a section within the plaque resulting from vasoconstriction in the wall of the vessel surrounding the plaque.

The abrupt interruption of the blood supply to the myocardium supplied by the occluded coronary artery results in an ischemic cascade of metabolic and biochemical events. The lack of oxygen inhibits the aerobic pathway for fatty acid metabolism. This in turn leads to accumulation of fatty acids within the cytoplasm. Simultaneously, there is an augmentation of carbohydrate metabolism, with glycogen breakdown and glucose availability. The cytoplasmic accumulation of fatty acids limits transport mechanisms across the mitochondrial membrane. Ischemia not only inhibits this oxidative metabolic pathway, but also contributes to the development of acidosis. Although the anaerobic pathway for glucose metabolism can be augmented, the inhibition of the shuttle system for inwardly transporting the hydrogen due to reduced nicotinamide adenine dinucleotide (NADH) across the mitochondrial membrane further contributes to the ischemic result. The ATP generated within the mitochondria may be compartmentalized owing to the inhibition condition of the translocase enzyme, which facilitates transport of adenosine diphosphate (ADP) into and ATP out of the mitochondria. Water and sodium move into the cells, and potassium and cellular myocardial enzymes move outward.

Ischemic myocardium may be salvaged initially, but after 20 to 40 minutes the damage probably cannot be repaired. Initially, the most vulnerable area of myocardium is the subendocardium, which is exposed to the highest stress within the myocardial wall and jeopardized by the terminal arterial branches from the occluded coronary artery. The ischemic and injured myocardium may extend from the endocardium to the middle and outer portions of the free wall. The rapidity and extent of collateral development and flow from other coronary vessels determine the extent of the damage to the myocardium.

Anatomic findings in the coronary arterial tree in patients with acute myocardial infarction typically reveal an atherosclerotic lesion underlying the recent thrombotic occlusion. However, coronary artery spasm in a patient exposed to cocaine may produce an infarction without underlying coronary artery atherosclerosis. After successful thrombolytic therapy for acute myocardial infarction, 85% of individuals demonstrate greater than 70% residual stenosis of the infarction-related coronary artery,[4] an atherosclerotic plaque that existed before the development of thrombus within the vessel. Furthermore, 50 to 75% of patients with acute myocardial infarction have significant atherosclerotic lesions in the remaining coronary arterial tree. Thus, the anatomic findings in patients with acute myocardial infarction consist of (1) a significant atherosclerotic plaque,

(2) thrombus, and (3) a high prevalence of diffuse atheromatous changes in the coronary arteries.

Disturbances in cardiac rhythm in acute myocardial infarction can be attributed to the infarction, to myocardial ischemia, to compensatory neurohumoral changes, and additionally, to drugs administered for treatment of the infarction. Rhythm disturbances and changes in heart rate can include either tachycardia or bradycardia, varying degrees of atrioventricular block with slowing of the ventricular response, and irregular rhythms such as atrial fibrillation, ventricular ectopy, or ventricular fibrillation.

Sinus tachycardia, a regular rate greater than 100 beats/min, can be due to pain or anxiety or can occur as a compensatory mechanism to left ventricular failure to maintain cardiac output. Slowing of the heart rate below 60 beats/min can occur as a result of the increased vagal influence that can accompany an inferior or posterior wall myocardial infarction. Degrees of atrioventricular block or complete heart block can develop in the acute phase of infarction. Drugs administered to the patient can modify the basic rate; nitrate drugs and other vasodilator agents can increase heart rate, whereas morphine, beta adrenergic-blocking and certain calcium channel-blocking drugs can decrease the heart rate.

Atrial flutter and atrial fibrillation, due to atrial ischemia or atrial infarction, can complicate inferior wall infarction. Accelerated junctional rhythms with rates approaching 100 beats/min can develop in inferior infarction. Atrioventricular conduction disturbances occur more frequently in inferior than anterior infarction. Increased vagal tone, as well as ischemic injury, may impair conduction; less frequently, actual necrosis develops in the atrioventricular node and His bundle. Atrioventricular block associated with anterior myocardial infarction usually results from extensive necrosis of the His bundle and branches.

Premature ventricular contractions are encountered in the majority of patients presenting with acute myocardial infarction; whether the pathogenesis relates to ischemia or to actual necrosis remains incompletely understood. Ventricular tachycardia or ventricular fibrillation often occurs soon (minutes or hours) after acute infarction; these serious rhythm disturbances develop before necrosis can be documented histologically.

Finally, rhythm disturbances can accompany successful thrombolysis and reperfusion of the infarcted myocardium. The most frequent disturbance is an idioventricular rhythm with rates varying from 60 to 100 beats/min. However, this ventricular rhythm has been reported with similar frequency in patients with failed thrombolysis without reperfusion. Partial reperfusion through collateral vessels could contribute to the genesis of an idioventricular rhythm in the absence of thrombolysis of the occluded artery.

Disturbances in ventricular function are frequent in acute myocardial infarction. Elevation of the left ventricular filling pressure, the most sensitive measure of ventricular function, can be abnormal in 75% of patients without any clinical evidence of heart failure. In 25% of patients with clinically uncomplicated infarction, the cardiac index may be abnormally reduced.

The earliest mechanical abnormality of the infarcted left ventricle is an alteration in diastolic function, manifesting as impaired filling. This indicates an abnormality in the elastic properties or diastolic compliance of the left ventricle. The next disturbance is decreased wall motion of the area supplied by the occluded coronary artery. The final hemodynamic event after acute coronary artery occlusion is a rise in the left ventricular end-diastolic pressure.

Global ventricular function in acute myocardial infarction has been evaluated by ventricular function curves. A ventricular function curve is constructed by relating a change in a diastolic parameter, such as left ventricular filling pressure, to a systolic parameter, such as cardiac index. The ventricular function curve can be created by incremental infusion of low-molecular-weight dextran into the pulmonary artery, relating changes in the left ventricular filling pressure or pulmonary artery end-diastolic pressure to changes in the cardiac index (Fig. 3-1). The slope of the ventricular function curve suggests the myocardial reserve and reflects the size of the myocardial infarction. Thus, a small infarction would display a steep ventricular function curve and a more extensive infarction would lead to a function curve with a flat or a depressed slope.

Serial hemodynamic observations in acute myocardial infarction reveal a gradual decline in the left ventricular filling pressure, accompanied by a measurable increase in cardiac index, during the first 3 or 4 days after acute infarction (Fig. 3-2). Since these observations have been documented in patients in the absence of specific treatment, the hemodynamic improvement would suggest spontaneous improvement in the global contractile state of the myocardium. This improvement could result from the development of collateral circulation to the ischemic area and diminution of the myocardial edema. Thus, disturbances in the left ventricular mechanical function can be documented with use of the Swan–Ganz catheter; serial observations have demonstrated improvement in the elevated filling pres-

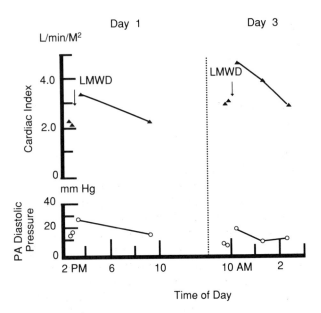

Fig. 3-2. Hemodynamic changes produced by low-molecular-weight dextran (LMWD) on day 1 and day 3 in a patient with acute myocardial infarction. The same volume of LMWD was infused each time, yet the cardiac index increased more on day 3 than on day 1. (From Rackley et al,[13] with permission.)

sure and an increase in the cardiac index. Akinesis due to either acute or chronic scarring can impose an additional burden for oxygen consumption on the viable myocardium.

LEFT VENTRICULAR DYSFUNCTION

Transient Impairment

Coronary artery occlusion results in myocardial damage that can range from reversible ischemia to irreversible necrosis. Since the marginal ischemic tissue may undergo necrosis or eventual restoration to the normal state, changes in left ventricular function reflect myocardial damage. Thus, the evolution of ischemic and infarcted myocardium during the initial 72 hours will influence changes in left ventricular filling pressure or pulmonary artery end-diastolic pressure (PAEDP) and cardiac index. Monitoring patients

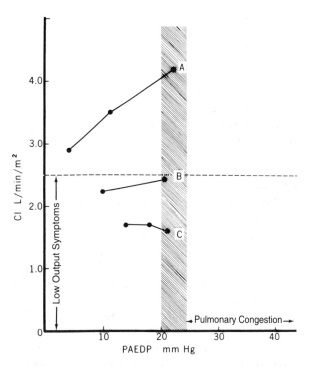

Fig. 3-1. Left ventricular function curves in three patients with acute myocardial infarction. Patient A sustained a small infarction, patient B had a previous plus a recent infarction, and patient C presented with a ventricular gallop and rales. The shaded area represents the range of optimal PAEDP for preload of the left ventricle. CI, cardiac index. (From Mantle et al,[12] with permission.)

hemodynamically during this period has shown a gradual decline in the PAEDP, accompanied by a concomitant increase in the cardiac index, even without pharmacologic intervention. Such changes, in the absence of therapeutic agents, suggest a gradual reduction in the size of the non-contracting myocardium and indicate that the marginal zone of ischemia has been restored to the normal contractile state. These spontaneous serial hemodynamic changes form an important basis with which to compare pharmacologic interventions.

In addition to hemodynamic measurements, wall motion abnormalities from noninvasive studies can confirm the reduction in size of the abnormally contracting segment in the ventricular wall and the increase in global mechanical performance or ejection fraction. Thus, segmental and global left ventricular function can be measured during the initial 72 hours of infarction and repeated at 1 week and months after the patient is discharged from the hospital.

Impact of Healing Infarction on Ventricular Function

Since an acute myocardial infarction can depress ventricular function to various degrees, re-placement of the damaged myocardium by fibrous tissue and scar will also influence the mechanical function of the ventricle. Angiographic studies performed after myocardial infarction provide a basis for measuring the size of the infarction as expressed by the percentage of the left ventricular diastolic silhouette that does not contract (Fig. 3-3). The expression "abnormally contracting segment" was introduced to quantitate the portion of the diastolic silhouette of the ventricle that remained noncontracting, akinetic, or dyskinetic in the systolic phase.[6] This technique permitted the size of the healed myocardial infarct to be correlated with the clinical course and hemodynamic abnormalities produced by the acute infarction.

In studies of patients within the year following acute myocardial infarction, the most sensitive measure of the abnormally contracting segment on ventricular function was diastolic compliance. A scar size of 8% (indicating that 8% of the diastolic silhouette was akinetic) produced abnormal stiffness of the ventricle following infarction (Table 3-2). When the scar size was 10% of the left ventricular surface, a measurable reduction in ejection fraction (less than the normal 50%) was observed. When the scar size approached 15% of the ventricle, left ventricular end-diastolic

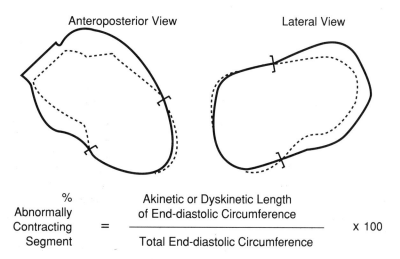

$$\frac{\%\ \text{Abnormally Contracting Segment}}{} = \frac{\text{Akinetic or Dyskinetic Length of End-diastolic Circumference}}{\text{Total End-diastolic Circumference}} \times 100$$

Fig. 3-3. Biplane left ventricular angiograms superimposed in a patient with a previous myocardial infarction. The solid line represents diastole, and the dashed line represents systole. The segments enclosed by the brackets indicate the site of the previous anterior myocardial infarction. (From Niess et al,[14] with permission.)

Table 3-2. Abnormally Contracting Segments in Postmyocardial Infarction

Size of Abnormally Contracting Segments[a]	Ventricular Function	Result
>8%	Compliance	↓
>10%	Ejection fraction	↓
>15%	LVEDP	↑
>17%	End-diastolic volume	↑
>17%	Left ventricular mass	↑
>23%	Clinical heart failure	
>40%	Cardiogenic shock	

[a] Size is related to abnormalities in left ventricular function in patients with previous myocardial infarctions.
(From Rackley et al,[15] with permission.)

pressure was elevated on a chronic basis; however, such an elevation was not sufficient to produce symptoms of pulmonary congestion or heart failure. When the scar size approached 17% within the first year after infarction, the end-diastolic volume increased abnormally and the left ventricular mass increased. Thus, the compensatory mechanisms of dilatation and hypertrophy were activated when the residual scar size was only 17% of the total surface of the left ventricle.

When the scar size became 23% of the left ventricle, patients often complained of dyspnea or orthopnea and exhibited pulmonary rales and a ventricular (S3) gallop. Finally, when the scar size was greater than 40%, patients usually had experienced cardiogenic shock during the acute infarction. This observation has been confirmed by autopsy, showing a greater than 40% loss of left ventricular myocardium in patients who had died of cardiogenic shock.

Thus, various invasive and noninvasive techniques for evaluating left ventricular function in patients with acute myocardial infarction can identify depression of ventricular function, monitor serial changes, predict the clinical course and complications of an infarction, and provide a physiologic basis for comparison of benefits from pharmacologic, mechanical, or surgical interventions.

COMPLICATIONS OF ACUTE MYOCARDIAL INFARCTION

Disturbances in Rhythm

Virtually all patients with acute myocardial infarction experience disturbances in cardiac rhythm. These rhythm disturbances can vary from sinus tachycardia, to ectopic beats, to ventricular fibrillation. The most serious arrhythmia is ventricular fibrillation, which is responsible for the majority of deaths from acute myocardial infarction. With collapse, cardiac arrest, and sudden cardiac death, ventricular tachycardia or fibrillation is usually the underlying arrhythmia. These rhythm disturbances occur most frequently within 1 hour after acute infarction and are responsible for 70% of early deaths.

Patients surviving for more than 1 hour after acute infarction generally manifest ectopy as premature ventricular complexes. Over 80% of patients hospitalized with acute infarction will exhibit enhanced ventricular irritability.

Disturbances in sinus rhythm can present as sinus tachycardia, with rates exceeding 100 beats/min or sinus bradycardia, with rates less than 60 beats/min. Sinus tachycardia may be the most serious of all rhythm disturbances, since the rapid heart rate reflects severe left ventricular impairment and is a compensatory mechanism for left ventricular failure. Sinus bradycardia, on the other hand, can occur with inferior wall myocardial infarction, which structurally damages a smaller percentage of the myocardium than does anterior infarction. Inferior infarctions are often associated with diminished sympathetic influence, resulting in enhanced vagal tone.

Disturbances in atrial rhythm may be due to atrial ischemia or infarction; they include atrial flutter and atrial fibrillation. Atrial fibrillation may be a more serious arrhythmic manifestation since it is associated with larger areas of myocardial damage. Increased vagal tone can produce variable atrioventricular block, from first degree (PR interval prolongation) to second and third degree. Second-degree heart block of the Wenckebach type is often associated with inferior wall infarction. Mobitz type II second-degree atrioventricular block can result from a large anterior infarction with greater structural damage to the conducting system. Finally, third-degree (complete) heart block can result from either of these mechanisms. In inferior wall infarction, any type of atrioventricular block, even complete heart block, may be transitory, whereas in anterior infarction the heart block is often permanent.

An idioventricular rhythm, ranging from 60 to 100 beats/min, is frequently observed when there is reperfusion of an occluded coronary artery. Reperfusion can occur through the body's own thrombolytic mechanisms or with development of collateral circulation. Currently this rhythm is most commonly encountered when pharmacologic thrombolysis is successful.

Any of these rhythm disturbances can occur or recur during the initial 72 hours of acute infarction, and they suggest either recurrent myocardial ischemia or extension of the infarction process. The ischemic mechanisms creating arrhythmias can be located in the peripheral zone of myocardial infarction or at more remote areas. Remote ischemia can be a complication of associated significant coronary stenotic lesions in the noninfarcted territory vessels. Recurrent postinfarction rhythm disturbances are related to the size of the initial myocardial infarction, residual myocardial ischemia, left ventricular dysfunction and, finally, the extent of the underlying coronary disease.

Impaired Mechanical Function

Theoretically, the loss of any contracting myocardium should diminish or impair global mechanical function of the ventricle. However, the

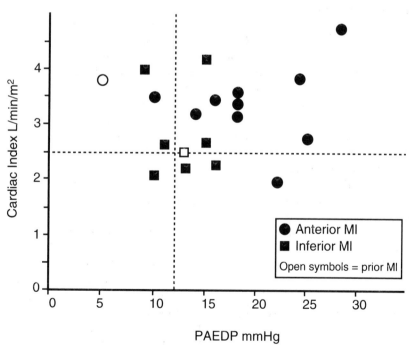

Fig. 3-4. Initial hemodynamic measurements of cardiac index (CI) and PAEDP in patients with uncomplicated acute myocardial infarctions. The normal CI is greater than 2.5 L/min/m^2, and the normal PAEDP less than 12 mmHg. (From Rackley et al,[16] with permission.)

sensitivity of available methods permits detection of impaired ventricular function only when there is a measurable amount of damaged myocardium. In patients with small myocardial infarctions who exhibit no clinical symptoms of left ventricular impairment, hemodynamic measurements with the Swan–Ganz catheter reveal that 75% of such individuals have an abnormally elevated left ventricular filling pressure, and 20% of such patients may have an abnormally depressed cardiac index (Fig. 3-4). Measurable deviations of the left ventricular filling pressure and the cardiac index from normal values at the time of acute myocardial infarction probably occur in all patients. Hemodynamic observations suggest that the majority of patients with acute myocardial infarction presenting without clinical symptoms of left ventricular failure exhibit measurable abnormalities in left ventricular function.

In addition to the baseline hemodynamic parameters such as left ventricular filling pressure and cardiac index, a mild stress imposed on the acutely infarcted left ventricle can demonstrate impairment of myocardial reserve.[7] Stress in the form of volume expansion with low-molecular-weight dextran can increase preload (Fig. 3-5). The changes in left ventricular filling pressure or preload can be related to alterations in the cardiac index. The relationship between a diastolic parameter, such as left ventricular filling pressure or preload, and a systolic parameter, such as the cardiac index, is the basis for construction of a ventricular function curve. In an acutely infarcted ventricle with minimal myocardial damage, volume expansion will elevate the filling pressure, and this increase in preload is associated with a significant increase in the cardiac index. Thus, the slope of the function curve relating changes in filling pressure or preload to changes in cardiac index describes a steep or ascending limb.

In the patient with a larger area of infarcted myocardium, volume expansion is attended by a greater increase in filling pressure or preload, with a relatively modest increase in the cardiac index. This creates a flat or depressed ventricular function curve. Finally, in the ventricle with a large area of infarcted myocardium, volume expansion will significantly increase the filling

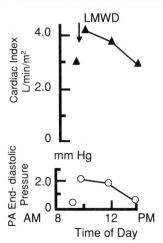

Fig. 3-5. Effect of infusion of low-molecular-weight dextran (LMWD) in a patient with acute myocardial infarction. Infusion elevated the PAEDP and increased the cardiac index. The hemodynamic changes persisted for 6 hours. (From Rackley et al,[17] with permission.)

pressure while the cardiac index can decline. This decline in cardiac index, accompanying an increase in filling pressure, is a manifestation of the descending limb of the ventricular function curve. Thus, in the infarcted left ventricle, the ventricular function curves can describe a steep or ascending limb, after which a plateau is reached in which further elevation of filling pressure produces no additional change in the cardiac index; and, finally, levels of left ventricular filling pressure can be achieved which result in a decline in the cardiac index.

Analysis of ventricular function curves in patients with acute myocardial infarction reveals a range of optimal left ventricular filling pressures associated with the peak or plateau of the ventricular function curve (Fig. 3-6). As shown in Fig. 3-6, a filling pressure between 20 and 24 mmHg is associated with a peak or plateau of the ventricular function curve. A left ventricular filling pressure less than 20 mmHg is associated with an ascending limb, whereas a filling pressure above 24 mmHg usually describes the descending limb of the ventricular function curve. Analysis and clinical application of the ventricular

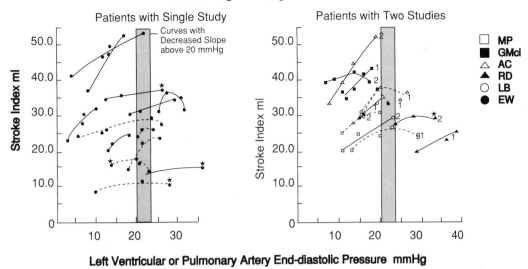

Fig. 3-6. Analysis of ventricular function curves in acute myocardial infarction showing the peak or plateau usually reached with a left ventricular end-diastolic pressure or PAEDP between 20 and 24 mm/Hg. (From Russell et al,[7] with permission.)

function curve concept to the patient with acute myocardial infarction provides a basis for optimizing the preload of the left ventricle. The optimal cardiac index can be achieved in the range of filling pressures from 20 to 24 mmHg. Thus, optimal preload can theoretically be achieved by raising the filling pressure with volume expansion or reducing the filling pressure with volume reduction through diuresis or the use of vasodilating agents.

CONGESTIVE HEART FAILURE

Clinical symptoms and signs of left ventricular heart failure indicate a significant loss of contracting myocardium. On the basis of the postinfarction studies and calculation of the residual scar size, 25% of the surface of the left ventricle must be akinetic before orthopnea develops and rales and a left ventricular gallop become audible. The presence of heart failure can influence the morbidity and mortality of patients with acute myocardial infarction. Patients with acute infarction often present with audible rales at the lung

bases as a result of cigarette smoking. In addition, the recumbent position in the emergency room, administration of narcotics that reduce respiratory rate, and elevation of the left ventricular filling pressure to a level exceeding the osmotic pressure of the plasma proteins can produce pulmonary rales. Furthermore, the cardiac output can remain within the normal range since systemic blood flow is maintained by compensatory changes in heart rate and stoke volume. Thus, the hemodynamic analysis of left ventricular failure must include considerations of preload or left ventricular filling pressure, afterload or systemic arterial blood pressure, inotropic or contractile state reflected as the ejection fraction, and heart rate. In addition to these basic determinants of the mechanical performance of isolated heart muscle, alterations in substrate utilization by the ischemic myocardium and the size of the infarcted area influence the function of the intact left ventricle.

Pulmonary congestion in patients with acute infarction can result from abnormal elevation of the filling pressure, which exceeds the oncotic pressure of plasma proteins in the presence of a normal ventricular ejection fraction and cardiac output. This can occur in individuals with underlying myocardial hypertrophy resulting from the pressure overload of hypertension, aortic stenosis, or extensive fibrosis within the ventricle. Abnormalities in preload thus result from changes in compliance of diastolic dysfunction of the infarcted ventricle. Under these conditions, pulmonary congestion as a manifestation of heart failure can occur despite a normal ejection fraction and cardiac output.

When 10% of the surface of the contracting left ventricle is akinetic, the ejection fraction is reduced below the normal value of 50%. Patients in left ventricular failure following myocardial infarction generally maintain ejection fractions less than 30%. Therefore, the range of values for the abnormally contracting segment for the total left ventricular surface area may range from 10 to 25% without significant reduction in ejection fraction. This is illustrated in Fig. 3-7, comparing ejection fraction with the size of the abnormally contracting segment. When the ejection fraction declines below 30%, the proportion of akinetic left ventricular myocardium usually exceeds 25%. Furthermore, it is important to appreciate the percentage of abnormal contracting myocardium that results from previous infarctions. Thus, when a patient experiences an initial infarction that destroys only 15% of the surface area of the left ventricle, residual left ventricular function may be sufficient to accommodate normal activities. However, a subsequent infarction with 10% loss of contracting myocardium can result in heart failure. Combination of the previous scar size of an infarction of 15% and the recent infarction of 10% results in a net loss of 25% of contracting myocardium. Thus, the history of a previous myocardial infarction is important in assessing the overall loss of contracting myocardium in any patient presenting with an acute myocardial infarction.

CARDIOGENIC SHOCK

Cardiogenic shock is the most serious complication of acute myocardial infarction since its mortality rate varies between 60 and 80%. The clinical syndrome of cardiogenic shock is composed of not only hypotension with a systolic blood pressure less than 90 mmHg, but also clinical evidence of impaired skin, renal, and central nervous system perfusion. Autopsy studies have estimated a loss of more than 40% of left ventricular myocardium by acute and/or previous infarctions. The majority of patients developing this complication have experienced previous myocardial infarctions, since occlusion of a single major coronary artery, excluding the left main coronary artery, will not result in a 40% loss of

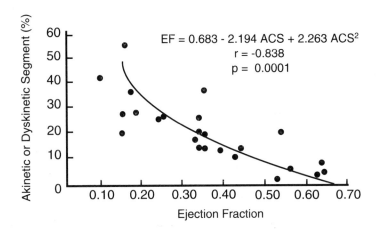

Fig. 3-7. Decrease in the left ventricular ejection fraction as the size of the akinetic segment increases in postinfarction patients. (From Feild et al,[6] with permission.)

contracting myocardium. However, hemodynamic measurements of left ventricular filling pressure and cardiac index have revealed a range of values in clinical cardiogenic shock (Fig. 3-8). With significant elevation of filling pressure and reduction in cardiac index, the mortality rate remains above 90%.[8] In patients with a reduced cardiac index and a filling pressure less than 15 mmHg, the extent of noncontracting myocardium is still large and the mortality rate approaches 65%. However, there is an unusual subset in cardiogenic shock in which the cardiac index may be maintained near normal and the filling pressure is normal or slightly elevated at 15 mmHg. This latter condition behaves in a manner hemodynamically similar to hypovolemic shock. In individuals with this condition, volume expansion with an agent such as low-molecular-weight dextran can raise the filling pressure to the optimal range of 20 to 24 mmHg and restore systemic blood pressure to an adequate level. Thus, understanding the hemodynamic changes and manifestations of cardiogenic shock not only permits an assessment of the degree of loss of contracting myocardium, but can also contribute to important therapeutic decisions and interventions.

MYOCARDIAL SALVAGE

Pharmacologic Methods

A pharmacologic panoply of agents is directed toward the management of acute myocardial infarction and correction of underlying physiologic disturbances. Narcotics and nitroglycerin compounds remain the initial drugs for relief of pain. Oxygen is beneficial for correcting the hypoxemia, and DC countershock can be administered for serious rhythm disturbances. Although these agents can provide immediate benefit to the patient and, in instances of hypotension and impaired ventricular function due to rhythm disturbances, can have a favorable effect on

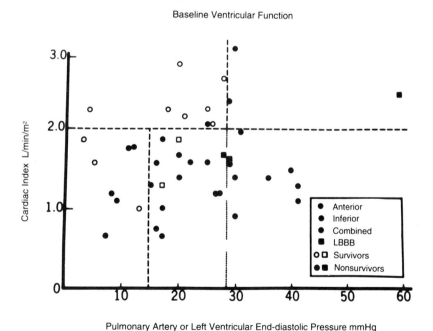

Fig. 3-8. Hemodynamic measurements for patients in cardiogenic shock. The open symbols denote survivors, and the solid symbols denote nonsurvivors. LBBB, left bundle branch block. (From Rackley et al,[18] with permission.)

myocardial damage, the major goal of treatment of acute myocardial infarction is to limit or reduce the size of damaged myocardium; this is important in influencing the ultimate morbidity and mortality.

During the past 20 years, pharmacologic treatments have been directed toward reducing the size of myocardial infarction. They have included anticoagulation, glucose-insulin-potassium (GIK) mixtures, nitrate drugs, beta-blocking drugs, calcium-blocking agents, and thrombolytic drugs. Although a measure of the infarction size can be derived from enzymatic estimates or expression of ventricular function and size of abnormal wall motion, these parameters can be influenced by various pharmacologic and mechanical interventions. Thus, any enhancement of blood flow to the infarcted area may contribute to enzyme washout and give a spuriously high estimate of the infarction size. On the other hand, subsequent measurements of the initially reduced ejection fraction and serial evaluations of wall motion can indicate salvage of infarcted myocardium. Nitrate drugs and beta-blocking drugs have been shown, in selected patients and studies, to reduce the size of the residual scar after myocardial infarction.

EVALUATION OF LEFT VENTRICULAR FUNCTION

The evaluation of left ventricular function in patients with acute myocardial infarction is crucial to the assessment of infarction size, evaluation of therapy, and prediction of future course. The acute loss of contracting myocardium due to necrosis and/or ischemia contributes to local and global abnormalities in left ventricular mechanical function. A broad approach to the assessment of ventricular function includes clinical symptoms, physical findings, radiographic evaluation, and additional procedures, both invasive and noninvasive. Invasive procedures include hemodynamic assessment with the use of the Swan–Ganz catheter and left ventriculography performed during diagnostic cardiac catheterization. Noninvasive approaches include echocardiogra-

phy and radionuclide techniques at rest and during exercise. Finally, assessment is important from the very first evaluation, during the initial 72 hours, and prior to hospital discharge.

One of the earliest clinical methods for assessing ventricular function was the Killip classification based on symptoms, physical findings, and radiographic interpretation (Fig. 3-9). The presence and/or absence of pulmonary rales, an audible ventricular gallop, diffuse pulmonary edema, and cardiogenic shock identified four categories with respective hospital mortality rates of 12, 18, 40, and 80%. Thus, this initial clinical assessment of ventricular function identified low- and high-risk patients from the time of admission to the coronary care unit.

An important development and contribution to the evaluation of left ventricular function in acute infarction was the development of the Swan–Ganz catheter. This invasive procedure provided measurements of left ventricular filling pressure, cardiac output, and derived parameters. The most sensitive abnormality of impaired left ventricular function is elevation of the left ventricular end-diastolic pressure. This pressure is reflected as mean left atrial pressure and ultimately pulmonary capillary pressure. Early experience with hemodynamic monitoring with the Swan–Ganz catheter demonstrated acceptable similarity of the PAEDP to the pulmonary capillary pressure. Thus, the PAEDP could be used to monitor changes in the left ventricular end-diastolic pressure, in the absence of mitral valve disease. The measurement of cardiac output basically estimated right ventricular output, which was assumed to be equal to left ventricular output. Additional indices of ventricular performance included calculation of stroke index, stroke work index, and stroke power index, by using measures of heart rate and systemic blood pressure.

The development of a variety of pharmacologic interventions for the treatment of acute myocardial infarction, in particular thrombolytic therapy, justified acute cardiac catheterization with coronary and left ventricular angiography. Quantitation of left ventricular volumes and wall thickness can provide estimates of end-diastolic volume, end-systolic volume, ejection fraction, and left ventricular mass. Superimposition of dia-

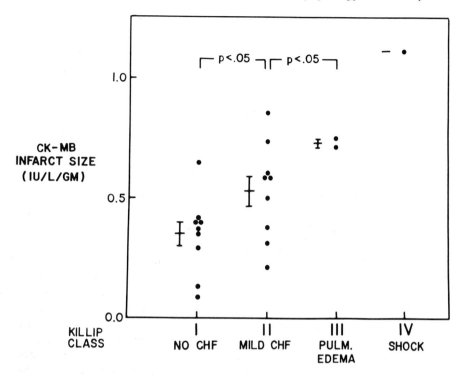

Fig. 3-9. Comparison of myocardial infarction size estimated by CK-MB enzymes with the Killip classification. CHF, congestive heart failure. The larger the infarction size, the greater the impairment of left ventricular function. (From Rackley et al,[16] with permission.)

stolic and systolic ventricular silhouettes can identify and quantify wall motion abnormalities. Thus, left ventricular angiography can provide a quantitative evaluation of the damage imposed by the infarction on wall motion as well as on global ventricular function. These invasive measurements provided a basis for calibration of the noninvasive approaches such as echocardiography and radionuclide angiography.

Echocardiography introduced a noninvasive approach to anatomic assessment of ventricular function in patients with acute myocardial infarction (see also Ch. 14). Initially, echocardiography generated estimates of chamber dimensions, ejection fraction, and cardiac output. With further refinement and advances in echocardiographic instrumentation, wall motion abnormalities could be identified. In addition to providing measures of chamber dimensions, ventricular function, and wall motion abnormalities, echocardiography has provided diagnostic informa-

tion on mechanical disturbances such as ruptured ventricular septum, papillary muscle rupture with mitral regurgitation, and pericardial tamponade.

Radionuclide techniques (see also Chs. 9, 15) can evaluate left ventricular chamber size and function in a similar way to their evaluation by quantitative ventriculography performed during diagnostic cardiac catheterization. The radionuclide techniques involve radioisotope labeling of red blood cells, thus enabling chamber size, global function, and wall motion abnormalities to be identified. Selective isotopes such as thallium and rubidium provide markers for myocardial perfusion in the specific areas of wall motion abnormalities.

Since a major goal in the treatment of acute myocardial infarction is to preserve damaged or ischemic myocardium, the invasive and noninvasive techniques to assess global and segmental wall motion abnormalities can document the results of treatment.

Pharmacologic Agents

Several pharmacologic agents such as nitroglycerin and beta-blocking drugs have reduced the mortality from acute myocardial infarction in patients participating in studies of these drugs. However, these studies were of selected groups, in which patients with the most severe complications such as hypotension and heart failure were excluded from analysis. Although this reduction in mortality suggests a reduction in infarction size, other mechanisms may have been involved such as reduction in afterload and stabilization of rhythm disturbances, both of which reduce myocardial oxygen demand without necessarily reducing infarction size. Although the calcium-blocking agents have been used to treat acute myocardial infarction, the only benefit has been the reduction in reinfarction of the so-called non-Q wave infarction, in the absence of ventricular dysfunction.[9] Calcium-blocking drugs have not been demonstrated to effect a reduction in infarction size.

Thrombolytic Drugs

Approximately 75% of clots responsible for Q-wave infarctions can be dissolved by intracoronary administration of a thrombolytic drug.[10] Several thrombolytic agents are capable of dissolving clots; they include streptokinase, tissue plasminogen activator (t-PA), urokinase, and anisolyated plasminogen-streptokinase activator complex (APSAC). Intravenous administration of these drugs within 4 to 6 hours of acute infarction is associated with a reduction in mortality form 12 to 9%, a 25% decrease (Table 3-3). Contraindications to thrombolytic drugs include a history of a cerebrovascular accident, surgery or resuscitation within 2 weeks, systolic blood pressure above 180 mmHg, or a risk of bleeding. To reduce the incidence of reocclusion after thrombolytic therapy, heparin is given simultaneously with the thrombolytic drug and continued for 2 to 3 days. An aspirin should also be given daily.

Mechanical Interventions

Since the process of acute myocardial infarction is caused by a thrombus superimposed on a significant atherosclerotic plaque, various mechanical efforts have been used to restore blood flow. One of the earliest was the use of emergency coronary bypass surgery to improve blood flow to the infarcted area; more recently, coronary angioplasty has been applied to the thrombosed artery. In selected patients and under specific circumstances, both surgery and angioplasty have been successful in improving blood flow. Surgery can reduce mortality during the hospital stay when performed within the first 4 to 6 hours after the infarction. Angioplasty can restore blood flow, but maintaining the patency of the infarct-related dilated artery remains a challenge. Combinations of angioplasty and surgery have been used in the high-risk condition of cardiogenic shock. One of the most beneficial hemodynamic devices has been the intra-aortic balloon pump, which augments diastolic perfusion of the coronary arteries. This intervention has been successfully used in both medical and surgical conditions to control the ischemia surrounding the infarcted zone. Even though the balloon assist device may not reduce the infarct size, it may limit extension of the infarct and may support marginal ischemic tissue.

Reperfusion Injury

Within minutes after coronary occlusion and diminution of myocardial blood supply and oxygen availability, metabolic and biochemical changes occur within the myocardial cell. The earliest change is an accumulation of fatty acids in the cytoplasm, enhancement of glucose metabolism, and a shift from aerobic to anaerobic metabolism within the cell to provide a metabolic source of ATP within the mitochondria. This shift in myocardial metabolism from aerobic to anaerobic pathways compensates for the energy requirements, but the potential for cellular insult persists. The perfusion of ischemic myocardium with blood containing a normal concentration of oxygen and increased free fatty acids and cate

Table 3-3. Effect of Thrombolytic Drugs on Mortality Rate

Drug	No. of Studies/ No. of Patients	Mortality ($\downarrow$ or $\uparrow$)
Acute Interventions		
Streptokinase, IC	9/1,000	$\downarrow$ 18%
Streptokinase, IV, <6 hr	31/25,000	$\downarrow$ 26%
Streptokinase, IV, >6 hr	31/11,000	$\downarrow$ 26%
t-PA, IV, <6 hr	5/6,500	$\downarrow$ 25%
APSAC, IV, <6 hr	9/2,000	$\downarrow$ 52%
Lidocaine	10/8,500	$\uparrow$ 11%
Beta-blocking drugs, IV	27/27,000	$\downarrow$ 13%
Nitrate drugs, IV	10/2,000	$\downarrow$ 35%
Calcium-blocking drugs	3/6,000	$\uparrow$ 10%
Anticoagulants	6/4,500	$\downarrow$ 22%
Aspirin	2/17,600	$\downarrow$ 21%
Long-Term Interventions		
Beta-blocking drugs	25/23,000	$\downarrow$ 22%
Antiplatelet drugs[a]	10/18,500	$\downarrow$ 11%
Calcium-blocking drugs	4/9,000	$\uparrow$ 6%

Abbreviations: IC, intracoronary; IV, intravenously.
[a] Aspirin, aspirin plus dipyridamole, or sulfinpyrazone.

cholamines can damage the cell membranes, the cytoplasm, and the myocardial metabolic pathways. Reperfusion injury is a recognized metabolic, biochemical, and pathologic condition in ischemic myocardium, and the potential of any pharmacologic or mechanical intervention to damage ischemic tissue must be considered. Increased collateral blood flow, drug-induced coronary vasodilation, and mechanical revascularization can improve the blood supply to ischemic myocardium. This metabolic benefit is threatened by the risk of temporary cell damage produced by oxygen radicals, excess fatty acids, and high concentrations of catecholamines. The effect of these latter substances must be considered in the process of reperfusion injury.

Metabolic and Biochemical Considerations

Optimization of preload, afterload, contractility, and heart rate for myocardial energy demands is also influenced by the size of the myocardial infarction and the shift from aerobic to anaerobic metabolism. During aerobic metabolism, the myocardium utilizes free fatty acids as the substrate for production of ATP, but ischemia induces a shift to glucose utilization, which re-

quires 10% less oxygen. This anaerobic shift to glucose metabolism creates an opportunity to use solutions of various composition to accompany pharmacologic and mechanical interventions to restore blood flow and preserve ischemic myocardium, with the ultimate goal of reducing the infarct size. Experience with reperfusion solutions have included the GIK solutions as well as addition of other potential metabolically active substances to assess the benefit of such metabolic solutions. Improvement in ventricular function, suppression of arrhythmias, and reduction in infarct size are appropriate goals, together with a reduction in mortality.

An early experience in the use of the metabolic approach to ischemic myocardium involved the use of a GIK solution with a goal of providing sufficient glucose to change the myocardial oxygen demands and the respiratory quotient from lipid to carbohydrate utilization (Fig. 3-10). A consistent concentration and infusion rate suppressed circulating free fatty acids in patients with acute myocardial infarction.[11] The mechanism of inhibiting fatty acid release involves the action of insulin on esterification of free fatty acids and glycerol to form triglycerides. Furthermore, the composition of the solution not only increased the glucose availability and the potassium content to combat the hypokalemia

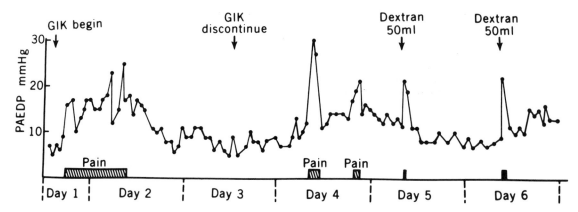

Fig. 3-10. Monitoring of the PAEDP in a patient with an acute infarction receiving a metabolic GIK solution. Chest pain recurred after the infusion had been discontinued. Dextran was infused to construct ventricular function curves. (From Rackley et al,[20] with permission.)

encountered with metabolically active solutions, but also improved the insulin availability, which stabilized the myocardial membranes and stimulated anaerobic pathways for energy production.

Hemodynamic measurements in patients with acute infarction who received the GIK solution showed beneficial changes in left ventricular filling pressure, preload, and cardiac index over the 72 hours of infusion (Fig. 3-11). In addition to hemodynamic improvement, infusion of the GIK solution suppressed ventricular irritability and

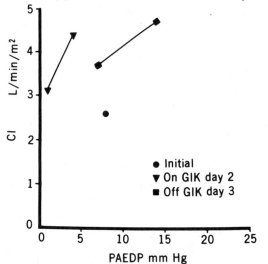

Fig. 3-11. Effect of GIK solution. In a patient receiving GIK the ventricular function curve was steeper on day 2 while receiving the solution than on day 3 off the solution. (From Rackley et al,[19] with permission.)

arrhythmias. Finally, studies of infarct size by using biplane ventriculography demonstrated a reduction in the size of the abnormal contracting zone. Patients with anterior infarction demonstrated greater reduction in infarct size than those with inferior infarction. Most importantly, a significant reduction in mortality (from approximately 12 to 6%) was observed in patients with acute myocardial infarction who were given the metabolic solution. The metabolic solution may stabilize ischemic myocardium and potentially prevent necrosis of myocardial cells. In clinical trials, the randomization of patients was based on symptoms and ECG changes, and patients assigned to receive the GIK solution had a lower incidence of enzymatically proven myocardial infarction than did control patients. One possible explanation was that the metabolic solution stabilized membranes in the ischemic myocardium and prevented the release of the enzymes that are used to confirm the presence of myocardial necrosis.

SUMMARY

The pathophysiology of coronary heart disease has been reviewed based on the pathogenesis of atheroma formation, mechanisms of myocardial ischemia, and the disturbances of the myocardial infarction process. The impact of myocardial ischemia and infarction on left ventricular function has been reviewed, and complications of myocardial infarction have been examined. Finally, methods of myocardial salvage based on interventions directed to control arrhythmias and support mechanical function have been discussed. These therapeutic efforts involve pharmacologic, mechanical, and surgical approaches. Review of available pharmacologic agents, thrombolytic drugs, and metabolic approaches is presented. By understanding the pathophysiology of coronary heart disease, one can appreciate the abnormalities produced by ischemia and infarction. Thus, the appropriate therapeutic interventions can be selected and objectively evaluated.

REFERENCES

1. Steinberg D, Parthasarathy S, Carew TE et al: Beyond cholesterol: Modifications of low-density lipoprotein that increase its atherogenicity. N Engl J Med 320:915, 1989

2. Ross R: Factors influencing atherogenesis. p. 877. In Hurst JW (ed): The Heart. 7th Ed. McGraw-Hill, New York, 1990

3. Rackley CE, Russell RO, Jr, Mantle JA, et al: Physiologic and clinical considerations for hemodynamic monitoring. p. 149. In Russell RO, Jr, Rackley CE (eds): Hemodynamic Monitoring in a Coronary Care Unit. 2nd Ed. Futura Publishing Co., Mt. Kisco, NY, 1981

4. Satler LF, Pallas RS, Bond OB et al: Assessment of the residual coronary arterial stenosis after thrombolytic therapy during acute myocardial infarction. Am J Cardiol 59:1231, 1987

5. Bartone AS, Hess OM, Gaglione A et al: Effect of intravenous propranolol on coronary vasomotion at rest and during dynamic exercise in patients with coronary artery disease. Circulation 81:1225, 1990

6. Feild BJ, Russell RO, Jr, Dowling JT et al: Regional left ventricular performance in the year following myocardial infarction. Circulation 46:679, 1972

7. Russell RO, Jr, Rackley CE, Pombo J et al: Effects of increase in left ventricular filling pressure in patients with acute myocardial infarction. J Clin Invest 49:1539, 1970

8. Ratshin RA, Rackley CE, Russell RO, Jr: Hemodynamic evaluation of left ventricular function in the shock complicating myocardial infarction. Circulation 45:127, 1972

9. Yusuf S, Wittes J, Freidman L: Overview of results of randomized clinical trials in heart disease. 1. Treatments following myocardial infarction. JAMA 260:2088, 1988

10. Antman RM, Braunwald E: Acute MI management in the 1990s. Hosp Pract 25:57, 1990

11. Rackley CE, Russell RO, Jr, Rogers WJ, et al: Clinical experience with glucose-insulin-potassium in acute myocardial infarction. Am Heart J 102:1038, 1981

12. Mantle JA, Russell RO, Jr, Rogers WJ et al: Recent advances in the evaluation and treatment of heart failure. p. 279. In Russell RO, Jr, Rackley CE (eds): Hemodynamic Monitoring in a Coronary Intensive Care Unit. 2nd Ed. Futura Publishing, Mt. Kisco, NY, 1981

13. Rackley CE, Russell RO, Jr, Mantle JA et al: Hemodynamic measurements in patients with uncomplicated myocardial infarctions. p. 181. In Russell RO, Jr, Rackley CE: Hemodynamic Monitoring in a Coronary Intensive Care Unit. 2nd Ed. Futura Publishing, Mt. Kisco, NY, 1981

14. Niess GS, Logic JR, Russell JO, Jr et al: Usefulness and limitations of thallium-201 myocardial scintigraphy in delineating location and size of prior myocardial infarction. Circulation 59:1010, 1979

15. Rackley CE, Russell RO, Jr, Mantle JA et al: Modern approach to the patient with acute myocardial infarction. p. 42. In Harvey WP (ed): Current Problems in Cardiology. Year Book Medical Publishers, Chicago, 1977

16. Rackley CE, Russell RO, Jr, Mantle JA et al: Modern approach to myocardial infarction: Determination of prognosis and therapy. Am Heart J 101:75, 1981

17. Rackley CE, Russell JO, Jr: Coronary Care: Invasive Techniques for Hemodynamic Measurements. American Heart Association, New York, 1973, p. 23

18. Rackley CE, Russell RO, Jr, Mantle JA et al: Cardiogenic shock in patients with myocardial infarction. p. 203. In Russell RO, Jr, Rackley CE (eds): Hemodynamic Monitoring in a Coronary Intensive Care Unit. 1st Ed. Futura Publishing, Mt. Kisco, NY, 1974

19. Rackley CE, Russell RO, Jr, Mantle JA et al: Recognition of acute myocardial infarction. p. 315. In Rackley CE, Russell RO, Jr (eds): Coronary Artery Disease: Recognition and Management. Futura Publishing, Mt. Kisco, NY, 1979

20. Rackley CE et al: Hemodynamic measurements of heart failure in patients with myocardial infarction. In Russell RO and Rackley CE (eds): Hemodynamic Monitoring in a Coronary Intensive Care Unit, 2nd. Ed. Futura, Mt. Kisco, NY, 1981

4

Risk Factors for the Progression of Coronary Heart Disease

Thomas E. Kottke, M.D.
Thomas G. Allison, Ph.D., M.P.H.
Ray W. Squires, Ph.D.

Fifty years ago the treatment of patients with an acute myocardial infarction was a minimum of 6 weeks of bed rest followed by a lifetime of iatrogenic disability.[1] Today the goal of treatment is early ambulation followed by appropriate physical activity within 2 weeks of the acute event. In the same manner, the attitude about risk factors (diet, serum lipid levels, smoking, blood pressure, physical activity, and coronary-prone behavior) has evolved from a belief that they have little to do with the prognosis and management of the patient with clinically manifest coronary heart disease (CHD)[2] to treatment of risk factors as the foundation of the long-term management of the patient with coronary heart disease. This chapter presents the evidence that this evolution of therapeutic strategy is based on scientific evidence, not just shifting custom.

METHODOLOGIC CONSIDERATIONS

Interpreting a field of research by simply summarizing the data is inadequate because a number of studies are based on faulty design and thus will have produced erroneous conclusions. To deal with this problem, recent literature reviews have focused on the highest-quality investigations, rather than reviewing all studies regardless of quality.[3-5] Likewise, expert panels have begun to provide an assessment of the quality of the evidence together with the evidence itself when making recommendations.[6,7] This chapter follows these conventions; it distinguishes between evidence based on observations and evidence based on clinical trials, and it considers only randomized controlled trials (RCTs) as "trial evidence." Although the RCT is considered prima facie evidence of a causal relationship, we also recognize that limiting all conclusions to evidence from randomized clinical trials can result in ignoring evidence that is compelling for other reasons. In cases such as these, we have used the guidelines for causality suggested by A. Bradford Hill.[8]

ATHEROGENIC DIET AND DYSLIPIDEMIA

Observations

Epidemiologic evidence that cornonary artery disease (CAD) could regress has been accumulating for over 60 years. Aschoff noted that war was associated with a decrease in the prevalence of aortic atherosclerosis observed at autopsy,[9] and a decline in deaths from atherosclerosis during World War II was observed in Norway.[10] In Finland, Vartiainen and Kanerva observed that atherosclerosis in the aorta and the coronary and cerebral vessels was 20 to 40% less common during the war years of 1940 to 1946 than in 1933 to 1938; the differences were most marked for complex atherosclerotic lesions in the 30- to 59-year age group.[11] Although these investigators suggested that the wartime change in nutrition was the cause of the change in death rates, their observations were subject to the limitations of all ecologic studies.

As the number of patients with more than one coronary angiogram accumulated, centers began to report that progression of coronary atherosclerosis was associated with uncontrolled risk factor levels in individual patients. For example, Campeau et al.[12] reported in 1984 that the new lesions developing in 67 of 82 patients reexamined 10 years after aortocoronary bypass grafting were in patients with higher levels of very low density lipoprotein (VLDL) and low-density lipoprotein (LDL) cholesterol and the lower levels of high-density lipoprotein cholesterol (HDL). Although there have been some reports to the contrary, the trend in the literature is that studies of this type with sufficient sample size and length of follow-up have found correlations between the risk factors for the development of CHD (smoking, blood pressure, and dyslipidemia) and the angiographically defined progression of coronary atherosclerosis.[13-16]

These observational studies were followed by diet trials without control groups. In the Leiden Intervention Trial, for example, Arntzenius et al.[17,18] treated 39 patients with stable angina pectoris with a vegetarian low-cholesterol diet for 2 years; this diet was associated with a slower than expected rate of growth in the coronary lesions observed at angiography. The linoleic acid-enriched diet lowered the total cholesterol level without affecting the HDL-cholesterol level. The investigators observed that increases in body weight were significantly and positively related to levels of total cholesterol and significantly and negatively related to levels of HDL cholesterol.

No coronary lesion growth was observed in patients with total/HDL-cholesterol ratios of less than 6.9, and regression of atherosclerosis was seen in 17% of all patients. Moreover, persistent angina pectoris and death in the 3.5 years of follow-up were significantly less frequent in the patient group with either no lesion progression or atherosclerotic regression.

Other lipoprotein components, particularly apoproteins (the protein moiety of lipoproteins), have been observed to correlate with the presence or absence of atherosclerosis.[19-21] However, longitudinal studies will be required to understand the cause-and-effect relationship between apoproteins and the progression of CHD.

Trials

The initial diet trials of lipid control after myocardial infarction were forced to rely on clinical endpoints (death or reinfarction) and were small; serum cholesterol levels in the intervention groups remained greater than 220 mg/dL. With the exception of the Oslo Diet-Heart Study,[22] the early randomized trials that reduced total fat in the diet[23] or increased the dietary polyunsaturated fat/saturated fat ratio[24,25] provided little or no evidence to support the hypothesis that either a fat-modified diet or serum cholesterol levels were important in the management of the patient after myocardial infarction.

The largest randomized trial of pharmacologic therapy to prevent recurrence of CHD events, the Coronary Drug Project, began to recruit subjects in 1966.[26] A total of 8,341 men, aged 30 through 64 years at entry, with verified evidence of one or more prior myocardial infarctions were randomized to five active-treatment groups (two different dosages of conjugated estrogen, clofibrate, dextrothyroxine, or niacin) and a control group that received a lactose placebo. The high-dose estrogen intervention was stopped early because of an excess of nonfatal cardiovascular events and because of the drug's lack of efficacy in reducing total mortality. The thyroxine and low-dose estrogen interventions were also discontinued prematurely because they were associated with excess deaths. Only the niacin and clofibrate interventions were continued for the planned duration of the study. The average total serum cholesterol level at entry for subjects in these two groups was 250 mg/dL. It declined to approximately 225 mg/dL in the niacin group and 235 mg/dL in the clofibrate group. At the end of an average of 6 years of follow-up, nonfatal myocardial infarction rates were modestly lower in the niacin group than in the control group, but neither clofibrate nor niacin altered total mortality or cardiovascular mortality rates. However, when the 15-year data were examined to determine whether there was a deleterious effect on all-cause mortality, an unexpected beneficial effect on all-cause mortality and mortality from CHD was observed[27] in patients treated with niacin.

After it became acceptable to perform coronary angiograms solely for purposes of clinical investigation, the angiographically defined progression or regression of coronary atherosclerosis could be used as a study endpoint. The National Heart, Lung, and Blood Institute (NHLBI) Type II Coronary Intervention Study was a randomized clinical trial designed to test the hypothesis that lowering the LDL cholesterol level in men with diet-resistant hyperlipidemia could arrest or retard the progression of CAD.[28,29] The intervention compared diet and cholestyramine (24 g/day) with diet and placebo. After initiation of the diet, but before initiation of drug treatment, the total serum cholesterol level was 293 mg/dL in the placebo group; it averaged 289 mg/dL over the 5-year study period. The average postdiet total serum cholesterol level for the intervention group was 310 mg/dL; it averaged 256 mg/dL over the 5-year treatment period. The average LDL cholesterol level during the trial was 219 mg/dL for the placebo group and 178 mg/dL for the intervention group. CAD progressed in 49% of the placebo-treated patients and 32% of the cholestyramine-treated patients. When the relationship between CAD progression and lipid changes was examined independent of the specific treatment group, a significant inverse relationship was found between progression and the combination of an increase in HDL cholesterol and a decrease in LDL cholesterol; changes in the HDL/total cholesterol and HDL/LDL ratios were the best predictors of CAD change.

The Cholesterol-Lowering Atherosclerosis Study (CLAS) randomized 188 nonsmoking men aged 40 to 59 with a history of coronary bypass surgery to placebo or the combination of colestipol and niacin.[30] Coronary angiograms were carried out before intervention and after 2 years of intervention. The intervention group achieved a 26% reduction in total cholesterol level (from 246 to 180 mg/dL), a 43% reduction in LDL cholesterol (from 171 to 97 mg/dL), and a 37% increase in HDL cholesterol (44.6 to 60.8 mg/dL). Lipid levels in the placebo group were 232 mg/dL for total cholesterol, 160 mg/dL for LDL cholesterol and 44.4 mg/dL for HDL cholesterol. Both groups experienced a net progression of lesions, but active drug treatment was associated with fewer new lesions, less progression of old lesions, and regression in 16% of the lesions that were present at the start of the study. The factors most strongly related to progression of atherosclerosis were LDL cholesterol and VLDL cholesterol levels in the placebo-treated group and the content of apoprotein C-III in high density lipoprotein in the drug-treated group.[31] (Apoprotein C-III is reported to inhibit lipoprotein lipase and retards hepatic uptake of triglyceride-rich lipoproteins and remanents).

Ornish et al.[32] randomized 28 patients with known CAD to treatment with a low-fat vegetarian diet, smoking cessation, stress management training, and moderate exercise. Twenty patients were randomized to a "usual-care" control group. Initial total serum cholesterol levels averaged 226 mg/dL among intervention group patients and 245 mg/dL among control group patients. After 12 months of intervention, the average total serum cholesterol level was 172 mg/dL for the intervention group and 230 mg/dL for the control group. On average, lesions in intervention group patients regressed, while lesions in control group patients progressed. There was also a dose–response relationship between adherence to the intervention and regression or progression of lesions, for both the experimental group and the entire study group.

Comment

In the intervention studies, an LDL cholesterol level of less than 100 mg/dL has been associated with regression and an LDL cholesterol level of 160 mg/dL has been associated with progression of atherosclerosis. The level of HDL cholesterol is inversely associated with progression. It appears that the goal of therapy should be to minimize or eliminate animal fat in the diet, lower the LDL cholesterol level to less than 100 mg/dL, and raise the HDL cholesterol level to the greatest extent possible.

HYPERTENSION

Observations
In the first 20 years of the Framingham study, 193 of the 2,336 male enrollees sustained their first myocardial infarction.[33] Among these 193 men, those who remained hypertensive had a fivefold-greater risk of mortality than did normotensive men. The men who had decreases in their systolic blood pressure of ≥ 10 mmHg as a result of their myocardial infarction had mortality rates 15 times higher than did normotensive men.

Analyzing the experience in Olmsted County, Connolly et al.[34] found that hypertension was a significant predictor of both short and long-term prognosis for the 1,069 patients who had their first manifestation of coronary disease between 1960 and 1975. Deaths within 30 days of infarction were less likely in treated than in untreated hypertensive patients. Adequate treatment, defined as reduction of the blood pressure from the definitely hypertensive range into either the borderline or normal range, was associated with a significantly better outcome than inadequately treated hypertension. Inadequate treatment, in turn, was associated with better outcome than no treatment at all.

Trials
No trials were designed exclusively to test the hypothesis that the intensity of treatment of hypertension affects the survival of patients after myocardial infarction. However, two trials, the Hypertension Detection and Follow-up Program (HDFP)[35,36] and the European Working Party on High Blood Pressure in the Elderly (EWPHE),[37] contained significant numbers of subjects with prior myocardial infarction. The EWPHE trial is discussed in the section on risk factors in the elderly.

The HDFP randomized participants to treatment with a "stepped-care" protocol that emphasized initial treatment with a diuretic, with addition of other agents if the blood pressure could not be controlled with a diuretic alone, or a "referred-care" protocol. Slightly over 1,000 ($n = 1,018$) subjects had a history of prior myocardial infarction. The group with prior myocardial infarction experienced both a greater relative benefit (about 20% reduction in risk) and absolute benefit (reduction in total mortality of 25/1,000 participants) from treatment than did the 9,922 subjects without a history of prior myocardial infarction (a relative benefit of 17% reduction in risk and an absolute benefit of 10/1,000 participants).

Comment
In subjects with ischemia (defined by electrocardiographic abnormalities), death rates from myocardial infarction are 5 to 7 events/1,000 person-years of treatment higher in the group whose diastolic blood pressure is lowered below 85 mmHg than in the group whose diastolic blood pressure is lowered to a lesser degree.[38–40] The implication is that "overtreatment" is one source of the difficulty in reducing death rates from myocardial infarction in hypertensive patients.

However, when considering patients with prior myocardial infarction, it should be remembered that the benefit from treatment in the HDFP subjects with prior myocardial infarction was three to five times the magnitude of the J-shaped curve described by Cruickshank.[38] Likewise, the benefit from giving beta-blocking drugs to patients after myocardial infarction appears at least twice as great as the potentially deleterious effect of overtreatment;[41] the benefit derived from giving angiotensin-converting enzyme (ACE) inhibitors to patients with class IV congestive heart failure is 30 times the magnitude of the potential J-shaped curve described by Cruickshank.[42] Although the data suggest that treatment benefits patients with hypertension after acute myocardial infarction, the clinician should be aware that the potential for "overtreatment" does exist.

SMOKING

Observations

Smoking affects several of the precursors of both atherosclerosis and thrombosis. It has been associated with low HDL-cholesterol levels, increased fibrinogen concentrations, elevated white blood cell counts, and elevated plasma catecholamine levels.[43] Stopping smoking is associated with an increase of 29% in HDL cholesterol levels.[44] For the same degree of coronary atherosclerosis, smokers are more likely than nonsmokers to have sustained a myocardial infarction.[45]

Patients who continue to smoke after myocardial infarction have death rates about twice as high as those in patients who stop smoking.[46–51] Continued smoking also increases the risk of recurrent sudden cardiac arrest.[52] Smoking is associated with left ventricular dysfunction, independent of a history of myocardial infarction and amount of myocardium supplied by the left anterior descending coronary artery.[53] Continued smoking after coronary angioplasty has been reported to be associated with increased restenosis.[54] Stopping smoking after myocardial infarction is also associated with a delay in the onset of angina,[55] and patients who stop smoking after coronary artery bypass experience more benefit than patients who continue to smoke.[56]

Trials

There are no randomized clinical trials of the effects of smoking cessation on mortality among patients with clinically manifest CHD. However, short-term trials have demonstrated that smoking causes silent ischemia,[57] blocks the increase in coronary blood flow normally associated with exercise,[58] reduces the antianginal efficacy of propranolol, atenolol, and nifedipine,[59] and triggers coronary spasm and abnormal segmental diffuse narrowing of the coronary arteries.[60]

Comment

It is generally accepted that smoking increases the risk of death from several causes. It is therefore doubtful that the hypothesis that smoking affects the long-term survival of patients after myocardial infarction will ever be tested. Even in the absence of trial data, it appears most prudent to clearly, unequivocally, and continuously encourage and help patients stop smoking. Because relapse is a major problem for all smokers, continued reinforcement of the benefits of not smoking is also an essential component of the intervention.

PHYSICAL INACTIVITY

Observations

Epidemiologic studies have demonstrated a strong inverse relationship between the incidence of CHD and physical activity, whether measured as habitual occupational activity,[61,62] leisure-time physical activity,[63–65] or physical fitness.[66] Powell et al.[67] analyzed 47 epidemiologic studies of physical activity and CHD and found a strong (relative risk [RR], 1.9), consistent, inverse relationship between routine physical activity and the incidence of CHD.

These relationships appear to persist after the onset of CHD. For example, Paffenbarger and Hyde,[64] in an observational study of Harvard alumni, assessed habitual physical activity in 782 alumni with known CHD. During an approximately 12-year study period, the more active subjects (who expended at least 2,000 kcal in total energy output per week) had a coronary event rate that was 30% lower than the rate for the less active alumni. The beneficial effect persisted after adjustment for cigarette smoking, blood pressure, body weight, family history of CHD, and age.

Trials

Experimental exercise effects in animals include increased coronary artery diameter,[68] overall coronary tree size,[69] and myocardial capillary density.[70–72] For example, Kramsch et al.[73] demonstrated that for nonhuman primates, regular aerobic exercise training (1 hour of jogging three times per week) reduced the severity of CHD in the setting of diet-induced hypercholesterolemia and resulted in increased epicardial coronary artery caliber. Not all studies have shown such improvements with training of healthy animals.[74–76]

Factors that may help explain these inconsistent results include species-specific effects (dogs are less likely to show improvement than rats, swine, or primates); age at training, especially in rats;[71] assessment techniques;[77] and the length and severity of the exercise training program.[71] Animal studies have shown an increase in myocardial perfusion from enhanced coronary collateral flow following exercise training after experimentally induced infarction or ischemia.[78–82] At least one study[83] failed to show this effect.

The physiologic effects of exercise training on human coronary patients in the first few months following myocardial infarction appear limited to increases in work capacity, maximal oxygen uptake, and HDL-cholesterol levels and are not different between high- and low-intensity training groups.[84] Typically, such studies have failed to demonstrate beneficial effects on myocardial perfusion, left ventricular function, or coronary collateral circulation.[85]

Longer-term, high-intensity exercise training may have more significant benefits for coronary patients, including improved left ventricular function,[86] stroke volume,[87,88] reversal of exertional hypotension,[89] reduced ST segment depression at a constant rate-pressure product,[90,91] and increased HDL-cholesterol levels.[91] One limited study suggested improved graft patency after coronary artery bypass graft surgery with early exercise intervention.[92] Exercise training has also been shown to reduce bothersome or limiting symptoms, improve oxygen transport, reduce objective evidence of myocardial ischemia, improve physical work capacity, reduce platelet aggregation, and benefit psychological function.[93] Benefits in improved work capacity and maximal oxygen uptake have been confirmed, even for patients with severe left ventricular dysfunction[94–95] and ventricular aneurysm.[96]

The National Exercise and Heart Disease Project[97] exemplifies the problems of trying to test the hypothesis that exercise affects survival. Initial planning called for 4,200 participants, but funding was limited to 651 men, who were randomized to exercise and control groups. Only 20 percent of the subjects entered the study within 2 to 6 months of their myocardial infarction. At the end of the 3-year trial, 23% of the exercise group were not attending the organized exercise program and claimed not be exercising elsewhere. Thirty-one percent of the control subjects reported regular exercise training. For the total sample, total mortality and recurrent myocardial infarction rate tended to favor the exercise group (7.3 versus 4.6% for total mortality and 7.0 versus 5.3% for recurrent myocardial infarction), but was not statistically significant. Among the subgroup of subjects with normal peak systolic blood pressures during graded exercise testing (>140 mmHg), total mortality was lower for the exercise group (6.2 versus 1.9%, $P < 0.05$).

Additional randomized trials of exercise training after myocardial infarction have been performed, although designs differed for the degree of modification of risk factors and education, in addition to the exercise component. Only one of the individual trials demonstrated a significant effect of exercise on subsequent cardiovascular mortality,[98] but trends were favorable in others.[99–104]

When these studies are combined through meta-analysis, favorable effects of exercise on the progression of CHD are evident. O'Connor et al.[5] combined 4,554 patients (most of them men) from 22 randomized trials, with an average follow-up interval of 3 years. In comparison with nonexercising control subjects, these patients experienced total mortality, cardiovascular mortality, and non-fatal reinfarction rates that were significantly reduced 20, 22, and 25% respectively. A second meta-analysis by Oldridge et al.[105] reported similar findings.

Comment

Although many salutary effects of exercise training have been appreciated for patients with CHD, the definitive single-factor trial of exercise training on secondary prevention of CHD is lacking and is unlikely to be performed because of cost and issues of feasibility and ethics. Habitual physical activity is a difficult behavior to isolate and evaluate, given its relationship to other atherogenic factors and behaviors. Patients cross over, and patients who begin an exercise program frequently make the decision to adopt "healthier" practices such as avoidance of tobacco, better compliance with medication schedules, a more prudent diet, and a more balanced outlook on life. Therefore, "proof" that exercise increases survival or prevents subsequent cardiac events must be acknowledged from indirect evidence[106] and from the meta-analyses that indicate a protective effect of exercise on the secondary prevention of CHD. However, most randomized studies included in the meta-analysis involved other coronary risk factor modifications in addition to exercise training.

Nevertheless, the 20 to 25% reduction in secondary coronary events as a result of exercise training and risk factor reduction is similar to that demonstrated with other, more expensive therapies including myocardial revascularization procedures, beta-adrenergic blocking drugs, lipid-lowering agents, and antihypertensive treatments. Except for orthopedic complications, the "side-effects" of exercise training are also more favorable than those of any of the medical therapies.[107,108] Exercise training should not be considered an alternative, but rather an adjunct, to medical or surgical therapy for CHD.

TYPE A BEHAVIOR

Observations
In 1959, Friedman and Rosenman introduced the concept of type A behavior.[109] This pattern of behavior is characterized by enhanced aggressiveness, ambitiousness, competitive drive, and hostility, and a chronic sense of time urgency. Among 3,154 subjects monitored for 8 to 9 years in the Western Collaborative Group Study, type A behavior, as measured by clinician-administered "structured interview," was strongly and independently associated with CHD incidence.[110] However, studies that measured type A behavior by questionnaire or with the structured interview administered by trained interviewers who were not clinicians rarely found an independent relationship between CHD events and type A behavior.[111]

Most observations about the relationship between type A behavior and the risk of recurrent events after myocardial infarction do not support the hypothesis that type A behavior is a risk factor for recurrent events. In fact, among the 231 men who sustained a myocardial infarction in the Western Collaborative Group Study and survived the event by more than 24 hours, the mortality rate from CHD was 19.1 per 1,000 person-years among 160 type A patients and 31.7/1,000 person-years among the 71 type B men.[112] Controlling for follow-up time, the type of initial coronary event, and levels of the traditional risk factors, the ratio of CHD-associated mortality among type A men compared with type B men was 0.58 (95% confidence limits [CL], 0.35 to 0.96).

A somewhat similar finding was reported by Barefoot et al.[113] in a cohort of all patients with documented coronary disease admitted to the Duke Medical Center between 1974 and 1980 (266 women and 1,201 men); type A behavior was related to survival only in patients with the most severe disease. Among the one-third of the patients with the most severe disease, those with type A behavior had a significantly *better* survival than patients with type B behavior. A number of other groups, using the Jenkins Activity Survey, have found either no relationship between type A behavior and cardiac mortality after a nonfatal coronary event[114,115] or an inverse relationship,[116] in contrast to the Friedman and Rosenman hypothesis.

Trials
To determine the ability of type A behavioral counseling to prevent recurrent events after myocardial infarction, Friedman et al.[117] randomized subjects to group cardiac counseling ($n = 270$) or to group cardiac counseling plus type A behavioral counseling ($n = 592$). (The unequal randomization was intentional because the investigators feared that a large number of the participants would drop out of the intervention group.) The initial diagnosis and assessment of type A behavior was determined by a videotaped clinical interview administered by an independent consultant, who was blinded to the group status of the patient. Repeat interviews were obtained at 3 and 4.5 years of follow-up for all participants.

There were no differences in the baseline average severity of CHD between the two groups, and the intervention resulted in a significant differential change in the intensity of type A behavior between the two groups. With the "intention to treat" rule applied to the analysis, the rate of recurrent coronary events was 21.2% in the control group and 12.9% in the active treatment group ($P < 0.005$). After the first year of the study, a significant difference in number of cardiac deaths was observed between the experimental and control groups during the remaining 3.5 years of the study ($P < 0.05$).

Comment

The investigators who conducted the postmyocardial infarction type A behavior intervention trial[117] believe that they were able to detect an intervention effect because their assessment of type A behavior was made by the *clinical examination* (original emphasis) of the subject, using physical signs and symptoms that can be observed in interview but cannot be captured by the paper questionnaire. They believe that they were able to produce an intervention effect because the members of the intervention team were *adequately trained and dedicated* (original emphasis) professional personnel. Significant differences in event rates between the two groups at the end of 3 years of intervention resulted in a special committee of the NHLBI advising that the study be stopped at 4.5 years rather than 5 years of intervention. Even so, the observation in 1981 that "fundamental uncertainties" exist in the characterization, assessment, impact, and treatment of type A behavior[118] remains true today.

RISK FACTORS FOR PROGRESSION OF CHD IN SPECIAL GROUPS

Elderly

Diet and dyslipidemia

In their autopsy study, Vartiainen and Kanerva[11] reported finding that the war years had little effect on the presence of atherosclerosis among the individuals over age 70. However, in this study, atherosclerosis in individuals over 70 was far less severe than for individuals in the age deciles between 40 and 69.

Until recently, Framingham data have been cited as evidence that serum lipid levels become unimportant as a risk factor after age 55.[119] However, as the Framingham data set matured, it became apparent that serum cholesterol level remains an important risk factor for development of CHD in individuals free of CHD at the time of their 65th birthday.[120] Likewise, the Hawaii Heart Study reported that the serum cholesterol level retains the same predictive relationship in older Hawaiian men (relative risk = 1.68 for total serum cholesterol level ≥ 6.20 mmol/L versus serum cholesterol level ≤ 4.92 mmol/L) as in younger Hawaiian men (relative risk = 1.71).[121] Because elderly persons, as a group, have higher CAD rates, the absolute difference in risk between high and low is greater for men 65 to 74 years of age (8/1,000 person-years) than for men 52 to 59 years of age (4/1,000 person-years); the effect of elevated serum cholesterol levels on coronary events in the elderly was of the same order of magnitude as the effect of elevated systolic blood pressure.

Smoking

Hermanson et al.[56] reported the experience of 1,086 individuals who had continued smoking and 807 who had quit in the Coronary Artery Surgery Study (CASS) registry. Continued smoking remained a risk factor for death (relative risk [RR], 1.6, 95% confidence limits [CL], 1.1 to 2.3) in the group aged 65 and older at entry, as it was for subjects 55 to 64 years of age (RR = 1.7 with 95% CL of 1.4 to 2.1) and subjects 35 to 54 years of age (RR = 1.6 with 95% CL of 1.4 to 1.9).

Hypertension

The EWPHE trial was a double-blind randomized trial involving patients over the age of 60 years (average, 72 ± 8 years) with sitting diastolic blood pressures on placebo treatment ranging from 90 to 119 mmHg diastolic and 160 to 239 mmHg systolic.[37] A total of 840 patients were randomized between 1972 and 1984, when the

Steering Committee reported that some of the trial endpoints had been reached. Mean diastolic blood pressure for the active treatment group was 101 mmHg during the randomization phase, 88 mmHg after 1 year, and 85 mmHg for the remaining 7 years of the trial. Stringent intention-to-treat analysis revealed a 9% decline (from 76/1,000 person-years) in total mortality ($P = 0.41$), a 38% decline (from 24/1,000 person-years) in cardiac mortality ($P = 0.036$), and 32% decline (from 16/1,000 person-years) in stroke mortality ($P = 0.16$). Analysis based on events during double-blind treatment revealed more favorable treatment effects.

Physical Activity

We are unaware of any trials of physical activity in elderly patients with CHD that have used either survival or recurrent events as the endpoint.

Comment

Although management of hypertension in the elderly has been an issue for more than a decade,[37] the "common knowledge" that cholesterol is not important for the elderly retarded investigation of the relationship between modification of serum cholesterol levels and progression of coronary disease in this age group of patients. An NHLBI pilot drug study to treat hypercholesterolemia in the elderly is now under way,[122] and further trials on the effects of treating elevated cholesterol in the elderly can be expected.

Women

Diet and dyslipidemia

Vartiainen and Kanerva[11] found that the war years in Finland affected atherosclerosis in women as it did in men. Likewise, Strøm and Jensen[10] reported that mortality from circulatory diseases declined for both men and women during World War II in Norway. In the Framingham study, the total serum cholesterol level predicted the onset of CAD for both men and women over age 65.[120]

Studies of the relationship between risk factors and the progression of atherosclerosis that include women at all usually contain only 10 to 20% of women subjects; few studies report the independent experience of women. The reported data, however, suggest that men and women share a common experience for progression of CAD; Campeau et al.[12] reported that CAD progression was slightly more frequent in men (58 of 69 [84%]) than in women (9 of 13 [69%]), but did not report whether these associations were independent of other coronary risk factors; Bourassa et al.[123] reported that disease progression in women after coronary bypass surgery did not differ from that in men. Moise et al.[13] reported that 29% of the women and 43% of the men in their series showed CAD progression. However, because of the small sample size, these differences were not statistically significant. The Leiden Intervention Trial[17] included only four women, and only five women participated in the Lifestyle Heart Trial.[32]

Smoking

Smoking appears as much a problem for women as it is for men. Studies reporting solely on women demonstrate that, for a given level of coronary atherosclerosis, women who smoke are more likely to have had a myocardial infarction.[45] Women who continue to smoke after a myocardial infarction have a significantly poorer long-term survival than women who stop smoking.[47,48] Studies of smoking that include women suggest that smoking-related problems for men are also problems for women who smoke.[14,53,54,58,60,124]

Hypertension

We are not aware of reports of the women in the Framingham cohort who had hypertension and subsequent myocardial infarction. The Olmsted County CHD incidence cohort included 230 women with hypertension, and the investigators reported that treatment was adequate in only 27% of these women;[34] however, they did not report the results by adequacy of treatment separately for women and men. Likewise, although data from the HDFP trial are reported by sex and for individuals with prior CHD, they are not reported with simultaneous stratification for these two variables.[36]

Type A behavior

The studies that were designed to observe the relationship between type A behavior and survival after the development of CHD included, on average, 10 to 20% women.[113–115] Only the Aspirin Myocardial Infarction Study[115] reported the experience of women apart from the experience of men. As measured by the Jenkins Activity Survey, type A behavior was associated with a trend to fewer recurrent events in the women who exhibited the strongest type A behavior. Ten percent of the participants in the Recurrent Coronary Prevention Project[117] were women; however, their experience is not reported independently of the experience of the men.

Exercise

One study documented similarly improved exercise tolerance in women to that in men with exercise cardiac rehabilitation, despite poorer compliance.[125] However, none of the clinical trials has satisfactorily addressed the effects of exercise training on collateral circulation, myocardial perfusion, cardiac function, or survival in female patients.

Estrogen replacement

The Lipid Research Clinics Program Follow-up Study included a cohort of 2,270 white women, aged 40 to 69 years at baseline.[126] After an average follow-up of 8.5 years, there were 44 deaths due to cardiovascular disease among the 1,677 nonusers of estrogens and 6 deaths due to cardiovascular disease among the 593 estrogen users. The age-adjusted relative risk of cardiovascular disease deaths in estrogen users compared with nonusers was 0.34 (95% confidence limits, 0.12 to 0.81) and the multivariable adjusted relative risk was 0.37 (95% confidence limits, 0.16 to 0.88). Statistical analyses suggest that much of the protective effect of estrogen replacement therapy arises from its tendency to raise HDL cholesterol levels and lower LDL cholesterol levels. However, the differences in serum lipids between estrogen users and nonusers do not fully explain the differences in event rates.

About 10% of the women had cardiovascular disease at baseline (defined as the occurrence of myocardial infarction, stroke, hypertension, hyperlipidemia, diabetes, or peripheral vascular disease). Four percent of both users ($n = 23$) and nonusers ($n = 60$) of estrogen replacement therapy reported a prior myocardial infarction or stroke. Although the group of women with only stroke or myocardial infarction is too small to calculate risk ratios, the experience of the larger group of women with any cardiovascular disease (a 13.8/10,000 cardiovascular disease death rate in estrogen users compared with 66.3/10,000 in nonusers) is consistent with the hypothesis that estrogen replacement therapy reduces death rates in women with CHD.

Sullivan et al.[127] examined the relationship between severity of atherosclerosis at cardiac catheterization, estrogen usage, and subsequent death in 2,268 women who underwent coronary angiography and were either over age 55 or had previously undergone bilateral oophorectomy. During the 10 years of follow-up, there was no significant difference in survival among patients initially free of coronary disease at angiography who had either never used ($n = 377$) or ever used ($n = 69$) estrogens. Among patients with mild to moderate coronary stenosis ($n = 644$), the 10-year survival of those who never used estrogens was 85.0% and that of the 99 who had ever used estrogen was 95.6% ($P < 0.03$). Survival was 60.0% among those with >70% coronary stenosis who had never used ($n = 1108$) estrogens and 97.0% among the 70 who had ever used estrogens. Even though those who had never used estrogens were older, had a lower proportion of cigarette smokers, and had a higher proportion of diabetes and hyperlipidemia, estrogen use had a significant independent beneficial effect on survival in women. The adjusted relative risk of death for estrogen use was 0.16 (confidence limits, 0.04 to 0.66).

Trials

There have been no randomized clinical trials of hypertension treatment, smoking cessation, treatment of hyperlipidemia, or estrogen replacement therapy to prevent recurrent CHD events in women.

Comment

The problem of lack of data for the relationship between survivors of myocardial infarction and risk factors for the development of CHD is amplified when women are considered independent of men. For hypertension, smoking, exercise, and hyperlipidemia, however, existing data are consistent with the hypothesis that the same physiologic processes act in the same manner in both men and women.

However, the effects of estrogen replacement appear very different in women and men. Although Coronary Drug Project[26] data suggest that estrogen therapy harms men, the data from the Lipid Research Clinics Prevalence Study[126] and the data of Sullivan et al.[127] suggest that the opposite is true for women. There is a major unanswered question regarding estrogen replacement therapy; because unopposed estrogen effect may be a risk factor for uterine and breast cancers,[128] it has become customary to give progestins when giving estrogen replacement therapy. It is not known whether the effects of progestins that are intended to offset the putative carcinogenic effects of estrogens also offset the cardioprotective effects of estrogens.

WHAT SHOULD THE CLINICIAN CONCLUDE FROM THE EVIDENCE?

The observations and trials reviewed in this chapter indicate that high-fat diet and dyslipidemia, hypertension, smoking, and physical inactivity are risk factors for the progression of CHD, just as they are risk factors for the onset of CHD (Table 4-1). The randomized controlled trial evidence that reducing coronary-prone behavior reduces the risk of recurrent coronary events cannot be ignored. Even if treating coronary-prone behavior does not reduce the risk of death or recurrent myocardial infarction, our clinical impression is that coronary-prone behavior has a significant negative impact on both patients and their families. Therefore, treatment of this

Table 4-1. Evidence That Risk Factors for Development of CHD also Predict Progression of the Disease

---

Atherogenic diet and dyslipidemia

There is consistent *epidemiologic* evidence that diet and dyslipidemia influence survival of individuals with CHD.[9–18] *Randomized trials* have demonstrated that lifestyle modification interventions that include vegetarian diets or pharmacologic treatment of hyperlipidemia can halt, slow, or reverse the progression of CHD.[30–32]

Hypertension

It has been *observed* that mortality rates after myocardial infarction are higher when hypertension is not treated.[34] Although there are no *randomized trials* of hypertension treatment after myocardial infarction, the experience from randomized trials that have included subjects with a history of myocardial infarction suggests that patients benefit from treatment.[35,37] Although patients without heart disease may have adverse effects when their diastolic blood pressure is lowered below 85 to 90 mmHg,[38–40] the positive effects of treatment with beta-blocking drugs after myocardial infarction[41] and ACE inhibitors when congestive heart failure is severe[42] far outweigh the potential harmful effects of overtreating elevated blood pressure levels.

Smoking

The effects of stopping smoking on survival after myocardial infarction have never been tested in a *randomized trial*. However, it has been *observed* that cessation of smoking is associated with a marked improvement in outcome when compared with continued smoking.[46–57] *Trials* on the short-term effects of smoking cessation demonstrate that smoking adversely affects coronary blood flow and reduces the efficacy of antianginal drugs.[58–60]

Physical inactivity

The need for a very large number of subjects makes non-feasible a single-factor *randomized trial* of the effect of exercise on survival. However, meta-analyses of *randomized trials* of coronary rehabilitation[5,105] suggest that exercise improves survival, not just cardiac function and physical work capacity.[84–91]

Type A behavior

There is *randomized trial* evidence that treatment of type A behavior after myocardial infarction improves survival.[117] However, measurement of type A behavior remains a problem, and the *association* between type A behavior and survival has been reported to be positive, negative, and nonexistent.[112–116]

---

condition is warranted as part of the coronary rehabilitation process.

There is no evidence that the course of CHD in the elderly is fundamentally different than in the young; neither is there is evidence that elderly patients with CHD do not respond to interventions that benefit the young. Therefore, coronary risk factors should be modified to the greatest extent tolerated by the elderly patient, and every attempt should be made to remobilize elderly patients to previous levels of activity. Elderly patients may justifiably be more oriented to the present than the future when compared with young patients, and treatments aimed at maximizing the length of life at a cost of compromising the present quality of life may be less valued by the elderly than the young patient. However, withholding the offer of treatment to a patient simply because of age is to be avoided.

Except for their response to estrogen replacement therapy, the bulk of the evidence suggests that, as with men, women with CHD benefit from risk factor control. What little evidence is available suggests that estrogen replacement is potentially a powerful intervention for the woman with CHD. Because of the lack of trial data, however, physicians may be justified in waiting for further evidence until estrogen replacement therapy is prescribed for all women with CHD.

In 1939 Mallory et al. advised that it was preferable to keep the coronary patient at strict bed rest for 8 weeks or more.[1] However, as the early studies of coronary rehabilitation demonstrated that remobilization of the patient before 6 to 8 weeks at bed rest was safe, programs began to report that patients not only were not harmed but appeared to be helped by increasing physical activity and controlling smoking, hypertension, diet, dyslipidemia, and coronary-prone behavior. The ideal way to remobilize the patient and provide risk factor management is through comprehensive coronary rehabilitation. All patients who are expected to survive the clinical manifestations of CHD, regardless of gender or age, have the potential to benefit from comprehensive coronary rehabilitation; because these patients tend to return to their old habits,[129] they will probably benefit from periodic booster sessions.

REFERENCES

1. Mallory GK, White PD, Salcedo-Salgar J: The speed of healing of myocardial infarction: A study of the pathological anatomy in seventy-two cases. Am Heart J 18:647, 1939
2. Meijler F: Contribution of the risk factor concept to patient care. J Am Coll Cardiol 1:13, 1983
3. Yusuf S, Wittes J, Friedman L: Overview of results of randomized clinical trials in heart disease. Part I. Treatments following myocardial infarction. JAMA 260:2088, 1988
4. May GS, Eberlein KA, Furberg CD et al: Secondary prevention after myocardial infarction: A review of long-term trials. Prog Cardiovasc Dis 24:331, 1982
5. O'Connor GT, Buring JE, Yusuf S et al: An overview of randomized trials of rehabilitation with exercise after myocardial infarction. Circulation 80:234, 1989
6. US Preventive Services Task Force: Guide to clinical preventive services: An assessment of the effectiveness of 169 interventions. p. 387. In: Report of the US Preventive Services Task Force. Williams & Wilkins, Baltimore, 1989
7. Report of a Task Force to the Conference of Deputy Ministers of Health: Periodic Health Examination Monograph. Canadian Publishing Center, Hull, Quebec, Canada, 1980
8. Hill AB: Principles of Medical Statistics. 9th Ed. Oxford University Press, New York, 1971
9. Aschoff L: Atherosclerosis. p. 131. In: Lectures in Pathology (delivered in the United States in 1924). Hoeber, New York, 1924
10. Strøm A, Jensen RA: Mortality from circulatory diseases in Norway 1940–1945. Lancet i:126, 1951
11. Vartiainen I, Kanerva K: Arteriosclerosis in wartime. Ann Med Intern Fenn 36:748, 1957
12. Campeau L, Enjalbert M, Lesperance J et al: The relation of risk factors to the development of atherosclerosis in saphenous vein bypass grafts and the progression of disease in the native circulation: A study 10 years after aortocoronary bypass surgery. N Engl J Med 311:1329, 1984
13. Moise A, Theroux P, Taeymans Y, Waters DD: Factors associated with progression of coronary artery disease in patients with normal or minimally narrowed coronary arteries. Am J Cardiol 56:30, 1985
14. Raichlen JS, Healy B, Achuff SC, Pearson TA: Importance of risk factors in the angiographic

progression of coronary artery disease. Am J Cardiol 57:66, 1986

15. Barth JD, Jansen H, Kromhout D et al: Progression and regression of human coronary atherosclerosis. The role of lipoproteins, lipases and thyroid hormones in coronary lesion growth. Atherosclerosis 68:51, 1987

16. Bruschke AV, Kramer JR Jr, Bal ET et al: The dynamics of progression of coronary atherosclerosis studied in 168 medically treated patients who underwent coronary arteriography three times. Am Heart J 117:296, 1989

17. Arntzenius AC, Kromhout D, Barth JD et al: Diet, lipoproteins and the progression of coronary atherosclerosis: The Leiden Intervention Trial. N Engl J Med 312:805, 1985

18. Arntzenius AC: Regression of atherosclerosis. Horm Metab 19:19, 1988

19. Murai A, Miyahara T, Fujimoto N et al: Lp(a) as a risk factor for coronary heart disease and cerebral infarction. Atherosclerosis 59:199, 1986

20. Reinhart RA, Gani K, Arndt MR, Broste SK: Apolipoproteins A-I and B as predictors of angiographically defined coronary artery disease. Arch Intern Med 150:1629, 1990

21. Rhoads GG, Dahlen G, Berg K et al: Lp(a) lipoprotein as a risk factor for myocardial infarction. JAMA 256:2540, 1986

22. Leren P: The Oslo diet-heart study. Eleven year report. Circulation 42:935, 1970

23. Medical Research Council: Low-fat diet in myocardial infarction. A controlled trial. Lancet ii:501, 1965

24. Rose GA, Thomson WB, Williams RT: Corn oil in treatment of ischaemic heart disease. Br Med J 1:1531, 1965

25. Medical Research Council: Controlled trial of soya-bean oil in myocardial infarction. Lancet ii:693, 1968

26. Coronary Drug Project Research Group: Clofibrate and niacin in coronary heart disease. JAMA 231:360, 1975

27. Canner P, Berge KG, Wenger NK: Fifteen year mortality in Coronary Drug Project patients: Long-term benefit with niacin. J Am Coll Cardiol 8:1245, 1986

28. Brensike JF, Levy RI, Kelsey SF et al: Effects of therapy with cholestyramine on progression of coronary atherosclerosis: Results of the NHLBI Type II Coronary Intervention Study. Circulation 69:313, 1984

29. Levy RI, Brensike JF, Epstein SE et al: The influence of changes in lipid values induced by cholestyramine and diet on progression of coronary artery disease: results of the NHLBI Type II Coronary Intervention Study. Circulation 69:325, 1984

30. Blankenhorn DH, Nessim SA, Johnson RL et al: Beneficial effects of combined colestipol-niacin therapy on coronary atherosclerosis and coronary venous bypass grafts. JAMA 257:3233, 1987

31. Blankenhorn DH, Alaupovic P, Wickham E et al: Prediction of angiographic change in native human coronary arteries and aortocoronary bypass grafts. Lipid and nonlipid factors. Circulation 81:470, 1990

32. Ornish D, Brown SE, Scherwitz LW et al: Can lifestyle changes reverse coronary heart disease? The Lifestyle Heart Trial. Lancet 336:129, 1990

33. Kannel WB, Sorlie P, Castelli WP, McGee D: Blood pressure and survival after myocardial infarction: the Framingham study. Am J Cardiol 45:326, 1980

34. Connolly DC, Elveback LR, Oxman HA: Coronary heart disease in residents of Rochester, Minnesota, 1950–1975. III. Effect of hypertension and its treatment on survival of patients with coronary artery disease. Mayo Clin Proc 58:249, 1983

35. Browner WS, Hulley SB: Effect of risk status on treatment criteria. Implications of hypertension trials. Hypertension, suppl I:I-51, 1989

36. Langford HC, Stamler J, Wassertheil-Smoller S, Prineas RJ: All-cause mortality in the Hypertension Detection and Follow-up Program: findings in the whole cohort and for persons with less severe hypertension, with and without other traits related to risk of mortality. Prog Cardiovasc Dis 29:29, 1986

37. Amery A, Birkenhager W, Brixko P et al: Mortality and morbidity results from the European Working Party on Hypertension in the Elderly Trial. Lancet i:1349, 1985

38. Cruickshank JM: Coronary flow reserve and the J curve relation between diastolic blood pressure and myocardial infarction. Br Med J 297:1227, 1988

39. Fletcher AE, Beevers DG, Bulpitt CJ et al: The relationship between a low treated blood pressure and IHD mortality: a report from the DHSS hypertension care computing project (DHCCP). J Hum Hypertension 2:11, 1988

40. Berglund G: Goals of anti-hypertensive therapy. Is there a point beyond which pressure reduction is dangerous? Am J Hypertension 2:586, 1989

41. Yusuf S, Peto R, Lewis J et al: Beta blockade dur-

ing and after myocardial infarction: an overview of the randomized trials. Prog Cardiovasc Dis 27:335, 1985

42. The CONSENSUS Trial Study Group: Effects of enalapril on mortality in severe congestive heart failure: results of the Cooperative North Scandinavian Enalapril Survival Study (CONSENSUS). N Engl J Med 316:1429, 1987

43. McGill HC: The cardiovascular pathology of smoking. Am Heart J 115:250, 1988

44. Stubbe I, Eskilsson J, Nilsson-Ehle P: High-density lipoprotein concentrations increase after stopping smoking. Br Med J 294:1511, 1982

45. Freedman DS, Gruchow HW, Walker JA et al: Cigarette smoking and non-fatal myocardial infarction in women: Is the relation independent of coronary artery disease? Br Heart J 62:273, 1989

46. Vlietstra RE, Kronmal RA, Oberman A et al: Effect of cigarette smoking on survival of patients with angiographically documented coronary artery disease: Report from the CASS registry. JAMA 255:1023, 1986

47. Perkins J, Dick TB: Smoking and myocardial infarction: Secondary prevention. Postgrad Med J 61:295, 1985

48. Johansson S, Bergstrand R, Pennert K et al: Cessation of smoking after myocardial infarction in women. Effects on mortality and reinfarctions. Am J Epidemiol 121:823, 1985

49. Wilhelmsson C, Vedin JA, Elmfeldt D et al: Smoking and myocardial infarction. Lancet i:415, 1975

50. Salonen JT: Stopping smoking and long-term mortality after acute myocardial infarction. Br Heart J 43:463, 1980

51. Mulcahy R: Influence of cigarette smoking on morbidity and mortality after myocardial infarction. Br Heart J 49:410, 1983

52. Hallstrom AP, Cobb LA, Ray R: Smoking as a risk factor for recurrence of sudden cardiac arrest. N Engl J Med 314:271, 1986

53. McKenzie WB, McCredie RM, McGilchrist CA, Wilcken DE: Smoking: A major predictor of left ventricular function after occlusion of the left anterior descending coronary artery. Br Heart J 56:496, 1986

54. Galan KM, Deligonul U, Kern MJ et al: Increased frequency of restenosis in patients continuing to smoke cigarettes after percutaneous transluminal coronary angioplasty. Am J Cardiol 61:260, 1988

55. Daly LE, Graham IM, Hickey N, Mulcahy R: Does stopping smoking delay onset of angina after infarction? Br Med J 291:935, 1985

56. Hermanson B, Omenn GS, Kronmal RA, Gersh BJ, et al: Beneficial six-year outcome of smoking cessation in older men and women with coronary artery disease: Results from the CASS Group Study Registry. N Engl J Med 319:1365, 1988

57. Deanfield JE, Shea MJ, Wilson RA et al: Direct effects of smoking on the heart: Silent ischemic disturbances of coronary flow. Am J Cardiol 57:1005, 1986

58. Winniford MD, Jansen DE, Reynolds GA et al: Cigarette smoking-induced coronary vasoconstriction in atherosclerotic coronary artery disease and prevention by calcium antagonists and nitroglycerin. Am J Cardiol 59:203, 1987

59. Deanfield J, Wright C, Krikler S et al: Cigarette smoking and the treatment of angina with propranolol, atenolol, and nifedipine. N Engl J Med 310:951, 1984

60. Maouad J, Fernandez F, Hebert JL et al: Cigarette smoking during coronary angiography: Diffuse or focal narrowing (spasm) of the coronary arteries in 13 patients with angina at rest and normal coronary angiograms. Cathet Cardiovasc Diagn 12:366, 1986

61. Morris JN, Heady JA, Raffle PAB et al: Coronary heart disease and physical activity of work. Lancet ii:1053, 1953

62. Paffenbarger RS, Jr, Laughlin ME, Gima AS, Black RA: Work activity of longshoremen as related to death from coronary heart disease and stroke. N Engl J Med 282:1109, 1970

63. Morris JN, Everitt MG, Pollard R et al: Vigorous exercise in leisure-time: Protection against coronary heart disease. Lancet ii:1207, 1980

64. Paffenbarger RS, Jr, Hyde RT: Exercise in the prevention of coronary heart disease. Prev Med 13:3, 1984

65. Leon AS, Connett J, Jacobs DR Jr, Rauramaa R: Leisure-time physical activity levels and risk of coronary heart disease and death: The Multiple Risk Factor Intervention Trial. JAMA 258:2388, 1987

66. Blair SN, Kohl HW, Paffenbarger RS et al: Physical fitness and all-cause mortality: A prospective study of healthy men and women. JAMA 262:2395, 1989

67. Powell KE, Thompson PD, Caspersen CJ, Kendrick JS: Physical activity and the incidence of coronary heart disease. Annu Rev Public Health 8:253, 1987

68. Haslam RW, Cobb RB: Frequency of intensive, prolonged exercise as a determinant of relative coronary circumference index. Int J Sports Med 3:118, 1982

69. Wyatt HL, Mitchell J: Influences of physical conditioning and deconditioning on coronary vasculature of dogs. J Appl Physiol 45:619, 1978

70. Tomanek RJ: Effects of age and exercise on the extent of the myocardial capillary bed. Anat Rec 167:55, 1970

71. Jacobs, TB, Bell RD, McClements JD: Exercise, age and the development of the myocardial vasculature. Growth 48:148, 1984

72. Rakusan K, Wicher P: Morphometry of the small arteries and arterioles in the rat heart: Effects of chronic hypertension and exercise. Cardiovasc Res 24:278, 1990

73. Kramsch DM, Aspen AJ, Abramowitz BM et al: Reduction of coronary atherosclerosis by moderate conditioning exercise in monkeys on an atherogenic diet. N Engl J Med 305:1482, 1981

74. Tharp GD, Wagner CT: Chronic exercise and cardiac vascularization. Eur J Appl Physiol 48:97, 1982

75. Kayer SR, Conley KE, Claassen H, Hoppeler H: Capillarity and mitochondrial distribution in rat myocardium following exercise training. J Exp Biol 120:189, 1986

76. Cohen MV, Steingart RM: Lack of effect of prior training on subsequent ischaemic and infarcting myocardium and collateral development in dogs with normal hearts. Cardiovasc Res 21:269, 1987

77. Laughlin MH, Tomanek RJ: Myocardial capillarity and maximal capillary diffusion capacity in exercise-trained dogs. J Appl Physiol 63:1481, 1987

78. Heaton WH, Marr KC, Capurro NL et al: Beneficial effect of physical training on blood flow to myocardium perfused by chronic collaterals in the exercising dog. Circulation 57:575, 1978

79. Koerner JE, Terjung RL: Effect of physical training on coronary collateral circulation of the rat. J Appl Physiol 52:376, 1982

80. Cohen MV, Yipintsoi T, Scheuer J: Coronary collateral stimulation by exercise in dogs with stenotic coronary arteries. J Appl Physiol 52:664, 1982

81. Bloor CM, White FC, Sanders TM: Effects of exercise on collateral development in myocardial ischemia in pigs. J Appl Physiol 56:656, 1984

82. Przyklenk K, Groom AC: Effects of exercise frequency, intensity, and duration on revascularization in the transition zone of infarcted rat hearts. Can J Physiol Pharmacol 63:273, 1985

83. Schaper W: Influence of physical exercise on coronary collateral blood flow in chronic experimental two-vessel occlusion. Circulation 65:905, 1982

84. Blumenthal JA, Rejeski WJ, Walsh-Riddle M et al: Comparison of high- and low-intensity exercise training early after acute myocardial infarction. Am J Cardiol 61:26, 1988

85. Nolewajka AJ, Kostuk WJ, Rechnitzer PA, Cunningham DA: Exercise and human collateralization: An angiographic and scintigraphic assessment. Circulation 60:114, 1979

86. Panigrahi G, Pedersen A, Boudoulas H: Effect of physical training on exercise hemodynamics in patients with stable coronary artery disease. The use of impedance cardiography. J Med 14:363, 1983

87. Patterson DH, Shephard RJ, Cunningham D et al: Effects of physical training on cardiovascular function following myocardial infarction. J Appl Physiol 47:482, 1979

88. Ehsani AA: Mechanisms responsible for enhanced stroke volume after exercise training in coronary heart disease. Eur Heart J (Suppl G.)8:9, 1987

89. Martin WH, Ehsani AA: Reversal of exertional hypotension by prolonged exercise training in selected patients with ischemic heart disease. Circulation 76:548, 1987

90. Raffo JA, Luksic IY, Kappagoda CT et al: Effects of physical training on myocardial ischaemia in patients with coronary artery disease. Br Heart J 43:262, 1980

91. Rogers MA, Yamamoto C, Hagberg JM et al: The effect of 7 years of intense exercise training on patients with coronary artery disease. J Am Coll Cardiol 10:321, 1987

92. Nakai Y, Kataoka Y, Bando M et al: Effects of physical exercise training on cardiac function and graft patency after coronary artery bypass grafting. J Thorac Cardiovasc Surg 93:65, 1987

93. Squires RW, Gau GT, Miller TD et al: Cardiovascular rehabilitation: Status 1990. Mayo Clin Proc 65:731, 1990

94. Hoffmann A, Duba J, Lengyel M, Majer K: The effect of training on the physical working capacity of MI patients with left ventricular dysfunction. Eur Heart J (Suppl. G)8:43, 1987

95. Sullivan MJ, Higginbotham MB, Cobb FR: Exercise training in patients with severe left ventricular dysfunction. Hemodynamic and metabolic effects. Circulation 78:506, 1988

96. Giordano A, Giannuzzi P, Tavazzi L: Feasibility of physical training in post-infarct patients with left ventricular aneurysm: A haemodynamic study. Eur Heart J (Suppl. F)9:11, 1988

97. Shaw LW: Effects of a prescribed supervised ex-

ercise program on mortality and cardiovascular morbidity in patients after a myocardial infarction. Am J Cardiol 48:39, 1981

98. Kallio V, Hamalainen H, Hakkila J et al: Reduction in sudden deaths by a multifactorial intervention programme after acute myocardial infarction. Lancet ii:1081, 1979

99. Sanne H: Exercise tolerance in physical training of non-selected patients after myocardial infarction. Acta Med Scand, suppl. 551:103, 1973

100. Wilhelmsen L, Sanne H, Elmfeldt D et al: A controlled trial of physical training after myocardial infarction: Effects on risk factors, nonfatal reinfarction, and death. Prev Med 4:491, 1975

101. Kentala E: Physical fitness and feasibility of physical rehabilitation after myocardial infarction in men of working age. Ann Clin Res, suppl. 4:S9, 1972

102. Harpur JE, Conner WT, Hamilton M et al: A controlled trial of early mobilisation and discharge from hospital in uncomplicated myocardial infarction. Lancet ii:1331, 1971

103. Bloch A, Maeder J-P, Haissly J-C et al: Early mobilization after myocardial infarction: a controlled study. Am J Cardiol 34:152, 1974

104. Groden BM: The management of myocardial infarction: a controlled study of the effects of early mobilization. Card Rehabil 1:13, 1971

105. Oldridge NB, Guyatt GH, Fischer ME, Rimm AA: Cardiac rehabilitation after myocardial infarction. Combined experience of randomized clinical trials. JAMA 260:945, 1988

106. Shephard RJ: Exercise in the tertiary prevention of ischemic heart disease: Experimental proof. Can J Sport Sci 14:74, 1989

107. Thompson PD: The benefits and risks of exercise training in patients with chronic coronary artery disease. JAMA 259:1537, 1988

108. Van Camp SP, Peterson RA: Cardiovascular complications of outpatient cardiac rehabilitation programs. JAMA 256:1160, 1986

109. Friedman M, Rosenman RH: Association of specific overt behavior pattern with blood and cardiovascular findings: Blood cholesterol level, blood clotting time, incidence of arcus senilis and clinical coronary artery disease. JAMA 169:1286, 1959

110. Rosenman RH, Brand RJ, Jenkins CD et al: Coronary heart disease in the Western Collaborative Group Study. Final follow-up experience of 8½ years. JAMA 233:872, 1975

111. Jenkins CD, Zyzanski SJ, Rosenman RH: Risk of new myocardial infarction in middle-aged men with manifest coronary heart disease. Circulation 53:342, 1976

112. Ragland DR, Brand JB: Type A behavior and mortality from coronary heart disease. N Engl J Med 318:65, 1988

113. Barefoot JC, Peterson BL, Harrell FE Jr et al: Type A behavior and survival: a follow-up study of 1,467 patients with coronary artery disease. Am J Cardiol 64:1427, 1989

114. Case RB, Heller SS, Case NB, Moss AJ: Multicenter post-infarction research group. Type A behavior and survival after acute myocardial infarction. N Engl J Med 312:737, 1985

115. Shekelle RB, Gale M, Norusis M: Type A score (Jenkins Activity Survey) and risk of recurrent coronary heart disease in the Aspirin Myocardial Infarction Study. Am J Cardiol 56:221, 1985

116. Dimsdale JE, Gilbert J, Hutter AM Jr et al: Predicting cardiac morbidity based on risk factors and coronary angiographic findings. Am J Cardiol 47:73, 1981

117. Friedman M, Thoresen CE, Gill JJ et al: Alteration of type A behavior and its effect on cardiac recurrences in post myocardial infarction patients: Summary results of the Recurrent Coronary Prevention Project. Am Heart J 112:653, 1986

118. Review Panel on Coronary-Prone Behavior and Coronary Heart Disease: Coronary-prone behavior and coronary heart disease: A critical review. Circulation 63:1199, 1981

119. Gordon T, Castelli WP, Hjortland MC et al: Predicting coronary heart disease in middle-aged and older persons. JAMA 238:497, 1977

120. Harris T, Cook EF, Kannel WB, Goldman L: Proportional hazards analysis of risk factors for coronary heart disease in individuals aged 65 or older. The Framingham Heart Study. J Am Geriatr Soc 36:1023, 1988

121. Benfante R, Reed D: Is elevated serum cholesterol level a risk factor for coronary heart disease in the elderly? JAMA 263:393, 1990

122. National Institutes of Health: HMG CoA Reductase Inhibitors in the Elderly: Pilot Study. Primary prevention trial. RFA NIH 89-HL-060H. National Institutes of Health, Bethesda, Md, 1990

123. Bourassa MG, Enjalbert M, Campeau L, Lesperance J: Progression of atherosclerosis in coronary arteries and bypass grafts: ten years later. Am J Cardiol 53:102C, 1984

124. Myers MG, Benowitz NL, Dubbin JD et al: Cardiovascular effects of smoking in patients with ischemic heart disease. Chest 93:14, 1988

125. O'Callaghan WG, Teo KK, O'Riordan J et al: Comparative response of male and female patients with coronary artery disease to exercise rehabilitation. Eur Heart J 8:649, 1984

126. Bush TL, Barrett-Connor E, Cowan LD et al: Cardiovascular mortality and noncontraceptive use of estrogen in women: Results from the Lipid Research Clinics Program Follow-up Study. Circulation 75:1102, 1987

127. Sullivan JM, Vander Zwaag R, Hughes JP et al: Estrogen replacement and coronary artery disease. Effect on survival in postmenopausal women. Arch Intern Med, 150:2557, 1990

128. Council on Scientific Affairs, American Medical Association: Estrogen replacement in the menopause. JAMA 249:359, 1983

129. Young DT, Kottke TE, McCall MM, Blume D: A prospective controlled study of in-hospital myocardial infarction rehabilitation. J Cardiac Rehab 2:32, 1982

RISK FACTORS AND CORONARY ATHEROSCLEROTIC HEART DISEASE

5

Efficacy of Risk Factor Change

Richard A. Carleton, M.D.

The concept of risk factors for coronary atherosclerotic heart disease (CHD) derives from early observations of the Framingham Heart Study.[1] In that study, and many others, myriad factors have been analyzed at a time of baseline observation, serially, or in retrospect. People with various traits (e.g., race, initial age, blood pressure level) have been monitored over time to observe who develops coronary atherosclerosis and CHD. Over the years, many factors have been identified that bear statistical associations with the development of coronary disease. Some, such as age and gender, are considered unmodifiable. Family history is a complex interplay of unmodifiable and modifiable factors, with the former including genetic composition[2] and the latter including factors such as smoking, eating, and physical activity patterns, influenced strongly by familial behavioral patterns.

Most interest has focused on the risk factors judged to be modifiable. These have been identified and confirmed in many studies.[3] These risk factors for the production of CHD have also been analyzed to characterize individuals at high risk, meriting application of treatment algorithms.[4]

In more recent years, a different use of the term "risk factor" has emerged. People who already have symptomatic CHD have two other factors, which become their major predictors of further morbidity or mortality: the extent, location and severity of coronary atherosclerosis itself, and the degree of impairment of ventricular function. However, traditional risk factors continue as predictors, and risk modification can provide benefit.

In this chapter, the focus will be on the individual with symptomatic coronary atherosclerosis and on the efficacy of efforts to retard, reduce, or reverse atherosclerosis or to improve survivorship and quality of life by influencing the major modifiable risk factors for CHD.

MAJOR MODIFIABLE CHD RISK FACTORS

Over the past four decades, beginning with the observations of the Framingham Heart Study,[1] many factors have been shown to be associated with CHD. Among these are socioeconomic factors, with a higher incidence rate of CHD in the less educated, less affluent segments of our society. This has been particularly true in recent years as the decline in CHD mortality rate has occurred,[5] particularly in the higher socioeconomic strata. Race, partly because of the higher prevalence of high blood pressure in blacks, is also associated with CHD. Certain personality or behavioral traits, sometimes referred to as type A or coronary-prone behavior,[6] have been variably associated with CHD. Elevated fibrinogen levels, high uric acid levels, and a variety of disorders in amount and/or composition of apoproteins[7] have all been shown in epidemiologic research to be associated with CHD. Among the most important predictors of CHD is a reduced level of high density lipoprotein (HDL) cholesterol. This factor is subject to limited change by modification of individual behavior; smoking cessation and the adoption of regular physical activity can be expected to produce small increases in HDL cholesterol. Dietary factors are also of importance; losing excess weight usually results in increased HDL cholesterol level. Although alcohol ingestion may raise the HDL cholesterol level, this is not a desirable approach. The limited efficacy of these efforts to change the HDL cholesterol level, however, has led to recommendations that HDL cholesterol be listed as a risk factor if the level is below 35 mg/dL and not be the primary target of therapeutic efforts.[4]

There is general consensus that five major modifiable risk factors are high blood pressure, cigarette smoking, obesity, a habitually sedentary lifestyle, and an elevated blood cholesterol level. Each of these five risk factors is associated with a tendency for premature coronary disease and a higher mortality rate from CHD. Some also bear important relationships to other diseases. High blood pressure is a powerful predictor of stroke, congestive heart failure, and renal failure. Cigarette smoking bears a particularly strong relationship to sudden cardiac death as an outcome of coronary atherosclerotic disease, to lung cancer, and to chronic obstructive-destructive pulmonary disease. Obesity is closely related to the prevalence of high blood pressure, non-insulin dependent diabetes mellitus, and degenerative joint disease. Regular exercise is an important source of protection from disabling osteopenia and also appears to reduce the severity of high blood pressure. The high-fat dietary intake that commonly accompanies elevated blood cholesterol levels in populations appears likely to increase the prevalence of carcinoma, particularly of the breast and colon.

Each of these additional effects of the major modifiable risk factors constitutes further reasons for efforts to change these risk factors in people both before and after CHD is manifest.

Risk Factors and Load Factors

Certain of these modifiable risk factors assume another role when cardiac damage exists. This role is that of circulatory loads. Increased circulatory load may be deleterious when it increases myocardial oxygen demand or decreases myocardial oxygen supply in the presence of obstructive coronary artery disease. Alternatively, cardiac load factors may make it more difficult for a left ventricle impaired by ischemia or infarction to carry out its tasks.

The most obvious of these is high blood pressure. Left ventricular afterload, that combination of forces that impede sarcomere shortening, is directly related to left ventricular systolic pressure and, therefore, to systemic blood pressure.

Cigarette smoking, apart from its effects on the lungs, significantly impairs the oxygen-delivering capacity of blood by the creation of carboxyhemoglobin. In addition, cigarette smoking increases the general bodily metabolic rate,[8] whereas nicotine and other substances increase heart rate and blood pressure. Thus, cigarette smoking increases both bodily and myocardial oxygen demand, while decreasing the oxygen-delivering capacity of the blood.

Obesity is also an obvious load factor. Adipose tissue has a somewhat lower metabolic rate than many other tissues. However, the average metabolic cost of maintaining an overweight body is greater than that of nurturing a body at ideal body weight. The most obvious manifestation of obesity appears when one considers the energetics of transporting bodily mass on level ground or up any elevation. The increased foot-pounds of work performed must be fueled by oxygen and nutrients delivered by an impaired heart and coronary arterial system.

Exercise, when considered under the heading of load, has mixed attributes. Obviously, the act of performing exercise involves increased bodily work that must be met by oxygen-nutrient delivery by the heart and circulation, as well as increased heart rate, blood pressure, and sympathetic nervous system activation. Thus, in the short term, exercise itself constitutes increased circulatory load. It is in the longer term that regular exercise has a net effect of reducing circulatory load at any given level of submaximal activity. Exercise is an important part of the strategy of controlling obesity. Habitual exercise is well known to reduce the heart rate both at rest and during equivalent exercise at submaximal workloads. This effect appears to reflect decreased sympathetic nervous system activation after exercise training. As a corollary, blood pressure is reduced. Accordingly, the pressure–rate product, a predictor of myocardial oxygen demand, is lower at the same level of exercise in physically trained individuals than in their sedentary counterparts. A direct manifestation of load reduction by habitual physical activity, as described in Chapter 6, is the improved ability of patients with angina pectoris to exercise without symptoms.[9]

Of the five major modifiable risk factors, only an elevated blood cholesterol level cannot also be considered an immediate load factor. Each of the others not only augments the likelihood of developing or facilitating progression of CHD, but also has the ability to aggravate the clinical manifestations of that disease through their second identity as load factors.

RISK FACTOR CHANGE AFTER SYMPTOMATIC CHD IS PRESENT

It had been widely believed that risk factors for CHD had done their damage once symptomatic disease was evident and that risk factor modification was of relatively little avail. As will be described below, there are now substantial grounds for optimism that modification of risk factors in patients with symptomatic CHD can produce substantial benefit. Each of five major modifiable factors will be dealt with in sequence.

High Blood Pressure

As described above, substantial evidence implicates high blood pressure in the pathogenesis of atherosclerosis. Perhaps as importantly, many studies, reviewed well by Yusuf et al.,[10,11] have shown that reducing high blood pressure prevents stroke, premature death, and myocardial in-

farction. Most of these trials have shown a lesser effect on myocardial infarction than would have been predicted on the basis of long-term longitudinal epidemiologic follow-up of population cohorts. The reason for this is not clear but may include adverse effects from specific antihypertensive agents (e.g., on lipids or on electrolytes). However, the overall mortality benefit of reducing high blood pressure has been confirmed in these studies and appears to persist even beyond the time of the formal study phase itself.[12] This persistent benefit is believed to be likely to represent a smaller degree of damage to end organs such as the heart and kidney during the phase of active pharmacologic intervention.

The proved efficacy of treating high blood pressure in hypertensive populations has led to a gratifying fact. There have been no formal trials of treating or not treating high blood pressure in patients with symptomatic CHD. There are other obvious benefits beyond the clearly established effects of control of high blood pressure. High blood pressure, as described above, is a dominant factor in left ventricular overload. High blood pressure, as expressed in the pressure–rate product, also sharply increases myocardial oxygen demand at any given external bodily workload.

A factor that has inhibited some clinicians from treating high blood pressure aggressively in the presence of symptomatic CHD has been consideration of coronary hemodynamics. Coronary blood flow occurs predominantly during ventricular diastole, when systolic wall tension compressing intramyocardial coronary arteries is low. A major factor contributing to coronary blood flow is, therefore, the intra-aortic pressure as it declines from the moment of aortic valve closure to the end of diastole. Although it is clear, from a hydraulic view, that flow across a coronary stenosis will be reduced if the driving pressure in the aorta is excessively low, this has not proved to be of clinical importance and should not serve as an impediment to treating high blood pressure. It should be remembered that the "diastolic pressure" determined by sphygmomanometry simply reflects the aortic end-diastolic pressure and not the pressure driving coronary flow throughout diastole. End-diastolic pressures in the normal physiologic range have never been shown to be a clinically important source of inadequate coronary flow.

Although there have been no formal randomized trials of treatment of hypertensive patients with symptomatic CHD, two categories of clinical trials have direct relevance.

The effect of beta-adrenergic blocking agents in patients with angina pectoris has been studied; they have been shown to have a directly beneficial effect. They lessen the frequency of angina pectoris at equivalent workloads and improve effort tolerance at the anginal threshold. This improvement reflects several actions of the beta-receptor blocking drugs. The heart rate is lower at rest and at any given workload. Myocardial contractility, and thereby oxygen demand, is reduced. Blood pressure is reduced. The beta-blocking agents are not pure antihypertensive drugs, so it is not feasible to dissect out the exact contribution from blood pressure reduction, but it is undoubtedly of some importance.

A second major application of beta-adrenergic blocking drug therapy has been its use after myocardial infarction. The data are overwhelmingly clear. Administration of beta-blocking drugs reduces sudden cardiac death, other forms of cardiac death, and nonfatal reinfarction. According to Yusuf et al.[10] over 27 trials, involving over 27,000 people, have been conducted to study the effect of intravenous beta-blocking agents after acute myocardial infarction. In these trials, highly significant reductions in total mortality and in recurrent myocardial infarction have been found.[13,14] The utilization of beta-blocking drugs for more protracted periods after myocardial infarction has been tested in 25 random-allocation trials involving over 23,000 patients, usually excluding patients in Killip classes 3 or 4. The death rate in treated patients was 7.6% and in control patients 9.4%; this represents an estimated 22% reduction in the risk of death, a highly significant figure. These reductions in mortality rates occur both within the first 7 days after myocardial infarction and in the subsequent months and years. Again, these trials, studying chronic effects, demonstrate benefit, particularly on sudden cardiac death but also on recurrent infarction and other forms of cardiac death. One can properly ask whether the effectiveness of beta-blocking drugs

reflects in any sense its effects on blood pressure. The answer is not available. Any or all of the major effects of beta-blocking drugs may play a role. Some data suggest that the combination of effects on heart rate, blood pressure, and myocardial contractility is associated with reduced infarct size when the drugs are administered very soon after acute myocardial infarction. Other benefits may relate to an antiarrhythmic influence of beta-blocking drugs. Although the role of blood pressure change is not known, it is likely that part of the effect is attributable to lowering the blood pressure in patients with symptomatic CHD.

A second type of clinical trial also relates to the theme of blood pressure modification in patients with symptomatic CHD. Again, these trials have not primarily targeted patients with high blood pressure, but they have had an effect on blood pressure. These have been trials of vasodilator or antihypertensive agents used to reduce left ventricular afterload in patients with congestive heart failure. Many of these patients have CHD. Others have had other causes of congestive heart failure. An important clinical trial centered at the University of Minnesota compared the effects of prazosin hydrochloride, isosorbide dinitrate plus hydralazine, and placebo in three groups made up of over 600 patients with congestive heart failure. Patients were monitored for approximately 2 years. The combination of isosorbide dinitrate and hydralazine was associated with a 12% reduction in mortality. One can postulate that this reflected a combined effect on left ventricular preload and left ventricular afterload, with the latter being mediated, in part, through a reduction in blood pressure. The group that received prazosin, an alpha-adrenergic blocking drug, showed no significant difference from the placebo group.[15]

More recently, angiotensin-converting enzyme (ACE) inhibitors, a class of powerful antihypertensive agents, have been studied to ascertain their efficacy in patients with congestive heart failure. Several of these important studies are continuing, but others have yielded promising results. The CONSENSUS Trial[16] studied over 200 patients with New York Heart Association Class IV congestive heart failure. The patients received enalapril or placebo with an average of 6 months of follow-up. A highly significant reduction in mortality attributable to the enalapril administration was found. Combined data for these trials suggest an approximately 33% reduction in mortality when ACE inhibitors are administered to patients with congestive heart failure.[11] Other similar trials are currently in progress.

As described above, the treatment of high blood pressure is so clearly beneficial that administration of placebo to hypertensive patients with symptomatic CHD is not ethically acceptable. Whether reduction of high blood pressure slows progression of coronary atherosclerosis or induces regression in humans may never be known. It is clear, however, that administration of drugs that reduce blood pressure, among other effects, benefits patients with angina pectoris, prior myocardial infarction, or the congestive heart failure that is so often a sequel of CHD.

Cigarette Smoking

The adverse health effects of cigarette smoking are so numerous and so well documented that it would be astonishing if the benefits of smoking cessation did not extend to patients with symptomatic CHD.

Epidemiologic observations have clearly incriminated cigarette smoking in the pathogenesis of atherosclerosis in the coronary and many other arteries. Cessation of cigarette smoking has been shown to reduce the rates of incidence of myocardial infarction and of death as soon as 1 year after cessation, with benefit continuing through 10 years, after which the death rate approximates that of those who have never been cigarette smokers. Some of the acute deleterious effects of cigarette smoking in patients with CHD have been described above. The chronic effects on the heart, lungs, and other organs are likely to be no less severe in patients with symptomatic CHD than in other people. For these reasons, there can never be a random allocation clinical trial to assess the effects of smoking cessation.

In its place, however, a compelling observational trial has been reported. The Coronary Artery Surgery Study (CASS) registered over 14,000 patients with angiographically proved CHD. The patients in the study included 4,886 people who were smoking at the time of registration, 6,719 former smokers, and 2,912 individuals who reported that they never had been smokers. Among these patients, Vlietstra et al.[17] defined two contrasting subgroups. The first included patients who were smoking at the time of entry into the CASS registry and who reported at each annual follow-up that they continued to smoke. The other group was composed of patients who had been smokers until the year before registration in the study, who had quit, and who reported at each annual follow-up that they were still not smoking. These two subgroups constituted 2,675 individuals who continued to smoke and 1,490 individuals who had quit smoking. Since this was not a random-allocation trial, differences between the groups at follow-up should be anticipated. In fact, it appears likely that those who quit smoking often did so because they were more ill. The quitters, indeed, had a small, but significantly higher average congestive heart failure score, left ventricular wall motion abnormality score, number of coronary artery segments with 50% or more stenosis, prevalence of prior coronary bypass surgery, average left ventricular end-diastolic pressure, and mean age. Each of these factors was associated adversely with survival, placing the group that quit smoking at higher risk than the group who continued smoking. Despite these differences, substantial benefits were associated with smoking cessation. Overall survival was highly significantly affected. The 5-year mortality rate was 20.5% among those who continued smoking and only 15.7% among those who had quit smoking. This represents approximately a 24% reduction in total mortality rate associated with smoking cessation. This difference is particularly notable given the higher values of important predictors of mortality for those who had quit smoking. Subdividing the causes of mortality, a significant reduction in cardiac mortality was seen and the mortality rate from myocardial infarction was nearly halved. Sudden cardiac death also declined significantly.

In a separate analysis, Hermanson et al.[18] studied 1,893 older men and women from the CASS registry. Each was 55 years of age or older and had angiographically documented CHD. Of these older people, 1,086 continued to smoke throughout 6 years of follow-up. Their outcome was compared with that of 807 individuals who quit smoking during the year before study enrollment and who did not smoke during the time of the study. As in the overall group, both the mortality rate and the rate of myocardial infarction were significantly reduced in those who stopped smoking. When death or myocardial infarction were combined as outcomes, a highly significant reduction in relative risk was found among those who quit smoking in individual age groups of 55 to 59 years, 60 to 64 years, 65 to 69 years, and 70 years and above. Advanced age is not an excuse to continue to smoke.

The data on the effects of smoking are incontrovertible. Smoking cessation is critical in all patients with symptomatic CHD (as well as in patients with asymptomatic CHD and documented silent ischemia). Lessened angina pectoris, fewer myocardial infarctions, and longer survival can all be anticipated. A variety of approaches is available. The role of health professionals in fostering cigarette smoking cessation is central.[19]

Obesity

As has been addressed above, obesity is widely considered a major modifiable risk factor. In addition, it is an important load factor. There is an important distinction associated with the different distributions of excess adipose tissue. Central-torso obesity is particularly related to a higher incidence of CHD.[20] This relationship probably reflects intrinsic genetic-metabolic factors that influence both adipose tissue distribution and propensity to atherosclerosis. It should be remembered that part, but probably not all, of the negative impact of obesity on coronary atherosclerosis derives from associated abnormalities. The obese have a higher prevalence of high blood pressure, a greater likelihood of elevated total blood cholesterol and low density lipoprotein (LDL) cholesterol levels, a high frequency of non-insulin dependent diabetes mellitus, and a relatively sedentary lifestyle. From this, it follows that control of obesity is an important adjunct in the management of high blood pressure,

of hypercholesterolemia, and of non-insulin dependent diabetes mellitus. An important strategy for control of obesity is to increase regular physical activity. Another is to reduce consumption of food energy (calories), particularly by reducing consumption of fat and saturated fatty acids, the most calorie-dense nutrient at 9 cal/g.

Perhaps it is simple logic that indicates that control of obesity is important in reducing the likelihood of atherosclerosis and of limiting the disabling impact of atherosclerosis. Perhaps it is the intrinsic difficulty of envisioning a clinical trial in which obesity alone is successfully controlled in one group and not in another. Perhaps it is the near impossibility of controlling obesity in an intervention group without influencing other important cardiovascular risk factors. For whatever reason, there has been no controlled clinical trial to study obesity in coronary patients. On the basis of all the available information, however, it is appropriate to recommend that all patients with CHD reach and maintain a desirable body weight and body fitness. The most widely used definition of desirable body weight is that set forth in the Metropolitan Relative Weight Tables.

Sedentary Lifestyle

Regular exercise has many benefits and some risks. The risks are predominantly orthopedic. There does appear to be a greater likelihood of sudden cardiac death during exercise, but when this risk is taken in the context of the reduced likelihood that individuals performing habitual exercise will develop symptomatic CHD, this risk becomes exceedingly small.[21] Habitual exercise favorably influences other cardiovascular risk factors including total blood cholesterol, HDL cholesterol, blood pressure, and, of course, body weight and fatness.

The physiologic effects of exercise training are considered elsewhere in this text (see Chs. 6 and 20). There are many, and they can reasonably be expected to favorably influence myocardial oxygen demand during submaximal exercise.

A number of randomized trials have assessed the effect of exercise on survival following myocardial infarction. Two of these trials were confounded because other interventions were also included (e.g., smoking cessation advice). When the results were pooled in a meta-analysis of about 4,300 patients,[11] there was a 9% death rate among the patients allocated to the exercise group, contrasting with a 15% death rate among those allocated to the control group, a statistically significant difference. Indeed, the order of magnitude of reduction in mortality compares favorably with that found with the administration of beta-blocking drugs following myocardial infarction.

In contrast, these nine trials of exercise following myocardial infarction did not demonstrate a significant change in the frequency of recurrent myocardial infarction. These trials did not investigate the frequency or intensity of angina pectoris. Many other studies have, however, demonstrated clear benefit on effort tolerance, frequency of angina pectoris, need for antianginal medication, and general perceived quality of life.[22]

On the basis of these data, it is clear that it is appropriate to recommend regular prescribed physical exercise (see Ch. 20) to patients with symptomatic CHD. Improvements in self-confidence, performance, and survival are realistic expectations.

Elevated Blood Cholesterol Levels

The enormous body of evidence relating dietary factors, blood cholesterol, and coronary atherosclerosis has been reviewed in detail.[23,24] It is clear that an elevated blood cholesterol level is a major risk factor for CHD. It is equally clear that, although genetic factors are important, modifiable dietary factors powerfully influence the blood cholesterol level.

Data supporting these conclusions concerning the potential for elevated blood cholesterol, particularly the LDL cholesterol component, to induce accelerated atherosclerosis come from many sources. These include extensive epidemiologic research, biochemical and genetic research, multispecies animal studies, metabolic ward research in humans, and clinical trials involving dietary

and/or pharmacologic intervention. This wealth of data has led to recommendations in the United States and other countries[23,25] that eating patterns be modified. Specific recommendations for the United States[23] have included a primary focus on saturated fatty acids, with the strong recommendation that all individuals above the age of 2 years derive an average of fewer than 10% of their daily calories from saturated fatty acids. Total fat intake has a less clear relationship to CHD than does saturated fatty acid intake. Despite this, it has been recommended that an average of 30% or less of calories be derived from total fat intake. There are several reasons for this, including facilitation of attaining the saturated fatty acid recommendation, greater ease of attaining and maintaining ideal body weight by limiting calorie-dense fat, and the probability of reducing the incidence of certain forms of cancer. Additionally, a recommendation to limit total fat intake may inhibit potentially harmful excesses (e.g., 20% of calories) from polyunsaturated fatty acids. The third nutrient recommendation concerns total energy intake; it is recommended that all U.S. adults reach and maintain a desirable body weight through a balance of energy intake (kilocalories) and expenditure involving a program of regular exercise. Lastly, dietary cholesterol is a targeted nutrient. Dietary cholesterol, in the overwhelming majority of studies, is a factor that elevates total blood cholesterol and LDL cholesterol. The effect is less dramatic than that of saturated fatty acids, but it is real and of importance. The recommendation is that all U.S. adults consume, on average, less than 300 mg of cholesterol daily.

A number of specific recommendations[23] concern eating patterns to facilitate attainment of these nutrient intakes. All U.S. adults are encouraged to eat a greater quantity and variety of fruits, vegetables, breads, cereals, and legumes such as bean and peas. These particularly provide the complex carbohydrates that are suitable and appropriate substitutes for saturated fatty acids and other forms of fat. All are encouraged to eat more low-fat high-calcium dairy products such as skim or low-fat milk or milk products in lieu of butterfat-rich products. Moderate amounts (up to 6 oz/day cooked) of trimmed, lean red meat, poultry without skin, or fish are recommended in place of foods high in saturated fatty acids. Egg yolks should be eaten only in moderation, but egg whites, which do not contain cholesterol, can be eaten often. The use of oils, margarines, and shortenings containing primarily unsaturated fatty acids rather than saturated fatty acids is recommended. The use of plant oils containing high proportions of saturated fatty acids, such as palm oil, palm kernel oil, and coconut oil, should be minimized. When choosing baked goods, it is recommended that those made with unsaturated vegetable oils and, at most, small amounts of egg yolk be selected. "Convenience foods" are commonplace in U.S. society, and it is recommended that all persons be guided by low saturated fatty acid, total fat, and cholesterol content in selecting such foods from the grocery shelf. Food labels contain valuable information, and it is recommended that food labels be read and used to guide choices of foods with smaller amounts or lower proportions of saturated fatty acids and/or total fat. It is recommended that, when preparing foods, the use of fats be kept to a minimum and low-fat alternatives be used as available. When eating out in restaurants and fast food outlets, information concerning saturated fatty acid, total fat, and cholesterol content should be requested from waiters and proprietors and foods low in these nutrients be selected in preference to foods high in these nutrients. Broadly, the recommendation to the United States is attainment of a habitual pattern of eating that is low in saturated fatty acids, total fat, and cholesterol. No single food or supplement serves as a "magic bullet." Specifically, fish oil supplementation or Omega-3 fatty acids are not effective means of reducing LDL cholesterol. Soluble dietary fiber may serve as an adjuvant, but does not alone suffice to adequately reduce blood cholesterol levels. Alcohol, in part because of its many negative health consequences, is not recommended as a means of dealing with elevated blood cholesterol levels.

Adoption of these recommendations to the U.S. population is to be facilitated by implementation of recommendations targeting other segments of society. Health professionals must both practice and advocate the recommended eating patterns. They should ensure that blood cholesterol is measured in their patients, that the result is prop-erly interpreted, and that appropriate counseling concerning diet is given. Health professionals should help ensure that future health professionals receive appropriate nutritional education. In addition, health professionals must work with industry, government, and health care agencies to encourage health-promoting nutrition. The food industry, including food scientists, must continue development of products low in the target constituent and also must assume an active role in professional and consumer education concerning the recommended eating patterns. The food industry should also provide clear information on food labels concerning cholesterol-elevating saturated fatty acid, total fat, cholesterol, and caloric intake to facilitate informed choices by consumers. Furthermore, the food industry must avoid misleading labeling or advertising such as "no cholesterol" on foods high in saturated fatty acids or for foods that never contain cholesterol or fats.

Government has important roles in influencing cardiovascular health. The Food and Drug Administration has the authority to require more detailed and precise food labeling in an informative, comprehensible format. Perhaps most importantly, the government has an opportunity, through the U.S. Department of Agriculture, the U.S. Department of Health and Human Services, and other agencies, to provide consistent, coordinated nutrition statements and policies emphasizing attainment of the recommended eating patterns.

Other recommendations concern the educational systems of our nation. Elementary through high school classes should incorporate curricula that promote recommended eating patterns. This is particularly important in vocational schools and culinary art schools that relate to food production, distribution, and preparation. Equally important are the agricultural and other food science schools so that the personnel of the food industry of the future understand health-promotive human nutrition. Other recommendations from the Population Panel concern an active role of mass media in disseminating appropriate information concerning recommended eating patterns; establishment of standards and recommendations concerning measurement of and counseling about blood cholesterol levels; and, finally, the need for ongoing research and surveillance of their impact on CHD, national blood cholesterol profile, and national food consumption patterns.

These recommendations clearly target the entire U.S. population with a particular focus on those who are ostensibly well, many of whom have asymptomatic coronary and other atherosclerotic vascular disease. One may hope that these recommendations will, in the future, reduce the societal burden of CHD and other atherosclerotic vascular diseases. At the same time, however, myriad individuals in the United States have symptomatic CHD; in most of them, an elevated blood cholesterol has played an important role. The question is—has the die been cast for these individuals? Or can existing atherosclerosis be influenced?

The remainder of this chapter will focus on the growing data base that gives hope that atherosclerosis may be reversible in humans. This hope is currently sufficiently well-developed to make control of LDL cholesterol levels an important priority in any patient with symptomatic CHD.

It has been known for many years that alteration of dietary lipids, particularly cholesterol, can induce atherosclerosis in many animal species. Perhaps more importantly, it has been shown that removal of dietary cholesterol can bring about regression of induced atherosclerotic lesions in several species.[26]

More recently, several studies have cast light on the same issue in humans. Brensike et al.[27] reported a small trial in which hyperlipidemic men with angiographically proved coronary lesions were randomly assigned to receive the bile sequestrant cholestyramine or placebo. Followup angiograms demonstrated marginally significant slowing of progression and a suggestion, in a small number of patients, that some coronary arterial lesions may have undergone slight regression. This work has been extended by Blankenhorn et al.[28] in a study of atherosclerosis both in native vessels and in saphenous vein bypass grafts in middle-aged men who had undergone previous coronary bypass surgery. Coronary angiograms were performed 2 years apart. Men were randomly assigned to colestipol plus niacin plus rigorous dietary intervention or to placebo

plus modest dietary intervention. The initial blood cholesterol levels ranged from 180 to 350 mg/dL. The results were equally striking for those with cholesterol levels below 240 mg/dL and those with levels above this value. After 2 years, the treatment group had significantly fewer new atherosclerotic lesions, significantly less lesion progression, and significantly less evidence of atherosclerosis in their coronary bypass vein grafts. Perhaps most remarkably, 16% of lesions in the treatment group, as assessed by blinded cinangiographic interpreters, showed mild but definite regression during the 2 years between angiograms.

Of the 188 men, 103 elected to remain in their treatment group for an additional 2 years after the initial report. These later data have subsequently been presented by Cashin-Hemphill et al.[29] After 4 years of treatment or placebo, the colestipol-plus-niacin group continued to have a significant reduction in progression of lesions both in their native coronary arteries and in their bypass grafts. More patients in the placebo group (40.4%) had new lesions than did those receiving colestipol and niacin (12.5%). Once again, regression was detected at significantly different rates in the two groups, with 17.9% of the treated group but only 6.4% of the placebo group demonstrating lesion regression.

A somewhat similar trial has been the subject of a report by Brown et al.[30] In this trial, men under the age of 62 with angiographically demonstrated CHD were counseled concerning their diet and then were assigned randomly to one of three groups: niacin plus colestipol, lovastatin plus colestipol, or "conventional therapy" consisting of placebo with or without colestipol. An average of 2.5 years elapsed between successive coronary angiograms. The conventional therapy group had a 9% reduction in LDL cholesterol and showed a 1.7% average increase in the degree of stenosis. Sixteen patients showed progression, and four demonstrated regression. The lovastatin-plus-colestipol group had a 48% reduction in LDL cholesterol level, a 14% increase in HDL cholesterol level, significantly fewer cardiovascular events than the conventional therapy group, and a mean decrease of 0.3% in the average percent lesion stenosis. Ten patients showed progression, and 13 showed regression. The best results appear to have occurred with the niacin-plus-colestipol group. In this group, the LDL cholesterol level declined by 34% while the HDL cholesterol level increased by 41%. A single cardiovascular event occurred, a highly significant difference from the conventional therapy group. The mean percent decrease in lesion stenosis was 0.9%. Only 9 patients showed lesion progression, whereas 15 showed lesion regression. Brown et al. concluded that coronary lesions and clinical course changes are mediated both by changes in LDL and in HDL cholesterol levels. Buchwald and colleagues,[31] using ileal bypass to control hypercholesterolemia, have also recently reported lesion regression in some patients.

These four studies demonstrate that the natural history of atherosclerotic coronary lesions can be modified. Furthermore, these studies provide substantial grounds for enthusiasm that atherosclerotic lesions can undergo regression in humans, especially if interventions are begun early. The optimal therapy to produce regression is unclear and will remain the subject of ongoing study, but early insights are apparent.

A number of additional studies involving angiographic documentation of lesion progression and/or regression are in progress. These include the ileal bypass surgery study by Buchwald et al.[31] and other pharmacologic studies designed to influence circulating lipid levels.

Other exciting work holds initial promise concerning the management of atherosclerotic lesions. Although not directly related to lifestyle modification of traditional cardiovascular risk factors, the common theme of directly altering atherosclerotic lesions is compelling. Calcium has been implicated in the atherosclerotic process for many years. Initially, extracellular calcium and calcium salts have been clear participants in the sclerotic process itself. More recently, many lines of investigation have suggested a role for intracellular calcium, particularly in the migration and modification of smooth muscle cells in the atherosclerotic process. Experimental studies with calcium antagonists in animals have suggested the potential of beneficial effects on atherosclerotic lesions. Recently, Lichtlen et al.[32] presented a preliminary report of a trial of nifedipine compared with placebo in patients with coronary artery lesions. Follow-up angiograms were done after an average interval of 3 years of therapy. Compliance was adequate. Of 148 patients receiving placebo, 73 developed 118 new atherosclerotic lesions, each producing greater than 20% coronary arterial stenosis. This was contrasted with the 134 patients receiving nifedipine, 55 of whom developed 79 new lesions, a significantly smaller number. In this preliminary report, no difference was seen in progression of existing lesions. One can currently postulate that nifedipine interferes with smooth muscle cell reactivity in the initiation of the atherosclerotic process, but plays little, if any, role in progression (or regression) of the disease.

Taken together, these studies provide significant optimism that clinical medicine will soon have within its power the management of atherosclerotic lesions, not simply the management of their sequelae. At present, it is clear that an appropriate recommendation is substantial reduction of LDL cholesterol, although to what level remains unclear. Studies currently in progress, funded by the National Institutes of Health, should provide guidance on this important question in the years to come.

In the meantime, the most widely supported set of recommendations for modification of circulating lipids in patients with symptomatic CHD are those presented by the Adult Treatment Panel of the National Cholesterol Education Program.[4] In these recommendations, for symptomatic individuals, aggressive therapeutic efforts to reduce the LDL cholesterol level below 130 mg/dL are forcefully presented. The first line of therapy is careful nutritional counseling, using the step 1 diet with less than 30% of calories from fat, less than 10% of calories from saturated fatty acids, and less than 300 mg of cholesterol daily. If the target LDL level is not achieved with careful nutritional counseling at this level, the step 2 diet, reducing saturated fatty acid calories to less than 7% and cholesterol to less than 200 mg per day should be vigorously pursued. If this is ineffective, supplemental pharmacologic therapy is appropriate. Therapies that are currently available and for which there are clear disease outcome data to support their utilization include cholestyramine, colestipol, niacin, gemfibrozil, and lovastatin. For patients with an HDL cholesterol level that itself constitutes a risk factor (less than 35 mg/dL), the use of niacin or gemfibrozil has a particular rationale, particularly if associated with an elevated blood triglyceride level. Combinations, as in the studies of Blankenhorn et al.[28] and Brown et al.[30] are rational if first-line single medication approaches do not work.

SUMMARY

The major modifiable cardiovascular risk factors have traditionally been believed to be of importance before the onset of symptomatic CHD. This review points out the burgeoning body of evidence indicating that five major modifiable risk factors are equally important targets of intervention after the onset of symptomatic CHD. Several are not only risk factors but also circulatory load factors, compounding the urgency for their management. There is substantial evidence indicating the importance of controlling high blood pressure in patients with angina or in patients who have experienced myocardial infarction. Cigarette smoking cessation is mandatory; accomplishment of that difficult task will significantly improve survivorship. Control of obesity facilitates the control of high blood pressure and high blood cholesterol. It also lessens the likelihood of or difficulty of control of non-insulin–dependent diabetes mellitus. Perhaps most importantly, having a desirable body weight facilitates moving the body around. Habitual exercise, similarly, favorably influences other modifiable risk factors while providing both health and life quality benefits of its own. Recent data have provided particular excitement about the prospects that the atherosclerotic lesion itself can be manipulated through aggressive modification of circulating lipid levels.

In all, risk factor modification no longer can be considered a closed chapter once symptoms of CHD begin. Symptomatic CHD simply opens a new chapter requiring aggressive management of each of the major modifiable coronary atherosclerotic risk factors.

REFERENCES

1. Kannel WB, Dawber TR, Kagan A, et al: Factors of risk in the development of coronary heart disease—six-year follow-up experience: The Framingham Study. Ann Intern Med 55:33, 1961
2. Brown NS, Goldstein JL: A receptor-mediated pathway for cholesterol homeostasis. Science 232:34, 1986
3. Pooling Project Research Group: Relationship of blood pressure, serum cholesterol, smoking habit, relative weight and ECG abnormalities to incidence of major coronary events: Final report of the Pooling Project. J Chron Dis 31:201, 1978
4. National Cholesterol Education Program: Report of the Expert Panel on Detection, Evaluation, and Treatment of High Blood Cholesterol in Adults. Bethesda, MD. U.S. Department of Health and Human Services, Public Health Service, National Institutes of Health, National Heart, Lung, and Blood Institute, NIH Pub. No. 88-2925, January, 1988
5. Goldman L, Cook EF: Reasons of the decline in coronary heart disease mortality: Medical interventions versus life-style changes. p. 67. In Higgins MW, Luepker RV (eds): Trends in Coronary Heart Disease Mortality. Oxford University Press, New York, 1988
6. Friedman M, Ulmer D: Coronary Prone Behavior: Treating type A behavior and your heart. Knopf-Random House, New York, 1985
7. Havel RJ: Origin, metabolic fate, and metabolic function of plasma lipoproteins. p. 117. In Steinberg D, Olefsky JM (eds): Hypercholesterolemia and atherosclerosis: Pathogenesis and prevention. Churchill Livingstone, New York, 1986
8. Perkins KA, Epstein LH, Marks BL et al: The effect of nicotine on energy expenditure during light physical activity. N Engl J Med 320:898, 1989
9. Borer JS, Brensike JF, Redwood DR et al: Limitations of the electrocardiographic response to exercise in predicting coronary-artery disease. N Engl J Med 293:367, 1975
10. Yusuf S, Wittes J, Friedman L: Overview of results of randomized clinical trials in heart disease: I. Treatments following myocardial infarction. JAMA 260:2088, 1988

11. Yusuf S, Wittes J, Friedman L: Overview of results of randomized clinical trials in heart disease: II. Unstable angina, heart failure, primary prevention with aspirin, and risk factor modification. JAMA 260:2259, 1988

12. Hypertension detection and follow-up program cooperative group: Persistence of reduction in blood pressure and mortality of participants in the hypertension detection and follow-up program. JAMA 259:2113, 1988

13. The MIAMI Trial Research Group: Metoprolol in acute myocardial infarction (MIAMI): A randomized placebo-controlled international trial. Eur Heart J 6:199, 1985

14. ISIS-1 Collaborative Group: Mechanisms for the early mortality reduction produced by beta-blockade started early in acute myocardial infarction. Lancet i:921, 1988

15. Cohn JN, Archibald DG, Ziesche S, et al: Effect of vasodilator therapy on mortality in chronic congestive heart failure. N Engl J Med 314:1547, 1986

16. The CONSENSUS Trial Study Group: Effects of enalapril on mortality in severe congestive heart failure. Results of the Cooperative North Scandinavian Enalapril Survival Study (CONSENSUS). N Engl J Med 316:1429, 1987

17. Vlietstra RE, Kronmal RA, Oberman A, et al: Effect of cigarette smoking on survival of patients with angiographically documented coronary artery disease: Report from the CASS registry. JAMA 255:1023, 1986

18. Hermanson B, Omenn GS, Kronmal RA, et al. Beneficial six-year outcome of smoking cessation in older men and women with coronary artery disease. Results from CASS Registry. N Engl J Med 319:1365, 1988

19. Ockene JK: Physician-delivered interventions for smoking cessation: Strategies for increasing effectiveness. Preven Med 16:723, 1987

20. Higgins ML, Kannel WB, Garrison RJ et al. Hazards of obesity: The Framingham experience. Acta Medica Scand 723:23, 1987

21. Thompson PD, Funk EJ, Carleton RA, Sturner WQ: Incidence of death during jogging in Rhode Island from 1975–1980. JAMA 247:2535, 1982

22. Haskell WL: Mechanisms by which physical activity may enhance the clinical status of cardiac patients. p. 276. In Pollock ML, Schmidt DH (eds): Heart Disease and Rehabilitation. John Wiley & Sons, New York, 1979

23. National Cholesterol Education Program: Report of the Population Panel. U.S. Department of Health and Human Services, Public Health Service, National Institutes of Health, National Heart, Lung, and Blood Institute, NIH Pub. No. 90-3046, November, 1990

24. National Research Council. Diet and Health: Implications for Reducing Chronic Disease Risk. National Academy Press, Washington, DC, 1989

25. Gyarfas I, Stanley K: Diet and chronic diseases: A global perspective. World Health Organization. In press

26. Fincham JE, Woodroof CW, vanWyk MJ et al. Promotion and regression of atherosclerosis in Vervet monkeys by diets realistic for westernized people. Atherosclerosis 66:205, 1987

27. Brensike JF, Levy RI, Kelsey SF et al: Effects of therapy with cholestyramine on progression of coronary arteriosclerosis: Results of the NHLBI Type II Coronary Intervention Study. Circulation 69:313, 1984

28. Blankenhorn DH, Nessim SA, Johnson RL et al: Beneficial effects of combined colestipol-niacin therapy on coronary atherosclerosis and coronary venous bypass grafts. JAMA 257:3233, 1987

29. Cashin-Hemphill L, Sanmarco ME, Blankenhorn DH et al: Augmented beneficial effects of colestipol-niacin therapy at four years in the CLAS Trial. Circulation (Suppl. II) 80:II-381, 1989

30. Brown G, Albers JJ, Fisher LD et al: Regression of coronary artery disease as a result of intensive lipid-lowering therapy in men with high levels of apolipoprotein B. N Engl J Med 323:1289, 1990

31. Buchwald H, Varco RL, Matts JP et al: Effect of partial ileal bypass surgery on mortality and morbidity from coronary heart disease in patients with hypercholesterolemia: Report of the program on the surgical control of the hyperlipidemias (POSCH). N Engl J Med 323:946, 1990

32. Lichtlen PR, Hugenholtz P, Rafflenbeul W et al: Retardation of the progression of coronary artery disease with nifedipine: Results of INTACT. Circulation (Suppl. II)80:II-382, 1989

II

Physiology of Exercise and Exercise Testing

6

Physiology of Exercise in Normal Individuals and Patients with Coronary Heart Disease

Gary J. Balady, M.D.
Donald A. Weiner, M.D.

The body's physiologic response to exercise involves a complex series of events that occur in concert to provide energy to working muscles while maintaining optimal conditions in organ beds not directly involved with the exercise itself. Nearly all organ systems, from the cardiovascular and neurologic to the integument, are involved in this process. Reactions that occur at the molecular level trigger a cascade of actions and interactions among organ systems to allow muscular work to be performed. How these systems respond depends on the type of exercise being performed—specifically, the muscle groups involved, the body position, and whether the work being done is predominantly static or dynamic. Furthermore, these physiologic events may vary with the age, sex, and general health conditions of the individual.

Various parameters are currently measured in the assessment of these responses at both the molecular and systemic levels. Such measurement is important in many areas, including the clinical evaluation of an individual to ensure that systems are operating normally, the assessment of the body's response to an altered condition (e.g., change in ambient environment, effect of a med-ication, impairment of an organ system by disease), and further elucidation of the numerous responses during exercise that remain poorly understood or undefined. Of particular interest are measurements that can be made easily and noninvasively. Since respiratory gas exchange measurements are among the most readily obtained, a clear understanding of their use and significance is essential.

Exercise is an increasingly integral part of the lives of many individuals. No longer reserved for those involved in competitive athletics, routine exercise is now used both recreationally and therapeutically. "Fitness" for many has become a way of life, and the core of this lifestyle is a program of regular exercise. The physiologic responses to regular (or long-term) exercise are thus important, because they promote morphologic and functional changes that have major clinical implications. This is especially true for the cardiovascular adaptations to exercise training that may, in fact, affect the pathophysiology of atherosclerotic coronary heart disease (CHD).

This chapter explores the physiology of exercise with a particular focus on the acute and chronic responses of the cardiovascular system.

103

TYPES OF EXERCISE

Much of this chapter addresses the physiologic responses to exercise, so it is important to define the different types of exercise, as each will evoke specific acute and chronic responses. Practically speaking, exercise can be divided into two main types:

Dynamic

Dynamic exercise involves high-repetition movements against a low resistance; this is also referred to as isotonic exercise, implying that, although there is muscle shortening, the muscle tension remains constant throughout the movement. Actually, muscle tension does vary throughout the contraction, so that the term "isotonic" is not entirely correct.[1,2] Dynamic exercise is best represented by rhythmic activity as performed during cycling, running, or swimming. This type of exercise involves relaxation between contractions, allowing for increases in blood flow to the working muscles, while venous blood is pumped back to the heart during the multiple muscular contractions. Routine dynamic exercise training is often termed "endurance training" as it leads to improvement in an individual's functional capacity for prolonged bouts of dynamic exercise.

Static

Static exercise primarily involves low-repetition movements against a high resistance. Such exercise involves isometric contractions in which tension develops without muscle shortening, although there is some dynamic component to most static exercise routines. Static exercise causes the development of increased muscle tension, with a restriction of blood flow to exercising muscle during the contraction. Static exercise training programs are also referred to as "power training" or "strength training" and are best represented by activities such as weight lifting.

The physiologic responses to acute and chronic static or dynamic exercise should be viewed with the understanding that most exercise activities are a combination of both types of exercise, with a predominance of either one or the other.

SKELETAL MUSCLE PHYSIOLOGY

Contraction–Relaxation

The central theme of all exercise physiology is that exercise requires contraction of skeletal muscle and that this contraction and subsequent relaxation are energy-dependent processes. The skeletal muscle acts as a machine that transforms chemical energy into mechanical energy[2] through a series of interactions between muscle proteins (actin, myosin, troponin, and tropomyosin) and calcium. Since the motor nerves stimulate the muscle, the muscle cell membrane depolarizes, resulting in a release of calcium from the sarcoplasmic reticulum into the sarcoplasm. The calcium then binds to troponin, causing a change in the troponin–tropomyosin–actin complex, allowing interaction between the myosin head and actin. Utilizing adenosine tryphosphate (ATP), the actin filaments move along the myosin filaments. Actin activates myosin ATPase to hydrolyze ATP into adenosine diphosphate (ADP) and free phosphate. After this scheme of contraction, additional ATP is utilized to dissociate myosin from actin. Calcium is then released from troponin and is transported, by an energy-dependent process, back into the sarcoplasmic reticulum. This process requires the hydrolysis of one ATP molecule per two calcium ions. The troponin–tropomyosin–actin complex then resumes its original conformation. These events are repeated as long as the muscle is stimulated.[3] ATP is thus utilized in actin–myosin interaction during contraction, actin–myosin detachment, and calcium uptake into the sarcoplasmic reticulum during relaxation.

Muscle Fiber Types and Exercise Performance

Although various classification systems are used and nomenclature is at times confusing, it is generally agreed that humans have at least three different skeletal muscle fiber types. It is useful to review these fiber types as their distinct biochemical and ultrastructural properties translate to differences in the capacity of an individual to perform specific kinds of exercise.

Previously, muscles were classified into "red" and "white" on the basis of their color, or "fast" and "slow" twitch, depending on the time it takes the fibers to reach peak tension (fast twitch, less than 40 msec; slow twitch, approximately 80–100 msec).[3] More recently, muscle fibers have been classified into two broad categories on the basis of histochemical staining for myofibrillar ATPase: type I (light staining), which has low ATPase activity, and type II (dark staining), which has high ATPase activity.[3–5] Note that high ATPase activity appears to be associated with increased contractility. Type II fibers are further subdivided into type IIA (fast-twitch red) and type IIB (fast-twitch white).[5] The characteristics of these fiber types are outlined in Table 6-1.

Type I fibers are red and slow-contracting, with a high respiratory capacity (large number of mitochondria) and myoglobin content, but a low capacity for glycogenolysis and a low myofibrillar ATPase activity. Type IIB fibers are white and fast contracting, with a low respiratory capacity (fewer mitochondria), high capacity for glycogenolysis, low myoglobin, and high myofibrillar ATPase activity. Type IIA fibers vary considerably among individuals. These are fast-twitch red fibers with high respiratory capacity, high glycogenolytic capacity, high myoglobin content,

and high myofibrillar ATPase activity. Type I and IIA fibers are very similar in endurance-trained athletes, whereas type IIA and IIB fibers are similar in sedentary individuals. Although the average human skeletal muscle contains approximately 50% slow-twitch and 50% fast-twitch fibers, there is great variability among individuals. This distribution is, at least in part, genetic. Type I and IIA fibers are stimulated by small motor neurons and are recruited for low- and moderate-intensity work. Type IIB fibers are stimulated by large motor neuron units, when excitatory input to motor neurons is high, as during heavy exercise. Type IIB fibers are also recruited when types I and IIA are fatigued. Type I and IIA fibers are involved with prolonged muscular activity with minimal lactate production, whereas type IIB fibers are involved with short bursts of activity with increased lactate production.[5] Myoglobin increases the rate of oxygen diffusion through the sarcoplasm to the mitochondria and thus may facilitate oxygen utilization for aerobic generation of ATP in the mitochondria. Therefore, the myoglobin content of specific muscle fiber types will affect their capacity for different types of work.

Long-term endurance exercise increases the mitochondrial number in skeletal muscle in the fast type IIA fibers more than in the type I fibers. Therefore, mitochondrial enzyme levels in type I and IIA fibers become very similar. The increase in mitochondrial number appears to be muscle specific, such that runners will have higher mitochondrial levels in their leg muscles than in the skeletal muscles of other body parts. Endurance training also affects the content of enzymes required in fuel metabolism, as will be discussed below.[4] Additionally, there is an increase in the capillary density of skeletal muscle beds after training. This facilitates the exchange of nutrients between the vascular and the extravascular spaces, decreases the diffusion path for oxygen, and increases red blood cell transit time in muscle beds.[6] Such adaptations facilitate aerobic metabolism for ATP generation and thus improve the capacity for prolonged endurance exercise.

The effects of static exercise in skeletal muscle are less well documented and appear limited to increased muscle cell hypertrophy via the syn-

Table 6-1. Human Skeletal Muscle Fiber Types

Property	Type I	Type IIA	Type IIB
Color	Red	White	White
Shortening velocity	Slow	Fast	Fast
Motor neuron size	Small	Large	Large
Myofibrillar ATPase	Low	High	High
Mitochondrial enzyme capacity	High	Medium	Low
Glycogenolytic capacity	Low	High	High
Myoglobin content	High	Medium	Low

thesis of increased contractile protein and thickening of connective tissues.[1]

FUELS FOR EXERCISE

Although skeletal muscle is approximately 50% of total body weight, it accounts for only 15 to 30% of resting energy expenditure. The amount of energy utilized is reflected in the amount of oxygen consumed during a given activity ($\dot{V}o_2$). During exercise, $\dot{V}o_2$ can increase up to 15- to 20-fold over resting values, most of which is consumed by exercising skeletal muscle.[5,7] The energy is produced in the form of ATP, which is involved in both contraction and relaxation of skeletal muscle.

ATP is produced by three main mechanisms.

The first is creatine phosphate, which, via creatine kinase, yields creatine plus ATP. This reaction is anaerobic (does not require oxygen) and contributes a small and finite amount of energy. The second is glycolysis; the degradation of glucose or glycogen can be either aerobic or anaerobic and yields either pyruvate plus ATP or lactate plus ATP, respectively. If oxygen is available to accept hydrogen ions from pyruvate metabolism, further production of ATP will take place in the mitochondria, with the final products being ATP and water (Fig. 6-1). The third mechanism is the Krebs cycle and electron transport; the aerobic metabolism of glucose, fat, or protein via the Krebs cycle in the mitochondria yields ATP and water (Fig. 6-1).[7] Most fatty acids originate from adipose tissue. They are mobilized by hydrolysis, released into the bloodstream, and taken up by active muscles.[9]

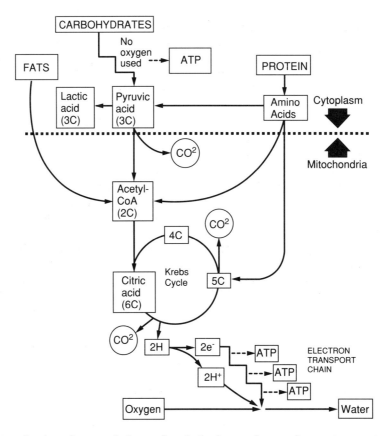

Fig. 6-1. Steps involved in the metabolism of carbohydrates, fats, and proteins to yield ATP. (From Astrand and Rodahl,[8] with permission.)

The selection of the particular substrate or muscle fuel for energy generation depends on the relative intensity and duration of exercise. The first several minutes of exercise are fueled primarily by anaerobic metabolism of creatine phosphate and glucose. As exercise continues, predominantly aerobic metabolism of glucose and fatty acids occurs. When heavy work is performed (greater than 60% $\dot{V}o_2$max) there is a shift toward anaerobic metabolism of glucose. The contribution of fatty acids to total energy production at this level of exercise can vary between 10 and 40% depending, in part, on the training state of the individual. Glycolysis is inhibited by fatty acid oxidation, probably by the accumulation of citrate, which inhibits phosphofructokinase. Thus, glycogen stores are maintained. However, when work becomes so intense that ATP is utilized above the capacity of muscle to generate ATP from oxidative metabolism (e.g., decreased oxygen presence to accept hydrogen ions to form water and ATP), lactate production is increased from the anaerobic metabolism of glucose. This causes a drop in pH, which in turn inhibits phosphofructokinase and turns off glycolysis. Thus, fatigue ensues and exercise ceases.[5] Heavy exercise can be maintained, providing the lactate concentration does not exceed 4 to 6 mmol/L.[9]

Endurance exercise training increases the enzyme capacity for fatty acid and glucose metabolism primarily in type I and IIA fibers.[10] At the same relative exercise intensity (similar percentage of $\dot{V}o_2$max), there is a greater amount of energy derived from fatty acid metabolism,[4,5] a decrease in lactate production, and the resultant sparing of glycogen. As glycogen stores are maintained, endurance (exercise duration) is increased. There is evidence that exercise training increases the sensitivity of adipocytes to epinephrine-mediated lipolysis, thus increasing the availability of free fatty acids for oxidative metabolism.[11]

Although the metabolism of 1 g of fat yields 9 kcal and 1 g of carbohydrate yields 4 kcal, it requires more oxygen to release each kilocalorie from fat. Therefore, carbohydrate supplies more kilocalories per liter of oxygen consumed than does fat (5.05 versus 4.69 kcal/L respectively). Conveniently stated, for each liter of oxygen consumed, approximately 5 kcal of energy is generated. Note that proteins are not used as a major substrate for energy production during exercise and are thus not important in this analysis.[12]

RESPIRATORY RESPONSES TO EXERCISE

The respiratory system responds to exercise by providing a continued supply of ambient oxygen to the circulatory system for delivery to working muscles, as well as providing a mechanism for the excretion of metabolic by-products of fuel metabolism (namely, CO_2). Minute ventilation ($\dot{V}E$) is the volume of air flowing through the pulmonary system in 1 minute. It is the product of the breathing frequency (breaths per minute) and the tidal volume (volume of air per breath). As shown in Fig. 6-2, $\dot{V}E$ increases with increasing work rate rectilinearly, together with breathing frequency and tidal volume, until a certain point is reached. At this level, $\dot{V}E$ increases curvilinearly and steeply, primarily as a result of increases in breathing frequency.[13,14]

Respiration is modulated by a complex system involving central and peripheral mechanisms. The respiratory center at the cerebral medulla is regulated by both neural and humoral stimulation. Mechanoreceptors in exercising muscles, as well as chemoreceptors, both centrally and peripherally, alter ventilation to maintain a normal pH, Po_2, and Pco_2 in arterial blood.

The etiology of the sudden and sharp rise in $\dot{V}E$ with increasing work rates is an area of continued controversy and is not yet fully understood. It is probably due to many factors that influence the respiratory center, including pH and afferent impulses from exercising muscles. (1) During anaerobic metabolism of heavy exercise, lactate production increases, causing a drop in pH; this stimulates central and peripheral chemoreceptors, leading to an increase in ventilation. (2) Afferent impulses travel from exercising muscles to the central nervous system and back to the respiratory muscles via a spinal reflex. Since this level of exercise at which $\dot{V}E$ abruptly increases usually occurs at a time when lactate

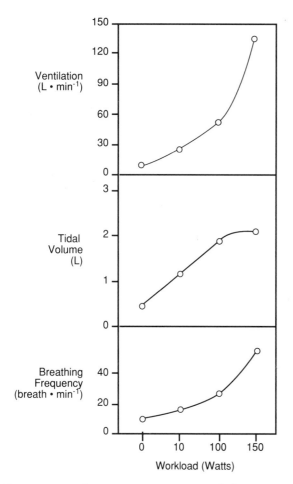

Fig. 6-2. Ventilatory responses to graded exercise. (From Durstine and Pate,[14] with permission.)

begins to accumulate, it has been termed the "anaerobic threshold." The concept of anaerobic threshold is discussed in detail below.

CARDIOVASCULAR RESPONSES TO ACUTE EXERCISE

Hemodynamic Changes

The cardiovascular system responds in several ways and via many mechanisms to meet the metabolic needs of exercising muscles. The complex interactions between the heart, peripheral vessels, neurohumoral influences, and local stimuli in muscle beds work together to (1) ensure an adequate supply of oxygen to exercising muscles; (2) remove metabolic by-products and heat released during muscular exercise; and (3) transport regulatory hormones to target tissues to assist in neurohumoral control of organ system responses. In normal individuals, cardiac output during maximal dynamic exercise can increase by four to five times its resting value. An increased cardiac output serves to increase blood flow (and hence oxygen delivery) to exercising muscle beds and facilitate removal of lactate, CO_2, and heat. Cardiac output increases as a result of an augmentation of both stroke volume and heart rate.[14] Stroke volume, which is the volume of blood ejected per ventricular contraction, increases until about 50% of maximal exercise capacity is reached. At that point, the increase in stroke volume plateaus and any further increases in cardiac output are due solely to increases in heart rate. Stroke volume augmentation is influenced by sympathetic stimulation, circulating epinephrine and norepinephrine, and the Frank-Starling mechanism. Increases in venous return, which occur when a greater volume of blood is pumped from the capacitance vessels in exercising muscle beds, lead to an increase in left ventricular end-diastolic volume. As in skeletal muscle, this stretching of muscle leads to a greater tension and contractility and hence an increase in stroke volume up to 1.3 to 1.5 times resting levels.[14-16]

Heart rate can increase during exercise up to 2 to 2.5 times resting levels. This rise in heart rate is influenced by central neural stimulation, withdrawal of vagal influences, and an increase in autonomic sympathetic tone, as well as by circulating epinephrine and norepinephrine.[17] Total peripheral resistance is determined primarily by the balance of vasoconstrictor and vasodilator forces at the arteriolar level. Peripheral resistance drops during dynamic lower extremity exercise, owing to the vasodilatation that occurs in the arterioles of exercising muscles. The by-products of metabolism cause a drop in local pH, a rise in P_{CO_2}, and an increase in lactate and thus lead to vasodilatation that overrides the vasoconstrictor influences of the heightened sympathetic tone. Therefore, diastolic blood pressure, which is an indicator of peripheral resistance, usually decreases during dynamic exercise. Systolic blood pressure rises despite the decline in vascular resistance, primarily as a result of the augmentation of cardiac output.[14]

It is important to note that cardiac output increases linearly in response to total-body oxygen consumption ($\dot{V}O_2$). The rise in cardiac output is influenced primarily by the relative percentage of maximal oxygen consumption that can be achieved (termed $\dot{V}O_2$max). This, in turn, is a product of the work rate and active exercising muscle mass.[16] Cardiac output during exercise is also related to body position, age, gender, fitness level, and underlying cardiac status.[18]

The effects of muscle mass and body position on cardiac output are best demonstrated by analyzing the cardiorespiratory responses to arm and leg exercise. Dynamic arm exercise, at any given submaximal work rate, is typified by a higher $\dot{V}O_2$, $\dot{V}E$, systolic blood pressure, heart rate, and cardiac output. Peripheral vascular resistance is greater during arm work, since relatively less vasodilation occurs, owing to the smaller vascular area in arm muscles, while relatively greater vasoconstriction occurs in the extensive vascular beds of the nonexercising muscles. Therefore, diastolic blood pressure during arm exercise is higher than during leg exercise at matched submaximal work rates. Heart rate rises more steeply, at least in part as a result of differences in sympathetic response, while stroke volume augmentation is small, as a result of the relatively small amount of blood being pumped back to the heart by the smaller muscle mass of the exercising upper extremities. During arm and leg exercises at similar work rates, $\dot{V}O_2$ is greater with arm work, owing to the additional muscle mass recruited for stabilization of body position.[16,19-23] This point is well illustrated by the greater $\dot{V}O_2$ when performing work with the arms in the overhead position than when performing work with arms at horizontal (or bench) level. Of note, heart rate, systolic and diastolic blood pressures, and $\dot{V}E$ are also greater during overhead arm work than at bench level.[22] The added isometric work of back, buttock, and leg muscles probably accounts for these observed differences.

Stated differently, at similar submaximal $\dot{V}O_2$ levels cardiac output during arm and leg work is the same, although this occurs at relatively lower work rates of arm exercise than leg exercise. The maximal heart rate achieved during both types of exercise is also similar, although peak oxygen consumption during arm exercise is usually only 70% of that during leg exercise.[23]

Most investigators agree that during low-level supine dynamic leg exercise, cardiac output increases mainly as a function of heart rate since there is little to no change in exercise stroke volume. However, during high levels of supine exercise, an augmentation of left ventricular diastolic volume results in a small but definite increase in stroke volume (up to 20%). This is probably due to the Frank-Starling mechanism.[18]

Myocardial Oxygen Demand and Coronary Circulation

During exercise, myocardial oxygen demand increases in response to the rise in total body oxygen demand. The need for oxygenated blood by the myocardium is related to heart rate, blood pressure, left ventricular contractility, and left ventricular wall stress.[16] Alterations in any of these factors—many of which are interdependent and all of which are increased during dynamic exercise—can affect the myocardial demand for oxygen. Of these, heart rate and blood pressure are the easiest to measure and monitor. The product of heart rate and systolic blood pressure, termed the rate–pressure product, is a very reliable index of myocardial oxygen demand[24] and is widely used clinically. The coronary circulation responds to these increases in oxygen demand by augmenting coronary flow. This flow depends on coronary perfusion pressure, coronary lumen diameter, and resistance in the distal coronary vessel. Ninety percent of coronary vascular resistance occurs at the level of the arterioles, which can dilate fourfold.[25] Local changes in the vasomotor tone of coronary vascular smooth muscle can influence flow and affect the delivery of oxygenated blood to the myocardium. Coronary vasomotor tone is affected by a complex interplay between neuromodulation and endothelial control. In the normal coronary artery, alpha-adrenergic stimulation causes coronary vasoconstriction, while beta-adrenergic activation produces direct coronary vasodilation. Sympathetic stimulation of the normal coronary artery, however, produces a net vasodilation. The endothelium is now recognized as an important and complex regulator of coronary smooth muscle tone. Its release of numerous vasoactive substances, particularly endothelium-derived relaxing factor (EDRF), can affect coronary vasomotion. Many substances trigger its release. Increases in epinephrine and in vascular wall shear stress, as occur during exercise, can release EDRF and induce vascular smooth muscle relaxation.[26,27] Together, these responses serve to increase coronary flow to meet the demands of the myocardium during exercise.

Coronary vasculature that is affected by atherosclerosis has an impaired response to myocardial oxygen demand, which may result in the development of ischemia during exercise. Most commonly, flow is compromised by the presence of an atherosclerotic plaque within the lumen of the coronary artery. Many factors influence the significance of a given luminal stenosis, including the degree and length of luminal obstruction, the dynamic properties of the stenosis, the number and size of functioning collateral vessels, the autoregulatory capacity of the distal vascular beds, and the magnitude of the mass of myocardium being supplied.[28] A 50 to 70% reduction in luminal area will impair peak reactive hyperemia, as might occur during exercise.[29] Additionally, sympathetic stimulation in the presence of a coronary stenosis may lead to a net coronary vasoconstriction.[30] This latter observation is probably due in part to the fact that damaged and diseased endothelium cannot release EDRF. The underlying vascular smooth muscle is then exposed to vasoconstrictor substances, which serve to decrease myocardial perfusion.[26]

Shifts in Regional Blood Flow

Major shifts in regional blood flow occur during exercise as a result of the changes in arteriolar resistance in different organ beds in response to neurohumoral and local influences on peripheral vascular tone.[16,31] Upright dynamic leg exercise appears to cause marked shifts in blood volume from the legs and abdominal organs to the heart and lungs. These changes in regional blood volume are closely related to increasing oxygen consumption during exercise, as demonstrated in Fig. 6-3.

Cerebral blood flow remains either constant or increases,[16] while lung volume increases as much as 18% and cardiac end-diastolic volume increases by 10%. Despite the significant rise in blood flow to exercising muscles, exercising-leg volume decreases as much as 32%. This is probably due to the movement of blood from venous capacitance vessels in the legs back to the heart, via the pumping action of contracting muscles. Vasoconstriction in splanchnic beds leads to a 24% decrease in renal blood volume, an 18% decrease in hepatic blood volume, and a 46% decrease in splenic blood volume.[31] Thus, it appears that the augmentation of heart and lung blood volumes at low exercise work rates occurs due to the redistribution of exercising-leg-blood volume, but that at higher work rates it is due to the shift of blood from abdominal organ beds.

These blood volume shifts facilitate the increased cardiac output required to meet the increased systemic oxygen demands during exercise. Blood flow to the skin is influenced by the interaction between sympathetic stimulation and reflexes related to thermoregulation. Skin blood flow initially decreases during exercise, but increases later at submaximal levels of exercise. During maximal exercise, skin blood flow again decreases, even in hot environments.[16]

Neurohumoral Responses and their Relation to the Cardiovascular Response

The central and reflex neurohumoral mechanisms that orchestrate the cardiovascular response to exercise involve a series of actions and interactions among the exercising muscles, the central nervous system, peripheral receptors, the adrenal medulla, the heart, and the peripheral vasculature. Peripheral-receptor control is mediated through baroreceptors, chemoreceptors, cardiopulmonary stretch receptors, and ergore-

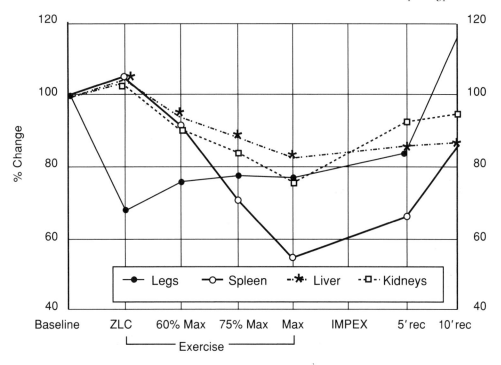

Fig. 6-3. Percent change of thorax and organ blood volumes before, during, and immediately after (IMPEX) exercise and during recovery from exercise. (From Flamm et al.,[31] with permission.)

ceptors of contracting muscles.[15] With the onset of exercise, neuroinputs are received from both ergoreceptors in exercising muscle and central command input from the motor areas of the brain, as shown in Fig. 6-4.

The mechanical and metabolic alterations in exercising muscle activate ergoreceptors, whose afferent impulses are conducted to the spinal cord, where they ascend to the central cardiovascular areas. As a result, the parasympathetic activity to the heart decreases and is often referred to as a withdrawal of vagal tone. Sympathetic activity to the heart, peripheral blood vessels, and adrenal medulla increases. Adrenal stimulation results in secretion of epinephrine into the circulation. Baroreceptors in the carotid sinus and aortic arch respond to increased arterial blood pressure and modify, possibly via vagal efferent impulses, the increases in blood pressure. Cutaneous veins dilate as a result of withdrawal of sympathetic outflow to these areas; while splanchnic, renal, and nonexercising muscle ar-

terioles constrict.[33] The central and reflex mechanisms overlap and may be redundant.

Responses in the Elderly

The cardiovascular responses during exercise are altered in the elderly individual, primarily owing to morphologic and functional changes in the cardiovascular and neurologic systems. With aging, there is a progressive decline in the amount of elastic tissue in the vascular media, with an associated increase in the amount of collagen. These changes in structure translate into an increase in vascular stiffness, resulting in an increase in arterial blood pressure. Left ventricular hypertrophy, which occurs in response to the elevated blood pressure, together with an increase in the amount of intercellular myocardial connective tissue, results in a reduction in left ventricular compliance. Thus, the increase in end-diastolic volume that occurs during dynamic

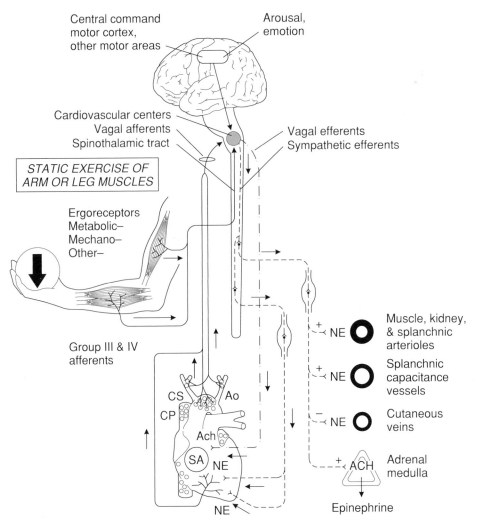

Fig. 6-4. Neurologic pathways and factors involved in the cardiovascular response to exercise. CS and Ao, mechanical receptors of carotid sinus and aortic arch; SA, sinoatrial node; NE, norepinephrine; Ach, acetylcholine. (From Shepherd et al.,[32] with permission.)

exercise may lead to a significant rise in end-diastolic pressure. This may provoke exercise-induced dyspnea at relatively low work loads.[34] Although resting cardiac output remains constant in healthy elderly persons, there is a progressive decline with age in the augmentation of cardiac output during exercise. This is a result of a decreased adrenergic responsiveness, which leads to a reduction in the maximal heart rate that can be achieved during exercise, as well as diminished left ventricular contractility. These factors yield a lower maximal cardiac output, which, in part, contributes to the decline in the maximal exercise capacity observed in older individuals.[35,36]

Responses in Patients with Atherosclerotic Coronary Heart Disease (CHD)

The acute effects of exercise among patients with atherosclerotic coronary artery narrowing, without underlying damaged myocardium, relate to the supply–demand imbalance for oxygenated blood to the myocardium that may develop during exercise. The severity of this imbalance, which translates into myocardial ischemia, depends on the relative increases in myocardial oxygen demand and the response of the coronary circulation to provide an adequate supply of oxygenated blood. The factors that determine this relationship are outlined above. The functional significance of ischemia depends on the degree of impairment of myocardial function and the development of angina during exercise. Symptoms of angina alone may limit exercise tolerance. Myocardial dysfunction can occur without symptoms of angina,[28] yet lead to increased diastolic stiffness. This results in an increase in left ventricular end-diastolic pressure, with associated dyspnea; and/or a reduction in myocardial contractility, which limits stroke volume and cardiac output during exercise. The latter may diminish the supply of oxygenated blood to exercising muscles, leading to fatigue.

In patients with damaged myocardium due to myocardial infarction, resting systolic function may be reduced, leading to congestive heart failure. These patients usually demonstrate abnormal cardiovascular responses to exercise that may, in part, lead to impaired exercise tolerance, although the exact mechanisms responsible for this impairment are not completely understood. The heart rate response to exercise is blunted, and stroke volume does not increase. This translates to a reduction in cardiac output. The $\dot{V}_E$ response to exercise is exaggerated. The systolic blood pressure response is blunted, yet total peripheral resistance is high. Thus, blood pressure is maintained by elevated systemic resistance (rather than reduced, as in normal individuals) in the presence of an attenuated cardiac output at a given submaximal level of exercise. This heightened peripheral vascular resistance occurs because resistance vessels fail to dilate in response to exercise.[17,37] Only a small portion of cardiac output appears to be delivered to exercising muscles, as limb vascular resistance also remains abnormally high. There is increased muscular anaerobic activity and acidosis. Whether this is related to reduced muscle blood flow or to an intrinsic abnormality in muscle metabolism remains unclear. This muscular acidosis may lead to fatigue and cessation of exercise.[17,38,39]

Earlier investigators stressed the importance of exercise-induced elevation of pulmonary wedge pressure with resulting pulmonary congestion in the pathogenesis of exercise-limiting dyspnea. However, several factors argue against this theory: (1) most patients with congestive failure claim that fatigue rather than dyspnea limits effort; (2) pulmonary wedge pressure in these patients rises to the same levels during submaximal and maximal exercise (exhaustion); and (3) arterial oxygen saturation remains unchanged even during maximal symptom-limited exercise in patients with congestive heart failure.[39] Continued investigation is needed to further elucidate the factors that allow patients with similar impairment in left ventricular systolic function to have, at times, vastly different levels of exercise tolerance.

ENERGY EXPENDITURE AND FITNESS AS ASSESSED BY RESPIRATORY GAS ANALYSIS

The discussion thus far has focused on the ways in which the various organ systems respond to the body's increased need for oxygen during exercise. Measurements of oxygen consumption during exercise can provide valuable information in the assessment of the functional status of an individual. An understanding of the terminology used in this assessment is important.

During exercise, a major portion of total body oxygen consumption ($\dot{V}_{O_2}$) is related to the utilization of oxygen by exercising muscles. The $\dot{V}_{O_2}$ during exercise correlates closely with the rate at which work is being performed (also called power output). Oxygen consumption is also linearly related to cardiac output:

$$\dot{V}_{O_2} = \text{cardiac output} \times \text{A–V}_{O_2}$$
$$\text{(arteriovenous oxygen) difference}$$

$$= \text{stroke volume} \times \text{heart rate}$$
$$\times \text{A–V}_{O_2} \text{ difference}$$

The *A–Vo2 difference* reflects the extraction of oxygen from the blood by the peripheral tissues. It is the difference between the oxygen content of arterial blood and mixed venous blood. The arterial blood contains about 20 mL of O_2/100 mL and the average A–Vo2 difference at rest is 5 mL/100 mL. However, during maximal exercise, it can increase to 16 mL/100 mL. Thus, during maximal exercise, approximately 85% of the oxygen content of arterial blood is removed by peripheral exercising tissues.[14] The maximal oxygen uptake of an individual, termed $\dot{V}_{O_2}max$, is the best indicator of aerobic work capacity and fitness. $\dot{V}_{O_2}$ can be easily and noninvasively assessed by using a metabolic measurement cart which analyzes the gas content of an individual's expired air obtained at rest and during exercise. The $\dot{V}_{O_2}max$ is defined as the level of oxygen consumption that does not increase despite increases in work rate. It can also be assessed as the point at which $\dot{V}_{O_2}$ increases less than 150 mL/min despite an increase in work rate.[40]

$\dot{V}_{O_2}$ is usually expressed in milliliters per minute (mL/min) or milliliters per kilogram of body weight per minute (mL/kg/min). Individuals with greater muscle mass (i.e., greater lean-body mass) will have a higher resting $\dot{V}_{O_2}$ (mL/min). A convenient method of expressing $\dot{V}_{O_2}$ at a given work rate is by use of the *MET* system. One MET is defined as the amount of oxygen consumed by an awake individual at rest and is equal to 3.5 mL/kg/min. Thus, any given $\dot{V}_{O_2}$ measured during activity can be indexed against resting $\dot{V}_{O_2}$, by dividing that $\dot{V}_{O_2}$ (mL/kg/min) by 3.5. Note that the MET values are less reliable in those with low lean-body mass (obese individuals) or muscular individuals with high-lean body mass, since their true resting $\dot{V}_{O_2}$ will not approximate 3.5 mL/min/kg.[14]

The *oxygen pulse* is a noninvasive index of the efficiency of oxygen transport from the heart to the peripheral tissues:

$$\text{Oxygen pulse} = \dot{V}_{O_2}/\text{heart rate} =$$
$$\text{stroke volume} \times$$
$$\text{A–V}_{O_2}\text{ difference}^{41}$$

The oxygen pulse is higher in trained individuals than in untrained,[42] while patients with coronary heart disease have a lower than normal oxygen pulse.[43]

Mechanical efficiency refers to the ratio of the work done (power output) to the energy costs ($\dot{V}_{O_2}$). The body is only about 20% efficient, wasting about 80% of its energy as heat. Mechanical efficiency can be increased by previous experience with a particular exercise activity and can be decreased by obesity and neuromuscular disorders that affect motor coordination.[41,44]

The *respiratory exchange ratio* (RER), called *respiratory quotient* (RQ) at the cellular level, is a measure of the volume of CO_2 production per volume of oxygen utilized:

$$\text{RER} = \dot{V}_{CO_2}/\dot{V}_{O_2}$$

The RER serves as an indicator of substrate utilization. When fats are the primary fuel, the RER is 0.70, whereas when carbohydrates are being used, the RER is 1.0. The RER measured during exercise reflects the fuel being utilized at that specific time of exercise and is directly related to the percentage of $\dot{V}_{O_2}max$ at which the individual is working. At work rates lower than 60% of $\dot{V}_{O_2}max$, the RER is below 1.0, since fatty acids are the main energy source. However, at heavy work rates (greater than 60% of $\dot{V}_{O_2}max$), the RER equals or exceeds 1.0, as glucose is the main fuel substrate. An RER that exceeds 1.0 indicates that energy metabolism is predominantly anaerobic, yielding an increased volume of CO_2 from the buffering of lactate by bicarbonate. Thus, the RER is useful in estimating the relative percentage of maximal effort at which an individual is exercising.

Another index of relative work effort is the *anaerobic threshold*. This is a highly reproducible point during exercise at which ventilation abruptly increases despite linear increases in work rate. Shortly beyond the anaerobic threshold, fatigue usually ensues and work ceases. The term *anaerobic threshold* is based on the hypothesis that, at a given work rate, the oxygen supply does not meet the oxygen requirement. This imbalance increases anaerobic glycolysis for energy generation, yielding lactate as a metabolic by-product.[45] Although the anaerobic threshold is a defined endpoint that can be established by several different methods, the actual cause of the observed abrupt rise in $\dot{V}E$ remains controversial. In favor of the above hypothesis is that the measured lactate level increases at the point at which $\dot{V}E$ begins its curvilinear relationship to work rate. However, whether muscle hypoxia is a main stimulus for increased lactate production is not yet clear. It appears that increases in muscle lactate occur despite indices which indicate that muscle oxygenation is adequate (muscle venous P_{O_2} and myoglobin saturation).[46] Whether lactate is a stimulus for the increase in $\dot{V}E$ also remains unsettled, since patients with McArdle's disease, who lack muscle phosphorylase and hence the ability to produce lactate, also demonstrate an abrupt increase in $\dot{V}E$ at approximately 70% of $\dot{V}O_2max$.[41]

The anaerobic threshold usually occurs at 47 to 64% of $\dot{V}O_2max$ in healthy untrained persons, but is noted at 70 to 90% of $\dot{V}O_2max$ in highly trained subjects.[12] Despite the uncertainty in its cause, the anaerobic threshold is determined by several easily recognized measurements that can be obtained during respiratory gas analysis. These are illustrated in Fig. 6-5 and include (1) a departure of linearity in $\dot{V}E$ and $\dot{V}CO_2$ with increasing work rates and an abrupt increase in the RER and fraction of O_2 in expired air (Fe_{O_2}); (2) an increase in $\dot{V}E/\dot{V}O_2$ without an increase in $\dot{V}E/\dot{V}CO_2$, and an increase in Fe_{O_2} without a decrease in the fraction of CO_2 in expired air; (3) the lowest $\dot{V}E/\dot{V}O_2$ value measured during exercise; and (4) a curvilinear increase in $\dot{V}E$ and $\dot{V}CO_2$ with a linear increase in $\dot{V}O_2$.[41]

Finally, the anaerobic threshold is an important functional demarcation during exercise, since above this point metabolic acidosis occurs; exercise endurance is reduced; and $\dot{V}E$ increases disproportionately to the metabolic requirement, resulting in tachypnea. Below the anaerobic threshold, $\dot{V}O_2$ reaches a steady state by 2 to 3 minutes of exercise at a given work rate. However, above the anaerobic threshold, oxygen kinetics are slowed such that steady state is delayed.[47]

Energy costs during exercise are most easily assessed by using measurements of $\dot{V}O_2$, where for each liter of oxygen consumed, approximately 5 kcal of energy is used.[12] $\dot{V}O_2$ is directly related to the work rate or power output of a given ex-

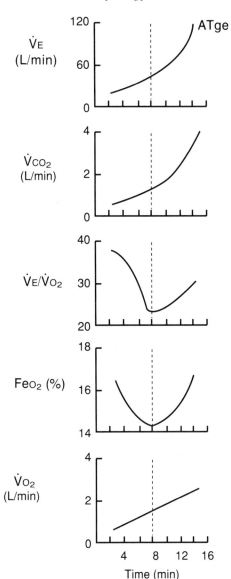

Fig. 6-5. Measurements used to determine the gas exchange anaerobic threshold (ATge). $\dot{V}E$, minute ventilation; $\dot{V}CO_2$, carbon dioxide production; $\dot{V}O_2$, oxygen uptake; Fe_{O_2}, fraction of expired air that is oxygen. (From Sullivan and Froelicher,[41] with permission.)

ercise. Although direct measurement of $\dot{V}O_2$ is relatively easy, the process is time-consuming and not always readily available. Therefore, estimates of $\dot{V}O_2$ during common types of exercise, including walking, bicycling, and arm cycle ergometry, can be calculated on the basis of regression equations from data obtained in normal healthy individuals.[48–50] Work rate is a product of force, distance, and a reciprocal of time. Work rate during walking exercise is dependent on body weight, which is the major component of the moving force. $\dot{V}o_2$ during walking or treadmill exercise is thus usually expressed in terms relative to body weight (i.e., mL/kg/min). At the same work rate, individuals of different body weights will have similar $\dot{V}o_2$ (in mL/kg/min or METs). However, during ergometry exercise (bicycle or arm cycle), the work rate is related primarily to an external weight applied to the flywheel apparatus, moving through the flywheel circumference × the reciprocal of time. Most of the body weight is supported and thus is much less of a factor in $\dot{V}o_2$. Since $\dot{V}o_2$ during ergometry is usually expressed in mL/min, body weight must be measured to calculate $\dot{V}o_2$ in mL/kg/min. Therefore, during ergometry exercise, $\dot{V}o_2$ (in mL/kg/min or METs) is greater in the lighter individual than in the heavier person exercising at the same work rate.[12,48,50]

CARDIOVASCULAR RESPONSES TO CHRONIC EXERCISE: EFFECTS OF TRAINING

Cardiac Morphology and Function

Studies of the cardiac adaptations to long-term exercise have concentrated mostly on highly trained athletes. Significant increases in left ventricular dimension, wall thickness, and mass have been noted in both endurance-trained and power-trained athletes.[51–58] The echocardiographic data from a composite analysis of 25 separate studies of healthy athletes with regard to chamber dimensions and mass are outlined in Table 6-2. Endurance-trained athletes who are subject to high volumes of venous return during exercise demonstrate larger left ventricular volumes than power-trained athletes. Conversely, chronic exposure to elevations in systemic vascular resistance, and hence elevated systolic blood pressure during power training, yields greater left ventricular wall thickness in these

athletes than in those who are endurance-trained. Both groups demonstrate marked increases in left ventricular mass, although the left ventricular mass/lean-body mass ratio in power-trained athletes is normal, whereas that in endurance-trained athletes is significantly elevated.[58] Therefore, the increase in left ventricular mass observed from predominantly static exercise training is proportional to increases in skeletal muscle mass.

Left ventricular wall stress measured at rest among athletes involved in dynamic exercise training is normal. Resting wall stress measured in power-trained athletes is low, owing to the differences in wall thickness relative to chamber dimensions observed between both types of athletes.[59]

Despite the increased wall thickness that occurs after prolonged exercise training, diastolic function as measured by using echo-Doppler parameters of left ventricular wall motion and filling are normal in both endurance-trained[60] and power-trained[61,62] athletes. Some studies suggest that diastolic relaxation during exercise is superior in athletes compared with nonathletes.[63] Systolic function in well-trained individuals, at rest and during exercise, is probably normal, although the data remain somewhat controversial. This is due at least in part to the different methods and parameters that are used to analyze systolic function. Most researchers agree that ejection fraction or echocardiographically derived fractional shortening at rest is normal,[59,63–65] although others have found the ejection fraction at rest and during exercise to decrease after training.[66,67] Stroke volume in athletes, however, is greater than in nonathletes. With the greater left ventricular end-diastolic volume of the trained heart, a similar ejection fraction results in a greater volume of ejected blood.[59,67]

After prolonged periods of high-intensity exhaustive endurance exercise, left ventricular systolic function, as measured by fractional shortening or ejection fraction, decreases and later recovers within days.[68–71] This observation has been termed "cardiac fatigue."[72] The precise mechanism for this reduction in systolic function is not yet understood.

The cessation of exercise training for as brief a

Table 6-2. Ventricular Dimensions in Athletes and Nonathletes as Assessed by Echocardiography

Echocardiographic Variable	Nonathlete Controls		Athletes		Percent Difference[a]
	Mean Value	Number of Subjects	Mean Value	Number of Subjects	
Ventricular septal thickness (mm)	9.1	313	10.4	461	+14.3
Posterior free wall thickness (mm)	9.0	439	10.7	740	+18.9
LV end-diastolic dimension (mm)	49.1	394	53.7	701	+9.8
Estimated LV mass (g)	175	252	256	381	+46.3
RV internal transverse dimension (mm)	17.7	146	22.0	147	+24.3

[a] Percent change of the dimension in athletes, as compared with nonathlete control subjects.
Abbreviations: LV, left ventricular; RV, right ventricular.
(From Maron,[51] with permission.)

period as 3 weeks leads to changes in left ventricular dimensions and stroke volume.[73,74] Reductions in left ventricular mass by 20% have been observed (Fig. 6-6). Significant decreases in left ventricular diastolic dimension and stroke volume (measured in the upright position) have also been noted in athletes after deconditioning (Fig. 6-7). These findings have been attributed to the loss of the augmented cardiac filling that occurs during training. This lowering of preload leads to a reduction in left ventricular diastolic dimension and (via the Frank-Starling mechanism) a decrease in stroke volume.

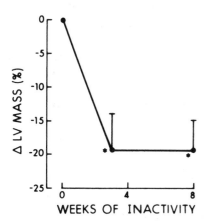

Fig. 6-6. Percent change in left ventricular (LV) mass as a function of duration of inactivity. *$P < 0.05$ compared with results for subjects when they were in the trained state. (From Martin et al.,[74] with permission.)

Coronary Circulation

Exercise training has been shown to increase myocardial capillary density and enlarge surface coronary vessels in experimental animals. Studies in humans have been limited primarily to patients with atherosclerotic CHD. These studies have failed to demonstrate increases in coronary blood flow (as measured by using coronary sinus flow) or increases in angiographically determined coronary collateral circulation after training.[75] However, several provocative studies have demonstrated a reduction in the ischemic response at a given heart rate–blood pressure product after training compared with the pretrained state. The findings that angina,[76] ST segment depression,[77–79] and thallium perfusion defects[80] are decreased at a similar level of myocardial oxygen demand suggest an improvement in myocardial oxygen supply after training. These findings are not conclusive and remain unexplained, although there are several possible mechanisms. Various parameters that regulate coronary smooth muscle tone may be affected by exercise training. A blunting of alpha-adrenergic vasoconstrictor responses has been observed in the coronary arteries of dogs after training.[81] Whether this also occurs in humans is not known. Alterations in blood rheology may play a role in increased myocardial perfusion. A decrease in blood and plasma viscosity,[82–84] a decrease in red blood cell aggregability, and an increase in blood cell filterability[82] have been demonstrated in human

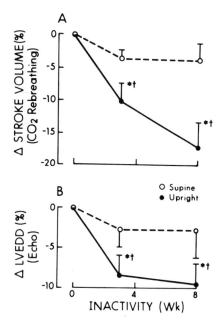

Fig. 6-7. **(A)** Percent change in the exercise stroke volume in both the upright and supine positions as a function of duration of inactivity. **(B)** Percent change in left ventricular end-diastolic dimension (LVEDD) during exercise in the upright and supine positions as a function of duration of inactivity. *$P < 0.005$ compared with results for subjects when they were in the trained state. †$P < 0.05$ upright compared with supine posture. Echo, echocardiographically determined. (From Martin et al.,[74] with permission.)

subjects after training. Alterations in these parameters may also be important in the coronary circulation, particularly when affected by atherosclerosis.

Neurohumoral Responses to Chronic Exercise

Exercise training produces different types of responses in many tissues. Neurohumoral and receptor mechanisms play a key role in mediating these responses. Two main features of the cardiovascular response to chronic exercise are (1) reduced heart rate at rest and (2) reduced heart rate at any given submaximal work rate. Although various mechanisms contribute to this response, alterations in the balance of sympathetic and

parasympathetic stimulation of the cardiovascular system are important. The bradycardia at rest and exercise are attributed to an increased vagal (parasympathetic) tone and a decreased sympathetic tone.

The changes in vagal tone appear to be modulated by an increased neural input rather than by a change in muscarinic receptor activity.[10] Available evidence also demonstrates that decreased sympathetic nerve activity, rather than a change in beta-adrenergic receptors, is responsible, particularly for the attenuated heart rate response to submaximal exercise. Lower plasma levels of catecholamines have been observed in response to exercise in well-trained individuals.[85] These individuals do not appear to have an altered responsiveness to beta-adrenergic agonist infusions[86,87] compared with healthy controls. Moreover, direct analysis of beta-adrenergic receptors in cardiac tissue of trained individuals does not reveal different biochemical properties from these receptors in sedentary individuals. Neither beta-adrenergic receptor number nor receptor sensitivity in myocardial tissue appears to change with training. Conversely, increases in alpha-adrenergic receptor affinity and number have been noted in animal models, but the physiologic significance of this finding is not yet known.[10,81]

Summary of Adaptations to Chronic Exercise

A complex interrelationship among cardiovascular, skeletal muscle, and neurohumoral adaptations to chronic exercise occur to yield a variety of outcomes which are responsible for the "training effect," that is, the ability of an individual, after a period of exercise training, to reach a higher peak work rate and demonstrate a blunted heart rate response to each submaximal level of exercise. These include (1) changes in parasympathetic and sympathetic tone with resultant effects on the cardiovascular system; (2) changes in heart size and stroke volume; (3) changes in skeletal muscle characteristics (myoglobin, mitochondrial number, and capillary density); and (4) alteration in fuel metabolism, yielding a decrease in lactate production at given submaximal work rates.

Whether the central cardiac adaptations play an important role among patients with atherosclerotic CHD remains controversial. Although some studies demonstrate no improvement in cardiac output or stroke volume with exercise training[88-90] and indicate that peripheral adaptations are entirely responsible for the training effect, others have clearly demonstrated central cardiac changes.[91-94] The discrepancies in these findings probably relate to the heterogeneity in patient populations with respect to the severity of atherosclerotic CHD and underlying left ventricular dysfunction, training intensity and duration, and the testing modalities used to demonstrate effects on cardiac size and function.

REFERENCES

1. Sharkey B: Specificity of exercise. p. 55. In Resource Manual for Guidelines for Exercise Testing and Prescription. American College of Sports Medicine. Lea & Febiger, Philadelphia, 1988
2. Asmussen E: Similarities and dissimilarities between static and dynamic exercise. Circ Res 48 (suppl. I):I-3, 1981
3. Astrand P, Rodahl K: Textbook of Work Physiology. 3rd Ed, p. 12. McGraw-Hill, New York, 1986
4. Holloszy JO, Coyle EF: Adaptations of skeletal muscle to endurance exercise and their metabolic consequences. J Appl Physiol 56:831, 1984
5. Holloszy JO: Muscle metabolism during exercise, Arch Phys Med Rehabil 63:231, 1982
6. Terjung RL: Peripheral adaptations in skeletal muscle induced by exercise training. Heart Failure 4:93, 1988
7. Powers SK: Fundamentals of exercise metabolism. p. 40. In Resource Manual for Guidelines for Exercise Testing and Prescription. American College of Sports Medicine. Lea & Febiger, Philadelphia, 1988
8. Astrand P, Rodahl K: Textbook of Work Physiology. 3rd Ed., p. 18. McGraw-Hill, New York, 1986
9. Karlsson J: Metabolic adaptations to exercise: a review of potential beta-adrenoceptor antagonist effects. Am J Cardiol 55:48D, 1985
10. Lash JM, Sherman WM: Adaptations of skeletal muscle to training. p. 65. In Resource Manual for Guidelines for Exercise Testing and Prescription. American College of Sports Medicine. Lea & Febiger, Philadelphia, 1988
11. Williams RS: Role of receptor mechanisms in the adaptive response to habitual exercise. Am J Cardiol 55:68D, 1985
12. Franklin BA, Gordon S, Timmis GC: Fundamentals of exercise physiology: Implications for exercise testing and prescription. p. 1. In Franklin BA, Gordon S, Timmis G (eds): Exercise in Modern Medicine. Williams & Wilkins, Baltimore, 1989
13. Astrand P, Rodahl K: Textbook of Work Physiology. p. 209. McGraw-Hill, New York, 1986
14. Durstine JL, Pate RR: Cardiorespiratory responses to acute exercise. p. 48. In Resource Manual for Guidelines for Exercise Testing and Prescription. American College of Sports Medicine. Lea & Febiger, Philadelphia, 1988
15. Shepherd JT: Circulatory responses to exercise and health. Circulation 76 (suppl. VI):VI-3, 1987
16. Clausen JP: Circulatory adjustments to dynamic exercise and effects of physical training in normal subjects and in patients with coronary artery disease. Prog Cardiovasc Dis 18:459, 1976
17. Francis GS: Hemodynamic and neurohumoral responses to dynamic exercise: Normal subjects vs. patients with heart disease. Circulation 76 (suppl. VI):VI-11, 1987
18. Higginbotham MB: Cardiac performance during submaximal and maximal exercise in healthy persons. Heart Failure 4:68, 1988
19. Franklin BA, Vander L, Wrisley D, Rubenfire M: Aerobic requirements for arm ergometry: implications for exercise testing and training. Physician Sports Med 11:81, 1983
20. Pendergast DR: Cardiovascular, respiratory, and metabolic responses to upper body exercise. Med Sci Sports Exercise 21(suppl.):S121, 1989
21. Miles DS, Cox MH, Bomze JP: Cardiovascular responses to upper body exercise in normals and cardiac patients. Med Sci Sports Exercise 21 (suppl.):S126, 1989
22. Astrand I, Goharray A, Wahren J: Circulatory responses to arm exercise with different arm positions. J Appl Physiol 25:528, 1968
23. Vander LB, Franklin BA, Wrisley D, Rubenfire M: Cardiorespiratory responses to arm and leg ergometry in women. Physician Sportsmed 12:101, 1984
24. Kitamura K, Jorgensen CR, Gobel FL et al: Hemodynamic correlates of myocardial oxygen consumption during upright exercise. J Appl Physiol 32:516, 1972

25. Brown BG, Smith BH: Regulation of myocardial perfusion in ischemic heart disease. p. 16. In Singh BN (ed): Silent Myocardial Ischemia and Angina. Pergamon Press, New York, 1988

26. Griffith TM, Lewis MJ, Newby AC, Henderson AH: Endothelium derived relaxing factor. J Am Coll Cardiol 12:797, 1988

27. Vanhoutte PM: The endothelium-modulator of vascular smooth muscle tone. N Engl J Med 319:512, 1989

28. Herzil HO, Leutwyler R, Krayenbuhl HP: Silent myocardial ischemia: hemodynamic changes during dynamic exercise in patients with coronary artery disease despite absence of angina pectoris. J Am Coll Cardiol 6:275, 1985

29. Maseri A, Davies G, Hackett D: Pathogenesis of myocardial ischemia. p. 28. In Singh BN (ed): Silent Myocardial Ischemia and Angina. Pergamon Press, New York, 1988

30. Marcus M: Regulation of myocardial perfusion in health and disease. Hosp Pract 22:105, 1988

31. Flamm SD, Taki J, Moore R et al: Redistribution of regional and organ blood flow volume and effect on cardiac function in relation to upright exercise intensity in healthy human subjects. Circulation 81:1550, 1990

32. Shepherd JT, Blomqvist CG, Lind AR et al: Static (isometric) exercise: retrospection and introspection. Circ Res 48 (suppl. I):I-179, 1981

33. Mitchell JH: Cardiovascular control during exercise: central and reflex neural mechanisms. Am J Cardiol 55:34D, 1985

34. Lakatta EG, Mitchell JH, Pomerance A, Rowe GG: Human aging: changes in structure and function. 18th Bethesda Conference Report. Cardiovascular Disease in the Elderly. J Am Coll Cardiol 10:42A, 1987

35. Lakatta EG: Determinants of cardiovascular performance. Modification due to aging. J Chronic Dis 36:15, 1983

36. Harris R: Cardiovascular disease in the elderly. Med Clin N Am 67:379, 1983

37. Zelis R, Longhurst J, Capone RJ, Mason DT: A comparison of regional blood flow and oxygen utilization during dynamic forearm exercise in normal subjects and patients with congestive heart failure. Circulation 50:137, 1974

38. Roubin GS, Anderson SD, Shen W et al: Hemodynamic and metabolic basis of impaired exercise tolerance in patients with severe left ventricular dysfunction. J Am Coll Cardiol 15:986, 1990

39. Engel PJ: Effort intolerance in chronic heart failure: what are we treating? J Am Coll Cardiol 15:995, 1990

40. Taylor HL, Buskirk E, Heschel A: Maximal oxygen intake as an objective measure of cardiorespiratory performance. J Appl Physiol 8:73, 1955

41. Sullivan MA, Froelicher V: Maximal oxygen uptake and gas exchange in coronary heart disease. J Cardiac Rehabil 3:549, 1983

42. Karlsson J, Astrand PO, Ekblom B: Training of the oxygen transport system in man. J Appl Physiol 22:1061, 1967

43. McDonough JR, Danielson RA, Willis RE, Vine DL: Maximal cardiac output during exercise in patients with coronary artery disease. Am J Cardiol 33:23, 1974

44. Whipp BJ: Dynamics of pulmonary gas exchange. Circulation 76:(suppl. VI):VI-18, 1987

45. Wasserman K: Dyspnea on exertion—is it the heart or the lungs? JAMA 248:2039, 1982

46. Graham TE: Lactate metabolism during submaximal and maximal exercise. Heart Failure 4:77, 1988

47. Wasserman K: Determinants and detection of anaerobic threshold and consequences of exercise above it. Circulation 76 (suppl. VI):VI-29, 1987

48. American College of Sports Medicine: Guidelines for Exercise Testing and Prescription. 3rd Ed. p. 157. Lea and Febiger, Philadelphia, 1986

49. Roberts JM, Sullivan MA, Froelicher VF et al: Predicting oxygen uptake from treadmill testing in normal subjects and coronary artery disease patients. Am Heart J 108:1454, 1984

50. Balady GJ, Weiner DA, Rose L, Ryan TJ: Physiologic responses to arm ergometry exercise relative to age and gender. J Am Coll Cardiol 16:130, 1990

51. Maron BJ: Structural features of the athletic heart as defined by echocardiography. J Am Coll Cardiol 7:191, 1986

52. Longhurst JC, Kelly AR, Gonyea WJ, Mitchell JH: Chronic training with static and dynamic arm exercise: cardiovascular adaptations and response to exercise. Circ Res (suppl I):48:I-171, 1988

53. Huston TP, Puffer JC, Rodney WM: The athletic heart syndrome. N Engl J Med 313:24, 1985

54. Graettinger WF: The cardiovascular response to chronic physical exertion and exercise training: An echocardiographic review. Am Heart J 108:1014, 1984

55. Morganroth J, Maron BJ, Henry W et al: Comparative left ventricular dimensions in trained athletes. Ann Intern Med 82:521, 1975

56. Hauser AM, Dressendorfer RH, Vos M et al: Symmetric cardiac enlargement in highly trained endurance athletes: a two-dimensional echocardiographic study. Am Heart J 109:1038, 1985

57. Ikaheimo MJ, Palatsi I, Takkunen JT: Noninvasive evaluation of the athletic heart syndrome: sprinters vs. endurance runners. Am J Cardiol 44:24, 1979

58. Longhurst JC, Kelly AR, Gonyea WJ, Mitchell JH: Echocardiographic left ventricular masses in distance runners and weightlifters. J Appl Physiol 48:154, 1980

59. Colan SD, Sanders SP, Borow KM: Physiologic hypertrophy: Effects on left ventricular systolic mechanics in athletes. J Am Coll Cardiol 9:776, 1987

60. Pearson AC, Schiff M, Mrosek D et al: Left ventricular diastolic function in weight lifters. Am J Cardiol 58:1254, 1986

61. Finkelhorr S, Hanak LJ, Bahler RC: Left ventricular filling in endurance trained subjects. J Am Coll Cardiol 8:289, 1986

62. Colan SD, Sanders SP, MacPherson D, Borow KM: Left ventricular diastolic function in elite athletes with physiologic cardiac hypertrophy. J Am Coll Cardiol 6:545, 1985

63. Fagard R, Vandenbroek E, Amery A: Left ventricular dynamics during exercise in elite marathon runners. J Am Coll Cardiol 14:112, 1989

64. Fagard R, Aubert A, Lysens R et al: Noninvasive assessment of seasonal variations in cardiac structure and function in cyclists. Circulation 167:896, 1983

65. Granger CB, Karimeddini MD, Smith BE et al: Rapid ventricular filling in left ventricular hypertrophy. I. Physiologic hypertrophy. J Am Coll Cardiol 5:862, 1985

66. Rerych SK, Scholz PM, Sabiston DC, Jones RH: Effects of exercise training on left ventricular function in normal subjects: A longitudinal study by radionuclide angiography. Am J Cardiol 45:244, 1980

67. Fizman E, Frank AG, Ben-Ari E et al: Altered left ventricular volume and ejection fraction responses to supine dynamic exercise in athletes. J Am Coll Cardiol 15:582, 1990

68. Carrio I, Serra-Grima R, Berna L et al: Transient alterations in cardiac performance after a six-hour race. Am J Cardiol 65:1471, 1990

69. Niemela KO, Palatsi AJ, Ikaheimo J et al: Evidence of impaired left ventricular performance after uninterrupted competitive 24-hour run. Circulation 70:350, 1984

70. Upton MT, Rerych SK, Roebach JR et al: Effect of brief and prolonged exercise on left ventricular function. Am J Cardiol 45:1154, 1980

71. Seals DA, Rogers MA, Yamamoto C et al: Left ventricular dysfunction after prolonged strenuous exercise in healthy subjects. Am J Cardiol 61:875, 1988

72. Douglas PS, O'Toole ML, Hiller DB et al: Cardiac fatigue after prolonged exercise. Circulation 76:1206, 1987

73. Ehsani AA, Hagberg JM, Hickson RC: Rapid changes in left ventricular dimensions and mass in response to physical conditioning and deconditioning. Am J Cardiol 42:52, 1978

74. Martin WH, Coyle EF, Bloomfield SA, Ehsani AA: Effects of physical deconditioning after intense endurance training on left ventricular dimensions and stroke volume. J Am Coll Cardiol 7:982, 1986

75. Scheuer J: Effects of physical training on myocardial vascularity and perfusion. Circulation 66:491, 1982

76. Ben-Ari E, Kellermann JJ, Rothbaum DA et al: Effect of prolonged intensive vs. moderate leg training in the untrained arm exercise response in angina pectoris. Am J Cardiol 59:231, 1987

77. Rogers MA, Yamamoto C, Hagberg JM et al: The effect of seven years of intense exercise training in patients with coronary artery disease. J Am Coll Cardiol 10:321, 1987

78. Ades PA, Grunvald MH, Weiss RM, Hanson JS: Usefulness of myocardial ischemia as predictor of training effect in cardiac rehabilitation after acute myocardial infarction or coronary artery bypass grafting. Am J Cardiol 63:1032, 1989

79. Raffo JA, Luksic IY, Kappagoda CT et al: Effects of physical training on myocardial ischemia in patients with coronary artery disease. Br Heart J 43:262, 1980

80. Schuler G, Schierf G, Wirth A et al: Low fat diet and regular supervised physical exercise in patients with symptomatic coronary artery disease: reduction of stress induced myocardial ischemia. Circulation 77:172, 1988

81. Bove AA, Dewey JD: Proximal coronary vasomotor reactivity after exercise training in dogs. Circulation 71:620, 1985

82. Ernst EEW, Matrai A: Intermittent claudication, exercise and blood rheology. Circulation 76:1110, 1987

83. Letcher RL, Pickering TG, Chien S et al: Effects of exercise on plasma viscosity in athletes and sedentary controls. Clin Cardiol 4:172, 1981

84. Eichner ER: Coagulability and rheology: hematologic benefits from exercise, fish and aspirin. Implications for athletes and nonathletes. Physician Sportsmed 14:102, 1986

85. Cooksey JD, Reilly P, Brown S et al: Exercise training and plasma catecholamines in patients

with ischemic heart disease. Am J Cardiol 42:372, 1978

86. Williams RS, Eden RS, Moll M et al: Mechanisms of training bradycardia: Studies of beta adrenergic receptors in man. J Appl Physiol 51:1232, 1981

87. Mann SJ, Krakoff OR, Felton K, Yeager K: Cardiovascular responses to infused epinephrine: effect of the state of physical conditioning. J Cardiovasc Pharmacol 6:339, 1984

88. Varnauskas E, Bergman H, Houk P, Bjorntorp P: Hemodynamic effects of physical training in coronary patients. Lancet ii:8, 1966

89. Detry JM, Rousseau M, Vandenbroucke G et al: Increased arterial venous oxygen difference after physical training in coronary heart disease. Circulation 44:109, 1971

90. Lec AP, Ice R, Blessey R, Sanmarco NE: Long term effects of physical training on coronary patients with impaired ventricular function. Circulation 56:375, 1987

91. Ehsani AA, Biello DR, Schultz J et al: Improvement of left ventricular contractile function by exercise training in patients with coronary artery disease. Circulation 74:350, 1986

92. Hagberg JM, Ehsani AA, Holloszy JO et al: Effect of 12 months of intense exercise training on stroke volume in patients with coronary artery disease. Circulation 67:1194, 1983

93. Paterson DH, Shephard RJ, Cunningham D et al: Effects of physical training on cardiovascular function following myocardial infarction. J Appl Physiol 47:482, 1979

94. Sullivan MA, Higginbotham MB, Cobb FR: Exercise training in patients with severe left ventricular dysfunction. Circulation 778:506, 1988

7

Excercise Testing: Basic Principles*

Barry A. Franklin, Ph.D.
Herman K. Hellerstein, M.D.
Seymour Gordon, M.D.
Gerald C. Timmis, M.D.

Exercise tests have immediate value in assessing functional capacity and the safety of physical exertion, as well as long-term prognostic significance in regard to morbidity and mortality.[1] The results may be used to determine the effects of interventions such as coronary artery bypass surgery (CABG), percutaneous transluminal coronary angioplasty (PTCA), medications, or physical training. Recent studies also indicate that success or failure of exercise training may be accurately predicted on the basis of clinical information, psychosocial data, and exercise-testing variables of cardiac dysfunction and physical fitness.[2]

The objective of exercise tests is to evaluate quantitatively the following variables: aerobic capacity of the body, i.e., the peak or maximal oxygen uptake ($\dot{V}o_2$max); hemodynamic changes as assessed by the heart rate and systolic and diastolic blood pressure responses; limiting clinical signs or symptoms (e.g., angina pectoris); and associated changes in the electrical function of the heart, especially supraventricular and ventricular arrhythmias and ST segment displacement.[3] Additional exercise-related parameters of function are presented in other chapters: myocardial perfusion (Ch. 9); myocardial metabolism (by positron emission tomography), magnetic resonance imaging (Ch. 15); wall movement, global and regional function, and ejection fraction by radionuclide-based exercise testing (Ch. 9), and exercise echocardiography (Ch. 10).

From the viewpoint of a World Health Organization (W.H.O.) Expert Committee on Rehabilitation, "the primary purpose of an exercise test is to determine the responses of the individual to efforts at given levels and from this information to estimate probable performance in specific life and occupational situations."[4] Exercise tests, although not necessarily predictive of circulatory responses in the world of work at equivalent energy levels, provide reasonable information about somatic and myocardial aerobic capacity and tolerance to increases in heart rate and blood pressure. However, some recreational and occupational situations may impose demands greater than those produced by peak effort in an exercise laboratory.

Clinical variables that should be monitored during exercise testing include blood pressure, heart rate, and multiple-lead electrocardiograms (ECGs), which increase sensitivity but may reduce specificity. Although the monitoring of 12 or more leads is recommended by some clinicians, we have found that recording 3 ECG leads is adequate for most situations and favor the precordial leads V_1 or V_2, V_5 or CM_5, and aVF—an approximate orthogonal lead system, equivalent to the Z, X, and Y vector leads, respectively. How-

* Supported in part by grants from the William Beaumont Hospital Research Institute (B.A.F.); grants from Mr. and Mrs. Leo Demsey, Mr. and Mrs. Harry E. Figgie, Jr., Dr. and Mrs. Benjamin Harlan, Mr. and Mrs. David Kangesser, Mr. and Mrs. Donald Krush, and Mr. and Mrs. Harry Mann; and grants from the U.S. Public Health Service to the Clinical Heart Center of Western Reserve University (HE 06304) and from the Rehabilitation Service Administration, Department of Health, Education and Welfare (grant 13-P-5738) and National Heart Institute (grant HE 07216) (H.K.H.).

ever, a single lead (V_5 or CM_5) will reveal ST segment depression in about 80% of all instances that have been detected with a multiple-lead system.[5] Unfortunately, there is no reliable relationship between the specific ECG leads that show ST segment depression and the anatomic localization of coronary artery stenosis. Thus, ST segment depression in the inferior leads, II, III, and aVF, does not necessarily reflect right coronary artery or circumflex artery stenosis.[6]

Other parameters of function include Borg's perceived-exertion ratings[7]; cardiac output determination by CO_2 rebreathing, nitrous oxide, impedance or other methods; the direct measurement of expired gases for submaximal and maximal oxygen uptake (Fig. 7-1); and gas exchange anaerobic threshold (AT) determinations.[8,9] The AT, signifying the peak work load or oxygen consumption at which oxygen demands

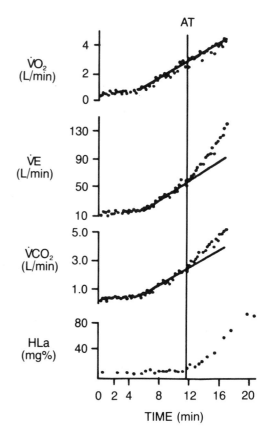

Fig. 7-2. Relationship between intensity of exercise (oxygen consumption, $\dot{V}O_2$) and simultaneous, abrupt nonlinear increases in serum lactate (HLa), CO_2 production ($\dot{V}CO_2$), and minute ventilation ($\dot{V}E$) occurring at the anaerobic threshold (AT). Exercise was initiated at minute 4. (Modified from Davis et al.,[10] with permission.)

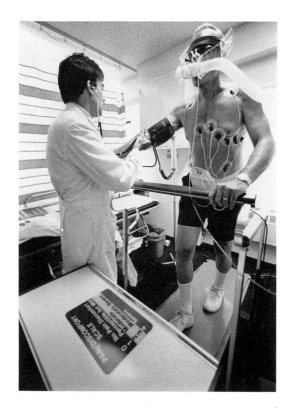

Fig. 7-1. Determination of oxygen consumption during exercise testing, using an automated metabolic measurement system (Medical Graphics 2001 CAD-NET).

exceed the circulation's ability to sustain aerobic metabolism, can be measured by detecting the work rate or oxygen consumption just below the disproportionate increase in minute ventilation ($\dot{V}E$) or CO_2 production ($\dot{V}CO_2$) (Fig. 7-2).[10] An increase in the ventilatory equivalent for oxygen ($\dot{V}E/\dot{V}O_2$) during exercise, without a corresponding change in the ventilatory equivalent for CO_2 ($\dot{V}E/\dot{V}CO_2$), has also been reported to be a sensitive and reliable noninvasive technique for determining the AT (Fig. 7-3).[11]

Informed consent prior to the exercise test, safety precautions, trained personnel, a defibrillator, and emergency equipment are essential

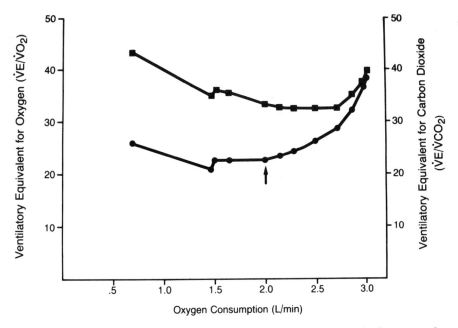

Fig. 7-3. Ventilatory equivalent for oxygen (●) and carbon dioxide (■) as a function of oxygen consumption for one subject. Arrow indicates ventilatory threshold, which occurred at 67% of the maximal oxygen consumption.

when evaluating the patient with documented or suspected coronary heart disease (CHD). The purpose of the consent form is to ensure that the patient is aware of the risk of complications (albeit small) during exercise testing (see Ch. 32 appendixes). Following performance of the exercise test, the subject should not leave the premises until the heart rate, blood pressure, and ECG variables have returned to a "normal" range, based on pretest levels.

DIAGNOSTIC EXERCISE TESTING

Recently, the need for submaximal[12] or maximal exercise testing as a screening procedure before asymptomatic adults undertake exercise has been questioned. Sox et al.[13] suggested that exercise testing might be justifiable for screening asymptomatic adults who have at least one coronary risk factor or a total cholesterol/HDL cholesterol ratio greater than 6.0. However, Ekelund et al.[14] reported that abnormal results at exercise testing, even in a hypercholesterolemic popula-

tion, still had a very low predictive value. A joint report by the American College of Cardiology and the American Heart Association[15] states that "exercise testing is of little or no value, inappropriate, or contraindicated" for "asymptomatic, apparently healthy men or women with no risk factors for CAD [coronary artery disease]." The report further states that there are no conditions, in apparently healthy individuals, in which "there is general agreement that exercise testing is justified." Critics emphasize that the cost of mass screenings of all sedentary adults in the United States (60 to 70 million persons) would be prohibitive and that the incidence of exercise-related cardiovascular complications in presumably healthy adults is extremely low.[16,17] Moreover, false-positive exercise tests are not uncommon in asymptomatic populations. Consequently, diagnostic exercise tests should be administered and interpreted on the basis of knowledge about the prevalence of CHD in that population.

Bayes' theorem states that the likelihood that a positive test represents true disease is directly related to the prevalence of the disease in the population being evaluated. Accordingly, in populations in which the actual prevalence of CHD is low, for example in relatively young, asymptomatic persons with no coronary risk factors, an abnormal (positive) test is much more likely to be a false-positive test than is a truly abnormal test in a population with a high prevalence of disease (e.g., older men with multiple risk factors or with chest pain). It is important, therefore, to assess the patient's pretest likelihood of having CHD.

Estimating the Pretest Likelihood of CHD

Clinicians now use three variables, age, sex, and symptoms, to estimate a person's pretest risk of CHD.[18] The likelihood of disease may be even further defined by complementary information regarding blood pressure, smoking status, and serum cholesterol profile.

In general, the risk of CHD increases with advancing age. Moreover, at any age, men are at a higher risk than are women. Persons who have anginal symptoms also have a greater pretest probability of CHD than those who are free of symptoms. For example, an asymptomatic 45-year-old woman has only a 1% chance of having significant CHD (Table 7-1).[18] A 55-year-old man with chest pain atypical for angina pectoris has a 59% pretest probability of CHD, whereas a 65-year-old man with typical angina pectoris has a very high (94%) pretest risk of CHD.

Determining the Post-test Likelihood of CHD

The results of the exercise test are considered together with the pretest risk to determine the post-test likelihood of CHD. When a person's pretest risk of CHD is either very high or very low, a normal or abnormal exercise ECG response will have little impact on the post-test likelihood of coronary disease. Thus, for the above-referenced 45-year-old woman or 65-year-old man, an exercise ECG would be of limited additional value in the diagnosis of CHD. On the other hand, when a person's pretest risk of CHD is in the intermediate range (i.e., in the 30 to 70% range of pretest probability), the exercise test result may substantially alter the post-test likelihood of coronary disease.[19] For example, the 55-year-old man with chest pain atypical for angina pectoris has an approximately 59% likelihood of having significant CHD before any testing is done ("pretest likelihood of disease"). After an exercise ECG, his likelihood of having significant CHD ("post-test likelihood of disease") changes to about 90% if the ECG is abnormal, demonstrating significant ST segment depression, and to about 30% if the ECG is normal (Fig. 7-4).[20] Thus, by applying Bayesian analysis to the conventional exercise ECG, the need for additional diagnostic studies (e.g., coronary angiography) can be more intelligently defined.

Guidelines for Preliminary Screening of Physically Active Adults

Although moderate exercise (intensity of 40 to 60% of $\dot{V}o_2max$) is safe for most individuals, it is desirable for some persons to have at least a limited health appraisal, physical examination, or both, before starting a vigorous (intensity of >60% of $\dot{V}o_2max$) exercise regimen. For many adults, the pretraining evaluation can be done by

Table 7-1.   Pretest Likelihood (%) of CHD in Patients by Age, Sex, and Symptoms

Age (yrs)	Asymptomatic		Nonanginal Chest Pain		Atypical Angina		Typical Angina	
	Men	Women	Men	Women	Men	Women	Men	Women
35	1.9	0.3	5.2	0.8	21.8	4.2	69.7	25.8
45	5.5	1.0	14.1	2.8	46.1	13.3	87.3	55.2
55	9.7	3.2	21.5	8.4	58.9	32.4	92.0	79.4
65	12.3	7.5	28.1	18.6	67.1	54.4	94.3	90.6

(Adapted from Diamond and Forrester,[18] with permission.)

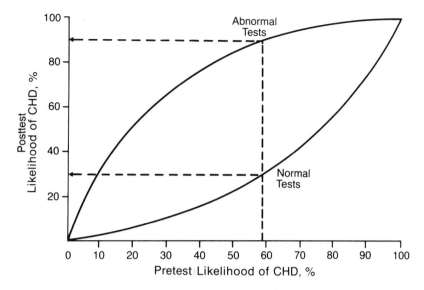

Fig. 7-4. Impact of 59% likelihood of CHD on post-test likelihood of disease when exercise ECG is normal (30%) or abnormal (90%). The sensitivity of the exercise ECG is 75% and its specificity is 85%. (Modified from Epstein,[20] with permission.)

allied health professionals in nonmedical settings. On the other hand, a medical evaluation generally includes three major components: the medical history, physical examination, and laboratory tests. Age, sex, health (disease) status, presence of symptoms and/or major coronary risk factors, and intensity characteristics of the planned exercise program are factors that determine the extent of evaluation required and the need for exercise testing.

To provide general guidance on preliminary screening procedures for participation in an exercise program, the American College of Sports Medicine[21] suggests that it is desirable for some individuals to have a medical examination and diagnostic exercise test (Table 7-2). This guideline applies to apparently healthy persons at or above age 40 for men and age 50 for women, or higher-risk individuals of any age, who plan to begin vigorous exercise. These screening pro-

Table 7-2.   Guidelines for Preliminary Screening for Exercise Participation

	Apparently Healthy		Higher Risk[b]		
	Younger[a]	Older	No symptoms	Symptoms	With Disease[c]
Medical examination and diagnostic exercise test recommended prior to:					
Moderate exercise[d]	No[e]	No	No	Yes	Yes
Vigorous exercise[d]	No	Yes[e]	Yes	Yes	Yes

[a] Men ≤40 years; women ≤50 years.
[b] Persons with two or more major coronary risk factors or symptoms.
[c] Persons with known cardiac, pulmonary, or metabolic disease.
[d] Moderate exercise: exercise intensity, 40 to 60% $\dot{V}O_2max$; vigorous exercise: exercise intensity, >60% $\dot{V}O_2max$.
[e] The "no" responses indicates that a medical examination and diagnostic exercise test are generally "not necessary"; however, it does not mean that these procedures should not be done. A "yes" response means that preliminary screening is recommended.
(Adapted from American College of Sports Medicine,[21] with permission.)

cedures are also advocated for symptomatic high-risk individuals who plan to initiate moderate intensity exercise. A thorough medical evaluation is recommended before starting any physical training program, regardless of the anticipated exercise intensity, for all individuals with known cardiovascular, pulmonary, or metabolic disease.

CONTRAINDICATIONS TO EXERCISE TESTING

Exercise testing is warranted (in the absence of contraindications) when it is clinically important to obtain quantitation of cardiovascular status, including associated changes in electrical functions of the heart, from the early stages of a coronary event (e.g., a few days following acute myocardial infarction) to later in convalescence and recovery.

There are, however, certain patients for whom the risks of exercise testing may outweigh the potential information that might be gained. Accord-

Table 7-3.   Absolute Contraindications to Exercise Testing

A recent significant change in the resting ECG suggesting myocardial infarction or other acute coronary events

Recent complicated myocardial infarction

Unstable angina pectoris

Uncontrolled ventricular arrhythmia

Uncontrolled atrial arrhythmia that compromises cardiac function

Third-degree atrioventricular block (without pacemaker)

Acute congestive heart failure

Severe aortic stenosis

Suspected or known dissecting aortic aneurysm

Active or suspected myocarditis or pericarditis

Thrombophlebitis or intracardiac thrombi

Recent systemic or pulmonary embolus

Acute infection

Significant emotional distress (psychosis)

(Adapted from American College of Sports Medicine,[21] with permission.)

ingly, patients with absolute contraindications (Table 7-3)[21] should not be tested, unless the test is conducted to determine the need for or potential benefit of additional immediate interventions, such as cardiac catheterization or drug therapy. For example, exercise testing of the convalescing patient with "uncomplicated" myocardial infarction is now used not only to assess a patient's functional status, but also as a diagnostic, prognostic, and therapeutic guide. Relative contraindications to exercise testing, such as resting systolic or diastolic hypertension (>200 mmHg or >120 mmHg respectively), moderately severe valvular heart disease, cardiomyopathy, electrolyte abnormalities (e.g., hypokalemia, hypomagnesemia), serious supraventricular or ventricular arrhythmias, left main coronary arterial obstruction, uncontrolled metabolic disease (e.g., diabetes, thyrotoxicosis), and chronic infectious disease (e.g., mononucleosis, hepatitis) can be superseded under certain circumstances, if appropriate precautions are taken.

ECG RESPONSES TO EXERCISE TESTING

ECG responses to exercise tests should be interpreted according to the type and degree of ST segment displacement and the presence of supraventricular and ventricular arrhythmias. Recent studies indicate that computer analysis of ECG ST segment depression may significantly increase the diagnostic and prognostic accuracy of exercise test results.[22] Other aspects of the exercise ECG that merit attention range from U wave inversion, which may indicate myocardial ischemia and significant stenosis of the left anterior descending coronary artery,[23] to an increase of R wave amplitude.[24] Such information is useful in evaluating the effects of selected clinical interventions, for example, CABG, PTCA, medications, or physical training.

ST Segment Depression

The interpretation of exercise-induced myocardial ischemia has historically relied on the presence of three types of ST segment depression: horizontal (Fig. 7-5), down-sloping, and slowly up-sloping. However, normal (or negative) tests are often considered "inconclusive" when the peak heart rate achieved is less than 85% of the predicted maximum, because of inadequate cardiac stress.[25]

Current consensus considers an abnormal ECG response as 1.0 mm or more of horizontal or down-sloping ST segment depression at 80 msec beyond the J point. In a meta-analysis of 22 years of research data from laboratories worldwide, the mean sensitivity of this criterion was 68% and the specificity was 77%.[26] For detection of multivessel coronary disease, the sensitivity was 81% and the specificity was 66%. In contrast, slowly up-sloping ST segment depression is considered a weaker indicator of myocardial ischemia and may

be classified as normal or abnormal by several methods of assessing ST segment displacement.[1,3]

Methods of Assessing ST Segment Displacement

ST segment displacement can be quantitated manually or more precisely with the aid of a computer. Four methods are commonly used to assess its magnitude: ST junction (STJ) and ST segment method; ST segment index; ST depression 80 msec after STJ; and the ST area displacement method. The methodology for each technique is described below, with specific citation of measurement criteria and categorization of normal and abnormal responses. In addition, two as yet not validated methods designed to improve the diagnostic accuracy of ST depression analysis by using heart rate adjustment are also presented, i.e., ST/heart rate slope[27] and ST/heart rate index.[28]

STJ and ST Segment Method.   In an STJ and ST slope plot,[29] the STJ displacement is measured in millimeters from the reference level of the end of the P-R segment of two consecutive beats. The slope of the first 80 msec of the ST segment is expressed in millivolts per second. Lester et al.[29] plotted the slope and STJ displacement and classified zones of normal, borderline, and abnormal responses (Fig. 7-6). Normal responses show a marked increase in ST slope that exceeds the STJ with increasing levels of effort. Abnormal STJ displacement is 0.1 mV or more with a zero or negative slope. The responses during multistage exercise tests can be plotted to determine the levels of effort at which borderline or abnormal responses occur. The ECGs of follow-up tests can be evaluated in the same manner and comparison made for the same leads at identical workloads. Deterioration of exercise ECGs can be judged by a change in category.

ST Segment Index.   The ST segment index is the algebraic sum of the STJ depression in millimeters and the ST slope in millivolts per second (mV/sec). To determine the ST segment index, a baseline ECG is first established from three consecutive QRS complexes in which the P-R interval is on the same isoelectric line.[30] The ST slope and depression can be calculated manually using

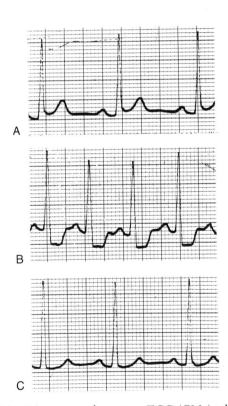

Fig. 7-5. **(A)** A patient's resting ECG (CM$_5$) taken before exercise testing. **(B)** ECG obtained after several minutes of an exercise test showing significant ST segment depression (3 to 4 mm). **(C)** Resting ECG recorded 6 minutes after exercise, representative of a "normal" configuration.

ST Segment Slope
mV/sec

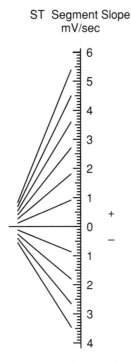

Fig. 7-6. Transparent overlay used to quantitate ST segment slope (millivolts per second, mV/sec) and depression (millimeters). (Modified from Lester et al.,[29] with permission.)

the transparent overlay shown in Figure 7-6.[29,31] ST segment depression is the distance in millimeters from the baseline to the J point. The ST slope is measured by forming a tangent from two points: the J point and 80 msec past the J point. The tangent is extended 2.5 cm (1 second) from the intersect, and the slope is read in millivolts per second. An ST segment index of zero or less is considered to be abnormal, assuming that the magnitude of the ST segment depression is at least 1.0 mm (Fig. 7-7).[30]

ST Segment Depression 80 msec after STJ. Technical problems in obtaining noise-free ECG recordings may make it difficult to obtain quantitative measurements of the ST slope. An alternative method that attains acceptable accuracy is measurement of the magnitude of ST depression at 0.08 seconds after the J junction. Degrees of ST segment depression can be classified as 0.5 mm, ≥1.0 mm, ≥1.5 mm, ≥2.0 mm, and so forth.

In sinus tachycardia, the duration of the ST segment is reduced so that ST displacement at 80 msec after STJ falls on the ascending limb of the T wave. In such cases, the displacement of the end of the ST segment, that is, before the onset of the T wave, can be used. This has been designated the "ST bar" and has been found to occur at approximately one-eighth of the R-R interval from the onset of the QRS complex. The same criteria for abnormality of the ST bar apply as in ST depression 80 msec after STJ.

ST Area Displacement Method. The area below the reference level can be measured precisely by computer; it can be measured less precisely, but still adequately, by estimating the number of millimeter squares in the area below the reference level (Fig. 7-8). Each millimeter square equals 4 μV-sec. An ST-T area of approximately 8 μV-sec or more is considered abnormal.[32]

Characteristics of Exercise-Induced ST Segment Depression that Increase the Likelihood of CHD

The degree and type of ST segment depression, as well as its time of onset, persistence, and accompanying symptoms, all appear to have diagnostic value. Silent ischemia (ST segment depression without angina) carries a better long-term prognosis than does ST segment depression with concomitant angina pectoris.[33,34] In general, the more pronounced the exercise-induced ST segment depression, the greater the likelihood of significant CHD. Moreover, downsloping ST segment depression is associated with a higher incidence of subsequent coronary events than either the horizontal or up-sloping pattern. A graver prognosis is also evident when the ST segment depression evolves into a down-sloping pattern during recovery than when the ST abnormality becomes up-sloping. Significant ST segment depression that occurs early in a test protocol (i.e., Bruce stage I or II), at relatively low heart rates (e.g., less than 130 beats/min), and/or that persists several minutes into recovery is also suggestive of severe coronary disease and an unfavorable prognosis.[35,36]

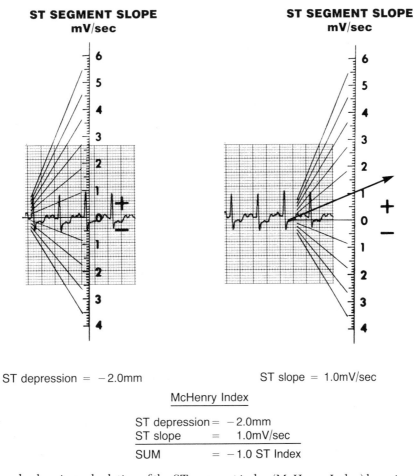

Fig. 7-7. Example showing calculation of the ST segment index (McHenry Index) by using a transparent overlay to determine the ST segment slope and depression. Abnormal ECG response with up-sloping ST segment depression is shown.

Relating ST Segment Depression to Heart Rate

Although simple measurement of the magnitude of exercise-induced ST segment depression has been the traditional diagnostic benchmark, several recent studies[27,37–39] have claimed that the ST segment/heart rate (ST/HR) slope, a method that normalizes the degree of exercise-induced ST segment depression for corresponding increases in heart rate, more accurately reflects the balance between myocardial oxygen supply and demand than does the ST segment index or 1.0-mm ST segment depression relative to rest. This physiologic approach seems justified in that there appears to be little reason why 1.0 mm of ST seg-

ment depression in a patient who exercises to a peak heart rate of 160 beats/min should be taken as a reflection of more ischemia than 0.5 mm of ST segment depression occurring in another patient who achieves a peak heart rate of only 80 beats/min.

Analysis of the rate-related change in exercise-induced ST segment depression, the ST/HR slope, has significantly improved the accuracy of the exercise ECG. Kligfield et al.[37], using an ST/HR slope value of 11 mm/bpm/1,000 (1.1 μV/bpm) as an upper limit of normal, improved the exercise test sensitivity from 57 to 91% in patients with stable angina pectoris, while preserving the specificity of the test at more than 90%.

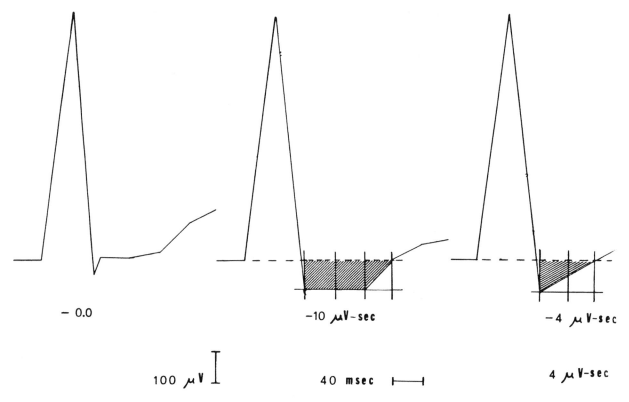

Fig. 7-8. ST-T area displacement method. On the left there is no depression of the ST interval. In the center there is a depressed ST area of exactly 2.5 squares, corresponding to 2.5 units on standard chart paper. At 4 μV-seconds per square unit, this equals − 10 μV-seconds. On the right there is a depressed ST area equal to exactly half of 2 square units (equal to − 4 μV-seconds). (From Sheffield et al.,[32] with permission.)

In addition, an ST/HR slope value of 60 mm/bpm/1,000 (6.0 μV/bpm) was found to partition patients with and without three-vessel CHD with a sensitivity of 78%, a specificity of 97%, a positive predictive value of 93%, and an overall test accuracy of 90%. In contrast, Lachterman et al.[28] found that the ST/HR index did not improve the diagnostic accuracy of the exercise ECG for identifying the presence or severity of CHD relative to standard visual criteria, 1.0 mm ST segment depression relative to rest. The change in heart rate, delta heart rate (ΔHR) was calculated as the standing preexercise heart rate subtracted from the maximal heart rate value during exercise.[28] The ST segment measurements were made at the J junction. The J junction was used to avoid overlap with the T wave at high heart

rates, although little change in classification occurred between the J point and at 70 msec later.[40] Furthermore, Kligfield et al.[41] showed only an insignificant difference between the results of the ST/HR slope and the ST/HR index method of Lachterman et al.[28]

In a thoughtful editorial on the academic life cycle of a noninvasive test, Pryor commented that "refinement in exercise testing techniques that solve all clinical problems in evaluating patients with coronary disease should be greeted with appropriate skepticism by practicing clinicians."[42] Wise advice has been given that clinicians should not replace standard proven criteria with a measurement whose performance has not been definitively demonstrated to provide improvement.[43] New techniques, such as ST/HR index or

ST/HR slope, must be validated before they are given widespread application.[43,44]

Uninterpretable ST Segment Depression

In the context of digitalis therapy, left ventricular hypertrophy, left bundle branch block, or preexcitation (Wolff-Parkinson-White [WPW]) syndromes, ST segment abnormalities that develop during exercise are often uninterpretable as evidence of myocardial ischemia.[45,46] Other conditions that preclude reliable diagnostic ECG information from exercise testing include physiologic rate-adaptive pacing and, in some cases, extensive anterior wall myocardial infarction.[21] Additional factors that may contribute to spurious ST segment depression are anemia, hypokalemia, alkalosis, mitral valve prolapse, and selected other valvular and congenital heart diseases.[47] Diuretic drugs (because of their potential to cause hypokalemia),[48] digitalis preparations,[49] and estrogen therapy,[50] may also cause "positive tests" in the absence of significant CHD. Although exercise-induced ST segment changes in the inferior and right precordial leads are difficult to interpret in the presence of right bundle branch block, the lateral precordial leads (V_4 to V_6) may provide a reliable indication of myocardial ischemia.[51] When substantial ST segment depression is present at rest, an additional 1.0 mm of depression is required as evidence of myocardial ischemia.[52]

Influence of Medications

For initial diagnostic exercise testing, it is helpful to have the patient discontinue the use of prescribed cardiovascular medications if there are no anticipated adverse effects from so doing. Beta-blocking drugs and other antianginal medications often prevent the patient from attaining the desired level of cardiac work, resulting in a reduced peak rate–pressure product and a higher prevalence of false-negative responses.[53] Patients who take intermediate- or high-dose beta-blocking agents should taper their medication over several days to minimize hyperadrenergic withdrawal responses.[21] However, it is generally recom-

mended that a beta-blocking agent not be withdrawn in patients with significant CHD.

Although the effect of a single morning dose of a "long-acting" beta-blocking drug may persist throughout the day, the reduction in exercise heart rate and blood pressure is not necessarily uniform over time. Atenolol, for example, has a maximal effect between 2 and 4 hours after ingestion. Consequently, early-morning exercise testing may result in attenuated hemodynamic and ECG responses relative to those obtained during the late afternoon. To test this hypothesis, Timmis et al.[54] subjected 18 coronary patients (mean age, 54 years) receiving a low dose (25 to 50 mg) of atenolol daily (in the morning) to morning and late afternoon exercise tests (Bruce protocol). The mean peak exercise duration for these tests was similar, 11.2 and 11.5 minutes, respectively; however, peak exercise heart rates were uniformly higher for afternoon testing (range, 5 to 35 beats/min, mean, 19 beats/min). Moreover, 5 of the 18 patients (28%) demonstrated at least 1 mm of ST segment depression, anginal symptoms, or both, only during afternoon testing (Fig. 7-9A and B). The authors concluded that discordant ischemic responses to afternoon and morning exercise testing may occur in patients on once-daily beta-blocking drugs.

Calcium channel-blocking[55] and nitrate drugs[56] may increase the exercise duration or work load required to elicit abnormal ST segment depression or angina pectoris; in some cases, such drugs may prevent the appearance of these signs and symptoms. If the purpose of the test is to establish a diagnosis of CHD, these drugs should be withheld, if clinically feasible, for at least 12 hours.

In patients taking digoxin, it is best to discontinue the drug for at least 10 to 14 days before "diagnostic" exercise testing, provided there are no clinical contraindications.[45]

ST Segment Elevation

Exercise-induced ST segment elevation in leads displaying evidence of a previous Q wave infarction almost always reflects an aneurysm or a wall motion abnormality.[57] In the absence of

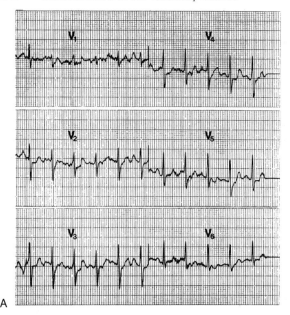

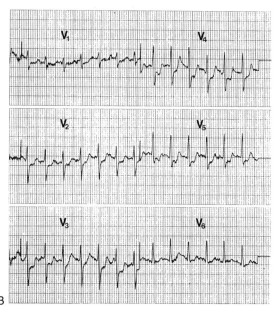

significant Q waves or Prinzmetal's angina, exercise-induced ST segment elevation is often associated with a fixed, high-grade coronary stenosis corresponding to the site of ischemia seen on ECG.[25] In addition, this finding appears to represent more severe ischemia than ST segment depression, reflecting transmural as opposed to subendocardial myocardial ischemia.[58]

Changes in R Wave Amplitude with Exercise

An increase in the R wave amplitude with exercise has been suggested as indicative of myocardial ischemia in patients with CHD. Failure of the ischemic ventricular myocardium to decrease its volume during exercise has been thought to account for the increase of the R wave (Brody effect).[59] Normal subjects generally show an increase in R wave amplitude during submaximal exercise, with a decrease at maximal exercise.[60] In contrast, increases of more than 1 mm in the R waves of multiple ECG leads after exercise have been reported in a large percentage of patients with CHD.[61] Recent studies, however, involving several lead systems, sympathetic stimulation or beta blockade,[62] different clinical subsets of patients, and varied classification criteria suggest that numerous factors can affect the R wave amplitude response to exercise.[60] Thus, this finding does not appear to have diagnostic significance, except perhaps in the interpretation of equivocal ST segment depression or as an indicator of myocardial ischemia in left bundle branch block.[21]

Supraventricular and Ventricular Arrhythmias

Isolated atrial or ventricular ectopic beats and short runs of supraventricular tachycardia commonly occur during exercise testing and do not appear to have diagnostic or prognostic significance for CHD. Moreover, frequent or repetitive exercise-induced ventricular ectopic beats in older, asymptomatic individuals without apparent heart disease do not predict increased cardiac

Fig. 7-9. (A) Precordial leads in a 55-year-old coronary patient (receiving 50 mg of atenolol once a day in the morning) who was asymptomatic at maximal exertion during morning exercise testing. The peak heart rate was 125 beats/min, and the ECG revealed no significant ST segment depression. **(B)** Precordial leads at maximal exercise for the same patient, 3 days later, at the identical maximal work load and exercise duration during late afternoon testing. The peak heart rate was 153 beats/min. The patient reported moderate chest pain; significant ST segment depression is apparent.

morbidity or mortality and therefore do not require antiarrhythmic drug therapy.[63] Ventricular arrhythmias during exercise increase as a function of age (15 to 35% of men younger than 35 years have such rhythms, compared with 50 to 60% of men between 45 and 55 years).[64] Califf et al.[65] showed that the suppression of resting ventricular arrhythmias during exercise does not exclude the presence of underlying CHD; conversely, premature ventricular beats that increase in frequency, complexity, or both, do not necessarily signify underlying CHD. On the other hand, frequent paired or multiform ventricular premature beats, salvos, or ventricular tachycardia occur more commonly in coronary patients and at significantly lower heart rates than in persons without heart disease.[66] *Such complex forms of ventricular ectopy are more likely to be associated with significant CHD and a poor prognosis if they occur in the presence of ischemic ST segment depression.*[25,36] Since these high-grade ventricular arrhythmias may be harbingers of ventricular fibrillation, exercise should be terminated and antiarrhythmic therapy should be considered.

HEMODYNAMIC RESPONSES

Although the ST segment response was once the primary, and often the sole, criterion for assessing effort-induced myocardial ischemia, evaluation of hemodynamic responses (i.e., heart rate and blood pressure) during exercise has been shown to enhance the predictive value of exercise testing.[67]

Heart Rate

The "normal" heart rate response to progressive exercise is a relatively linear increase, corresponding to 8 to 12 beats/MET for sedentary subjects.[68] A patient with a markedly blunted heart rate response to exercise is said to have "chronotropic incompetence" or "sustained relative bradycardia." This is identified by a peak exercise heart rate that is two standard deviations

or greater below the age-predicted maximal heart rate for normal subjects.[69-71] Chronotropic incompetence during exercise, even in the absence of significant ST segment depression, has been related to left ventricular dysfunction, multivessel CHD, and a higher incidence of subsequent coronary events.[72]

The age-predicted maximal heart rate can be estimated in one of the following two ways: $220 - $ age in years or $215 - (0.66 \times$ age in years).[73] Since the maximal heart rate normally decreases with age, impairment of chronotropic capacity due to heart disease and/or medications can be calculated by the following formula:

$$\text{Percent chronotropic impairment} = \frac{a - b}{a} \times 100$$

where a is age-predicted maximal heart rate and b is heart rate attained at peak or maximal effort.

Blood Pressure

There is a linear increase in the systolic blood pressure with increasing levels of dynamic exercise, approximating 8 to 12 mmHg/MET, with maximal values typically reaching 180 to 220 mmHg.[68] At peak exercise, however, systolic blood pressure often levels off or even declines. Maximal systolic blood pressure values may vary considerably depending on age, weight, medications, fitness, and gender. For example, many young adult women show normal peak systolic blood pressure values of 160 mmHg or less. In contrast, diastolic pressure usually falls slightly or remains unchanged; thus, pulse pressure increases in direct proportion to the intensity of exercise. An exercise-induced increase of more than 15 mmHg in diastolic pressure, using the disappearance of sound—the fifth Korotkoff—rather than the fourth muffling sound, is associated with a greater prevalence and severity of CHD and left ventricular dysfunction, independent of ischemic ST segment depression.[74] The mechanism underlying the increase in diastolic pressure with exercise is unknown.

Although patients with hypertension generally

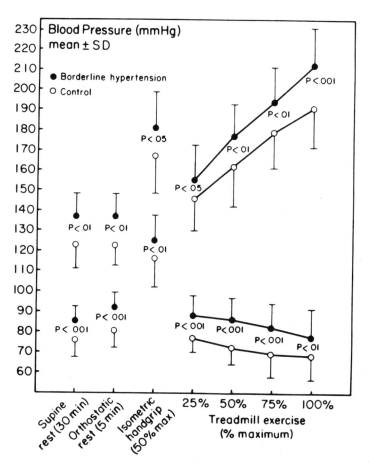

Fig. 7-10. Systolic and diastolic blood pressure responses in normal and borderline hypertensive young men during supine rest, orthostatic stress, isometric exertion, and increasing percentages of maximum treadmill exercise capacity. (From Hanson et al.,[78] with permission.)

show higher than normal systolic and diastolic blood pressure values during exercise, most studies report no difference in the relative blood pressure increase from rest between subjects with mild hypertension and normotensive control subjects.[75–77] In other words, it appears that blood pressure is simply "reset" and maintained at higher levels, regardless of whether the subject is at rest, or performing isometric handgrip or treadmill exercise at varying percentages of maximal capacity (Fig. 7-10).[78] Other patients with mild hypertension may demonstrate a normalization of blood pressure during exercise compared with resting values. This phenomenon is presumably attributable to metabolic vasodila-

tion, which transiently lowers an elevated resting peripheral resistance.

The peak systolic blood pressure achieved during exercise appears to be prognostically significant. In a cohort of 1,586 men with CHD, Irving and associates[79] showed a negative correlation between the maximal systolic blood pressure during exercise and the annual rate of sudden cardiac death (Table 7-4). Others have confirmed that exertional hypotension, defined as an exercise-induced decrease in systolic blood pressure (≥ 10 mmHg) or a failure of systolic pressure to rise above 130 mmHg with exercise, is associated with abnormal left ventricular contractility, myocardial ischemia or prior myocardial infarction,

Table 7-4. Relation between Maximal Exercise Systolic Pressure and Annual Rate of Sudden Cardiac Death

Maximal Systolic Pressure (mmHg)	Annual Rate of Sudden Death (per 1,000)
<140	97.0
140–199	25.3
>200	6.6

(From Irving et al.,[79] with permission.)

and a 3.2-fold increased risk of coronary events at 2-year follow-up.[80–87]

The postexercise systolic blood pressure response has also been proposed as a highly sensitive and specific index for diagnosing CHD. Amon et al.[83] reported that some patients have recovery values of systolic blood pressure that exceed those measured at peak exercise. In their study, ratios of early-recovery systolic blood pressure to peak-exercise systolic blood pressure were more sensitive than were ECG changes and angina in identifying patients with severe angiographically documented CHD. Moreover, Kato et al.[84] reported that an abnormal postexercise systolic blood pressure response was the strongest predictor of subsequent cardiac mortality in persons surviving an acute myocardial infarction. Patients with an abnormal hemodynamic response to treadmill exercise testing, defined as a systolic blood pressure recovery ratio greater than 0.9, were more likely to have exercise-induced myocardial ischemia, left ventricular dysfunction, and extensive coronary artery lesions. On the other hand, with bicycle ergometer exercise testing, ST segment depression seems more accurate than the systolic blood pressure ratio in diagnosing CHD.[85]

Myocardial Aerobic Impairment

The percent of myocardial aerobic impairment (MAI) can be calculated by relating the product of the individual's heart rate (HR) and systolic blood pressure (SBP) (HR × SBP) at peak effort to values for healthy individuals of the same age and sex.[86]

The experience of Bruce et al.[87] was that age-predicted maximal $[(HR \times SBP)/100](Y)$ can be calculated from the formula $Y = 364 - (0.58 \times$ age in years).

Percentage MAI =

$$= \frac{\text{age-predicted maximal } (HR \times SBP)}{-\text{ attained maximal } (HR \times SBP)} \times 100$$

For example, if a 50-year-old man develops a peak heart rate of 145 beats/min and a systolic blood pressure of 180 mmHg at symptom-limited peak exercise performance, with a $\dot{V}O_2max$ of 24.5 ml/kg/min, his functional aerobic impairment (FAI) is 31.2%; i.e., $[(35.6 - 24.5)/35.6] \times 100$. His percent MAI is 22.1%, i.e., $[(335 - 261)/335] \times 100 = 22.1\%$. This degree of MAI becomes more meaningful when his maximal $(HR \times SBP)/100$ double product or calculated myocardial oxygen consumption $(M\dot{V}O_2)$, expressed as milliliters of oxygen per 100 grams of left ventricle per minute, is related to body $\dot{V}O_2$ and to that of a healthy man his age, that is, a $\dot{V}O_2max$ of 35.6 ml/kg/min. Myocardial oxygen consumption is estimated from two of its major hemodynamic determinants, HR and SBP, where $M\dot{V}O_2 = (0.14 \times HR \times SBP) - 6.3$ $(r = 0.92)$.[88,89] The ratio of the maximal $(HR \times SBP)/100$ product to $\dot{V}O_2$ of the patient is $261/24.5 = 10.7$, and that of a healthy man his age is $335/35.6 = 9.4$. The ratios of calculated $M\dot{V}O_2/\dot{V}O_2$ are $30.24/2.45 = 12.3$ and $40.6/3.56 = 11.4$, respectively.

RATING OF PERCEIVED EXERTION

Because of the considerable variance in maximal heart rate for any given age (standard deviation, ± 10 beats/min), it is helpful to evaluate perceived effort during exercise testing to assess whether maximal physical exertion is being approached. This may be even more important if patients are taking medications that attenuate the chronotropic response to exercise (e.g., beta-blocking drugs). The concept of perceived effort during exercise was first introduced by Borg,[7] who subsequently developed the category and category-ratio perceived exertion scales illustrated in Figure 7-11 to quantify subjective exercise intensity.[90]

The category scale includes 15 progressive numeric levels, ranging from 6 to 20, with descriptive "effort ratings" at every odd number. Numerous studies have shown the rating of perceived exertion (RPE) to be highly correlated with several exercise variables such as power output, oxygen uptake, and heart rate, particularly when these variables are expressed as percent-ages of their respective maxima.[91] Among healthy young individuals, the RPE often approximates 1/10 of the heart rate response to exercise.

During most exercise tests, the category RPE scale provides a valid and reliable index of impending fatigue. Most individuals rate the anaerobic or ventilatory threshold (~70% $\dot{V}O_2$max) as "somewhat hard" to "hard" (RPE, 13 to 16) and reach volitional fatigue at perceived exertion ratings of 17 to 19 ("very hard" to "very, very hard").[3,21] However, in clinical experience, 5 to 10% of persons unfamiliar with the scale, as well

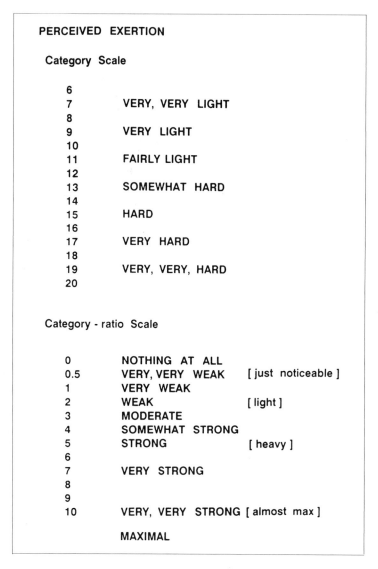

Fig. 7-11. Perceived exertion scales with descriptive "effort ratings." (From Borg,[90] with permission.)

as those with certain personality types (e.g., extreme "type A" individuals), tend to suppress RPE below expected levels. Maximal exercise ratings of 13 to 16 ("somewhat hard" to "hard") are not uncommon for such persons, despite severe fatigue and physiologic evidence that true maximal effort has been achieved (e.g., a respiratory exchange ratio > 1.15, a heart rate that exceeds the maximal predicted value).

Although category ratings are appropriate for most exercise tests, in some situations it may be desirable to use Borg's newer category scale with ratio properties.[90] This scale is based on the fact that biochemical and cardiorespiratory responses to intense exercise appear to increase exponentially, rather than in a linear fashion. As the exercise intensity rises, the individual may select any higher number rating in proportion to 10 that describes the relative increase in intensity. Accordingly, if a work rate feels 50% harder than it did at a rating of 10, the RPE would be 15.

To reduce problems of misinterpretation of RPE for persons with and without heart disease, it is important to preface the exercise test RPE with a standardized set of instructions. Individuals should be cautioned not to overemphasize any one sign or symptom, such as leg fatigue or dyspnea, but to try to assess their overall feeling of exertion and physical fatigue. The following instructions are recommended for explaining the RPE scale:

> During the graded exercise test we want you to pay close attention to how hard you *feel* the work rate is. This feeling should be your total amount of exertion and fatigue, combining all sensations of physical stress, effort, and fatigue. Don't concern yourself with any one factor such as leg pain, shortness of breath or exercise intensity, but try to concentrate on your *total, inner* feeling of exertion. Don't underestimate or overestimate, just be as accurate as you can.[21]

The concept of perceived exertion appears to be valid even for patients whose heart rates are attenuated by propranolol, since similar RPEs are obtained at a given percentage of maximal heart rate reserve, regardless of the beta-blocking drug dosage or the peak heart rate.[92] However, there are limitations in using RPE alone to gauge exercise intensity. Although the subjective rating correlates well with heart rate, oxygen uptake, minute ventilation, and power output, ischemic ST segment depression and serious ventricular arrhythmias can occur without symptoms at low ratings of perceived exertion.[93]

SYMPTOMS

It is critical that the clinician learn all symptoms that occur during and after the exercise test. Dyspnea may be a dominant exercise symptom in patients with severe CHD, particularly when it is accompanied by poor exercise tolerance and a hypotensive blood pressure response.[21] Especially important are symptoms that may represent classic angina pectoris such as substernal pressure radiating across the chest and/or down the left arm; or back, jaw, stomach, or lower neck pain or discomfort. Such symptoms can be subjectively rated by the patient on a scale of 1 to 4; where 1 is perceptible but mild; 2 is moderate; 3 is moderately severe; and 4 is severe. Ratings of more than 2 should generally be used as endpoints for exercise testing.

Although patients with marked ST segment abnormalities are often asymptomatic, when angina pectoris occurs in conjunction with ST segment displacement, the likelihood that the ECG changes are due to CHD is significantly increased.[94] Moreover, exercise-induced angina pectoris alone is now considered an "independent" variable that identifies a subset of patients at higher risk of subsequent coronary events.[95]

SAFETY OF EXERCISE TESTING

Pathophysiologic information suggests that exercise testing may precipitate cardiac arrest or myocardial infarction in certain persons, particularly individuals with latent or overt CHD. By increasing myocardial oxygen consumption and simultaneously shortening diastole and hence coronary perfusion time, exercise may evoke a transient oxygen deficit in the subendocardial myocardium, which can be exacerbated by a decrease in venous return secondary to abrupt cessation of activity. Subendocardial ischemia can contribute to disturbances in the automaticity of myocardial conducting tissue, triggering serious ventricular arrhythmias and, in extreme cases, cardiac arrest. In addition, intracellular sodium/potassium imbalance, catecholamine excess, and increased circulating free fatty acids may be arrhythmogenic (Fig. 7-12).[96]

In the widely quoted survey by Rochmis and Blackburn,[97] involving 170,000 exercise tests from 73 medical centers, the mortality rate of exercise testing was found to be 1 death per 10,000 tests (0.01%) and the combined morbidity/mortality to be 4 per 10,000 tests (0.04%). A more recent report of 518,448 exercise tests conducted in 1,375 centers revealed a 50% lower mortality rate, 0.5 death per 10,00 tests (0.005%), but a higher combined complication rate, 8.86 per 10,000 tests (0.09%).[98] In a retrospective review of 71,914 maximal exercise tests conducted at a single medical facility, Gibbons et al.[99] encountered six major cardiovascular complications, including one death. The overall event rate in this population of men and women with a low pretest likelihood of CHD was only 0.8 complication per 10,000 tests (0.008%). Although the complications associated with exercise testing appear to be relatively low, the ability to maintain a high degree of safety depends on knowing when not to perform an exercise test, when to terminate the test, and being prepared for any emergency that might arise.

Young et al.[100] reviewed exercise-related complications in 263 patients with *serious ventricular arrhythmias* who underwent a total of 1,377 maximal treadmill tests. Complications occurred in 24 patients (9%) during 32 tests; however, there were no deaths or myocardial infarctions. Clinical variables previously considered to confer increased risk during exercise, such as poor left ventricular function, high-grade ventricular arrhythmias (Lown grade 4A or 4B), exertional hypotension, and ST segment depression, were not predictive of complications. The authors concluded that maximal exercise testing can be safely conducted in patients with malignant arrhythmias.

Supervision of Exercise Testing

The use of maximal or sign/symptom-limited exercise testing has expanded greatly to help guide decisions regarding medical management and surgical therapy in a broad spectrum of pa-

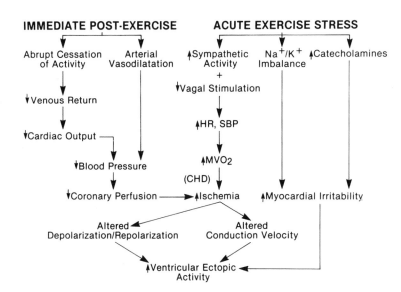

Fig. 7-12. Physiologic alterations accompanying acute exercise and recovery and their possible sequelae. (From Franklin,[96] with permission.)

tients. More than a decade ago, the American Heart Association Subcommittee on Rehabilitation endorsed the concept that exercise testing may, in some instances, be delegated to "experienced paramedical personnel."[101] Contemporary cost containment issues and time constraints on physicians have also encouraged more extensive use of specially trained health care professionals (e.g., nurses, physician assistants, exercise physiologists, physical therapists) to directly supervise exercise tests, with a physician immediately available for emergencies that may arise.[102]

The degree of supervision can range from assigning monitoring of the test to a properly trained nonphysician for the testing of apparently healthy younger persons (younger than 40 years) to the physician who directly monitors the patient's blood pressure and ECG responses throughout exercise and recovery.[60,103] Recently, the latter has been endorsed for the testing of all coronary patients and those at increased risk for exercise-induced complications.[21,60] Despite this recommendation, there is disagreement as to whether direct physician supervision of exercise tests in individuals with known cardiovascular disease is routinely needed. Critics argue that specially trained paramedical specialists can make an effective interpretation of ancillary signs and symptoms, terminating an exercise test at an appropriate intensity level.[102,104,105] This premise is supported by available data showing that the incidence of cardiovascular complications is no higher with "experienced paramedical personnel" than with physician supervision of exercise tests.[106] Moreover, some contend that general medical supervision of exercise tests is neither cost-effective nor necessary.

Although exercise tests are usually directly or indirectly supervised by a cardiologist, general internists and family practice physicians with adequate training and experience are also qualified to conduct the tests. Recent guidelines suggest that a medical resident should perform at least 50 such tests to qualify to do this testing in private practice and that physicians should perform at least 10 exercise tests per year to maintain clinical competence.[103,107] However, we recommend that physicians do two or three times as many tests in each category to provide optimal testing.

REFERENCES

1. Hellerstein HK, Franklin BA: Evaluating the cardiac patient for exercise therapy: Role of exercise testing. p. 371. In Franklin BA, Rubenfire M (eds): Cardiac Rehabilitation. WB Saunders, Philadelphia, 1984
2. van Dixhoorn J, Duivenvoorden HJ, Pool J: Success and failure of exercise training after myocardial infarction: Is the outcome predictable? J Am Coll Cardiol 15:974, 1990
3. Hellerstein HK, Franklin BA: Exercise testing and prescription. p. 197. In Wenger NK, Hellerstein HK (eds): Rehabilitation of the Coronary Patient. 2nd Ed. John Wiley & Sons, New York, 1984
4. Hellerstein HK, Banerja JC, Biorck G et al: Rehabilitation of patients with cardiovascular diseases. WHO Tech Rep Ser 270, 1964
5. Chaitman BR, Hanson JS: Comparative sensitivity and specificity of exercise electrocardiographic lead systems. Am J Cardiol 47:1335, 1981
6. Mark DB, Hlatkey MA, Lee KL et al: Localizing coronary obstructions with the treadmill test. Ann Intern Med 106:53, 1988
7. Borg G: Perceived exertion as an indicator of somatic stress. Scand J Rehabil Med 2:92, 1970
8. Newberg GW, Friedman SH, Weiss MB et al: Cardiopulmonary exercise testing: The clinical value of gas exchange data. Arch Intern Med 148:2221, 1988
9. Keyser RE, Mor D, Andres FF: Cardiovascular responses and anaerobic threshold for bicycle and arm ergometer exercise. Arch Phys Med Rehabil 70:687, 1989
10. Davis JA, Vodak P, Wilmore JH et al: Anaerobic threshold and maximal aerobic power for three modes of exercise. J Appl Physiol 41:544, 1976
11. Davis JA, Frank MH, Whipp BJ et al: Anaerobic threshold alterations caused by endurance training in middle-aged men. J Appl Physiol Respir Environ Exercise Physiol 46:1039, 1979
12. Siscovick DS, Ekelund LG, Johnson JL et al: Sensitivity of exercise electrocardiography for acute cardiac events during moderate and strenuous physical activity: The Lipid Research Clinics Coronary Primary Prevention Trial. Arch Intern Med 151:325, 1991

13. Sox HC, Jr, Littenberg B, Garber AM: The role of exercise testing in screening for coronary artery disease. Ann Intern Med 110:456, 1989

14. Ekelund LG, Suchindran CM, McMahon RP et al: Coronary heart disease morbidity and mortality in hypercholesterolemic men predicted from an exercise test: The LRC Coronary Primary Prevention Trial. J Am Coll Cardiol 14:556, 1989

15. American College of Cardiology/American Heart Association: Guidelines for exercise testing. Circulation 74:653A, 1986

16. Vander L, Franklin B, Rubenfire M: Cardiovascular complications of recreational physical activity. Physician Sportsmed 10:89, 1982

17. Malinow M, McGarry D, Kuehl K: Is exercise testing indicated for asymptomatic active people? J Cardiac Rehabil 4:376, 1984

18. Diamond GA, Forrester JS: Analysis of probability as an aid in the clinical diagnosis of coronary-artery disease. N Engl J Med 300:1350, 1979

19. Franklin BA, Hollingsworth V, Borysyk LM: Additional diagnostic tests: Special populations. p. 223. In American College of Sports Medicine: Resource Manual for Guidelines for Exercise Testing and Prescription. 1st Edition. Lea & Febiger, Philadelphia, 1988

20. Epstein SE: Implications of probability analysis on the strategy used for non-invasive detection of coronary artery disease. Am J Cardiol 46:491, 1980

21. American College of Sports Medicine: Guidelines for Graded Exercise Testing and Exercise Prescription. 4th Ed. p. 1. Lea & Febiger, Philadelphia, 1991

22. Haskell W, Brachfeld N, Bruce RA et al: Task Force II: Determination of occupational working capacity in patients with ischemic heart disease. J Am Coll Cardiol 14:1025, 1989

23. Scholl JM, Wagniart P, Morice MC et al: Elimination of isolated exercise-induced U wave inversion after successful percutaneous transluminal coronary angioplasty of left anterior descending artery. Am Heart J 114:166, 1987

24. Ellestad MH: The mechanism of exercise-induced R wave amplitude changes in coronary heart disease—still controversial. Arch Intern Med 142:963, 1982

25. Fuller T, Movahed A: Current review of exercise testing: Application and interpretation. Clin Cardiol 10:189, 1987

26. Gianrossi R, Detrano R, Mulvihill D et al: Exercise-induced ST depression in the diagnosis of coronary artery disease. A meta-analysis. Circulation 80:87, 1989

27. Ameisen O, Kligfield P, Okin PM et al: Effects of recent and remote infarction on the predictive accuracy of the ST segment/heart rate slope. J Am Coll Cardiol 8:267, 1986

28. Lachterman B, Lehmann KG, Detrano R et al: Comparison of ST segment/heart rate index to standard ST criteria for analysis of exercise electrocardiogram. Circulation 82:44, 1990

29. Lester FM, Sheffield LT, Reeves JT: Electrocardiographic changes in clinically normal older men following near-maximal and maximal exercise. Circulation 36:5, 1967

30. McHenry PL, Phillips JF, Knoebel SB: Correlation of computer-quantitated treadmill exercise electrocardiogram with arteriographic location of coronary artery disease. Am J Cardiol 30:747, 1972

31. Radke JE, Hellerstein HK, Salzman SH et al: The quantitative effects of physical conditioning on the exercise electrocardiogram of subjects with arteriosclerotic heart disease and normal subjects. p. 168. In Brunner D, Jokl E (eds): Physical Activity and Aging. S Karger AG, Basel, Switzerland, 1970

32. Sheffield LT, Holt JH, Lester FM et al: On-line analysis of the exercise electrocardiogram. Circulation 40:935, 1969

33. Froelicher VF, Dubach P: Recent advances in exercise testing. Cardio (May):41, 1990

34. Bonow RO, Bacharach SL, Green MV et al: Prognostic implications of symptomatic versus asymptomatic (silent) myocardial ischemia induced by exercise in mildly symptomatic and in asymptomatic patients with angiographically documented coronary artery disease. Am J Cardiol 60:778, 1987

35. McNeer JF, Margolis JR, Lee KL et al: The role of the exercise test in the evaluation of patients for ischemic heart disease. Circulation 57:64, 1978

36. Ellestad MH, Cooke BM, Greenberg PS: Stress testing: Clinical application and predictive capacity. Prog Cardiovasc Dis 21:431, 1979

37. Kligfield P, Okin PM, Ameisen O et al: Evaluation of coronary artery disease by an improved method of exercise electrocardiography: The ST segment/heart rate slope. Am Heart J 112:589, 1986

38. Okin PM, Ameisen O, Kligfield P: Detection of anatomically severe coronary artery disease by the ST/HR slope. Chest 91:584, 1987

39. Sato I, Keta K, Aihara N et al: Improved accuracy of the exercise electrocardiogram in detection of

coronary artery and three-vessel coronary disease. Chest 94:737, 1988

40. Savvides M, Ahnves S, Bhargava V, Froelicher VF: Computer analysis of exercise-induced changes in electrocardiographic variables: Comparison of methods and criteria. Chest 84:699, 1983

41. Kligfield P, Ameisen O, Okin PM: Relation to the exercise ST/HR slope to simple heart rate adjustment of ST segment depression. J Electrocardiol 20:135, 1987

42. Pryor DB: The academic life cycle of a noninvasive test. Circulation 82:302, 1990

43. Froelicher VF, Lachterman B: Reply. The academic life cycle of a noninvasive test. Circulation 82:2285, 1990

44. Kligfield P, Okin PM: Letter to the Editor. The academic life of a noninvasive test. Circulation 82:2284, 1990

45. Schlant RC, Blomqvist CG, Brandenburg RO et al: Guidelines for exercise testing. Circulation 74:653A, 1986

46. Laslett LJ, Amsterdam EA: Management of the asymptomatic patient with an abnormal exercise ECG. JAMA 252:1744, 1984

47. Bruce RA: Editorial. Values and limitations of exercise electrocardiography. Circulation 50:1, 1974

48. Georgopoulos AJ, Proudfit WL, Page IH: Effect of exercise on electrocardiogram of patients with low serum potassium. Circulation 23:567, 1961

49. Sketch MH, Mooss AN, Butler ML et al: Digoxin-induced positive exercise tests: Their clinical and prognostic significance. Am J Cardiol 48:655, 1981

50. Jaffe MD: Effect of oestrogens on postexercise electrocardiogram. Br Heart J 38:1299, 1977

51. Tanaka T, Friedman MJ, Okada RD et al: Diagnostic value of exercise-induced ST segment depression in patients with right bundle branch block. Am J Cardiol 41:670, 1978

52. Chaitman BR: The changing role of the exercise electrocardiogram as a diagnostic and prognostic test for chronic ischemic heart disease. J Am Coll Cardiol 8:1195, 1986

53. Gianelly RE, Treister BL, Harrison DC: The effect of propranolol on exercise-induced ischemic ST segment depression. Am J Cardiol 24:161, 1969

54. Timmis GC, Franklin BA, Borysyk L et al: Failure of once-daily atenolol to prevent an ischemic response to exercise late in the afternoon. Chest 92:71S, 1987

55. Subramanian B, Bowles M, Lahiri A et al: Long-term antianginal action of verapamil assessed with quantitated serial treadmill stress testing. Am J Cardiol 48:529, 1981

56. Russek HI, Funk EH Jr: Comparative responses to various nitrates in the treatment of angina pectoris. Postgrad Med 31:150, 1962

57. Chaitman BR, Waters DD, Theroux P et al: S-T segment elevation and coronary spasm in response to exercise. Am J Cardiol 47:1350, 1981

58. Yasue H, Omote S, Takizawa A et al: Comparison of coronary arteriographic findings during angina pectoris associated with S-T elevation or depression. Am J Cardiol 47:539, 1981

59. Brody DA: A theoretic analysis of intracoronary blood mass influence on the heart lead relationship. Circ Res 4:731, 1956

60. Fletcher GF, Froelicher VF, Hartley LH et al: Exercise standards: A statement for health professionals from the American Heart Association. Circulation 82:2286, 1990

61. Berman JL, Wynne J, Cohn PF: Multiple-lead QRS changes with exercise testing. Circulation 61:53, 1980

62. Boudoulas H, Dervenagas S, Lewis RP et al: Adrenergic stimulation and R-wave magnitude. J Cardiopulmonary Rehabil 1:108, 1981

63. Busby MJ, Shefrin EA, Fleg JL: Prevalence and long-term significance of exercise-induced frequent or repetitive ventricular ectopic beats in apparently healthy volunteers. J Am Coll Cardiol 14:1659, 1989

64. McHenry PL, Morris SN, Kavlier M et al: Comparative study of exercise-induced ventricular arrhythmias in normal subjects and patients with documented coronary artery disease. Am J Cardiol 37:609, 1976

65. Califf RM, McKinnis RA, McNeer JF et al: Prognostic value of ventricular arrhythmias associated with treadmill exercise testing in patients studied with cardiac catheterization for suspected ischemic heart disease. J Am Coll Cardiol 2:1060, 1983

66. McHenry PL, Fisch C: Clinical applications of the treadmill exercise test. Mod Concepts Cardiovasc Dis 46:21, 1977

67. Kozlowski JH, Ellestad MH: The exercise test as a guide to management and prognosis. p. 395. In Franklin BA, Rubenfire M (eds): Cardiac Rehabilitation. WB Saunders, Philadelphia, 1984

68. Naughton J, Haider R: Methods of exercise testing. p. 79. In Naughton JP, Hellerstein HK, Mohler IC (eds): Exercise Testing and Exercise Training in Coronary Heart Disease. Academic Press, San Diego, 1973

69. Chin CF, Messenger JC, Greenberg PS et al: Chronotropic incompetence in exercise testing. Clin Cardiol 2:12, 1979

70. Wiens RD, Lafia P, Marder CM et al: Chronotropic incompetence in clinical exercise testing. Am J Cardiol 54:74, 1984

71. Hinkle LE, Carver ST, Plakum A: Slow heart rates and increased risk of cardiac death in middle-aged men. Arch Intern Med 129:732, 1972

72. Ellestad MH, Wan MKC: Predictive implications of stress testing. Follow-up of 2700 subjects after maximum treadmill stress testing. Circulation 51:363, 1975

73. Bruce RA: Principles of exercise testing. p. 45. In Naughton JP, Hellerstein HK, Mohler IC (eds): Exercise Testing and Exercise Training in Coronary Heart Disease. Academic Press, San Diego, 1973

74. Sheps DS, Ernst JC, Briese FW et al: Exercise-induced increase in diastolic pressure: Indicator of severe coronary artery disease. Am J Cardiol 43:708, 1979

75. Bronson L, Wasir H, Sannerstedt R: Hemodynamic effects of static and dynamic exercise in males with arterial hypertension of varying severity. Cardiovasc Res 12:269, 1978

76. Chrysant SG: The value of grip test as an index of autonomic function in hypertension. Clin Cardiol 5:139, 1982

77. Sannerstedt R, Julius S: Systemic hemodynamic responses in borderline arterial hypertension: Responses to static exercise before and under the influence of propranolol. Cardiovasc Res 6:398, 1972

78. Hanson P, Ward A, Painter P: Exercise training for special patient populations. J Cardiopulmonary Rehabil 6:104, 1986

79. Irving JB, Bruce RA, DeRouen TA: Variations in and significance of systolic pressure during maximal exercise (treadmill) testing: Relation to severity of coronary artery disease and cardiac mortality. Am J Cardiol 39:841, 1977

80. Comess KA, Fenster PE: Clinical implications of the blood pressure response to exercise. Cardiology 68:233, 1981

81. Fisman EZ, Pines A, Ben-Ari E et al: Left ventricular exercise echocardiographic abnormalities in apparently healthy men with exertional hypotension. Am J Cardiol 63:81, 1989

82. Dubach P, Froelicher VF, Klein J et al: Exercise-induced hypotension in a male population. Criteria, causes, and prognosis. Circulation 78:1380, 1988

83. Amon KW, Richards KL, Crawford MH: Usefulness of the postexercise response of systolic blood pressure in the diagnosis of coronary artery disease. Circulation 70:951, 1984

84. Kato K, Saito F, Hatano K et al: Prognostic value of abnormal postexercise systolic blood pressure response: Prehospital discharge test after myocardial infarction in Japan. Am Heart J 119:264, 1990

85. Acanfora D, De Caprio L, Cuomo S et al: Diagnostic value of the ratio of recovery systolic blood pressure to peak exercise systolic blood pressure for the detection of coronary artery disease. Circulation 77:1306, 1988

86. Bruce RA: Progress in exercise cardiology. In Yu PN, Goodwin JF (eds): Progress in Cardiology. Lea & Febiger, Philadelphia, 1974

87. Bruce RA, Fisher LD, Cooper NM et al: Separation of effects of cardiovascular disease and age on ventricular function with maximal exercise. Am J Cardiol 34:757, 1974

88. Kitamura K, Jorgensen CR, Gobel FL et al: Hemodynamic correlates of myocardial O_2 consumption during upright exercise. J Appl Physiol 32:516, 1972

89. Nelson RR, Gobel FL, Jorgensen CR et al: Hemodynamic predictors of myocardial oxygen consumption during static and dynamic exercise. Circulation 50:1179, 1974

90. Borg G: Psychophysical bases of perceived exertion. Med Sci Sports Exercise 14:377, 1982

91. Ekblom B, Goldbarg AN: The influence of physical training and other factors on the subjective rating of perceived exertion. Acta Physiol Scand 83:399, 1971

92. Pollock ML, Foster C: Exercise prescription for participants on propranolol (abstract). J Am Coll Cardiol 1:624, 1983

93. Williams MA, Fardy PS: Limitations in prescribing exercise. J Cardiovasc Pulmonary Technol 8:36, 1980

94. Weiner DA, McCabe C, Hueter D et al: The predictive value of chest pain as an indicator of coronary disease during exercise testing (abstract). Circulation 54 (suppl. II):II-10, 1976

95. Cole JP, Ellestad MH: Significance of chest pain during treadmill exercise: Correlation with coronary events. Am J Cardiol 41:227, 1978

96. Franklin BA: The role of electrocardiographic monitoring in cardiac exercise programs. J Cardiopulmonary Rehabil 3:806, 1983

97. Rochmis P, Blackburn H: Exercise tests. A survey of procedures, safety and litigation experience in

approximately 170,000 tests. JAMA 217:1061, 1971

98. Stuart RJ Jr, Ellestad MH: National survey of exercise stress testing facilities. Chest 77:94, 1980

99. Gibbons L, Blair SN, Kohl HW et al: The safety of maximal exercise testing. Circulation 80:846, 1989

100. Young DZ, Lampert S, Graboys TB et al: Safety of maximal exercise testing in patients at high risk for ventricular arrhythmia. Circulation 70:184, 1984

101. Ellestad MH, Blomqvist CG, Naughton JP: Standards for adult exercise testing laboratories. Circulation 59:421A, 1979

102. DeBusk RF: Exercise test supervision: Time for a reassessment. Exercise Stand Malpract Rep 2:65, 1988

103. Schlant RC, Friesinger GC, Leonard JJ: Clinical competence in exercise testing: A statement for physicians from the ACP/ACC/AHA task force on clinical privileges in cardiology. Circulation 82:1884, 1990

104. Blessey RL: Exercise testing by non-physician health care professionals: Complication rates, clinical competencies and future trends. Exercise Stand Malpract Rep 3:69, 1989

105. Cahalin LP, Blessey RL, Kummer D et al: The safety of exercise testing performed independently by physical therapists. J Cardiopulmonary Rehabil 7:269, 1987

106. Shephard RJ: Safety of exercise testing—the role of the paramedical exercise specialist. Clin J Sports Med 1:8, 1991

107. Wigton RS, Nicolas JA, Blank LL: Procedural skills of the general internist. A survey of 2500 physicians. Ann Intern Med 111:1023, 1989

8

Excercise Testing: Methods and Protocols*

Barry A. Franklin, Ph.D.   *Seymour Gordon, M.D.*
Herman K. Hellerstein, M.D.   *Gerald C. Timmis, M.D.*

HYPERVENTILATION TEST

Before undergoing an exercise evaluation, the subject usually performs a hyperventilation test. While in the same position in which the multistage exercise test will be conducted, the person is instructed to breathe rapidly and deeply for 30 seconds, but not as vigorously as in a maximal-breathing test. A continuous recording is made, using the electrocardiographic (ECG) leads that will be employed during the exercise test, before, during, and for 30 seconds after hyperventilation.

Interpretation

Normal responses to hyperventilation include a feeling of lightheadedness, slight hypotension, tachycardia, and ECG changes of peaking of the P waves, prolongation of electrical systole, and a lowering of the amplitude of the T waves. Abnormal responses include tightness in the chest, confusion, persistence of the aforementioned symptoms and signs for longer than 5 minutes, arrhythmias, ST-T displacement, bundle branch block, or variable degrees of atrioventricular block. The ECG changes produced by hyperventilation are probably due to changes in acid–base balance, hypocapnia, and associated intracellular shifts of potassium, rather than to the oxygen cost of the effort of hyperventilation or to a significant reduction in coronary blood flow. Studies of the

---

* See footnote in Chapter 7, page 123.

oxygen cost of ventilation have suggested that no more than 250 to 350 mL of oxygen is expended during 30 seconds of hyperventilation.[1] This is less than the oxygen requirement of the first stage of most exercise test protocols. Nevertheless, changes that are elicited by the hyperventilation test should be taken into consideration when evaluating ST segment responses during peak or maximal effort.

EXERCISE TESTING OF THE LOWER EXTREMITIES

Standard lower-extremity exercise tests, employing either the treadmill or cycle ergometer, have the advantage of reproducibility and quantitation of physiologic responses to known external work loads. For cycle ergometer exercise testing, the seat height should first be positioned to ensure that the patient's knees remain slightly flexed at maximal pedal downstroke.

Treadmill Testing Versus Leg Cycle Ergometry

Treadmill exercise and cycle ergometry have an essential difference: on a treadmill the work performed during each stage is dependent on body weight, whereas cycle ergometry is weight independent.[2] Bicycle exercise testing should, ideally, be adjusted for body weight so that different subjects perform similar relative work at each stage.[3] Most existing cycle ergometer protocols fail to take this into account, since standardized increases of 150 to 300 kilogram-meters per minute (kg·m/min) (25 to 50 watts [W]) every 2 to 3 minutes are generally used. During treadmill exercise, the patient has to carry his or her own weight, so the work load progression is automatically standardized.

Both modalities have advantages and disadvantages in evaluating patients with and without heart disease. Many patients who are unable to perform treadmill walking because of ambulatory instability or orthopedic limitations can often complete a cycle ergometer exercise test. The cycle ergometer requires less space, makes less noise, and generally costs less than does the treadmill. It also minimizes movement of the torso and upper extremities, which facilitates better-quality ECG recordings; and blood pressure measurements are easier to obtain.[4] If provisions are taken to avoid isometric handgrip on the handlebars during measurement of blood pressure, erroneously high systolic blood pressure readings can be avoided. Its main disadvantage is that cycling is an unfamiliar method of exercise to many in the United States, often resulting in limiting localized muscle fatigue.[5] Treadmill testing, on the other hand, provides a more common form of physiologic stress (i.e., walking) during which subjects are more likely to attain a slightly higher maximal oxygen uptake ($\dot{V}o_2$max) and peak heart rate.[6] Foster et al.[7] demonstrated a consistent relationship between aerobic capacity on the treadmill and the cycle ergometer and suggested a method for predicting treadmill aerobic capacity, expressed as METs (1 MET = 3.5 mL/kg/min), from cycle ergometer functional capacity by using the equation:

Treadmill METs =
    0.98 (cycle ergometer METs) + 1.85

Despite the potential of treadmill exercise to elicit a higher $\dot{V}o_2$max and peak heart rate than cycle ergometry, it remains unclear whether there is a clinically significant difference between the two test modalities in evoking ischemic signs or symptoms. Ford et al.[8] found that chest pain and ischemic ST segment depression occurred less frequently with cycle ergometer ex-

ercise than with treadmill exercise, despite a significantly higher rate–pressure product with the former. However, Wicks et al.[9] reported a close relationship between the magnitude of ST segment changes induced by maximal exercise testing with the treadmill and the cycle ergometer in patients following myocardial infarction.

Treadmill Testing Versus Jogging in Place

Papazoglou et al.[10] compared jogging in place with the Bruce treadmill protocol in 141 patients (mean age ± SD, 55 ± 7 years) who had a wide spectrum of recurring chest complaints. Agreement between the tests for the presence or absence of ECG evidence of ischemia, manifested as significant ST segment displacement (≥1 mm at 80 msec from the J point) or U wave inversion, was observed in 128 (91%) of the patients. No adverse effects or cardiovascular complications were documented during either test. The investigators concluded that this simplified evaluation can be recommended as a safe and valid alternative to established multistage treadmill exercise protocols for any diagnostic or screening test application. Since quantification of fitness cannot be determined by this test, its limitations are the inability to facilitate risk stratification or to provide serial comparisons.

Methods and Protocols

Regardless of the equipment used, several features are desirable for any exercise protocol or test:

1. The protocol and procedures of the test should be explained in simple and straightforward language. Many patients are anxious before exercise testing. Their anxiety can be reduced or eliminated by a careful preliminary explanation, which should include a demonstration of how to perform the test (e.g., stepping on and off the treadmill).
2. The exercise test should not be performed sooner than 2 hours after a light meal, unless

the additive effects of food are being evaluated. The same proscription applies to alcohol, tobacco, and beverages containing caffeine (e.g., tea, coffee, cola drinks).

3. The test protocol should be selected to accommodate the individual patient's ability to perform lower-extremity exercise. Patients with severe peripheral vascular disease or musculoskeletal limitations who are unable to perform treadmill or cycle ergometer exercise may, alternatively, be evaluated by arm crank ergometry,[11] atrial pacing,[12] or adenosine or dipyridamole infusion at rest (see Ch. 9).

4. The exercise test should begin at an intensity level considerably below the anticipated peak or symptom-limited capacity and increase gradually in 2- or 3-minute stages, with observations (e.g., heart rate, blood pressure, perceived exertion) made at each progressive stage. Even the most severely limited patient should be able to exercise for at least 3 minutes, which necessitates starting at a low work load.[13]

5. The protocol must not be too long, lest fatigue and boredom become limiting factors. An average duration of 10 minutes has been suggested,[14,15] and all patients should reach their peak performance by 15 minutes.[14] A brief self-administered questionnaire to determine functional capacity (The Duke Activity Status Index) may be used to help guide the selection of the exercise test protocol.[16]

6. Blood pressure should be measured at least once during each stage and more frequently (e.g., at 30- to 60-second intervals) in the presence of hypo- or hypertensive readings. The use of an appropriately sized blood pressure cuff and a mercury manometer mounted at eye level is important to ensure accurate measurements.[17]

7. Contraindications to testing and indications for stopping exercise should be closely observed.

8. Monitoring should be continued for at least 6 minutes into recovery unless abnormal responses occur which necessitate a longer posttest observation period. In some laboratories, supine recovery is employed immediately after exercise. The resultant increase in venous return may produce additional left ventricular preload and aid in the detection of ischemic ST segment depression. On the other hand, a gradual cool-down (e.g., walking for an additional 3 to 5 minutes) after treadmill testing, rather than a sudden stop, has been suggested to decrease the risk of complications during recovery.[18] Abrupt cessation of exercise may significantly increase catecholamine levels, which could, in turn, increase ventricular arrhythmias and ischemia and precipitate cardiovascular complications.[19]

9. The temperature of the exercise-testing room should ideally be 22°C (72°F) or less, and the humidity should be below 60%.[2]

Figure 8-1 shows three commonly used multistage treadmill exercise protocols. Exercise stages are progressive in intensity; a duration at each stage of 2 minutes or more ensures that most cardiorespiratory variables reach a "steady-state" value. These protocols involve a constant "walking" speed (range, 2.0 to 3.4 mph) and standardized increases in grade or incline; nevertheless, the increments in aerobic requirements for each stage are identical, 1 MET.

The conventional Bruce[20] treadmill protocol (Fig. 8-2) is perhaps the most familiar and widely used protocol for which normative values for heart rate, blood pressure, and oxygen uptake have been established. A major advantage of the Bruce protocol is its relative brevity; most sedentary persons can complete only stage III (9 minutes; 9 to 10 METs). The protocol, however, has several limitations. The initial work load (stage I), corresponding to 1.7 mph at a 10% grade, has an aerobic requirement of 4 to 5 METs, equivalent to an oxygen uptake of 14.0 to 17.5 mL/kg/min; this exceeds the aerobic capacity of many cardiac, elderly, or deconditioned patients. Since the work load progression involves simultaneous increases in both speed and grade, it is difficult for many patients to adapt to the large work increments between stages, typically 2.5 to 3.0 METs. Consequently, patients often fail to attain a leveling off or plateau of physiologic responses, and delineation of the precise work load at the ischemic or anginal threshold is difficult. Researchers have also shown a significant error in estimating $\dot{V}o_2$ from the Bruce treadmill time.[2]

METS	1.6	2	3	4	5	6	7	8	9	10	11	12	13	14	15	16
Balke							3.4 Miles/hr									
				2	4	6	8	10	12	14	16	18	20	22	24	26
Balke				3.0 Miles/hr												
			0	2.5	5	7.5	10	12.5	15	17.5	20	22.5				
Naughton	1.0			2.0 Miles/hr												
	0	0	3.5	7	10.5	14	17.5									
METS	1.6	2	3	4	5	6	7	8	9	10	11	12	13	14	15	16
O$_2$,ml/kg/min	5.6	7		14		21		28		35		42		49		56
Clinical Status		Symptomatic Patients														
			Diseased, Recovered													
				Sedentary Healthy												
					Physically Active Subjects											
Functional Class	IV	III			II		I and Normal									

Fig. 8-1. Metabolic cost of selected treadmill test protocols. One MET signifies resting energy expenditure, equivalent to approximately 3.5 mL of oxygen uptake/kg of body weight/min (mL/kg/min). Unlabeled numbers refer to treadmill speed (top) and percentage grade (bottom).

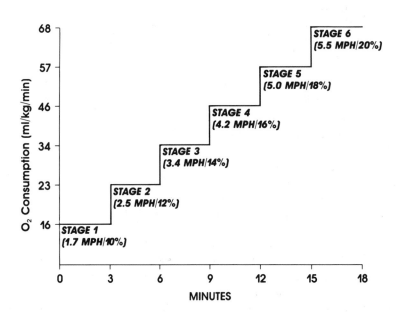

Fig. 8-2. The standard Bruce treadmill protocol showing progressive stages (speed, percent grade) and the corresponding aerobic requirement, expressed as mL/kg/min.

The inaccuracy is attributable primarily to rapid increases in speed and grade, which exceed the oxygen uptake kinetics of most coronary patients; and to the extensive use of treadmill handrails for support. In addition, the Bruce protocol is a walk–jog test with a variable transition point from walking to jogging at stage IV (9th to 12th minute), resulting in a variety of mechanical efficiencies at this stage with various oxygen costs. Finally, the ECG may be distorted by artifact caused by muscle movement and foot impact during jogging.

Consideration of these limitations, particularly in deconditioned patients, has resulted in the development of a "modified" Bruce protocol consisting of one or two preliminary 3-minute stages at 1.7 mph at a 0% grade and/or 1.7 mph at a 5% grade. A comparison of the Naughton and modified Bruce treadmill protocols for exercise testing after myocardial infarction revealed no significant differences in maximal heart rate, rate–pressure product, or work load achieved.[21] Although the Naughton protocol resulted in a significantly longer mean maximal exercise duration, 17.3 ± 5.0 versus 14.8 ± 2.8 minutes, the protocols were equally effective in detecting ischemic responses at 6 weeks after myocardial infarction.

Recently, Northridge et al.[3] described a new treadmill protocol that starts at a low work load (~ 2 METs) and increases by 15% of the previous stage every minute. The progression is accomplished by augmenting either the treadmill speed or elevation, but never both together. This is the first protocol to be based on exponential rather than linear increments in work load that is applicable to the wide range of patients' exercise capacities. The highest stage required to test even relatively fit patients is attained within 15 minutes. Table 8-1 shows the resulting standardized exponential exercise protocol (STEEP).

The STEEP test was applied to a cycle ergometer after adjusting for differences in body weight. This serves to reduce or eliminate the performance advantage that larger subjects have with most existing cycle ergometer protocols. Table 8-2 was derived to predict the power output (watts) to elicit the same relative oxygen consumption as the treadmill protocol for a given body weight. Figure 8-3 shows the oxygen consumption, expressed as mL/kg/min during each stage of the two STEEP tests.

Another recent advance in test methodology that can overcome many of the drawbacks of multistage exercise tests is ramping.[22] Ramp protocols involve a nearly continuous and uniform increase in energy cost that replaces the "staging" used in conventional exercise tests. With ramping, the gradual increase in demand allows a steady increase in cardiorespiratory responses. Protocols have been developed that provide for ramping increments appropriate to the wide range of patients' exercise capacities, for use with both the cycle ergometer and the treadmill.

Aerobic Requirements of Leg Ergometry

Because it is inconvenient to measure oxygen consumption directly, since this requires sophisticated equipment, technical expertise, and frequent calibration, clinicians have increasingly sought to predict or estimate $\dot{V}O_2max$ from the treadmill speed and percent grade (Figs. 8-1 and 8-2), or the cycle ergometer work load (kilogrammeters per minute, kg·m/min), corrected for body weight (Table 8-3).[2] The rationale is that the mechanical efficiency of treadmill walking or cycle

Table 8-1.   STEEP Treadmill Protocol

Work Load (stage [min])	1	2	3	4	5	6	7	8	9	10	11	12	13	14	15
Speed (mph)	1.5	2.0	2.0	2.0	2.5	2.5	2.5	3.0	3.0	3.0	3.5	3.5	3.5	4.2	5.0
Elevation (%)	0	0	1.5	3	3	5	7	7	9	11	11	13	16	16	16

(Adapted from Northridge et al.,[3] with permission.)

Table 8-2. STEEP Bicycle Protocol Showing the Work Load for Each of the 15 Stages of the Protocol as Determined by the Subject's Body Weight

Weight		Work Load (W)[a] at Stage (min)														
kg	lb	1	2	3	4	5	6	7	8	9	10	11	12	13	14	15
50	110	15	20	25	30	40	50	60	70	85	95	110	125	145	170	185
55	121	15	20	30	35	45	55	65	80	95	105	125	140	160	185	205
60	132	15	25	30	40	45	60	70	85	100	115	135	150	175	200	225
65	143	20	25	35	40	50	65	80	90	110	125	145	165	190	220	240
70	154	20	25	35	45	55	70	85	100	120	135	155	175	205	235	260
75	165	20	30	40	45	60	75	90	105	125	145	170	190	220	250	280
80	176	25	30	40	50	65	80	95	115	135	155	180	200	235	270	295
85	187	25	35	45	55	65	85	100	120	145	165	190	215	250	285	315
90	198	25	35	45	55	70	90	105	130	150	175	200	225	265	300	335
95	209	25	35	50	60	75	95	115	135	160	180	215	240	280	320	350
100	220	30	40	50	65	80	100	120	140	170	190	225	250	295	335	370

[a] For conversion of watts to kilogram·meters per minute, 1 W = 6.12 kg·m/min.
(Adapted from Northridge et al.,[3] with permission.)

ergometry is relatively constant in healthy persons. It should be emphasized, however, that a cardiac patient's oxygen uptake may be markedly overestimated when it is predicted from exercise time or peak work load.[23] Several explanations have been offered to account for this phenomenon.[24] The $\dot{V}O_2$ values presented in Figures 8-1 and 8-2 were obtained from healthy young adults and apply only when the subject has achieved steady-state conditions (i.e., completed the exercise stage). It has been suggested that depressed ventricular function may slow oxygen uptake kinetics, perhaps accounting for the fact that many coronary patients, especially those with chronic heart failure, often demonstrate lower submaximal and maximal oxygen uptake values

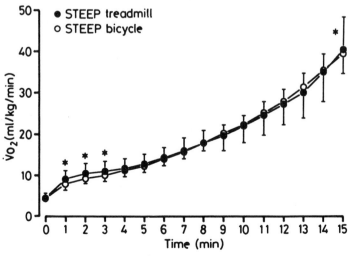

Fig. 8-3. Mean ± SD oxygen consumption ($\dot{V}O_2$) of 30 healthy men performing the two STEEP protocols. *$P < 0.05$. (From Northridge et al.,[3] with permission.)

Table 8-3.   Energy Expenditure During Bicycle Ergometry at Progressive Work Rates for Persons of Different Body Weights

Body Weight		Energy Expenditure (METs) at Work Rate (kg·m/min):						
kg	lb	300	450	600	750	900	1,050	1,200
50	110	4.4	6.1	7.9	9.6	11.3	13.0	14.7
60	132	3.9	5.3	6.7	8.1	9.6	11.0	12.4
70	154	3.4	4.7	5.9	7.1	8.3	9.6	10.8
80	176	3.1	4.2	5.3	6.4	7.4	8.5	9.6
90	198	2.9	3.9	4.8	5.8	6.7	7.7	8.6
100	220	2.7	3.6	4.4	5.3	6.1	7.0	7.9

(Adapted from American College of Sports Medicine,[2] with permission.)

and a larger oxygen debt for standard work loads.[25,26] Obstruction of the arterial circulation of the lower extremities as a result of peripheral vascular disease or experimental obstruction produced in normal subjects[27] may also affect the discrepancy between measured and estimated oxygen uptake values. Finally, beta-adrenergic blocking medications have been shown to result in a slower adaptation of oxygen consumption to steady-state submaximal work loads.[28]

Measured and estimated values of $\dot{V}o_2max$ can also vary widely among healthy individuals who perform any given maximal treadmill test.[29] Several groups of investigators using either the Balke or Bruce treadmill protocol, reported a wide range of measured oxygen consumptions for any particular maximal exercise time or work load.[23,30] For example, after 11 minutes of exercise using the Bruce protocol, equivalent to a work load of 4.2 mph at a 16% grade, the mean measured oxygen uptake was 44 mL/kg/min, but the range for the 95% confidence limit was 32 to 58 mL/kg/min.

Possible explanations for the wide range in measured oxygen consumption values at a given treadmill time include differences in exercise protocol intensity increments, variations in efficiency of treadmill walking, and the use of handrails for stability during treadmill testing.[24] Protocols that use large exercise intensity (work load) increments, creating a considerable oxygen deficit, are likely to be accomplished with a greater portion of the energy demand being met anaerobically. In such instances, the measured oxygen uptake may be significantly below the estimated value. Initial attempts at ergometric testing, awkward gait, or both, have also been associated with a disproportionate increase in oxygen uptake, reflecting a reduced mechanical efficiency. Finally, the use of handrails by the patient for balance and support, particularly while gripping tightly and pulling, has been shown to decrease the actual energy expenditure and to increase performance time, resulting in an overestimation of true aerobic capacity.[31]

Aerobic Capacity and Impairment

Maximal oxygen consumption may be expressed on an absolute basis in liters per minute, reflecting total body energy output and caloric expenditure, where each liter of oxygen consumed is equivalent to approximately 5 kcal. Because large persons usually have a large absolute oxygen consumption as a result of their large muscle mass, physiologists generally divide this value by body weight in kilograms to allow a more equitable comparison between individuals of different sizes. This variable, when expressed in milliliters of oxygen per kilogram of body weight per minute or as METs (1 MET = 3.5 mL/kg/min), is considered the single best index of physical work capacity or cardiopulmonary fitness.[32]

It is of value to express the $\dot{V}o_2max$ in milliliters per kilogram per minute (mL/kg/min) as compared with normative values. Bruce et al.[33] developed the concept of functional aerobic impairment (FAI) for this purpose. The FAI is the percent difference between the person's observed $\dot{V}o_2max$ and that predicted for a healthy person of the same age, sex, and habitual activity status. Average predicted values of $\dot{V}o_2max$, expressed as mL/kg/min, for active and sedentary men and women, are shown in Table 8-4.[20]

FAI and functional aerobic capacity (FAC) can be calculated from the following formulas:

$$\% \, FAI = \frac{predicted \, \dot{V}o_2max - observed \, \dot{V}o_2max}{predicted \, \dot{V}o_2max} \times 100$$

$$\% \, FAC = 100 - FAI$$

Table 8-4. $\dot{V}o_2max^a$ of Healthy Active and Sedentary Men and Women

Age (yr)	$\dot{V}o_2max$ of Men Active	$\dot{V}o_2max$ of Men Sedentary[b]	$\dot{V}o_2max$ of Women Active	$\dot{V}o_2max$ of Women Sedentary[b]
20	57.5	48.9	36.7	35.2
22	56.2	48.0	36.0	34.5
24	55.0	47.1	35.4	33.8
26	53.8	46.2	34.8	33.0
28	52.6	45.3	34.2	32.3
30	51.3	44.5	33.5	31.6
32	50.1	43.6	32.9	30.9
34	48.9	42.7	32.3	30.2
36	47.7	41.8	31.7	29.5
38	46.4	40.9	31.0	28.8
40	45.2	40.0	30.4	28.1
42	44.0	39.1	29.8	27.3
44	42.8	38.2	29.2	26.6
46	41.5	37.3	28.5	25.9
48	40.3	36.4	27.9	25.2
50	39.1	35.6	27.3	24.5
52	37.9	34.7	26.7	23.8
54	36.7	33.8	26.1	23.1
56	35.4	32.9	25.4	22.4
58	34.2	32.0	24.8	21.7
60	33.0	31.1	24.2	20.9
62	31.8	30.2	23.6	20.2
64	30.5	29.3	22.9	19.5
66	29.3	28.4	22.3	18.8
68	28.1	27.5	21.7	18.1
70	26.9	26.7	21.1	17.4

[a] Expressed as mL/kg/min.
[b] Subjects who do not exert themselves sufficiently to develop sweating at least once a week.
(Adapted from Bruce,[20] with permission.)

The normal value of the FAI is 0%; this indicates that the $\dot{V}o_2max$ is 100% of the age and sex-predicted value (FAC) and that there is no functional aerobic impairment. Negative values for FAI signify above-average fitness; i.e., the FAC is more than 100%. For the sake of convention, the degree of FAI can be categorized as mild (27 to 40%), moderate (41 to 54%), marked (55 to 68%), or extreme (>68%), equivalent to 73 to 60%, 59 to 46%, 45 to 32%, and less than 32% FAC, respectively.[20]

The concept of FAI or FAC is particularly useful in making serial evaluations of individuals as well as comparisons with peers. For example, a 46-year-old sedentary woman with a $\dot{V}o_2max$ of 18.0 mL/kg/min had an FAI [(25.9 − 18.0)/25.9] × 100 = 30.5%. In other words, her FAC was only 69.5% of the average normal expected value, corresponding to "mild" fitness impairment. Four years later her $\dot{V}o_2max$ had increased to 23.4 mL/kg/min as a result of participating in a supervised physical-training program. Although the increase in $\dot{V}o_2max$ was 5.4 mL/kg/min, equivalent to 30% [(5.4/18.0) × 100], the age-corrected FAI had improved from 30.5 to 4.5%. Accordingly, her FAC had increased from 69.5% at age 46 years to 95.5% at age 50 years.

Achievement of $\dot{V}o_2max$

There is considerable debate concerning the ability of the patient who is limited by angina pectoris to exercise to the cardiopulmonary limit, that is, to demonstrate a true physiologic $\dot{V}o_2max$. It is argued that the onset of chest pain or discomfort prevents achieving a plateau in oxygen consumption ($\dot{V}o_2$) at peak exercise. In contradiction, Eldridge et al.[34] found that 80% of patients limited by angina pectoris achieved a plateau in $\dot{V}o_2$ during the final 90 seconds of exercise, as compared with 77% of normal subjects. It should be emphasized that the plateau concept has been subjected to many different interpretations,[35] and that some researchers question or dismiss the notion that oxygen delivery always limits exercise capacity.[36] Moreover, recent studies suggest that the occurrence of a plateau may be random.[37]

ARM EXERCISE TESTING

Dynamic arm exercise testing provides a reproducible noninvasive method of evaluating cardiovascular function in subjects with neurologic, vascular, or orthopedic impairment of the lower extremities.[11] In addition, arm exercise testing appears to be the functional evaluation of choice for persons whose occupational and recreational physical activity is dominated by upper extremity efforts, since leg exercise testing suboptimally predicts arm performance capacity (Fig. 8-4) and vice versa.[38]

Arm crank ergometry has been shown to offer a satisfactory, but perhaps not equivalent, alternative to leg exercise testing for the ECG detection of myocardial ischemia, the provocation of angina pectoris, or both. Several investigators have examined the ischemic response to arm versus leg exercise; however, the results are conflicting. Schwade et al.[39] noted no difference in the sensitivity of arm compared with leg exercise in eliciting myocardial ischemia in 33 men with coronary heart disease (CHD). Similarly, Shaw et al.[40] found no difference in the ischemic response to arm ergometry compared with treadmill testing. In contrast, Balady et al.[41] reported that arm exercise testing was less sensitive than was leg exercise testing in detecting CHD. Of 30 symptomatic patients with angiographically proven CHD, only 12 (40%) developed ST segment depression or angina during symptom-limited arm ergometry as compared with 26 (86%) during maximal treadmill testing, despite a comparable peak rate–pressure product for both tests.

Recently, Goodman et al.[42] reported that arm

exercise, coupled with thallium-201 scintigraphy, may be an effective method of detecting myocardial ischemia in patients with peripheral vascular disease. Those who performed enough exercise to increase the heart rate to at least 75% of predicted values without ST segment changes or perfusion defects were at lower risk for the development of subsequent coronary events. Similarly, Balady et al.[43] found that arm ergometer testing, in conjunction with thallium scintigraphy, yielded a sensitivity of 83% and a specificity of 78% in the detection of CHD.

Methods and Protocols

Our studies of coronary patients used a modified conventional leg cycle ergometer (Fig. 8-5) for arm cranking; other investigators have found that the Monark Rehab Trainer works just as well. The arm ergometer is mounted on a table at a height of 68 to 70 cm, so that the subject can perform arm cranking while seated upright, with the feet flat on the floor.[23] It is generally recommended that the ergometer be adjusted so that the midpoint of the sprocket wheel is at shoulder level. However, there appears to be no difference in the physiologic responses to either submaxi-

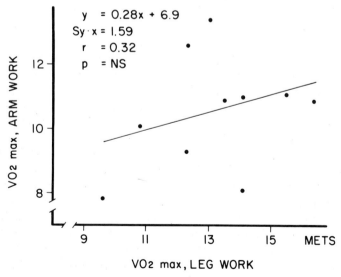

Fig. 8-4. The relationship between $\dot{V}o_2max$ (METs) during arm and leg ergometry using individual data. (From Franklin et al.,[38] with permission.)

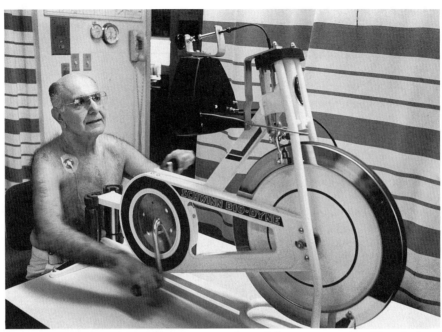

Fig. 8-5. The Schwinn Bio-Dyne cycle ergometer adapted for arm exercise. Bicycle handgrips have been fitted over the pedals, clamps secure the ergometer to a sturdy metal table, and a padded breast-plate helps to standardize the arm position.

mal or maximal arm cranking with the arms positioned above, at, or below heart level.[44] During cranking, the arms are alternately extended at right angles to the body, allowing for a slight bend at the elbow at maximal reach, analogous to the lower-limb extension in leg cycling, to facilitate maximal mechanical efficiency. The method of cranking most often used is of alternating the arms, as with leg ergometry; both arms, however, may pedal concurrently on a single shaft or fulcrum, with similar hemodynamic responses.[40]

Selection of an initial work load and work load increments for each stage must consider the disparity in cardiorespiratory and hemodynamic responses to arm versus leg exercise, as well as the subject's physical status. At a given submaximal work load, arm exercise is performed at a greater physiologic cost than is leg exercise (Fig. 8-6),[39] but maximal responses are generally lower during arm exercise. For example, $\dot{V}o_2max$ during arm exercise generally approximates only 70% ± 15% of the $\dot{V}o_2max$ during leg exercise.[11,45] Therefore, chronotropic and aerobic reserves,

relative to incremental loading, are attenuated for arm exercise as compared with leg exercise. Since a smaller muscle mass is used in arm cycle ergometer testing, and because many coronary patients are not physically conditioned for sustained upper-extremity exercise, there is a tendency to early fatigue. In cardiac, elderly, or symptomatic patients, clinical endpoints or fatigue often limit exercise to work loads at or below 300 kg·m/min. Consequently, low initial work loads and small work load increments per stage should be used when testing these patients.

Although the methodology of arm crank ergometry is now well established, certain technical limitations remain. Because of motion artifact, satisfactory diagnostic ECG records are more difficult to obtain during arm ergometer exercise than during treadmill or leg ergometer exercise testing. Pausing briefly between stages to obtain a high-quality 12-lead ECG recording will permit accurate quantitation of ST segment depression. In addition, it is difficult to assess blood pressure by the standard cuff method in an exercising arm.

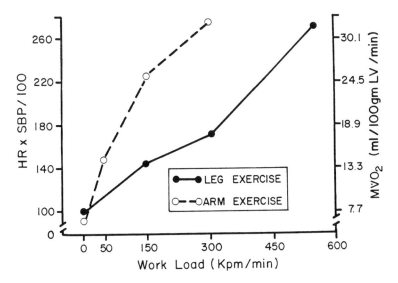

Fig. 8-6. Rate–pressure product (HR × SBP/100) and estimated myocardial oxygen consumption ($M\dot{V}o_2$) during arm and leg exercise in patients with ischemic heart disease. Mean values for the rate–pressure product at 600 kpm/min during leg work were not significantly different from mean values at 300 kpm/min during arm work. (Modified from Schwade et al.,[39] with permission.)

Consequently, blood pressure measurements during arm crank ergometry are generally obtained by one of two methods: measuring pressure in the inactive arm while the subject continues cranking with the other or having the subject crank with both arms and pause briefly between stages (i.e., immediately after cessation of exercise). Unfortunately, both methods have potential drawbacks. High work loads may be difficult to maintain with single-arm cranking, whereas the validity of immediate postexercise blood pressure measurements has been questioned. Our recent studies, using cuff occlusion techniques (Fig. 8-7) to obtain blood pressure values in the legs of exercising patients, indicate that systolic blood pressures taken by the standard cuff method immediately after arm crank exercise are likely to underestimate true physiologic responses (Fig. 8-8).[46]

A review of progressive multistage arm cycle ergometer exercise-testing protocols for patients with CHD is provided in Table 8-5, with specific reference to initial work loads and work load increments per stage, duration of discontinuous or continuous stages, cranking rate, and test endpoints. Exercise stages were 2 to 3 minutes in

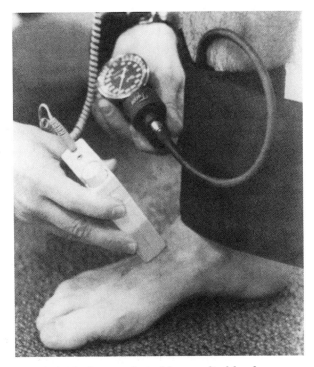

Fig. 8-7. Technique for ankle systolic blood pressure measurements by using a pneumatic cuff and an ultrasound Doppler stethoscope. (From Hollingsworth et al.,[46] with permission.)

Table 8-5. Arm Ergometer Exercise Testing Protocols

Study	Initial Work Load (kg·m/min)	Work Load Increment per Stage (kg·m/min)[a]	Duration of Stages (min)	Cranking Rate (rpm)	Discontinuous (D) or Continuous (C) Stages	Endpoints
Wahren and Bygdeman[47]	Individually determined	100–150	6	Not given	C	Angina
Shaw et al.[40]	200	100	3	40	C	Ischemic ECG; ≥90% HRmax; chest pain, dyspnea, or fatigue
Schwade et al.[39]	"Zero resistance"	150	3	50	D; 1-min rest period	Abnormal ECG or chest pain; fatigue or shortness of breath
Fardy et al.[45]	150	150	4	60	D; 2-min rest period	<60 rpm
Lazarus et al.[48]	100	Stage I = 150; 100 increments thereafter	3	60	C	Angina
DeBusk et al.[49]	150	150	3	Not given	D; 1-min rest period	Angina; dyspnea, fatigue or muscle discomfort; arrhythmias
Balady et al.[41]	215	150	3	Not given	C	Angina; dyspnea, fatigue, complex ventricular arrhythmias; ischemic ECG (>3 mm ST segment depression)
Balady et al.[51]	60	60	2	75–80	C	<75 rpm

[a] For conversion of kilogram meters per minute to watts, 1 W = 6.12 kg·m/min.

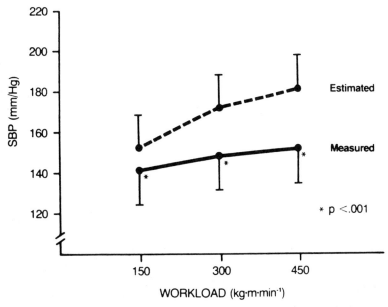

Fig. 8-8. Comparison of the postexercise measured and estimated systolic blood pressure for three progressive arm-crank ergometer work loads. Values are expressed as mean ± SD. (From Hollingsworth et al.,[46] with permission.)

duration; discontinuous protocols typically allowed 1 to 2 minutes of rest between stages, during which time high-quality ECG records and blood pressure measurements were obtained. The initial work load (warm-up) generally consisted of arm cranking at a power output of 200 kg·m/min (33 W) or less. Work load increments per stage averaged 100 to 150 kg·m/min, with cranking rates of 40 to 60 rpm. Peak effort was generally defined as the power output at which the subject was no longer able to maintain the designated pedal speed, notwithstanding encouragement, or the work load at which significant clinical signs or symptoms developed.

In contrast to the standard arm exercise-testing protocols summarized in Table 8-5, Williams et al.[52] designed a unique arm ergometer protocol in which the initial and incremental work loads are individually determined, based on the subject's body weight (Fig. 8-9). The protocol is conceptually analogous to the conventional treadmill exercise test protocols illustrated in Figure 8-1, in that the aerobic requirements at each stage can

be quantified in terms of METs, with 1-MET increments per stage.[50] The investigators have found it to be practical and easy to administer in the clinical setting, eliminating problems in the selection of an initial work load and work load increments per stage.

Aerobic Requirements of Arm Ergometry

Our early studies in men[38] showed that the regression of oxygen uptake ($\dot{V}O_2$) on power output during arm ergometry was $y = 3.06\,x + 191$ ($y = \dot{V}O_2$ in mL/min; x = power output in kg·m/min), where $r = 0.91$ and S (standard error of estimate)$y·x = 191.6$. Since absolute arm $\dot{V}O_2$ (mL/min) at a given work load demonstrated the smallest variability between subjects, Table 8-6 was constructed to predict arm $\dot{V}O_2$ in mL/kg/min, based on a constant absolute $\dot{V}O_2$ with a variable subject body weight (50 to 110 kg). More recently, Balady et al.[51] reported separate regression equa-

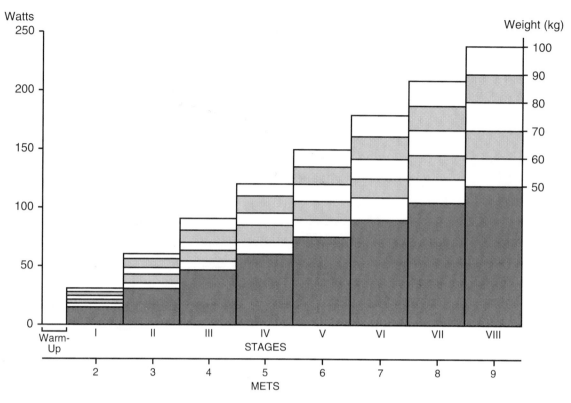

Fig. 8-9. Weight-adjusted arm ergometry protocol. Two-minute stages are used at a cranking rate of 60 rpm; 15-second pauses between stages permit accurate ECG and blood pressure recordings. (Modified from Williams et al.,[52] with permission.)

Table 8-6.   Aerobic Requirements of Arm Ergometry

Work Load[a] (kg/m/min)	150	300	450	600	750
$\dot{V}_{O_2}$ (mL/min)	648	1104	1,562	2,079	2,431

Body Weight						
lbs	kg	\multicolumn{5}{c}{Oxygen Consumption (mL/kg/min)}
110	50	13.0	22.1	31.2	41.7	48.7
132	60	10.9	18.6	25.9	34.7	40.6
154	70	9.1	15.8	22.4	29.8	34.7
176	80	8.1	13.7	19.6	25.9	30.5
198	90	7.4	12.3	17.5	23.1	27.0
220	100	6.7	11.2	15.8	20.7	24.2
242	110	6.0	10.2	14.4	18.9	22.1

[a] Table discontinued above 750 kg/m/min due to small sample size (n = 1).

(Adapted from Franklin et al.,[38] with permission.)

tions for predicting oxygen consumption from power output for healthy men and women. Oxygen uptake, minute ventilation, heart rate, systolic blood pressure, double product of heart rate and systolic blood pressure, and respiratory exchange ratios are significantly greater during arm exercise than during leg exercise at the same submaximal and maximal work loads.[45] Although the arm volume has been measured as being only 34% of the leg volume,[45] the $\dot{V}_{O_2}$max for arm exercise was 69% of that for leg exercise. When considered per milliliter of limb volume, $\dot{V}_{O_2}$max for arm exercise was twice that of the legs. A plausible explanation for this apparent discrepancy is that arm ergometry also utilizes muscle groups of the back, shoulders, and chest. When these muscle groups are added to the arm muscle volume, the muscle mass is greatly increased, and perhaps equilibrates oxygen utilization per unit of limb volume.[45]

ISOMETRIC EXERCISE TESTS

In addition to standardized, isotonic exercise testing of the upper and/or lower extremities, static exercise tests may be indicated for symptomatic or "high-risk" persons whose occupations entail sustained or intermittent isometric requirements (e.g., use of wrenches, saws, or levers; carrying weights; operating a jackhammer; carpentering) or for coronary patients with a hypersensitive carotid sinus reflex.[23] For example, the construction worker with atypical angina might be more appropriately evaluated by static isometric contractions, as in handgrip, weightlifting, or carrying, either alone or in combination with isotonic effort. Rather than arbitrarily proscribing such activities, the clinician should test the individual's responses to such predominantly isometric activities and give advice as to how to minimize adverse responses; for example, a yoke or shoulder strap for carrying heavy weights can avoid expiratory efforts with the glottis closed.[23]

Two of the most common static exercise tests involve the handgrip dynamometer and the Valsalva maneuver (Flack test).

Handgrip Contraction

Handgrip exercise testing can be performed by squeezing a handgrip dynamometer at some percentage of maximal voluntary contraction (e.g., 50%), maintaining the resistance over time. Changes in symptoms, heart rate and rhythm, and systolic and diastolic blood pressures should, as in conventional exercise testing, be monitored and recorded every 30 to 60 seconds.

Static exercise performed to the limit of fatigue produces a pressure load on the left ventricle and is reflected by an increased rate–pressure product that is disproportionate to the somatic oxygen uptake during the effort. Simultaneously, the ECG may show changes in rhythm and ST segment abnormalities that reflect a disparity between myocardial oxygen supply and demand. Subjects who regularly perform isometric exer-

tion in the course of their daily activities may develop significant ST-T displacement, ventricular arrhythmias, or both, and in coronary patients with hypersensitive carotid sinus reflexes, marked sinus bradycardia or even cardiac standstill may occur.

Valsalva Maneuver

The Valsalva maneuver is another type of static exercise used to measure cardiovascular function. It can elicit marked changes in heart rate and blood pressure, as well as ECG changes.[53,54] Cardiovascular responses to increased intrathoracic pressure and straining with a closed glottis are important in recreation and in occupations requiring sustained or intermittent isometric activity. This includes using wrenches and levers, playing wind instruments, and participating in body contact sports.

Equipment and Methods

The equipment required for measurement of the Valsalva maneuver consists of a standard aneroid or mercury manometer attached to a mouthpiece by connecting tubing. A needle placed in the tubing provides a small leak during the expiratory strain, which maintains the glottis open and thereby prevents subjects from maintaining the pressure with either cheek muscles or the tip of the tongue.

Subjects are studied in the semirecumbent or sitting position. They should be instructed in how to maintain an expiratory pressure of 40 mmHg for 10 to 15 seconds. The blood pressure should rise sharply at the onset and fall abruptly at the termination of the strain period. Following an appropriate orientation, each subject should perform two Valsalva maneuvers, separated by a rest period of at least 1 minute. Before and during each maneuver the heart rate should be recorded continuously, using an ECG recording throughout the strain period and for 15 seconds following release of the strain.

Hemodynamic Interpretation

In normal subjects the blood pressure rises and the heart rate slows reflexly with the onset of straining (phase 1); the blood pressure falls and the heart rate rises owing to sympathetic stimulation during the period of sustained straining (phase 2); with sudden release of straining (phase 3) the blood pressure drops and the heart rate increases; in phase 4 there is an overshoot of blood pressure that induces a marked reflex bradycardia, usually within five to nine beats. In the presence of severe myocardial disease, reduced myocardial reserve, or significant valvular obstruction, there is no increase in blood pressure and, hence, no bradycardia in phase 4. The heart rate changes induced by the Valsalva maneuver can be expressed as the Valsalva ratio (the ratio of maximal tachycardia to maximal bradycardia). The Valsalva ratio is calculated as the ratio of maximal R-R interval to minimal R-R interval; intervals associated with premature beats should be excluded. A Valsalva ratio of 1.50 has been suggested as a lower limit of normal. In one study, 96% of 200 normal subjects had ratios of 1.50 or higher.[54] The ratio is inversely related to left ventricular diastolic pressure and mean pulmonary wedge pressure.[54] The Valsalva ratio is significantly reduced in the presence of pulmonary congestion, obstructive mitral and aortic valvular disease, CHD, and cardiomyopathy. The Valsalva maneuver may elicit complex arrhythmias, reflex cardiac standstill, or syncope in patients with a hypersensitive carotid sinus reflex or chronic obstructive lung disease.

INDICATIONS FOR STOPPING AN EXERCISE TEST IN PROGRESS

Commonly used criteria for discontinuing a peak or symptom-limited exercise test include evidence of maximal performance (e.g., a respiratory exchange ratio > 1.15, hyperpnea, achievement of maximal predicted heart rate, subject's request to stop, perceived exertion greater than 17 [very hard]), evidence of excessive stress or potential hazard via the emergence of premonitory signs or symptoms, or failure of the ECG surveillance system.[2,23]

Clinical Signs and Symptoms

Abnormal clinical signs that warrant termination of an exercise test include marked dyspnea, pallor, cold sweating, cyanosis, nausea, or evidence of central nervous system dysfunction including ataxia, staggering, confusion in responding to questions, and head nodding. Physical signs that require discontinuation of exercise testing include exertional hypotension, defined as a significant decrease ($\geq$ 20 mmHg) in systolic blood pressure or failure of the systolic blood pressure to rise with increasing work loads; an excessive rise in blood pressure (systolic pressure > 250 mmHg; diastolic pressure > 120 mmHg); and ECG abnormalities, including serious ventricular arrhythmias, frequent multiform premature ventricular complexes (PVCs), "R-on-T phenomenon," recurring couplets, salvos or paroxysms or sustained supraventricular or ventricular tachycardias, exercise-induced left bundle branch block, onset of second- or third degree atrioventricular block, and ST-T displacement of more than 2 mm (0.2 mV). Symptoms include progressive angina (stop at 3+ level or earlier on a scale of 1+ [perceptible but mild] to 4+ [severe]), or leg pain or other pain or discomfort (with or without ECG changes), lightheadedness, dizziness, or indications that the subject can continue no longer.

Peak performances in such tests are improperly classified as maximal. A physiologic maximal test is defined as a test in which the subject is unable to increase oxygen uptake with further effort. These tests are more appropriately designated *symptom-limited* tests (by chest pain, excessive dyspnea, or volitional fatigue) or *signomatic tests* (prematurely terminated due to multiform ventricular ectopic rhythms, marked ST-T displacement, incoordination).[23] The external work that produces such responses is more properly designated peak performance or peak work load.

EXERCISE TESTING SOON AFTER MYOCARDIAL INFARCTION

Exercise testing of the convalescing patient after uncomplicated myocardial infarction is used not only to assess functional status, but also as a diagnostic, prognostic and therapeutic guide (see Chs. 11 and 14).[55] The test also serves to promote patient self-confidence, providing reassurance that various physical activities, including lifting, sexual intercourse, and physical exertion in general, can be undertaken safely.[56,57] Since the risk of predischarge exercise testing is low,[58] it is now widely administered to many patients after myocardial infarction, except those with overt heart failure, persistent chest pain or unstable angina, hemodynamic instability, second- or third-degree atrioventricular block, or serious ventricular arrhythmias.[5] In a recent survey[59] involving 151,945 "early" exercise tests, no significant difference was noted between the rate of major cardiovascular complications occurring during testing less than 15 days after acute myocardial infarction versus testing performed between 15 and 28 days after the coronary event.

Methods and Protocols

Early postinfarction exercise tests, as compared with conventional diagnostic exercise tests, generally begin at a lower exercise intensity (e.g., ≤2.5 METs), proceed with smaller increments of work per stage, and often employ reduced peak work loads. The timing of such low-level exercise testing varies widely, from 3 days (i.e., before hospital discharge) to 4 weeks after infarction. Although the intensity of the test generally is lower than the first several stages of conventional exercise tests, the same recording methods, supervision procedures, and safety precautions are indicated. The modified protocol is designed to simulate and slightly exceed the somatic and myocardial aerobic requirements of activities that will be encountered at home during convalescence. For this reason, these tests typically impose peak work loads of up to 5 METs, equal to a body oxygen uptake of 17.5 mL/kg/min; however, a test may, in the absence of signs and symptoms, safely continue to peak or symptom-limited work loads.[60,61]

Whether the predischarge exercise test should be symptom-limited, or stopped when an arbitrary "submaximal" heart rate or work load is achieved, remains controversial. A recent survey[62] showed that the majority of physicians still preferred "low-level" exercise testing soon after acute myocardial infarction. The mean test endpoint reported was 123 beats/min or 72% of the age-predicted maximal heart rate, while the mean MET level achieved was 5.2. DeBusk and Haskell[63] compared protocols limited by heart rate or symptoms and found them to be equally safe and effective for eliciting both evidence of myocardial ischemia and arrhythmias soon after an uncomplicated myocardial infarction. On the other hand, Starling et al.[64] found that the symptom-limited exercise test was superior, yielding a higher frequency of ischemic signs or symptoms, without increasing the risk of the test. Hamm et al.[62] administered a symptom-limited exercise test to postinfarction patients an average of 12 days after the acute event and compared the diagnostic yield with data obtained during low-level testing limited to 4.6 METs. The symptom-limited test resulted in a 2.5-fold higher incidence of angina pectoris and 3.4-fold higher incidence of ischemic ST segment depression than the low-level test, confirming the observations of Starling et al.[64]

Figure 8-10 presents several protocols that are commonly used for low-level exercise testing.[23] The two most commonly used treadmill protocols are the modified Bruce[65] and the Naughton[66] protocols, starting at 1.7 mph at a 0% grade, and 2.0 mph at a 0% grade, respectively. Both tests employ a constant treadmill speed and increase the grade or incline every 3 minutes. The cycle ergometer protocol consists of pedaling at 50 or 60 rpm for 3 to 4 minutes at each of two or three progressive work loads, adjusted for body weight, to impose peak loads of up to 5 METs.

Guidelines for Stopping Early Postinfarction Exercise Tests

The criteria for discontinuing exercise tests soon after infarction are often more conservative than those for terminating fatigue-limited or symptom-limited exercise tests. Accordingly, one of three "submaximal" endpoints may be used: (1) heart rate; (2) work load; or (3) perceived exertion rating. Such tests are generally terminated

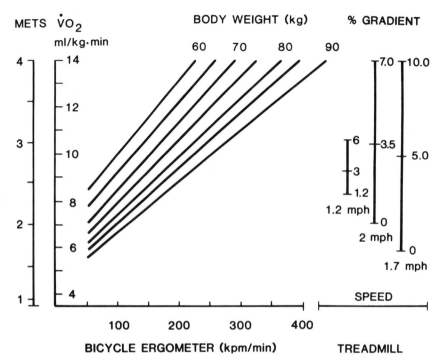

Fig. 8-10. Estimated oxygen consumption and MET requirements for four low-level exercise protocols suitable for testing of the convalescing patient with uncomplicated myocardial infarction. (From Hellerstein and Franklin,[23] with permission.)

once a predetermined heart rate response is reached (70 to 75% of the age-predicted maximal heart rate [60% with beta blockade]); a heart rate of 120 to 140 beats/min; or a peak rate of at least 30 beats/min above resting level, a work load (usually up to 5 METs), or a perceived exertion rating (usually "somewhat hard" to "hard") is attained.[4,67]

Interpretation of Results

The responses to exercise testing soon after myocardial infarction provide objective information about the functional capacity, the need for additional diagnostic studies (coronary angiograms, exercise radionuclide studies), and therapeutic strategies (including medications, interventional techniques or surgery) for the patient. Delaying discharge from the hospital or retesting after administration of cardiac medications may

be indicated for patients who demonstrate significant arrhythmias, ischemic ST segment depression, or angina pectoris.

Certain responses to early postinfarction exercise testing have been shown to be prognostically useful. *The presence of exercise-induced ST segment depression appears to be the most reliable prognostic indicator, identifying patients at increased risk for sudden cardiac death and recurrent infarction.*[4,55,67] Exercise-induced angina pectoris, with or without concomitant ST segment depression, is also prognostically valuable;[68] coronary angiography performed in patients with these abnormalities reveals a high incidence of residual multivessel disease. Exercise-induced ST segment elevation is also associated with a larger infarct size, transmural extension, prevalence of abnormal Q waves, higher peak creatine kinase values, lower ejection fraction, persistent thallium-201 defects, increased lung uptake of thallium-201, a greater number of akinetic or dyskinetic segments, and a poorer prognosis.[69,70] In contrast, ventricular arrhythmias, systolic hypotension (a relatively common response), and poor exercise capacity have been reported as inconsistent predictors of posthospital mortality.[71,72]

EXERCISE TESTING SOON AFTER CORONARY ARTERY BYPASS SURGERY (CABG) OR CORONARY ANGIOPLASTY (PTCA)

Low-level treadmill or cycle ergometer exercise testing has proved to be valuable in safely assessing the functional status and recurrence of stenosis (Chs. 17 and 18) and in prescribing levels of physical activity in the posthospital phase after CABG surgery (usually 3 to 5 weeks) or after PTCA (1 to 2 weeks). On the other hand, arm ergometer exercise testing within 3 to 5 weeks after CABG may be uncomfortable because of midsternal incisional pain, but usually is well tolerated at 6 to 8 weeks postoperatively.[2] The overall testing procedures are similar to those after acute myocardial infarction, i.e., indications, contraindications, guidelines for stopping the test, interpretation of results, and treatment of significant arrhythmias. Although the method of testing is similar, the average peak oxygen consumption and work load attained are often slightly greater than after acute myocardial infarction.[23] The results of the exercise test, coupled with information about the patient's activities of daily living, facilitate individualized prescriptions for medications and physical activities and lead to better control of the pace of convalescence before return to work.

EXERCISE TESTING FOR RISK STRATIFICATION

Identification, soon after myocardial infarction, of patients who are at increased risk for subsequent coronary events offers two major benefits:

(1) patients at moderate to high risk can be evaluated for more intensive pharmacotherapy, interventional cardiac catheterization, or surgery, and (2) patients at low risk can be spared early cardiac catheterization and unwarranted restriction of their vocational and recreational activities.[55]

DeBusk et al.[73] emphasized in their risk stratification algorithm (Fig. 8-11) that the degree of left ventricular dysfunction and residual resting or exercise-induced myocardial ischemia determine the risk of future coronary events. Using this algorithm, by 3 weeks after hospitalization, 100 survivors of documented acute myocardial infarction were distributed as follows: 50 patients were at low risk (less than 2% annual mortality) because of an absence of severe resting or exercise-induced myocardial ischemia and severe left ventricular dysfunction; 30 patients were at moderate to high risk (10 to 25% first-year mortality) because of severe resting or exercise-induced ischemia in the presence of moderate to good left ventricular function; and 20 patients were at high risk (greater than 25% first-year mortality) because of clinically evident severe pump failure or severe left ventricular dysfunction.

Although nearly half of the patients who will have reinfarction or die within the first year after acute myocardial infarction can be identified on the basis of severe ischemia or pump failure during the first 5 days of hospitalization, there is a need to identify additional patients at increased risk who do not demonstrate these abnormalities. Exercise testing soon after myocardial infarction provides a means of detecting residual myocardial ischemia. Abnormal findings suggest that additional areas of myocardium are perfused by stenosed coronary vessels and remain in jeopardy. According to this risk stratification algorithm, approximately 30% of all survivors of acute myocardial infarction demonstrate resting or exercise-induced ST segment depression, angina pectoris, or both, signifying a cohort of patients who are at moderate to high risk for a future coronary event. Such individuals are appropriate candidates for coronary angiography to evaluate for PTCA or CABG surgery.[73]

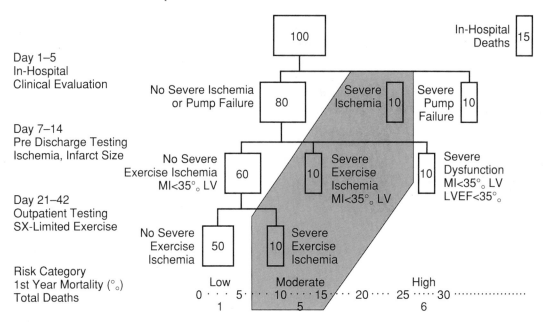

Fig. 8-11. Risk stratification algorithm for patients soon after acute myocardial infarction. The size of each patient subset (number in boxes) in the algorithm is approximate and will vary according to the patient population. Stratification of patients into the three main risk categories (low, moderate, and high) is based on the extent of myocardial ischemia (MI) and left ventricular (LV) dysfunction. A variety of clinical observations and tests may be used to detect these abnormalities at various times after acute myocardial infarction. Patients in the shaded area are those most likely to experience a reduction in mortality from coronary revascularization. LVEF, left ventricular ejection fraction; SX, symptom-limited. (From DeBusk et al.,[73] with permission.)

Prognostic Value of Multiple Exercise Variables

McNeer et al.[74] demonstrated that the ST segment response, duration of exercise (a correlate of fitness or aerobic capacity), and maximal heart rate identified low- and high-risk subgroups more accurately than coronary artery anatomy alone. Nearly half of their cohort of 1,472 patients were taking beta-blocking drugs at the time of testing, yet the significance of these findings remained valid. Over 97% of their patients who showed ≥1 mm ST segment depression at relatively low work loads (i.e., Bruce stages I or II) had significant CHD. Of these patients, more than 60% had three-vessel disease and over 25% had significant stenosis (≥50%) of the left main coronary artery. A more recent report from the Coronary Artery Surgery Study confirms these findings.[75]

Bruce and DeRouen[76] analyzed multiple hemodynamic and clinical variables and found three non-ECG parameters that were related to increased mortality in coronary patients. These were cardiomegaly, a systolic blood pressure less than 130 mmHg at peak exercise, and an exercise duration under 3 minutes (Bruce protocol), corresponding to an aerobic capacity below 5 METs. Dagenis et al.[77] also found that survival decreased with decreasing duration of exercise in asymptomatic patients who exhibited marked (>2 mm) horizontal or downsloping ST segment depression during treadmill exercise testing.

Recently, several computer scores have been derived that use multiple exercise variables and statistical techniques for predicting prognosis and disease severity.[22] For example, the Duke treadmill score[78] utilizes exercise time (minutes), ST segment displacement (millimeters), and an angina index (0, none; 1, occurring during treadmill test; 2, reason for terminating test):

Treadmill score = exercise time −

(5 × ST displacement) − (4 × angina index)

This combination of exercise variables accurately identifies patients at low (≥5 points), intermediate (−10 to +4), and high (≤ −11) risk.

Relation Between Fitness and All-Cause Mortality

A recent study by Blair et al.[79] identified a low level of aerobic fitness as an important risk factor for all-cause mortality. The investigators prospectively studied 10,224 men and 3,120 women who were given a preventive medical examination and a maximal treadmill exercise test to assess their functional capacity. Over an average follow-up of slightly more than 8 years, there were 240 and 43 deaths among the men and women, respectively. In general, the higher the initial level of fitness, the lower the subsequent mortality rate from cancer and heart disease (Fig. 8-12). This relationship held up to a slightly above-average fitness level for both men and women. Interestingly, there appeared to be no additional benefit associated with even higher levels of fitness (i.e., the "excellent" category). Moreover, the greatest reduction in risk for both men and women occurred with progression from the lowest level of fitness (poor) to the next lowest level (below average), suggesting that even a modest improvement in fitness among the most unfit confers a substantial health benefit. The fitness levels associated with a plateau in death rates, corresponding to 9 to 10 METs, can be attained by most men and women who simply walk briskly for 30 minutes or more each day.

SUMMARY

Exercise testing appears to play an important role in the medical management and rehabilitation of patients with CHD. Multistage exercise testing provides invaluable information in assessing the patient's functional capacity, formulating a safe and effective exercise prescription, and evaluating the effect of various interventions. Moreover, the results have long-term prognostic significance in regard to morbidity and mortality.

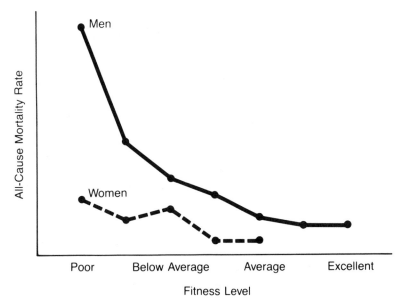

Fig. 8-12. Age-adjusted, all-cause mortality rates by physical fitness categories in men and women. (Modified from Blair et al.,[79] with permission.)

Although the principles of exercise testing should be developed as scientifically as possible, the exercise test procedure should be adapted to the patient, rather than the patient to the procedure.

REFERENCES

1. Levison H, Cherniak RM: Ventilatory cost of exercise in chronic obstructive pulmonary disease. J Appl Physiol 25:21, 1968
2. American College of Sports Medicine: Guidelines for Graded Exercise Testing and Exercise Prescription. p. 1. 4th Ed. Lea & Febiger, Philadelphia, 1991
3. Northridge DB, Grant S, Ford I et al: Novel exercise protocol suitable for use on a treadmill or a bicycle ergometer. Br Heart J 64:313, 1990
4. Fuller T, Movahed A: Current review of exercise testing: Application and interpretation. Clin Cardiol 10:189, 1987
5. Kozlowski JH, Ellestad MH: The exercise test as a guide to management and prognosis. p. 395. In Franklin BA, Rubenfire M (eds): Cardiac Rehabilitation. WB Saunders, Philadelphia, 1984
6. Franklin BA, Hellerstein HK, Gordon S, Timmis GC: Cardiac patients. p. 45. In Franklin BA, Gordon S, Timmis GC (eds): Exercise in Modern Medicine. Williams & Wilkins, Baltimore, 1989
7. Foster C, Pollock ML, Rod JL et al: Evaluation of functional capacity during exercise radionuclide angiography. Cardiology 70:85, 1983
8. Ford D, Maddahi J, Berman D et al: Differing ability of treadmill and upright bicycle exercise testing to induce clinical and electrocardiographic myocardial ischemia in patients with coronary artery disease (abstract). J Am Coll Cardiol 1:650, 1983
9. Wicks JR, Sutton JR, Oldridge NB et al: Comparison of electrocardiographic changes induced by maximum exercise testing with treadmill and cycle ergometer. Circulation 57:1066, 1978
10. Papazoglou N, Kolokouri-Dervou E, Fanourakis I et al: Jogging in place: Evaluation of a simplified exercise test. Chest 96:840, 1989
11. Franklin BA: Exercise testing, training and arm ergometry. Sports Med 2:100, 1985
12. Heller GV, Aroesty JM, Parker JA et al: The pacing stress test. Thallium-201 myocardial imaging after atrial pacing: Diagnostic value in detecting coronary artery disease compared with exercise testing. J Am Coll Cardiol 3:1197, 1984
13. Redwood DR, Rosing DR, Goldstein RE et al: Importance of the design of an exercise protocol in the evaluation of patients with angina pectoris. Circulation 43:618, 1971
14. Buchfuhrer MJ, Hansen JE, Robinson TE et al: Optimizing the exercise protocol for cardiopulmonary assessment. J Appl Physiol 55:1558, 1983
15. Webster MWI, Sharpe DN: Exercise testing in angina pectoris: The importance of protocol design in clinical trials. Am Heart J 117:505, 1989
16. Hlatky MA, Boineau RE, Higginbotham MD et al: A brief self-administered questionnaire to determine functional capacity (The Duke Activity Status Index). Am J Cardiol 64:651, 1989
17. American Heart Association: Recommendations for Human Blood Pressure Determination by Sphygmomanometers. American Heart Association, Dallas, 1980
18. Gibbons L, Blair SN, Kohl HW et al: The safety of maximal exercise testing. Circulation 80:846, 1989
19. Dimsdale JE, Hartley H, Guiney T et al: Postexercise peril: Plasma catecholamines and exercise. JAMA 251:630, 1984
20. Bruce RA: Principles of exercise testing. p. 45. In Naughton JP, Hellerstein HK, Mohler IC (eds): Exercise Testing and Exercise Training in Coronary Heart Disease. Academic Press, San Diego, 1973
21. Handler CE, Sowton E: A comparison of the Naughton and modified Bruce treadmill exercise protocols in their ability to detect ischaemic abnormalities six weeks after myocardial infarction. Eur Heart J 5:752, 1984
22. Froelicher VF, Dubach P: Recent advances in exercise testing. Cardio (May):41, 1990
23. Hellerstein HK, Franklin BA: Exercise testing and prescription. p. 197. In Wenger NK, Hellerstein HK (eds): Rehabilitation of the Coronary Patient, 2nd ed. John Wiley & Sons, New York, 1984
24. Franklin BA: Pitfalls in estimating aerobic capacity from exercise time or workload. Appl Cardiol 14:25, 1986
25. Weber KT, Janicki JS: Cardiopulmonary testing for the evaluation of chronic cardiac failure. Am J Cardiol 55:22A, 1985
26. Sullivan M, McKirnan MD: Errors in predicting functional capacity for postmyocardial infarction patients using a modified Bruce protocol. Am Heart J 107:486, 1984
27. Asmussen E, Christiansen EH, Nielsen M: Die O_2-Aufnahme der ruhenden und der arbeitenden Skellett Muskeln. Skand Arch Physiol 82:212, 1939

28. Hughson RL, Smyth GA: Slower adaptation of $\dot{V}o_2$ to steady state of submaximal exercise with beta-adrenergic blockade. Eur J Appl Physiol 52:107, 1983

29. Froelicher VF, Brammell H, Davis G et al: A comparison of the reproducibility and physiologic response to three maximal treadmill exercise protocols. Chest 65:512, 1974

30. Froelicher VF, Thompson AJ, Noguera I et al: Prediction of maximal oxygen consumption: Comparison of the Bruce and Balke treadmill protocols. Chest 68:331, 1975

31. Ragg KE, Murray TF, Karbonit LM et al: Errors in predicting functional capacity from a treadmill exercise stress test. Am Heart J 100:581, 1980

32. Buskirk E, Taylor HL: Maximal oxygen intake and its relation to body composition, with special reference to chronic physical activity and obesity. J Appl Physiol 2:72, 1957

33. Bruce RA, Kusumi F, Hosmer D: Maximal oxygen intake and nomographic assessment of functional aerobic impairment in cardiovascular disease. Am Heart J 85:546, 1973

34. Eldridge JE, Ramsey-Green CL, Hossack KF: Effects of the limiting symptom on the achievement of maximal oxygen consumption in patients with coronary artery disease. Am J Cardiol 57:513, 1986

35. Taylor HL, Buskirk E, Henschel A: Maximal oxygen intake as an objective measurement of cardiorespiratory performance. J Appl Physiol 8:73, 1955

36. Noakes TD: Implications of exercise testing for prediction of athletic performance: A contemporary perspective. Med Sci Sports Exercise 20:319, 1988

37. Myers J, Walsh D, Buchanan N et al: Can maximal cardiopulmonary capacity be recognized by a plateau in oxygen uptake? Chest 96:1312, 1989

38. Franklin BA, Vander L, Wrisley D et al: Aerobic requirements of arm ergometry: Implications for exercise testing and training. Physician Sportsmed 11:81, 1983

39. Schwade J, Blomqvist CG, Shapiro W: A comparison of the response to arm and leg work in patients with ischemic heart disease. Am Heart J 94:203, 1977

40. Shaw DJ, Crawford MH, Karliner JS et al: Arm-crank ergometry: A new method for the evaluation of coronary artery disease. Am J Cardiol 33:801, 1974

41. Balady GJ, Weiner DA, McCabe CH et al: Value of arm exercise testing in detecting coronary artery disease. Am J Cardiol 55:37, 1985

42. Goodman S, Rubler S, Bryk H et al: Arm exercise testing with myocardial scintigraphy in asymptomatic patients with peripheral vascular disease. Chest 95:740, 1989

43. Balady GJ, Weiner DA, Rothendler JA et al: Arm exercise-thallium imaging testing for the detection of coronary artery disease. J Am Coll Cardiol 9:84, 1987

44. Cummins TD, Gladden LB: Responses to submaximal and maximal arm cycling above, at, and below heart level. Med Sci Sports Exercise 15:295, 1983

45. Fardy PS, Webb D, Hellerstein HK: Benefits of arm exercise in cardiac rehabilitation. Physician Sportsmed 5:30, 1977

46. Hollingsworth V, Bendick P, Franklin B et al: Validity of arm ergometer blood pressures immediately after exercise. Am J Cardiol 65:1358, 1990

47. Wahren J, Bygdeman S: Onset of angina pectoris in relation to circulatory adaptation during arm and leg exercise. Circulation 44:432, 1971

48. Lazarus B, Cullinane E, Thompson PD: Comparison of the results and reproducibility of arm and leg exercise tests in men with angina pectoris. Am J Cardiol 47:1075, 1981

49. DeBusk RF, Valdez R, Houston N et al: Cardiovascular responses to dynamic and static effort soon after myocardial infarction: Application to occupational work assessment. Circulation 58:368, 1978

50. Hellerstein HK, Franklin BA: Evaluating the cardiac patient for exercise therapy: Role of exercise testing. p. 371. In Franklin BA, Rubenfire M (eds): Cardiac Rehabilitation. WB Saunders, Philadelphia, 1984

51. Balady GJ, Weiner DA, Rose L et al: Physiologic responses to arm ergometry exercise relative to age and gender. J Am Coll Cardiol 16:130, 1990

52. Williams J, Cottrell E, Powers SK et al: Arm ergometry: A review of published protocols and the introduction of a new weight adjusted protocol. J Sports Med Phys Fitness 23:107, 1983

53. Elisberg EI: Heart rate response to the Valsalva maneuver as a test of circulatory integrity. JAMA 186:120, 1973

54. Levin AB: A simple test of cardiac function based upon the heart rate changes induced by the Valsalva maneuver. Am J Cardiol 18:90, 1966

55. Fein SA, Klein NA, Frishman WH: Prognostic value and safety of exercise testing soon after uncomplicated myocardial infarction. Cardiovasc Clin 13:279, 1983

56. Cohn PF: The role of noninvasive cardiac testing

after an uncomplicated myocardial infarction. N Engl J Med 309:90, 1983

57. Ewart CK, Taylor CB, Reese LB et al: The effects of early post infarction exercise testing on self perception and subsequent physical activity. Am J Cardiol 51:1076, 1983

58. Epstein SE, Palmeri ST, Patterson RE: Evaluation of patients after acute myocardial infarction: Indications for cardiac catheterization and surgical intervention. N Engl J Med 307:1487, 1982

59. Hamm LF, Crow RS, Stull GA et al: Safety and characteristics of exercise testing early after acute myocardial infarction. Am J Cardiol 63:1193, 1989

60. Topol EJ, Juni JE, O'Neill WW: Exercise testing three days after onset of acute myocardial infarction. Am J Cardiol 60:958, 1987

61. Topol EJ, Burek K, O'Neill WW: A randomized controlled trial of hospital discharge three days after myocardial infarction in the era of reperfusion. N Engl J Med 318:1083, 1988

62. Hamm LF, Stull GA, Serfass RC et al: Prognostic endpoint yield of high-level versus low-level graded exercise testing. Arch Phys Med Rehabil 69:86, 1988

63. DeBusk RF, Haskell W: Symptom-limited versus heart rate-limited exercise testing soon after myocardial infarction. Circulation 61:738, 1980

64. Starling MR, Crawford MH, O'Rourke RA: Superiority of selected treadmill exercise protocols predischarge and six weeks postinfarction for detecting ischemic abnormalities. Am Heart J 104:1054, 1982

65. Bruce RA, Hornsten TR: Exercise stress testing in evaluation of patients with ischemic heart disease. Prog Cardiovasc Dis 11:371, 1969

66. Naughton J, Sevelius G, Balke B: Physiological responses of normal and pathological subjects to a modified work capacity test. J Sports Med 3:201, 1963

67. Weiner DA: Predischarge exercise testing after myocardial infarction: Prognostic and therapeutic features. Cardiovasc Clin 15:95, 1985

68. Cole JP, Ellestad MH: Significance of chest pain during treadmill exercise: Correlation with coronary events. Am J Cardiol 41:227, 1978

69. Bruce RA, Fisher LD, Pettinger M et al: ST segment elevation with exercise: A marker for poor ventricular function and poor prognosis. Coronary Artery Surgery Study (CASS) confirmation of Seattle Heart Watch results. Circulation 77:897, 1988

70. Haines DE, Beller BA, Watson DD et al: Exercise-induced ST segment elevation two weeks after uncomplicated myocardial infarction: Contributing factors and prognostic significance. J Am Coll Cardiol 9:996, 1987

71. Starling MR, Crawford MH, Kennedy GT et al: Exercise testing early after myocardial infarction: Predictive value for subsequent unstable angina and death. Am J Cardiol 46:909, 1980

72. Weld FM, Chu KL, Bigger JT Jr, et al: Risk stratification with low-level exercise testing 2 weeks after acute myocardial infarction. Circulation 64:306, 1981

73. DeBusk RF, Blomqvist CG, Kouchoukos NT et al: Identification and treatment of low-risk patients after acute myocardial infarction and coronary-artery bypass graft surgery. N Engl J Med 314:161, 1986

74. McNeer JF, Margolis JR, Lee KL et al: The role of the exercise test in the evaluation of patients for ischemic heart disease. Circulation 57:64, 1978

75. Weiner DA, Ryan TJ, McCabe CH et al: Prognostic importance of a clinical profile and exercise test in medically treated patients with coronary artery disease. J Am Coll Cardiol 3:772, 1984

76. Bruce RA, DeRouen TA: Exercise testing as a predictor of heart disease and sudden death. Hosp Pract 13:69, 1978

77. Dagenais GR, Rouleau JR, Hochart P et al: Survival with painless strongly positive exercise electrocardiogram. Am J Cardiol 62:892, 1988

78. Mark DB, Hlatky MA, Harrell FE et al: Exercise treadmill score for predicting prognosis in coronary artery disease. Ann Intern Med 106:793, 1987

79. Blair SN, Kohl HW, Paffenbarger RS et al: Physical fitness and all-cause mortality: A prospective study of healthy men and women. JAMA 262:2395, 1989

9

Radionuclide-Based Exercise Testing

George A. Beller, M.D.

The prognosis in survivors of acute myocardial infarction is related to the degree of global left ventricular dysfunction, the presence and extent of residual myocardial ischemia, and the presence of complex ventricular ectopy. Myocardial perfusion imaging performed in association with exercise testing or in conjunction with dipyridamole or adenosine infusion has proven to be useful for stratification of uncomplicated postinfarction patients into high- and low-risk subsets. Both the extent of irreversible myocardial damage and the amount of myocardium that is viable but jeopardized can be assessed by this radionuclide approach. Exercise radionuclide angiography is an alternative nuclear cardiology procedure, which has also been demonstrated to be effective in separating high- and low-risk subgroups of patients who have experienced a recent myocardial infarction. The extent of left ventricular dysfunction documented during exercise correlates with subsequent outcome. Positron emission tomography (PET) can also be employed for evaluation of myocardial perfusion and viability after acute infarction.

Decision-making with respect to selection of postinfarction patients who might benefit from invasive evaluation and subsequent myocardial revascularization has been aided by radionuclide imaging of perfusion and function. Low-risk patients as assessed by radionuclide testing should have an excellent 1-year survival and can enter a comprehensive program of coronary exercise rehabilitation and risk factor modification soon after hospital discharge. Patients with high-risk radionuclide findings on exercise might first undergo angiography and appropriate coronary revascularization before enrolling in a coronary rehabilitation exercise program.

TECHNICAL CONSIDERATIONS

Exercise Thallium-201 Scintigraphy

After the intravenous injection, the early myocardial uptake of thallium-201 is directly proportional to regional myocardial blood flow and the extraction of thallium by the myocardium.[1,2] At high myocardial blood flows, extraction of thallium diminishes. There is little effect on thallium extraction with acidosis, hypoxemia, digitalis administration, and propranolol therapy.[2,3] Extraction of thallium is unaltered in "stunned" myocardium, characterized by postischemic dysfunction after reperfusion (Fig. 9-1).[4] Similarly, a chronic low-flow state resulting in ischemic dysfunction (hibernating myocardium) is associated with preserved extraction and intracellular thallium-201 washout.[5] These data suggest that uptake of thallium by myocardial cells is not appreciably diminished until irreversible membrane injury occurs. Therefore, in the absence of necrosis, defects observed on myocardial thallium-201 scintigrams reflect abnormalities in regional blood flow rather than metabolic cellular dysfunction or abnormalities in membrane transport.

Following the initial myocardial uptake phase

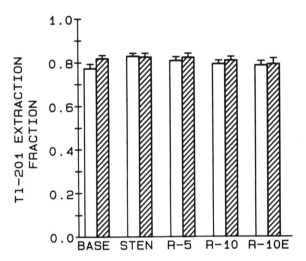

Fig. 9-1. Thallium-201 extraction fraction after intracoronary thallium-201 administration in stunned (open bars; n = 13) and control (crosshatched bars; n = 6) dogs. Stunning was produced by 10 five-minute transient occlusions of the left anterior descending coronary artery, each interspersed by 10 minutes of reperfusion. No significant difference in extraction fraction was seen between the two groups. Abbreviations: BASE, baseline; STEN, after creation of the coronary stenosis; R-5, after reperfusion 5 in stunned dogs; R-10, after reperfusion 10 in stunned dogs; R-10E, 40 minutes after reperfusion 10. (From Moore et al.,[4] with permission.)

after intravenous thallium-201 injection, there is continuous exchange of the tracer between the myocardium and the blood pool.[6,7] Thallium-201 is continually being washed out of normally perfused myocardium and being replaced by recirculating thallium-201 from residual activity in the blood pool. This process of continuous exchange forms the basis of delayed thallium-201 "redistribution." In clinical imaging parlance, redistribution is defined as total or partial delayed defect resolution following exercise-induced underperfusion or even during a chronic reduction in myocardial blood flow ("rest redistribution").[8] Figure 9-2 is a scintigram of a patient with a septal thallium-201 defect that exhibited delayed redistribution.

Delayed redistribution is also observed after dipyridamole-induced flow heterogeneity and is comparable in extent and severity to redistribution defects observed during exercise in the same patients.[9] However, during dipyridamole or adenosine infusion, there may be a transmural coronary steal in the stenotic region where flow decreases in subendocardial layers associated with a minimal increase of flow in subepicardial zones.[10]

Some patients may have defects that appear persistent at 2.5 to 4 hours after thallium-201 injection, but demonstrate late redistribution at 24 hours after thallium-201 administration.[11,12] This observation is of clinical relevance since such myocardial zones which demonstrate little redistribution at 2 to 4 hours may actually represent viable myocardium rather than scar or recent necrosis. Recently, the ability to distinguish between ischemia and scar by thallium scintigraphy has been enhanced by the administration of a second resting dose of thallium-201 after redistribution images have been obtained.[13]

Single photon emission computed tomography (SPECT) imaging offers several important advantages over planar imaging in assessment of myocardial perfusion and viability in postinfarction patients. The extent of perfusion abnormalities can be quantitated better by this tomographic approach than by three-view planar scintigraphy.[14] This permits a more accurate evaluation of infarct size as well as the extent of myocardium still in jeopardy. However, the specificity of SPECT thallium-201 scintigraphy is somewhat lower than that of planar imaging.[15] This may be due to the artifacts that can occur on SPECT images and that may be misconstrued as perfusion abnormalities.

In patients with chronic chest pain syndromes, the sensitivity and specificity of exercise thallium-201 scintigraphy for coronary heart disease (CHD) detection is in the range of 85 to 90%.[16] The detection of individual coronary stenoses in patients with underlying multivessel disease is enhanced by quantitative scan analyses.[17] In patients with chest pain who are evaluated for the presence or absence of CHD, the presence of thallium-201 redistribution is associated with a significantly worse prognosis during follow-up.[18] Figure 9-3 depicts the percentage of patients free from events if redistribution was present or absent on symptom-limited exercise scintigraphy.[18]

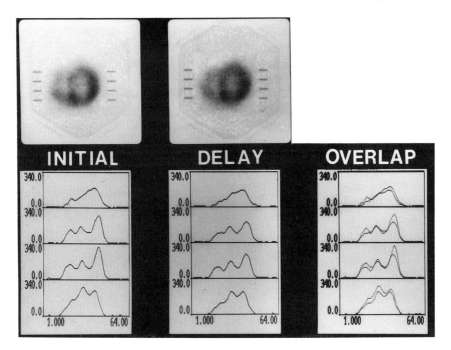

Fig. 9-2. Initial postexercise and 2.5-hour delayed thallium-201 scintigrams in 45° left anterior oblique projection. There is a septal defect postexercise that shows partial redistribution. The quantitative count profiles show normal thallium-201 washout from the posterolateral wall with abnormal washout from the septum. The overlap panel depicts the superimposition of exercise and rest count profiles.

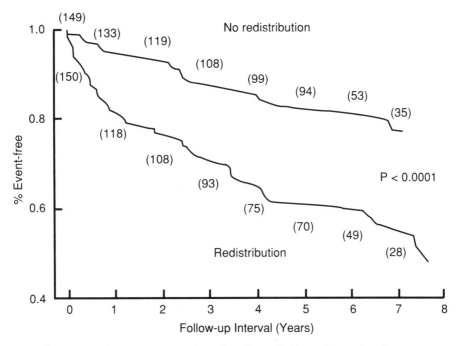

Fig. 9-3. Event-free survival in patients with and without thallium-201 redistribution on exercise imaging for evaluation of chest pain. (From Kaul et al.,[18] with permission.)

The exercise thallium-201 scintigram is more sensitive than exercise electrocardiography alone for detection of myocardial ischemia in patients undergoing exercise testing.[16] Also, there are many patients who have persistently abnormal resting electrocardiographic changes after myocardial infarction that preclude accurate interpretation of changes during exercise. In these patients, the addition of radionuclide imaging to conventional treadmill exercise testing improves the specificity of the test for detection of ischemia within and remote from the infarct zone.

Exercise Technetium-99m Isonitrile Imaging

The technetium-labeled isonitriles are lipophilic cationic technetium-99m complexes that, like thallium-201, are taken up by the myocardium in proportion to regional myocardial blood flow.[19,20] One of these agents, technetium-99m sestamibi, does not redistribute after transient myocardial ischemia and requires separate injections during exercise and rest to distinguish between myocardial ischemia and myocardial scar. Although the first-pass myocardial extraction of technetium-99m sestamibi is less efficient than that of thallium-201, the ultimate myocardial uptake of both tracers is similar under physiologic flow conditions.[21]

The precise mechanism of cellular uptake and sequestration of the technetium-99m isonitriles is unknown. However, ischemic or stunned myocardium still takes up this tracer in proportion to blood flow and viability, even in the presence of severe systolic dysfunction.[5] Thus, like thallium-201, technetium-99m sestamibi imaging can be used in postinfarction patients to identify viable but ischemic myocardium. It has been particularly effective in demonstrating the efficacy of thrombolytic therapy.[22,23]

Preliminary studies have demonstrated that the sensitivity and specificity for CHD detection is comparable between technetium-99m sestamibi and thallium-201 imaging.[24] However, image quality seems to be enhanced when the isonitrile is used as the perfusion tracer. Because of the high count rates achieved with technetium-99m sestamibi, perfusion images can be obtained in the gated mode, allowing for simultaneous assessment of perfusion and regional function. Likewise, one can perform first-pass exercise radionuclide angiography soon after injection of technetium-99m sestamibi at rest or during exercise. One then obtains the perfusion images from the same injected tracer dose 45 minutes later. This is another approach to simultaneously assessing myocardial function and perfusion in the same setting.

Exercise Radionuclide Angiography

Rest radionuclide angiography can be used after myocardial infarction to assess global and regional function and indirectly estimate the extent of myocardial injury. Zones of myocardial viability on rest radionuclide angiography most often demonstrate hypokinetic wall motion rather than akinesis or dyskinesis. However, soon after thrombolytic therapy, the presence of akinesis or even dyskinesis does not exclude the possibility of residual myocardial viability. This is because of the "stunning" phenomenon that is characterized by postischemic dysfunction after coronary reperfusion. Such postischemic asynergy may last from days to weeks following the acute event.

Exercise radionuclide angiography has been performed in patients with CHD to evaluate prognosis.[25,26] One can expect the left ventricular ejection fraction in normal subjects to increase by 5% or more during exercise.[27] In patients with significant underlying CHD, exercise-induced ischemia results in a fall in the exercise left ventricular ejection fraction at peak effort compared with the resting value. The magnitude of the fall in left ventricular ejection fraction reflects the underlying anatomic severity of disease and extent of ischemic asynergy. Figure 9-4 shows the 2-year survival and total coronary event-free survival as a function of the exercise left ventricular ejection fraction in medically treated patients with CHD.[25]

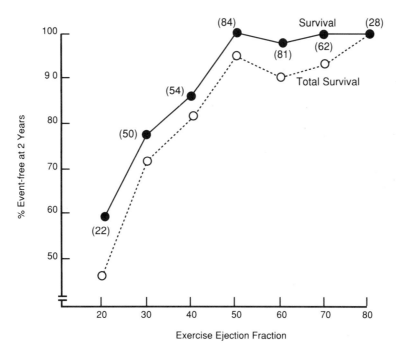

Fig. 9-4. Percentage of patients free from events at 2 years related to the value of the exercise ejection fraction in patients with CHD who are medically treated. (From Pryor et al.,[25] with permission.)

Dipyridamole or Adenosine Myocardial Perfusion Imaging

As mentioned above, dipyridamole or adenosine can be substituted for exercise to detect physiologically important CHD and to assess prognosis.[28,29] Dipyridamole or adenosine thallium scintigraphy may be uniquely of value in patients who are unable to exercise because of such noncardiac disorders as disabling arthritis, low back pain, cerebral vascular disease, and other orthopedic abnormalities. Dipyridamole has been approved by the Food and Drug Administration (FDA) for clinical use, but intravenous adenosine for imaging is still pending approval. The sensitivity of dipyridamole thallium-201 imaging for CHD detection is comparable to the sensitivity of exercise thallium scintigraphy. In a pooled analysis from 12 published studies comprising 616 patients with angiographically documented CHD and 206 patients with angiographically normal coronary arteries, the sensi-

tivity and specificity of dipyridamole thallium-201 scintigraphy for detection of CHD were 85.3 and 90.4%, respectively.[30] As with exercise imaging, dipyridamole thallium-201 imaging has been used successfully to differentiate between myocardial ischemia and myocardial scar in determining the presence of residual myocardial viability in patients demonstrating regional wall motion abnormalities. In a study by Okada et al.,[31] redistribution defects in dipyridamole thallium-201 scans were most often associated with normal rest and exercise left ventricular ejection fractions and preservation of regional wall motion.

One can infuse adenosine directly via the intravenous route as a substitute for dipyridamole as an agent for vasodilator stress.[29] Results have been comparable between the two agents, but side effects may be greater with adenosine infusion. A potential advantage of adenosine is that it has such a short half-life that mere cessation of the infusion is all that is required when side effects are encountered. This precludes the necessity of intravenous aminophylline (an adenosine antagonist) administration to reverse such side effects as hypotension, chest pain, or atrioventricular block.

PREDISCHARGE RISK STRATIFICATION UTILIZING EXERCISE RADIONUCLIDE IMAGING

Exercise and Dipyridamole Perfusion Imaging

Patients with myocardial infarction who have experienced uncomplicated clinical courses during hospitalization without evidence of clinical heart failure, serious ventricular arrhythmias, or recurrent rest or low-level exertional angina are eligible for predischarge treadmill or bicycle exercise testing for further prognostication. High-risk variables on myocardial perfusion scans in postinfarction patients include (1) failure to reach at least 4 METs or to achieve a target heart rate of 120 beats/min (in the absence of medications which decrease heart rate); (2) an abnormal blood pressure response, with failure to increase systolic blood pressure by 10 mmHg or more; (3) exercise-induced ventricular arrhythmias; (4) exercise-induced ST segment elevation; (5) exercise-induced ST segment depression of more than 1.0 mm; (6) the concomitant development of angina at less than 4 METs associated with ST segment depression; (7) multiple perfusion defects in more than one coronary supply region; (8) delayed redistribution in the infarct zone in patients with non-Q wave infarction; (9) an abnormal increase in lung thallium-201 uptake with a lung/heart ratio greater than 0.52; and (10) exercise-induced transient left ventricular dilatation as observed on initial anterior projection images.

In a study performed at the University of Virginia, the ability of predischarge quantitative exercise thallium-201 scintigraphy to predict future coronary events was evaluated prospectively in 140 consecutive patients with uncomplicated

myocardial infarction who were under 65 years of age.[32] By 15 ± 12 months, 50 of the 140 patients sustained a coronary event: 7 died, 9 experienced reinfarction, and 34 were rehospitalized with class III to IV angina. In this study, the patients whose sole abnormality was that of persistent defects in only one vascular region, with no evidence of redistribution or lung uptake, had only a 6% event rate during follow-up. There was one death in this group. In contrast, 15 of the 16 patients who either died or experienced a reinfarction had one of the high-risk thallium-201 scintigraphic findings. In this study, thallium-201 scintigraphy was more effective than exercise electrocardiography and coronary angiography in separating high- from low-risk patients (Fig. 9-5).

An explanation for the superiority of exercise thallium scintigraphy over exercise electrocardiography alone in risk stratification after myocardial infarction relates to its capacity for enhanced identification of underlying multivessel CHD. Several studies have shown that multiple defects in more than one coronary supply region are present in approximately 60% of patients with underlying multivessel CHD.[33,34] In contrast, only approximately 10% of patients with a myocardial infarction and underlying single-vessel disease will demonstrate multiple perfusion abnormalities in more than one coronary supply region.

High-risk patients with non-Q wave infarction can also be identified by demonstration of residual thallium redistribution on predischarge exercise scintigraphy.[35] The prevalence and extent of thallium redistribution within the zone of infarction were greater in patients with non-Q wave infarction (60%) than in those with Q wave infarction (36%).[35] The patients with non-Q wave infarction who subsequently died or sustained reinfarction or recurrent unstable angina had a significantly higher incidence of residual infarct zone ischemia by thallium-201 scan criteria than did patients who sustained no coronary events.

Dipyridamole thallium-201 scintigraphy has been evaluated in postinfarction patients to determine its prognostic utility. Gimple et al.[36] reported that dipyridamole-induced thallium-201 redistribution outside the infarct zone had a 63% sensitivity and 75% specificity for predicting sub-

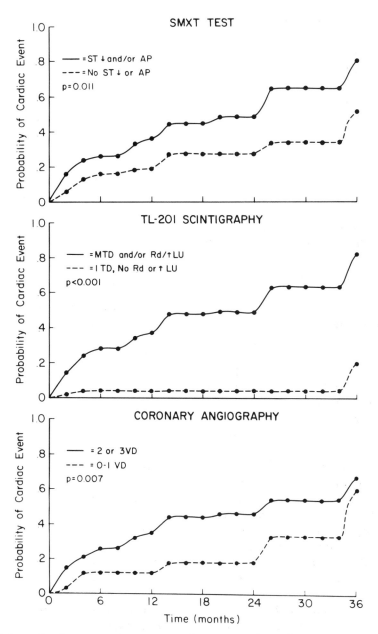

Fig. 9-5. Probability of a future coronary event after uncomplicated myocardial infarction based on results of the submaximal exercise electrocardiographic test (SMXT) (top), the exercise thallium-201 scintigram (middle), and coronary angiography (bottom). Abbreviations: ST↓, ST segment depression of ≥1.0 mm; AP, angina pectoris; MTD, multiple thallium-201 defects in more than one vascular region; Rd, thallium-201 redistribution; ↑LU, increased lung thallium-201 uptake; VD, vessel disease on angiography defined as ≥50% stenosis. (From Gibson et al.,[32] with permission.)

sequent coronary events. Leppo et al.[37] reported that the mere presence of a defect with delayed redistribution on dipyridamole scintigrams performed prior to discharge was the best predictor of subsequent coronary events in patients with uncomplicated infarction. Hendel et al.[38] examined the prognostic utility of dipyridamole thallium-201 imaging in 516 consecutive patients undergoing testing. This group reported that, by logistic regression analysis, an abnormal scan was an independent and significant predictor of subsequent infarction or death and increased the relative risk of an event more than threefold. The combination of diabetes mellitus, congestive heart failure, and an abnormal dipyridamole thallium-201 scintigraphic study resulted in the highest predicted probability of subsequent infarction or death and raised the relative risk of sustaining one or more of these events more than 26-fold.

Exercise Radionuclide Angiography

Exercise radionuclide angiography can be performed prior to hospital discharge to separate high- and low-risk patients after uncomplicated myocardial infarction. Patients who subsequently experience cardiac death or nonfatal infarction have a higher prevalence of an abnormal ejection fraction or abnormal end-systolic volume response to exercise at predischarge testing. Hung et al.[39] reported that low peak treadmill work load and the change in left ventricular ejection fraction during exercise were significant predictors of coronary events, as assessed by multivariate analysis, in men tested 3 weeks postinfarction. A peak treadmill workload of 4 METs or less, or a decrease in ejection fraction of 5% or more during submaximal exercise below the value at rest, distinguishes high- from low-risk subsets with 23 and 2% event rates, respectively.

Morris et al.[40] showed that exercise ejection fraction inversely correlated with subsequent mortality in 106 consecutive survivors of acute myocardial infarction. By Cox regression modeling, as the exercise ejection fraction fell below 45%, mortality increased dramatically. Similarly, Abraham et al. reported that when the exercise

ejection fraction fell to less than 50% compared with an ejection fraction of 50% or more, the 2-year event-free survival rate free of medical complications was 42% compared with 83%.[41]

In summary, the noninvasive radionuclide variables most predictive of an adverse outcome after myocardial infarction include multiple perfusion abnormalities, increased lung thallium-201 uptake, and a fall in left ventricular ejection fraction after exercise.

Invasive Versus Conservative Strategy

Following the in-hospital phase of acute myocardial infarction, a decision must be made whether to proceed with an invasive strategy characterized by coronary angiography with a view toward myocardial revascularization, or to follow a conservative strategy which comprises vigorous risk factor modification and appropriate prophylactic pharmacologic drugs. The latter may include oral beta-blockade therapy in patients who survive a Q wave infarction and diltiazem therapy for patients with non-Q wave infarction with preserved left ventricular function. Both groups of patients would be given aspirin. For medically treated patients, exercise therapy at the outset has been advocated as another effective means of reducing the risk of subsequent coronary events and enhancing physical performance, quality of life, and psychological well-being. For low-risk patients without extensive residual ischemia, it is safe to begin exercise therapy within 1 to 2 weeks after hospital discharge.

Predischarge exercise testing in association with radionuclide imaging can be used as a cost-effective means of determining which patients should undergo the invasive strategy and which should undergo the conservative strategy. As described above, patients with poor exercise tolerance and evidence for extensive residual ischemia are candidates for early angiography. If multivessel disease was evident, coronary bypass surgery or multivessel angioplasty may be appropriate revascularization approaches. In patients with single-vessel disease and residual ischemia, coronary angioplasty would be favored, but patients with small risk areas, particularly when associated with an inferior infarction, could be treated medically and by coronary rehabilitation measures alone.

Patients demonstrating low-risk exercise thallium-201 scintigraphic findings (neither redistribution nor increased lung thallium-201 uptake) would be treated medically unless symptoms subsequently develop. Such patients could immediately enter a prescribed exercise program with the goal of enhancing cardiovascular fitness and possibly reducing the risk of subsequent coronary events.

LONG-TERM FOLLOW-UP

Exercise myocardial perfusion imaging or radionuclide angiography are useful adjuncts to exercise electrocardiographic testing for evaluation of the efficacy of revascularization therapy or long-term medical management of survivors of an acute myocardial infarction. Patients who demonstrate redistribution thallium-201 defects preoperatively or prior to coronary angioplasty usually demonstrate improved myocardial perfusion after the procedure. This improvement in regional blood flow during exercise is usually accompanied by enhanced exercise tolerance.

Patients who develop graft occlusion or stenosis, restenosis of a dilated lesion after angioplasty, or stenosis of a previously uninvolved artery will usually demonstrate exercise ST segment depression and reappearance of redistribution thallium-201 scan abnormalities.[42,43] In several studies, the presence of thallium-201 redistribution was the single best predictor of restenosis and was more sensitive than exercise electrocardiographic changes. In a study by Briesblatt et al.,[44] the predictive accuracy of thallium-201 imaging for detection of restenosis after coronary angioplasty was evaluated in 121 asymptomatic patients. Of these asymptomatic patients, 25% had evidence of "silent" thallium-201 redistribution on scintigraphy 4 to 6 weeks after angioplasty. Evidence of restenosis was present by 6 months in 85% of these patients and by 1 year in 96%.

Myocardial perfusion imaging or exercise radionuclide angiography is probably not required as an adjunct to exercise testing for determining or adjusting the exercise prescription for postinfarction patients undergoing sustained exercise therapy. The exercise treadmill test alone is sufficient to determine the exercise prescription in such patients. The perfusion image or the exercise radionuclide angiogram is most useful in the initial assessment following myocardial infarction and also at 6 months or 1 year postdischarge. One would anticipate being able to monitor progression of CHD by symptoms and by periodic repeat radionuclide testing.

LIMITATIONS OF RADIONUCLIDE IMAGING

Thallium-201 Scintigraphy

There are several significant limitations of myocardial perfusion imaging with thallium-201. Interpretation of visual images can be difficult if the interpreter is not knowledgeable about image artifacts (e.g., breast attenuation, diaphragmatic attenuation) or variants of normal findings. These faulty interpretations will result in a high false-positive interpretation rate. Circumflex coronary lesions are less easily detected than left anterior descending or right coronary artery lesions. With SPECT imaging, patient motion can result in artifactual defects on the tomographic reconstruction. Other limitations of thallium-201 scintigraphy are the long time required to obtain serial postexercise images and the rather high cost of the procedure. Patients with left bundle branch block and normal coronary arteries often show septal abnormalities.[45] Unfortunately, absolute quantitation of myocardial blood flow in milliliters per minute per gram (mL/min/g) of myocardium cannot be obtained with thallium-201 and gamma camera imaging techniques. Cardiac PET has been shown to provide more quantitative estimates of regional myocardial perfusion.[46]

Exercise Radionuclide Angiography

There are some significant limitations to exercise radionuclide angiography as well. In certain patients with a high resting ejection fraction (>75%), one should not expect a further increase in the ejection fraction with exercise. Thus, such patients may have a "flat" ejection fraction response to exercise. The specificity of the exercise ejection fraction response for CHD is lower than that reported for thallium-201 scintigraphy. This is because noncoronary disorders such as hypertensive heart disease, idiopathic cardiomyopathy, scleroderma heart disease, and other entities will be associated with an abnormal response of the ejection fraction with exercise, but no associated CHD. Also, the specificity of the ejection fraction response in women is lower than in men.[47] Pretreatment with nitrate drugs or calcium-blocking drugs may prevent the abnormal left ventricular functional response to exercise. As with thallium scintigraphic studies, the sensitivity of exercise radionuclide angiography for CHD detection will be lower if patients are unable to achieve an adequate level of exercise.

SUMMARY

One of the major determinants of prognosis after myocardial infarction is residual myocardial ischemia induced by low-level exercise. Exercise testing with either myocardial perfusion imaging or radionuclide angiography is clinically useful for risk stratification and for identifying high-risk patients who would be candidates for coronary angiography and revascularization. Patients with underlying multivessel coronary artery disease who exhibit multiple thallium-201 redistribution defects and increased lung thallium-201 uptake at a low exercise heart rate or work load are at very high risk for a recurrent coronary event with medical therapy alone. Revascularization is indicated soon after testing, with subsequent planning for comprehensive risk reduction and exercise therapy. Patients with low-risk exercise radionuclide test findings are candidates for immediate structured coronary rehabilitation, which often includes exercise therapy as well as risk factor modification and administration of certain prophylactic medications.

REFERENCES

1. Strauss HW, Harrison K, Langan JK et al: Thallium-201 for myocardial imaging. Relation of thallium-201 to regional myocardial perfusion. Circulation 51:641, 1975
2. Weich HF, Strauss HW, Pitt B: The extraction of thallium-201 by the myocardium. Circulation 56:188, 1977
3. Leppo JA, Macneil PB, Moring AF, Apstein CS: Separate effects of ischemia, hypoxia and contractility on thallium-201 kinetics in rabbit myocardium. J Nucl Med 27:66, 1986
4. Moore CA, Cannon J, Watson DD et al: Thallium-201 kinetics in stunned myocardium characterized by severe postischemic systolic dysfunction. Circulation 81:1622, 1990
5. Sinusas AJ, Watson DD, Cannon JM et al: Effect of ischemia and postischemic dysfunction on myocardial uptake of technetium-99m-labeled methoxyisobutyl isonitrile and thallium-201. J Am Coll Cardiol 14:1785, 1989
6. Beller GA, Watson DD, Ackell P et al: Time course of thallium-201 redistribution after transient myocardial ischemia. Circulation 61:791, 1980
7. Grunwald AM, Watson DD, Holzgrefe HH Jr et al: Myocardial thallium-201 kinetics in normal and ischemic myocardium. Circulation 64:610, 1981
8. Pohost GM, Zir LM, Moore RH et al: Differentiation of transiently ischemic from infarcted myocardium by serial imaging after a single dose of thallium-201. Circulation 55:294, 1977
9. Varma SK, Watson DD, Beller GA: Quantitative comparison of thallium-201 scintigraphy after exercise and dipyridamole in coronary artery disease. Am J Cardiol 64:871, 1989
10. Beller GA, Holzgrefe HH, Watson DD: Effects of dipyridamole-induced vasodilation on myocardial uptake and clearance kinetics of thallium-201. Circulation 68:1328, 1983
11. Kiat H, Berman DS, Maddahi J et al: Late reversibility of tomographic myocardial thallium-201 defects: An accurate marker of myocardial viability. J Am Coll Cardiol 12:1456, 1988
12. Cloninger KG, DePuey EG, Garcia EV et al: Incomplete redistribution in delayed thallium-201

single photon emission computed tomographic (SPECT) images: An overestimation of myocardial scarring. J Am Coll Cardiol 12:955, 1988

13. Dilsizian V, Rocco TP, Freedman N et al: Enhanced detection of ischemic but viable myocardium by the reinjection of thallium after stress-redistribution imaging. N Engl J Med 323:141, 1990

14. Maddahi J, Van Train K, Prigent F et al: Quantitative single photon emission computed thallium-201 tomography for detection and localization of coronary artery disease: Optimization and prospective validation of a new technique. J Am Coll Cardiol 14:1689, 1989

15. DePasquale EE, Nody AC, DePuey EG et al: Quantitative rotational thallium-201 tomography for identifying and localizing coronary artery disease. Circulation 77:316, 1988

16. Beller GA: Nuclear cardiology: current indications and clinical usefulness. Curr Probl Cardiol 10:4, 1985

17. Berger BC, Watson DD, Taylor GJ et al: Quantitative thallium-201 exercise scintigraphy for detection of coronary artery disease. J Nucl Med 22:585, 1981

18. Kaul S, Lilly DR, Gascho JA et al: Prognostic utility of the exercise thallium-201 test in ambulatory patients with chest pain: Comparison with cardiac catheterization. Circulation 77:745, 1988

19. Okada RD, Glover D, Gaffney T, Williams S: Myocardial kinetics of technetium-99m-hexakis-2-methoxy-2-methylpropyl isonitrile. Circulation 77:491, 1988

20. Li Q, Frank TL, Franceschi D et al: Technetium-99m methoxyisobutyl isonitrile (RP-30) for quantification of myocardial ischemia and reperfusion in dogs. J Nucl Med 29:1539, 1988

21. Leppo JA, Meerdink DJ; Comparison of the myocardial uptake of a technetium-labeled isonitrile analogue and thallium. Circ Res 65:632, 1989

22. Wackers FJT, Gibbons RJ, Verani MS et al: Serial quantitative planar technetium-99m-isonitrile imaging in acute myocardial infarction: Efficacy for noninvasive assessment of thrombolytic therapy. J Am Coll Cardiol 14:861, 1989

23. Gibbons RJ, Verani MS, Behrenbeck T et al; Feasibility of tomographic 99mTc-hexakis-2-methoxy-2-methylpropyl-isonitrile imaging for the assessment of myocardial area at risk and effect of treatment in acute myocardial infarction. Circulation 80:1277, 1989

24. Kiat H, Maddahi J, Roy LT et al: Comparison of technetium 99m methoxyisobutyl isonitrile and thallium 201 for evaluation of coronary artery dis-

ease by planar and tomographic methods. Am Heart J 117:1, 1989

25. Pryor DB, Harrell FE, Lee KL et al: Prognostic indications from radionuclide angiography in medically treated patients with coronary artery disease. Am J Cardiol 53:18, 1984

26. Bonow RO, Kent KM, Rosing DR et al: Exercise-induced ischemia in mildly symptomatic patients with coronary-artery disease and preserved left ventricular function: Identification of subgroups at risk of death during medical therapy. N Engl J Med 311:1339, 1984

27. Borer JS, Bacharach SL, Green MV et al: Real-time radionuclide cineangiography in the noninvasive evaluation of global and regional left ventricular function at rest and during exercise in patients with coronary-artery disease. N Engl J Med 296:839, 1977

28. Iskandrian AS, Heo J, Askenase A et al: Dipyridamole cardiac imaging. Am Heart J 114:432, 1988

29. Verani MS, Mahmarian JJ, Hixson JB et al: Diagnosis of coronary artery disease by controlled coronary vasodilation with adenosine and thallium-201 scintigraphy in patients unable to exercise. Circulation 82:80, 1990

30. Leppo JA: Dipyridamole-thallium imaging. The lazy man's stress test. J Nucl Med 30:281, 1989

31. Okada RD, Dai Y, Boucher CA, Pohost GM: Serial thallium-201 imaging after dipyridamole for coronary disease detection: Quantitative analysis using myocardial clearance. Am Heart J 107:475, 1984

32. Gibson RS, Watson DD, Craddock GB et al: Prediction of cardiac events after uncomplicated myocardial infarction: A prospective study comparing predischarge exercise thallium-201 scintigraphy and coronary angiography. Circulation 68:321, 1983

33. Nygaard TW, Gibson RS, Ryan JM et al: Prevalence of high-risk thallium-201 scintigraphic findings in left main coronary artery stenosis: Comparison to patients with multiple- and single-vessel coronary artery disease. Am J Cardiol 53:462, 1984

34. Dunn RF, Freedman B, Bailey IK et al: Noninvasive prediction of multivessel disease after myocardial infarction. Circulation 62:726, 1980

35. Gibson RS, Beller GA, Gheorghiade M et al: The prevalence and clinical significance of residual myocardial ischemia 2 weeks after uncomplicated non-Q wave infarction: A prospective natural history study. Circulation 73:1186, 1986

36. Gimple LW, Hutter AM Jr, Guiney TE, Boucher

CA: Prognostic utility of predischarge dipyridamole-thallium imaging compared to predischarge submaximal exercise electrocardiography and maximal exercise thallium imaging after uncomplicated acute myocardial infarction. Am J Cardiol 64:1243, 1989

37. Leppo JA, O'Brien J, Rothendler JA et al: Dipyridamole-thallium-201 scintigraphy in the prediction of future cardiac events after acute myocardial infarction. N Engl J Med 310:1014, 1984

38. Hendel RC, Layden JJ, Leppo JA: Prognostic value of dipyridamole thallium scintigraphy for evaluation of ischemic heart disease. J Am Coll Cardiol 15:109, 1990

39. Hung J, Goris ML, Nash E et al: Comparative value of maximal treadmill testing, exercise thallium myocardial perfusion scintigraphy and exercise radionuclide ventriculography for distinguishing high- and low-risk patients soon after acute myocardial infarction. Am J Cardiol 53:1221, 1984

40. Morris KG, Palmeri ST, Califf RM et al: Value of radionuclide angiography for predicting specific cardiac events after acute myocardial infarction. Am J Cardiol 55:318, 1985

41. Abraham RD, Harris PJ, Roubin GS et al: Usefulness of ejection fraction response to exercise one month after acute myocardial infarction in predicting coronary anatomy and prognosis. Am J Cardiol 60:225, 1987

42. Robinson PS, Williams BT, Webb-Peploe MM et al: Thallium-201 myocardial imaging in assessment of results of aortocoronary bypass surgery. Br Heart J 42:455, 1979

43. Stuckey TD, Burwell LR, Nygaard TW et al: Quantitative exercise thallium-201 scintigraphy for predicting angina recurrence after percutaneous transluminal coronary angioplasty. Am J Cardiol 63:517, 1989

44. Breisblatt WM, Barnes JV, Weiland F et al: Incomplete revascularization in multivessel percutaneous transluminal coronary angioplasty: The role for stress thallium-201 imaging. J Am Coll Cardiol 11:1183, 1988

45. Rothbart RM, Beller GA, Watson DD et al: Diagnostic accuracy and prognostic significance of quantitative thallium-201 scintigraphy in patients with left bundle branch block. Am J Noninvasive Cardiol 1:197, 1987

46. Schelbert HR, Phelps ME, Hoffman E et al: Regional myocardial blood flow, metabolism and function assessed noninvasively with positron emission tomography. Am J Cardiol 46:1269, 1980

47. Higginbotham MB, Morris KG, Coleman RE, Cobb FR: Sex-related differences in the normal cardiac response to upright exercise. Circulation 70:357, 1984

10

Exercise and Other Stress Echocardiography

William F. Armstrong, M.D.

Early experience with exercise testing included analysis of symptoms and changes in the electrocardiogram (ECG) at the time of physical exercise. Throughout the early and mid-1970s it became apparent that analysis of symptoms and the ECG alone provided valuable but suboptimal accuracy, and that ancillary imaging enhanced accuracy as well as information regarding other functional manifestations of coronary heart disease.[1-3] More recently, echocardiographic imaging has been used during exercise and other stress testing to obtain analogous information.[2,4-11]

RATIONALE FOR EXERCISE AND OTHER STRESS ECHOCARDIOGRAPHY

The rationale behind the use of echocardiographic imaging is that myocardial ischemia, if induced by exercise or other stress, will result in abnormal wall motion, which can be detected with the two-dimensional echocardiogram. The relationship of ischemia to abnormal wall motion on echocardiography has been demonstrated in numerous studies, both in the animal laboratory[12] and in the clinical arena.[13,14] More recently, several investigators have documented that exercise or other stress-induced ischemia results in wall motion abnormalities which serve as an accurate marker for the presence of a coronary artery stenosis, although they may occur in noncoronary myocardial diseases as well.

ADVANTAGES AND DISADVANTAGES

As with other imaging techniques, exercise echocardiography has its own distinct advantages and disadvantages, which are listed in Table 10-1. A major advantage of echocardiographic imaging is its tremendous versatility. The routine two-dimensional echocardiogram can identify all four cardiac chambers, all four valves, and the great vessels and detect virtually any anatomic or functional abnormality. As such, information is available regarding the diagnosis of most forms of organic heart disease. Combined with Doppler techniques, accurate data can be obtained regarding the presence and effects of valvular, primary myocardial, pericardial, congenital, or cor-

Table 10-1. Advantages and Disadvantages of Exercise Echocardiography

Advantages
  Highly versatile
  Portable
  Minimal space requirements
  Low capital outlay/operational cost
  High resolution
  Detection of wall thickening
  Noninvasive and risk free
  Applicable to multiple exercise modalities
  Analysis at multiple exercise levels
Disadvantages
  Qualitative
  Technician/physician dependent
  Relatively limited success rates (90 to 95%)

onary heart disease. With the addition of imaging at the time of cardiovascular stress, additional information is obtained regarding inducible ischemia. Both the capital outlay and operational costs of echocardiography are lower than that for competing imaging techniques. Since the echocardiograph is portable, it can be used not only for exercise studies but also for routine studies in the echocardiography laboratory, emergency room, coronary care unit, and outpatient clinics. Modern echocardiography equipment has high resolution and is the only widely available mobile imaging technique capable of evaluation of abnormal myocardial thickening, which is a highly specific indicator of ischemia (Fig. 10-1). The technique is obviously noninvasive and free

of risk to the patient, operator, or pregnant women. Another advantage is that, unlike myocardial perfusion imaging, analysis can be undertaken at multiple exercise levels and the process is less cumbersome than many isotopic studies. Additionally, a very short period is required for its performance, typically extending the time required for a routine exercise test by no more than 30 minutes.

Balancing these advantages are several obvious disadvantages. Analysis of wall motion abnormalities remains a qualitative examination, which is highly dependent on the expertise of the technician recording the examination and the physician performing the interpretation. Satisfactory exercise echocardiograms may be difficult to

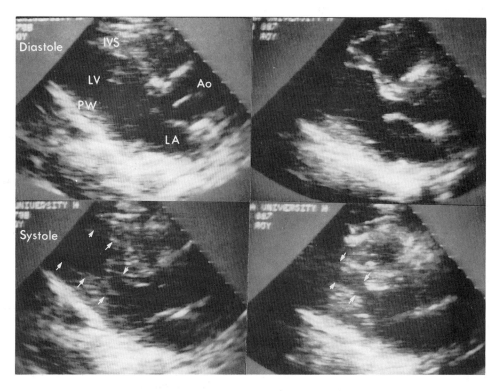

Fig. 10-1. Parasternal long-axis views in diastole (top) and systole (bottom) in a patient at the time of presentation with an acute anterior myocardial infarction (left panels) and 3 days following successful balloon angioplasty (percutaneous transluminal coronary angioplasty [PTCA]) of a critical left anterior descending coronary artery lesion (right panel). On the baseline study (before PTCA) the distal septum is dyskinetic in systole (upward-pointing arrows) while the more proximal septum moves normally. Following successful reperfusion there has been restitution of normal septal wall motion as seen in the lower right panel. Abbreviations: IVS, ventricular septum; LV, left ventricle; PW, posterior wall; LA, left atrium; Ao, aorta. (From Armstrong and Feigenbaum,[31] with permission.)

obtain; however, in most high-volume laboratories 90 to 95% of unselected patients are successfully studied.[5]

METHODOLOGY

Multiple forms of cardiovascular stress can be combined with echocardiographic imaging. These are listed in Table 10-2. The most common form of stress utilized is treadmill exercise[5,8,11] or bicycle ergometry.[4,9,10,11] It is not feasible to perform the echocardiographic examination in an upright walking patient, so that if treadmill exercise is utilized, imaging must be done immediately before and immediately after exercise. However, imaging can be obtained at each stage of exercise, including peak exercise, with supine or upright bicycle ergometry. The addition of imaging at peak exercise increases the sensitivity of the technique, but with a modest cost in specificity.[15] For patients unable to exercise, either pacing[16] or pharmalogic stress[17-19] can be undertaken. The greater experience has been with pharmacologic stress, with either dobutamine or dipyridamole infusions.[17,18]

Table 10-2. Types of Stress Used with Echocardiographic Imaging

Exercise
  Treadmill exercise
  Supine bicycle ergometry
  Upright bicycle ergometry
Pacing
  Transvenous atrial
  Esophageal atrial
  Postventricular
Pharmacologic
  Dobutamine
  Dopamine
  Isoproterenol
  Dipyridamole
  Adenosine
  Ergonovine
Other
  Cold pressor
  Mental stress

EXERCISE ECHOCARDIOGRAPHY

A typical exercise protocol involves scanning the patient's heart at rest in multiple tomographic planes by using two-dimensional echocardiography and then preparing the patient for routine exercise testing.[5,6] Either at the termination of each stage of exercise (with bicycle ergometry) or immediately after exercise (with treadmill exercise), images are repeated in as brief a time as possible. Acquisition of images in an abbreviated time frame is facilitated by digital acquisition systems, which allow capture of images and their playback in a continuous loop, with the rest and exercise counterparts displayed side by side.[6,11,15] In addition to echocardiographic imaging, these protocols preserve the integrity of the symptom and ECG analyses (Figs. 10-2 and 10-3).

Protocols are similar for pharmacologic stress, with the exception that the patient can remain in an optimal scanning position throughout the examination. Dipyridamole is typically infused in a fixed dose and scanning performed continuously throughout the infusion.[17,18] Dobutamine stress echocardiography involves incremental infusions ranging from 2.5 up to 3.5 μg/kg/min, in 3-minute stages.[19] The patient is continuously monitored with echocardiographic imaging as well as ECG recordings for heart rate and rhythm, blood pressure, and symptom analyses during the infusion.

Methods of Analysis

Irrespective of the type of stress utilized, the images are analyzed in a similar fashion. As mentioned above, availability of microcomputer-based programs for digitizing images and playback in a continuous-loop format, side by side, for comparison is advantageous and allows for detection of more subtle abnormalities. Wall motion can be analyzed at several different levels of complexity, ranging from a simple qualitative assessment of normal versus abnormal in any given region to calculation of ejection fraction, end-systolic pressure/volume ratios, end-systolic

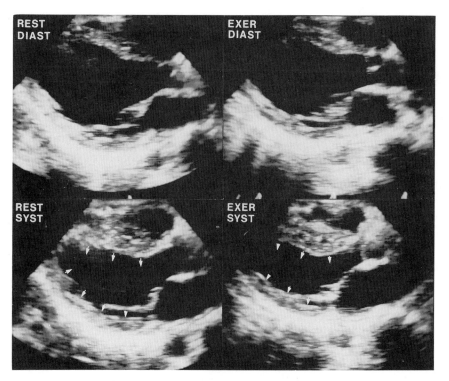

Fig. 10-2. Parasternal long-axis views from an exercise echocardiogram performed on a patient following an inferior myocardial infarction. The orientation is the same as in Fig. 10-1. At rest the proximal two-thirds of the inferoposterior wall is dyskinetic (downward-pointing arrows on the posterior wall). The ventricular septum moves normally. Immediately following exercise the ventricular septum has hyperdynamic wall motion and the inferoposterior wall remains dyskinetic (lower right). These findings imply isolated disease in either the right or left circumflex coronary artery system without ischemia in the anterior distribution. (From Ryan et al.,[32] with permission.)

stress, or detailed analysis of wall motion by using centerline chordal shortening or radian shrinkage methods, etc.[20] For clinical utility, creation of a wall motion score is highly advantageous and provides a semiquantitative number which then can be monitored serially after interventions.[21] The score is indexed to the number of myocardial segments visualized and is proportional to the magnitude and extent of the ischemic wall motion abnormality. Thus, the higher the score, the more abnormal the echocardiogram.

Diagnostic Accuracy

The accuracy of stress echocardiography for detection of coronary heart disease has been evaluated by several different groups of investigators (Table 10-3).[7,8,17,19,22,23] The earlier reports, using older-generation equipment without the benefit of digital acquisition, reported success rates of 75% or less and sensitivities for detection of coronary heart disease of 80% or less.[4] More recent larger studies, in high-volume laboratories and using state-of-the-art equipment, have resulted in higher success rates and increased accuracy. As a general rule, the addition of peak exercise imaging with bicycle ergometry increases sensitivity compared with postexercise imaging with treadmill testing, but at a cost of a reduced specificity.[15]

Several parallels can be drawn between the accuracy of stress echocardiography and that of competing nuclear medicine techniques, including a lower sensitivity for detecting patients with single-vessel coronary disease and reduced spec-

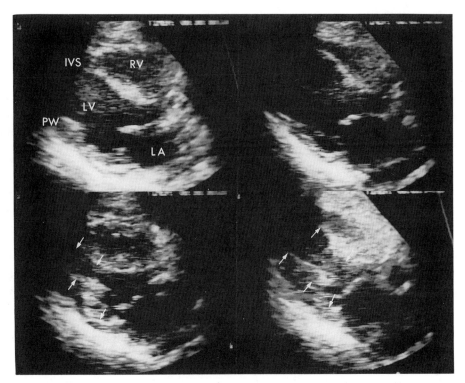

Fig. 10-3. Parasternal long-axis view in a patient following inferoposterior myocardial infarction. The orientation is the same as in Figure 10-1. The resting study is displayed on the left. The proximal inferoposterior wall is dyskinetic (lower left panel). Immediately following exercise the dyskinesis of the inferoposterior wall persists and a new wall motion abnormality develops in the distal ventricular septum. This implies disease in either the right or left circumflex coronary artery (responsible for the inferoposterior myocardial infarction) and additional disease in the left anterior descending coronary artery responsible for the septal ischemia.

Table 10-3. Accuracy of Echocardiography for Detection of Coronary Disease

Author	Stress[a]	Population	Number	Sensitivity (%) Overall	SV[b]	MV[c]	Specificity (%)
Armstrong et al.[7]	TME	General	123	87.3	80.9	93.2	86.4
		No MI[d]	51	78.4	72.4	86.4	
Limacher et al.[8]	TME	General	73	91	64	97	88
Spaccavento et al.[23]	TME	General	150	90	—	—	82
Sawada et al.[22]	Up-bike, TME	Women	57	86	—	—	86
Sawada et al.[19]	Dobutamine	General	71	92	—	—	87
Picano et al.[17]	Dipyridimole	General	93	74	50	85	100

[a] TME, treadmill exercise, postexercise imaging; Up-bike, Upright bicycle, peak imaging.
[b] SV, single-vessel coronary disease.
[c] MV, multivessel coronary disease.
[d] MI, myocardial infarction.

ificity for the precise identification of patients with multivessel disease. Additionally, there are limitations in the assignment scheme of coronary arteries to specific areas of the left ventricle, especially in the posterior circulation.[7] As such, the specific prediction of left anterior descending coronary artery disease is high with nuclear imaging; however, separation of right coronary from left circumflex coronary artery stenosis is less precise.

Clinical Utility of Stress Echocardiography

Since stress echocardiography increases the cost of a diagnostic evaluation, it is not a routine test, but rather should be used in specific settings. A major utilization is in the patient with a nondiagnostic treadmill response due to preexisting bundle branch block, ST segment abnormalities, or atypical exertional symptoms with an ambiguous ECG response to exercise. In this situation, the exercise echocardiogram provides additional information to that available from symptoms and changes in the ECG during exercise testing; 75% of the ambiguous treadmill responses can be correctly stratified by using exercise echocardiography.[6] Data from an Indiana University study also indicate that stress echocardiography in women has an accuracy for diagnosing coronary disease equivalent to that in male cohorts.[22] Its accuracy was unaffected by the ECG response or type of presenting symptoms, either atypical chest pain for ischemia or typical angina.

Assessment of Prognosis

In addition to diagnostic information, the stress echocardiogram can be used for assessing the prognosis. This has been evaluated for patients with stable angina pectoris and patients following myocardial infarction. In a study of 144 cardiac patients who had a normal exercise echocardiogram,[24] over a 2-year follow-up it was found that events occurred in only 5 patients and there were no deaths. These results for prognostic value of

stress echocardiography are similar to the larger experience with established nuclear medicine techniques. Corday et al.[25] have reported similar results; among 243 patients evaluated by exercise echocardiography, all clinical events occurred in the patients who had ischemic wall motion abnormalities on the exercise echocardiogram. The group without such abnormalities had a benign prognosis during a 19-month follow-up.

Three different groups of investigators have evaluated the use of exercise echocardiography in postinfarction patients.[26–28] Data from all three studies are concurrent and demonstrate that, in the convalescence period following myocardial infarction, patients with exercise-induced wall motion abnormalities (at submaximal levels of exercise) have a worse prognosis with respect to future events than do those without such abnormalities. The clinical outcome data from one study are presented in Table 10-4.[26] For this study, an abnormal exercise echocardiogram was defined as one in which a new wall motion abnormality developed (not related to the index myocardial infarction) or multiple abnormalities were present, at least one of which deteriorated following exercise. By definition, all these patients had myocardial infarction and, as such, at least one wall motion abnormality. A "normal"

Table 10.4. Predictive Value of Exercise Echocardiography to Identify Patients with Various Clinical Endpoints

Endpoint	New Wall Motion Abnormalities at Exercise Echocardiography[a]	
	Normal (−) (n = 23)	Abnormal (+) (n = 17)
Good outcome (n = 20)		
Asymptomatic	16	1
Mild angina	3	0
Poor outcome (n = 20)		
Unstable angina	4	10
Myocardial infarction	0	3
Cardiac death	0	3
Coronary artery bypass grafting	1	6

[a] Column totals are greater than n because some patients experienced more than one endpoint.

study allowed the presence of the abnormality related to the index infarction. Data from two additional studies are in agreement with these results and have shown that exercise echocardiography can identify a high-risk subset of patients following acute myocardial infarction.

Role After Interventions

Stress echocardiography may also have a valuable role following therapeutic interventions. Both exercise and pharmacologic stresses have been used following either coronary artery bypass grafting (CABG) surgery[29] or percutaneous balloon angioplasty (PTCA).[21,30] Stress echocardiography has been used to document recovery of function after these procedures. We have recently demonstrated that stress echocardiography may be used as a means of identifying patients following CABG who have either bypass graft stenosis, progression of native disease, or disease in nonrevascularized regions.[33]

Future Utilization

Other more investigational uses of stress echocardiography have included its use for stratification following thrombolytic therapy and for preoperative risk assessment for noncardiac surgery. Additionally, stress echocardiography has shown promise as a means of identifying stunned but viable myocardium and for providing valuable information for management of patients.

SUMMARY

Exercise and other stress echocardiography provide a noninvasive means of evaluating the functional significance of coronary heart disease. It can be used both for diagnostic purposes in patients presenting with chest pain of uncertain etiology and for prognostic purposes in patients with known coronary disease. Correlations can be made between the location of coronary lesions and their functional significance and can be used for serial follow-up of patients.

REFERENCES

1. Borer J, Brensike J, Redwood D et al: Limitations of the electrocardiographic response to exercise in predicting coronary-artery disease. N Engl J Med 293:367, 1975
2. Wasserman LA, Anerson GS, Hakki H et al: Merits of stress thallium-201 myocardial perfusion imaging in patients with inconclusive exercise electrocardiograms: Correlation with coronary angiograms. Am J Cardiol 46:553, 1980
3. Port S, Oshima M, Ray G et al: Assessment of single vessel coronary artery disease: Results of exercise electrocardiography, thallium-201 myocardial perfusion imaging and radionuclide angiography. J Am Coll Cardiol 6:75, 1985
4. Wann LS, Faris JV, Childress RR et al: Exercise cross-sectional echocardiography in ischemic heart disease. Circulation 60:1300, 1979
5. Robertson WS, Feigenbaum H, Armstrong WF et al: Exercise echocardiography: A clinically practical addition in the evaluation of coronary artery disease. J Am Coll Cardiol 12:1085, 1983
6. Armstrong WF, O'Donnell J, Dillon JC et al: Complementary value of two-dimensional exercise echocardiography to routine treadmill exercise testing. Ann Intern Med 105:829, 1986
7. Armstrong WF, O'Donnell J, Ryan TJ et al: Effect of prior myocardial infarction and extent and location of coronary disease on accuracy of exercise echocardiography. J Am Coll Cardiol 10:531, 1987
8. Limacher M, Quinones M, Roliner L et al: Detection of coronary artery disease with exercise two-dimensional echocardiography: Description of a clinically applicable method and comparison with radionuclide ventriculography. Circulation 67:1211, 1983
9. Ginzton L, Conant R, Brizendine M et al: Exercise subcostal two-dimensional echocardiography: A new method of segmental wall motion analysis. Am J Cardiol 53:805, 1984
10. Crawford M, Amon K, Vance W: Exercise two-dimensional echocardiography: Quantitation of left ventricular performance in patients with severe angina pectoris. Am J Cardiol 51:1, 1983
11. Sheikh K, Bengtson J, Helmy S et al: Relation of quantitative coronary lesion measurements to the

development of exercise-induced ischemia assessed by exercise echocardiography. J Am Coll Cardiol 15:1043, 1990

12. O'Boyle J, Parisi A, Neiminen M et al: Quantitative detection of regional left ventricular contraction abnormalities by two-dimensional echocardiography: Comparison of myocardial thickening and thinning and endocardial motion in a canine model. Am J Cardiol 51:1732, 1985

13. Kisslo J, Robertson D, Gilbert B et al: A comparison of real-time, two-dimensional echocardiography and cineangiography in detecting left ventricular asynergy. Circulation 55:134, 1977

14. Weiss J, Bulkley B, Hutchins G, Mason S: Two-dimensional echocardiographic recognition of myocardial injury in man: Comparison with postmortem studies. Circulation 63:401, 1981

15. Presti CF, Armstrong WF, Feigenbaum H: Comparison of echocardiography at peak exercise and after bicycle exercise in evaluation of patients with known or suspected coronary artery disease. J Am Soc Echocardiography 1:119, 1988

16. Chapman PD, Doyle TP, Troup PJ et al: Stress echocardiography with transesophageal atrial pacing: Preliminary report of new method for detection of ischemic wall motion abnormalities. Circulation 70:445, 1984

17. Picano E, Lattanzi F, Masini M et al: High dose dipyridamole echocardiography test in effort angina pectoris. J Am Coll Cardiol 8:848, 1986

18. Picano E, Lattanzi F, Masini M et al: Different degrees of ischemic threshold stratified by the dipyridamole-echocardiography test. Am J Cardiol 59:71, 1987

19. Sawada S, Segar D, Brown S et al: Dobutamine stress echocardiography for evaluation of coronary disease. Circulation 80 (suppl. II):II-66, 1989

20. Mann D, Gillam L, Weyman A: Cross-sectional echocardiographic assessment of regional left ventricular performance and myocardial perfusion. Prog Cardiovasc Dis 29:1, 1986

21. Broderick T, Sawada S, Armstrong WF et al: Improvement in rest and exercise-induced wall motion abnormalities after coronary angioplasty: An exercise echocardiographic study. J Am Coll Cardiol 15:591, 1990

22. Sawada S, Ryan T, Fineberg N et al: Exercise echocardiographic detection of coronary artery disease in women. J Am Coll Cardiol 14:1440, 1989

23. Spaccavento L, Houck P, Gonzalez V et al: Exercise echocardiography in the evaluation of coronary artery disease (abstract). J Am Coll Cardiol 9:216A, 1987

24. Sawada S, Ryan T, Conley M et al: Prognostic value of a normal exercise echocardiogram. Am Heart J 120:49, 1990

25. Corday S, Martin S, Areeda J et al: Prognostic value of treadmill echocardiography in patients with chest pain and positive stress ECG. Circulation 78 (suppl. II):II-272, 1988

26. Applegate R, Dell'italia L, Crawford M: Usefulness of two-dimensional echocardiography during low-level exercise testing early after uncomplicated acute myocardial infarction. Am J Cardiol 60:10, 1987

27. Jaarsma W, Visser C, Kupper A et al: Usefulness of two-dimensional echocardiography shortly after myocardial infarction. Am J Cardiol 57:86, 1986

28. Sawada S, Judson W, Ryan T et al: Upright bicycle exercise echocardiography after coronary artery bypass grafting. Am J Cardiol 64:1123, 1989

29. Labovitz A, Lewen M, Kern M et al: The effects of successful PTCA on left ventricular function: Assessment by exercise echocardiography. Am Heart J 117:1003, 1989

30. Picano E, Pirelli S, Marzilli M et al: Usefulness of high-dose dipyridamole echocardiography test in coronary angioplasty. Circulation 80:807, 1989

31. Armstrong WF, Feigenbaum HF: Echocardiography in patients with coronary artery disease. p. 5. In Pohost GM et al (eds): New Concepts in Cardiac Imaging 1988. Year Book Medical Publishers, Chicago, 1988

32. Ryan T, Armstrong WF, O'Donnell JA, Feigenbaum H: Risk stratification after acute myocardial infarction by means of exercise two-dimensional echocardiography. Am Heart J 114:1305, 1987

33. Sawada SG, Judson WE, Ryan T et al: Upright bicycle exercise echocardiography after coronary artery bypass grafting. Am J Cardiol 64:1123, 1989

III

Clinical Aspects of Coronary Heart Disease: Recognition and Management

11

Clinical Manifestations of Coronary Heart Disease and Guidelines for Management of the Patient

Anthony N. DeMaria, M.D.
Stephen Lenhoff, M.B., Ch.B.

Just as the pathology of coronary heart disease (CHD) may vary markedly from patient to patient, the clinical manifestations of this disorder may also be quite variable. Initial clinical manifestations of CHD include stable angina pectoris, unstable angina pectoris, acute myocardial infarction, and even sudden cardiac death. This chapter reviews these clinical manifestations with specific regard to definition, recognition, diagnosis, and therapy.

STABLE ANGINA PECTORIS

Pathophysiology

The pathophysiology of stable angina pectoris has been discussed in Chapter 3. Therefore, this topic is reviewed only briefly in the present discussion. Angina pectoris occurs when there is an imbalance between the supply of oxygen available to the myocardium and the demand for oxygen of that myocardium. Most often the imbalance in myocardial oxygen supply and demand occurs as a result of an increase in demand. Therefore, despite the presence of coronary ar-

tery obstructions, coronary blood flow is often adequate to meet the metabolic needs of the myocardium in the resting state. However, coronary blood flow reserve is lost with significant arterial stenoses, and the flow cannot be increased beyond resting levels. Accordingly, when myocardial oxygen demand is increased, the supply becomes inadequate and ischemia ensues. Since the principal determinants of myocardial oxygen demand are heart rate, contractility, and wall tension,[1] any intervention that augments these factors will increase the demand for coronary flow. Alternatively, an imbalance may occur as a result of a spontaneous decrease in the supply of oxygen to the myocardium. This is seen in its most dramatic form in coronary spasm, in which complete obstruction may be produced in an apparently totally normal coronary artery.[2]

Recently, it has become clear that the pathophysiology of angina pectoris is more complex than was initially thought. Specifically, it is now known that elements of both increased myocardial oxygen demand and decreased supply may be operative in the same patient.[3] Thus, in a given patient, a fixed coronary artery obstruction may be present that reduces the coronary flow reserve by 30%. However, an additional decrease in cross-sectional area may be superimposed upon this obstruction by an increase in coronary arterial vasomotor tone. This additional reduction of vessel cross-sectional area may result in an 80% loss of coronary reserve. Thus, both fixed and dynamic coronary obstructions may act in concert to limit coronary blood flow and thereby create an imbalance between myocardial oxygen supply and demand. Of significance, since coronary vasomotor tone is dynamic, this component may vary over time and may account for significant differences in the threshold for myocardial ischemia. The vasomotor component to coronary obstruction also presents a specific mechanism for treatment of angina.

Clinical Features

Regardless of the mechanism, when the myocardial oxygen demand exceeds supply, ischemia occurs and may be manifested by angina pectoris. The classic description of angina pectoris by Heberden[4] includes a dull pain in the chest, typically felt in the substernal region, radiating to the left or both arms or even the jaw. The discomfort characteristically abates within 5 minutes by removal of the inciting factor or administration of suitable pharmacologic agents. Often the chest discomfort is not perceived as a pain, but rather as a tightness or heavy sensation. The discomfort may be perceived in the abdomen, back, or mandible, and occasionally a pain equivalent such as shortness of breath may be experienced. In classic angina pectoris, the chest discomfort is provoked typically by exertion but often also by emotion or exposure to cold weather, and is relieved spontaneously within 5 to 10 minutes of termination of the provocation.

In some circumstances, myocardial ischemia may be silent or painless.[5] The mechanism by which myocardial ischemia produces pain in some patients but not in others is still uncertain. However, considerable evidence now exists to support the concept that electrocardiographic (ECG) changes (the typical manifestation of angina pectoris available in such patients) in the absence of chest discomfort are truly related to myocardial ischemia. In addition, a number of studies have demonstrated that painless myocardial ischemia has the same prognostic significance as angina pectoris and that most patients with silent ischemia also have painful episodes. At present, it is uncertain which patients should be screened for silent ischemia, which method should be used for the screening, and whether therapy should be administered on the basis of the presence or absence of this finding. Therefore, the remainder of this discussion will be confined to classic angina pectoris.

In general, the term *stable angina pectoris* relates to provoked chest pain that occurs at a predictable frequency with predictable stimulation and at a relatively constant level of intensity. Patients often learn which activities are apt to provoke the chest discomfort and subsequently avoid them. Nevertheless, considerable variation may exist in the frequency and ease of provocation of chest discomfort over time, and patients with stable angina pectoris may experience considerable variation in their pain syndromes.

Evaluation of the Patient

The basic factor underlying the evaluation of patients with angina pectoris is that patients may be totally free of symptoms and signs of myocardial ischemia between anginal episodes. Accordingly, the physical examination, the ECG, and results of other laboratory studies may be totally within normal limits in the intervals between myocardial ischemia. Moreover, episodes of myocardial ischemia may have variable manifestations, and no single physical or laboratory finding is 100% sensitive and specific in the recognition of CHD. Accordingly, the history plays a central role in the evaluation of the patient with angina pectoris. Furthermore, the assessment of chest pain or discomfort typically involves examination during the provocation of myocardial ischemia by some stimulus, such as exertion.

The onset of myocardial ischemia initiates a sequence of events involving the metabolic, mechanical, and electrical performances of the heart, as well as the appearance of symptoms. Thus, shortly after the initiation of myocardial ischemia, abnormalities of systolic and diastolic ventricular performance are observed.[6,7] Typically, these abnormalities result in segmental myocardial dysfunction. During the subsequent course of myocardial ischemia, ECG changes occur, primarily ST segment depression. After these two abnormalities, chest pain may appear. Thus, in addition to the metabolic abnormalities induced by myocardial ischemia and alterations in the mechanical and electrical characteristics of the heart, symptoms may occur that present the basis for the clinical manifestations of CHD.

The pathophysiologic consequences of myocardial ischemia also form the basis for detection of coronary atherosclerosis in the clinical setting. Thus, one may screen for evidence of left ventricular dysfunction, ECG abnormalities, or chest pain in the patients suspected of having coronary atherosclerosis. These disturbances will, of course, probably be absent during nonischemic intervals. However, if the opportunity arises to examine a patient during an episode of chest pain, one may seek physical findings compatible with the presence of left ventricular dysfunction including an S3 or S4 gallop, appearance of a mitral regurgitation murmur, or rales indicative of congestive heart failure. The ECG during the period of angina pectoris would be expected to manifest abnormalities, typically ST segment depression and/or T wave inversion.

It is unusual to have the opportunity to examine a patient with stable angina pectoris during an episode of ischemia. Therefore, a variety of maneuvers are used to provoke myocardial ischemia during monitoring for the contractile or electrical disturbances associated with ischemia. These diagnostic procedures are discussed in Chapters 7 through 10, 14, and 15 and will be outlined in this presentation.

Although a variety of pharmacologic agents and physical interventions (e.g., immersion in icewater) have been used to provoke myocardial ischemia, the usual method involves exercise stress.[8] The standard modality of exertion involves treadmill walking, although bicycle ergometry may also be used. Initially, the primary manifestation of myocardial ischemia sought during exercise testing was electrical, i.e., ST segment changes on the ECG. However, more recently a variety of imaging techniques have been added to exercise ECG to detect ischemia provoked by exertion. The imaging techniques provide data regarding ventricular mechanical dysfunction as well as information relating to myocardial perfusion and myocardial metabolism (see also Chs. 9, 10, 14, and 15).

The most common diagnostic maneuver used to recognize significant coronary atherosclerosis is the exercise ECG. Typically, the ECG is continuously monitored while the patient walks at progressively greater speeds and grades on a treadmill until the appearance of chest pain, ECG abnormalities, other disturbances, or fatigue. ECG abnormalities indicative of myocardial ischemia may be observed, but are not perfectly accurate in diagnosis. The sensitivity and specificity of treadmill exercise testing for the recognition of CHD in patients with chest pain syndromes is dependent on the ECG criteria used and the number and extent of coronary arteries with atherosclerotic obstructions.[9] Thus, certain ECG criteria, such as 0.5 mm of ST segment depression, may be extremely sensitive but are nonspecific in the detection of CHD, whereas more stringent criteria, such as 2.0 mm of ST segment depression, are much less sensitive but are substantially more specific. The optimal criterion consists of 1.0 mm of ST segment depression occurring for at least 80 msec following the J point of the ECG. With these specifications, the sensitivity of treadmill testing is approximately 60, 70, and 80% in patients with single, double, and triple-vessel disease, respectively, at angiography. The test may also have prognostic value. Data indicate that patients capable of completing stage 4 of a Bruce protocol without chest pain or ECG ST segment changes are at very low risk for myocardial infarction or death over one year of follow-up.

Graded exercise has been coupled with several radionuclide tracer studies to provide additional information regarding ventricular performance and myocardial perfusion with exertion (see also Ch. 9). Thallium-201 is a potassium analog isotope which is taken up by myocardial cells when injected intravenously. Following intravenous injection of thallium-201, recording of myocardial activity by a scintillation camera placed over the heart reveals uniform myocardial uptake in normal individuals. The failure of a region of the left ventricle to take up thallium during exertion creates a perfusion defect compatible with the presence of myocardial ischemia or infarction. These two conditions can be separated since ischemia but not infarction enables the affected area to take up thallium on a follow-up examination 4 hours later. In an alternative technique, red blood cells can be tagged with the isotope technetium 99M and a recording of left ventricular blood pool activity made before and immediately after exercise. The maximal and minimal radioactivity contained within the ventricle relate to end-diastolic and end-systolic left ventricular volumes, respectively, and hence permit the calculation of ejection fraction. Measurements derived from these blood pool studies reveal that ejection fraction increases with exertion in normal subjects but stays the same or decreases at peak effort in patients with myocardial ischemia. Reconstructed blood pool images may also reveal evidence of regional myocardial contractile abnormalities. Most recently, positron-emitting agents have been used in the detection of myocardial ischemia (see also Ch. 15). These agents decay with the release of two photons at 180° angles, thereby providing the potential for precise localizations of tracer and calculation of coronary blood flow by positron emission tomography (PET). Available evidence indicates that these radionuclide techniques permit enhanced sensitivity and specificity over exercise ECG. Thus, analysis of combined data in nearly 2,000 patients demonstrated that thallium-201 myocardial scintigraphy has a sensitivity of 91% and specificity of 82% for the detection of CHD versus 61% and 81%, respectively, by exercise ECG.[10]

Treadmill or bicycle exercise may also be coupled with echocardiography to detect CHD (see also Ch. 10). In the presence of myocardial ischemia, echocardiographic images reveal evidence of left ventricular contractile dysfunction by means of either reduced endocardial motion or diminished left ventricular wall thickening. In addition, the global left ventricular ejection fraction may become abnormal in patients with CHD. Echocardiographic exercise testing is a relatively new addition to the medical armamentarium, requires high technical proficiency, and may not yield technically adequate studies in some patients. Nevertheless, available data suggest that echocardiographic exercise testing is comparable to radionuclide exercise testing in the detection of CHD and that both are superior to exercise ECG alone.[11]

Several additional diagnostic modalities may have a role in some patients with angina pectoris (see also Ch. 14). Echocardiography without exercise may be used to evaluate left ventricular function and to assess the potential for nonischemic causes of cardiac chest pain such as mitral valve prolapse and hypertrophic cardiomyopathy. However, echocardiographic imaging at rest does not play a critical role in the evaluation of patients with classic angina pectoris who have not had evidence of myocardial infarction. The role of ambulatory ECG in patients with chest pain continues to be defined. Although painless ischemia as detected by ambulatory ECG recording has been shown to be of similar consequence to painful ischemia, the detection of such abnormalities by ambulatory ECG is difficult and not widely standardized. Ambulatory ECG may also be used in patients with angina pectoris in whom symptoms suggestive of arrhythmias, such as palpitations or syncope, are present.

Medical Management

Medical management of patients with stable angina pectoris is also discussed in Chapters 5, 16, and 20.

Medical management of these patients represents a comprehensive approach to reducing all factors capable of increasing myocardial oxygen demand, improving coronary blood flow with appropriate pharmacotherapy, and instituting measures designed to prevent the progression or induce the regression of the underlying atherosclerosis. Thus, general medical conditions that might increase myocardial oxygen demand or reduce oxygen supply, such as anemia, thyrotoxicosis, or hypertension, should be brought under control. The patient should be advised to attain and maintain optimal body weight, refrain from cigarette smoking, and adhere to a nonsedentary lifestyle. Dietary restriction of saturated fats and cholesterol should be rigorously maintained (see also Ch. 5). The weight of evidence suggests that low-dose aspirin consumption is valuable in preventing the conversion from stable angina pectoris to acute myocardial infarction or death. The value of a program of regular exercise training in reducing morbidity and mortality from CHD continues to be investigated. Moreover, there is considerable evidence indicating the value of exercise training in reducing determinants of myocardial oxygen demand.[12]

A variety of pharmacologic agents can be used to treat angina pectoris. Each agent has benefits and side effects, and the application of these drugs requires individualization for the patient. Antianginal agents may be used alone and in concert. The primary agents used in the medical treatment of stable angina pectoris include nitrates, beta-adrenergic blocking agents, and calcium-blocking drugs. A detailed discussion of these drugs is presented in Chapter 16.

Nitrates are the oldest class of agents used in the treatment of stable angina pectoris and are the drugs chosen first by most physicians. In optimal dosage they have little effect on the heart rate and contractile state, but reduce wall tension, particularly by diminishing left ventricular preload. They have demonstrated effectiveness as coronary artery vasodilators. Nitroglycerin tablets or spray suitable for sublingual administration for rapid effect is routinely indicated at the onset of chest pain in patients with stable angina pectoris. These drugs may also be used prophylactically before any activity that is likely to be associated with angina. Sublingual nitroglycerin has an onset of activity of less than 5 minutes and a duration of approximately 20 to 30 minutes. Long-acting nitrate preparations are available in tablet form, ointment, or sustained-release patches. Administration of nitroglycerin in this long-acting fashion has been demonstrated to be of value in reducing episodes of angina pectoris. However, long-acting nitrates may be associated with tolerance and therefore should not be applied any more frequently than every 8 hours, or

in conjunction with withholding of the agent during the evening or during sleep.[13]

Beta-adrenergic blocking agents have made a substantial contribution to the medical treatment of the patient with angina pectoris. They diminish the heart rate and myocardial contractility while having little effect on left ventricular wall tension and coronary blood flow. They have also been demonstrated to reduce the mortality rate following acute myocardial infarction. Unfortunately, beta-adrenergic blockade produces a number of undesirable side effects. Thus, nonselective beta-adrenergic blocking agents may be associated with bronchospasm in patients with obstructive airway disease, congestive heart failure in patients with marginal left ventricular function, and profound bradycardia and may exacerbate difficulties with peripheral vascular disease or diabetes mellitus. They may also induce easy fatigue. Abrupt withdrawal of these drugs has been associated with exacerbation of myocardial ischemic events, and their dosage should therefore be gradually tapered if they are to be discontinued.[14]

Calcium-blocking drug preparations are the newest class of pharmacologic agents for the treatment of angina pectoris. By blocking calcium entry, these agents are capable of interfering with electromechanical coupling, particularly in vascular smooth muscle. The agents therefore possess vasodilatory properties while mildly diminishing myocardial contractility. These drugs differ in their influence on heart rate, with verapamil and diltiazem slowing the sinoatrial rate by a direct action on the calcium channel and nifedipine potentially increasing the heart rate by virtue of an indirect response to its vasodilatory action. The calcium channel-blocking agents may be associated with side effects including gastrointestinal symptoms, dizziness, and edema.

Antianginal agents are frequently used in combination. In this regard, nitrates and beta-adrenergic blocking agents are very complementary: nitrates reduces wall tension while beta-blocking agents decrease heart rate and myocardial contractility. Moreover, the drugs are mutually protective against adverse effects on the determinants of myocardial oxygen demand. Calcium channel-blocking agents have been used in combination with both nitrates and beta-blocking agents, and these combinations have been demonstrated to yield superior antianginal efficacy over that of either drug alone.

Many physicians initiate antianginal therapy with nitrates because of their well-established effectiveness, low cost, and combined effect on myocardial oxygen demand (reduced wall tension) and myocardial oxygen supply (coronary vasodilation). Nitrates are often combined with beta-adrenergic blocking drugs in patients with effort angina because of their complementary effects. In patients with increased coronary vascular tone as evidenced by rest angina, or in whom contraindications to beta-adrenergic blockade are present, calcium channel blocking drugs provide effective combination therapy. Triple therapy with all three agents is often applied.

Indications for Cardiac Catheterization and Coronary Angiography

Guidelines for the application of cardiac catheterization with coronary angiography have been published by the American College of Cardiology/American Heart Association Task Force on Assessment of Diagnostic and Therapeutic Cardiovascular Procedures.[15] Cardiac catheterization with coronary angiography may be indicated in patients with stable angina pectoris for diagnostic purposes or to evaluate the need for and feasibility of revascularization therapy. Cardiac catheterization is the only test that provides definitive evidence for the presence, severity, or absence of coronary atherosclerosis, and it is unique in enabling the assessment of potential revascularization therapy. Coronary angiography is used for diagnostic purposes primarily in patients in whom the clinical evaluation is ambiguous. Thus, atypical chest pain in the presence of equivocal noninvasive test results often is addressed by angiographic assessment of coronary artery anatomy.

When the presence of CHD is firmly established, cardiac catheterization and coronary angiography are used primarily to assess the potential for myocardial revascularization. In this regard, revascularization is undertaken for three purposes: (1) to relieve angina pectoris, (2) to conserve myocardium, and (3) to prolong life. Accordingly, coronary angiography should be undertaken in any patient in whom angina pectoris presents life-restricting symptoms or asymptomatic severe myocardial ischemia despite aggressive medical therapy. The use of revascularization to prolong life is more complex. There is evidence that surgical revascularization prolongs life or reduces mortality in patients with left main coronary artery disease or multivessel coronary disease, particularly in association with left ventricular dysfunction.[16,17] Selection of patients for coronary angiography often revolves about identification of risk factors for early mortality. Thus, patients with left ventricular dysfunction, evidence of substantial inducible or spontaneous myocardial ischemia, and arrhythmias are known to be at risk for increased mortality and often are selected for angiography. In this regard, a markedly abnormal exercise test at low levels of effort or one in which the exertion produces hypotension is often taken as an indication for coronary angiography (see Chs. 7 and 8).

Indications for Myocardial Revascularization

Indications for myocardial revascularization are also discussed in Chapters 17 and 18.

Guidelines and indications for coronary artery bypass grafting (CABG) and percutaneous transluminal coronary angioplasty (PTCA) have been published by the American College of Cardiology/American Heart Association Task Force on Assessment of Diagnostic and Therapeutic Cardiovascular Procedures.[18,19] Standard CABG and PTCA have both been demonstrated to be effective in the reduction or elimination of angina pectoris. However, few data are available regarding the ability of PTCA to reduce morbidity or mortality in CHD. As indicated above, CABG may also be performed to prolong life. Successful CABG requires a vessel distal to an atherosclerotic obstruction that is sufficiently large to accommodate a bypass graft, as well as a viable area of myocardium subserved by that vessel. Significant risk factors for a less favorable outcome of CABG include female gender, left ventricular dysfunction, diabetes mellitus, and older age.

UNSTABLE ANGINA PECTORIS

Considerable debate has existed for many years regarding the prognostic significance and optimal treatment of unstable angina pectoris. The cause of much of this debate can be traced to the different definitions of this condition, as evidenced by its many titles, including preinfarction angina, acute coronary insufficiency, unstable angina, crescendo angina, and status anginosus. Patients with widely differing frequency, severity, duration, and ease of provocation of chest pain have all been described as having unstable angina. The uncertainty in the definition has resulted in the inclusion of heterogeneous patient groups and therefore in widely differing observations regarding prognosis and optimal therapy.

In a general sense, unstable angina pectoris may be described as an intermediate condition between stable angina pectoris and acute myocardial infarction. Similarly to stable angina pectoris, evidence of myocardial cell death is absent. However, in contrast to stable angina pectoris, and more clinically suggestive of acute myocardial infarction, chest pain is typically unprovoked, long-lasting, and poorly relieved by antianginal therapy. From a clinical vantage point, it is generally agreed that suitable criteria for unstable angina exist when the pain is not provoked, lasts 20 minutes or longer or occurs in recurrent episodes, and is only partially or not at all relieved by antianginal therapy. Abnormalities of the ST segment on ECG are usually, but not always, present; they signify a higher risk of ultimate infarction. Levels of cardiac enzymes are, of course, not elevated.

Several other clinical presentations are often classified as unstable angina pectoris. Among these is an abrupt increase in the frequency or ease of provocation of a previous pattern of stable angina. Unfortunately, sufficient variability exists in the anginal pattern in most patients that the distinction between stable and unstable angina pectoris on this basis is often blurred. Patients with persistent chest pain following myocardial infarction are often branded as having unstable angina pectoris. Similarly, patients in whom the initial onset of an anginal syndrome is prominent in terms of both the frequency and intensity of chest pain may be labeled as having unstable angina. These latter definitions of this condition clearly permit considerable leeway in observer interpretation in diagnosis.

Pathophysiology

The pathophysiology of unstable angina pectoris has puzzled cardiologists for many years. However, recent data support the concept that unstable angina pectoris typically occurs when there is a spontaneous reduction of myocardial oxygen supply. Reduced coronary blood flow may be produced by spontaneous platelet aggregates or coronary spasm or when a fixed atherosclerotic plaque fissures, ruptures, or undergoes an anatomic alteration such that thrombus is superimposed. Angioscopic evidence suggests that when a thrombus produces total occlusion of the vessel, myocardial infarction ensues, but when the thrombus results in incomplete occlusion of the vessel, unstable angina pectoris is the result.[20]

Clinical Evaluation

As is true of stable angina pectoris, the diagnosis of unstable angina pectoris is based primarily upon the clinical history. The symptom complex described above is of paramount importance in reaching the diagnosis. ECGs recorded during episodes of pain typically (but not always) reveal abnormalities. Cardiac enzyme levels are of great importance in ruling out the occurrence of myocardial infarction. In patients in whom low-level cardiac enzyme elevations are observed, the distinction between unstable angina pectoris and a small myocardial infarction becomes somewhat arbitrary.

Medical Management

The optimal approach to the medical management of unstable angina is comprehensive. First, the patient should be hospitalized in an intensive care unit and cardiac monitoring should be undertaken. The antianginal agents discussed in regard to stable angina pectoris are typically administered for unstable angina, with the choice of drugs being determined by the heart rate, blood pressure, and left ventricular function. Intravenous nitroglycerin has been found to be of particular value in patients with unstable angina.[21] In addition to antianginal drugs, antiplatelet drugs, specifically aspirin,[22] and anticoagulation with heparin have been determined to be valuable in treating patients with unstable angina.[23] The use of antiplatelet and anticoagulant agents is particularly appropriate in light of the recent demonstration of the importance of subacute vascular occlusion with thrombus in many patients with unstable angina.

In the era prior to PTCA, intra-aortic balloon pump (IABP) counterpulsation represented an intermediate therapeutic measure between medical and surgical therapy. IABP counterpulsation is most effective in producing relief of the anginal syndrome. Accordingly, the patient can be stabilized for subsequent coronary angiography and CABG on a more elective basis. Of importance, data suggest that the induction of anesthesia in patients with unstable angina undergoing CABG was safer with the support of IABP. Since the advent of PTCA, the role of IABP counterpulsation has been less prominent.

Indications for Cardiac Catheterization and Coronary Angiography

Cardiac catheterization and coronary angiography may be indicated acutely or electively in patients with unstable angina. For patients in whom medical therapy is unsuccessful in reducing the symptoms, urgent coronary angiography can delineate the lesions responsible and guide therapy by either PTCA or surgery. In patients in whom medical therapy successfully reduces the symptoms, the decision for coronary angiography is based primarily upon the assessment of prognosis. In this regard, studies have indicated that patients presenting with unstable angina pectoris have a higher rate of infarction and/or death in the ensuing 12 to 24 months than do patients with stable angina pectoris.[24,25] Accordingly, many physicians believe that cardiac catheterization is indicated in nearly all such patients who are successfully stabilized by medical therapy. The indications for myocardial revascularization either by catheter-based (PTCA) or operative (CABG) revascularization in patients with unstable angina pectoris are similar to those in patients with stable angina pectoris.

ACUTE MYOCARDIAL INFARCTION

After years of debate, it is now clear that acute coronary thrombus formation with total occlusion of a coronary artery is the mechanism of acute myocardial infarction in nearly all patients[26] (see also Ch. 2). The stimulus for thrombus formation is believed to involve disruption or dysfunction of the endothelium of the coronary plaque.[27] Thus, fissure of the plaque with subsequent exposure of the subendothelial layer to blood elements results in thrombus formation, which may be accentuated by the failure of the endothelium to produce vasodilator substances. Platelets adhere to the collagen-rich subendothelial layer, with subsequent release of vasoconstrictor substances and accumulation of fibrin to form a thrombus, with total vessel occlusion. The cessation of coronary blood flow produced by thrombosis results in cell death and coagulation necrosis in the area of myocardium perfused by the affected vessel. The necrosis may involve the full or partial thickness of the wall. With subsequent healing, the infarcted area is converted into a tensile thinned fibrous scar with impaired to absent contractile performance and potential paradoxic expansion during systole. Following myocardial infarction, a process of ventricular remodeling may occur involving overall ventricular dilatation and/or expansion of the infarct segment.[28]

Expansion of the infarct results from disruption and loss of tissue, with resulting thinning and lengthening of myocardium. Expansion occurs in approximately 30% of cases, primarily with Q wave (transmural) infarctions involving the anterior wall; the prognosis is poor.[29] Dilatation and altered function may also involve the noninfarcted segment.[30]

Clinical Features and Diagnosis

The classic presentation of acute myocardial infarction consists of chest pain of an anginal nature that begins spontaneously and continues uninterrupted for several hours. The pain is often accompanied by diaphoresis, nausea, and shortness of breath. In approximately 20% of patients, acute myocardial infarction may have an atypical presentation consisting not of chest pain, but rather of symptoms such as acute pulmonary edema, syncope, or mental confusion. Atypical presentations (silent or unrecognized myocardial infarction) are particularly common in elderly, hypertensive, and diabetic patients. The Framingham Study data indicated that one in four myocardial infarctions confirmed by ECG were detected at the time of a routine examination, and half of these were totally silent even with retrospective analysis.[31]

The physical examination in acute myocardial infarction primarily centers about the detection of left ventricular dysfunction. Thus, evidence of congestive heart failure manifested by lung rales or an S3 gallop, diastolic dysfunction manifested by an S4 gallop, severe pump dysfunction manifested by hypotension and hypoperfusion, or new-onset mitral regurgitation as evidenced by the appropriate murmur may be observed.

Laboratory evaluation, particularly by ECG, is central to the diagnosis of acute myocardial infarction. The earliest ECG findings consist of ST segment elevation in two or more contiguous leads, followed by a gradual loss of R wave amplitude, development of Q waves, and inversion of the T wave. The Q wave is the only definitive ECG indicator of acute myocardial infarction; and in patients in whom Q waves do not develop, the diagnosis rests on the clinical presentation and detection of an elevated cardiac serum enzyme level (non-Q wave infarction). It has been estimated that approximately one-third of acute myocardial infarctions are of the non-Q wave variety. Although it was initially thought that Q wave infarctions represented transmural necrosis, whereas non-Q wave infarctions indicated necrosis of the subendocardial layer, it is now clear that there is considerable overlap between the ECG nature of the infarction and the magnitude of myocardial damage within the ventricular wall.[32]

Necrosis of myocardial cells results in the liberation of intracellular enzymes and therefore provides a method for the diagnosis of infarction.[33] Over the years, a variety of enzymes have been analyzed for the detection of myocardial infarction; however, most were nonspecific and could be found at increased levels in other disorders. Currently, the diagnosis of myocardial infarction is based primarily on analysis of creatine kinase (CK) and lactic dehydrogenase (LDH). CK has three isoenzymes: BB, found predominantly in the brain; MM, localized predominantly to skeletal muscle; and MB, found in large proportion in the myocardium. Elevations of serum CK-MB can be detected 12 to 24 hours following acute myocardial infarction, and represent the most specific enzymatic marker of this condition. LDH has five isoenzymes, with LDH I being the most specific for myocardial damage. Increased LDH levels may be detected in the serum 24 to 72 hours following acute myocardial infarction and are of value in confirming CK measures or in detecting infarction that occurred 24 hours or longer prior to evaluation.

A variety of noninvasive imaging techniques may be of value in the evaluation of acute myocardial infarction. Myocardial perfusion may be assessed by the use of thallium-201 scintigraphy to detect myocardial infarction. Unfortunately, this technique may not distinguish between infarction and ischemia and is not currently applied frequently in the diagnosis of acute myocardial infarction. Echocardiography may be of value in the detection of infarction by virtue of the ability to identify abnormal myocardial contractile patterns. The portability and ease with which echocardiography can be performed have led to its increasing use in the assessment of chest pain syndromes, particularly in regard to decisions about the application of thrombolytic therapy.[34] Radionuclide blood pool scans (MUGA) may be used to assess left ventricular performance following myocardial infarction; however, these studies do not play a prominent role in diagnosis.

Emergency Management

The early emergency management of acute myocardial infarction has undergone significant change in the past several years, with the advent of thrombolytic therapy. The impetus for such therapy was derived from the studies of DeWood et al.,[26] which showed that acute thrombosis was the mechanism of myocardial infarction in the overwhelming majority of patients. Accordingly, the potential existed for drugs with the capability of dissolving clots to reestablish flow and interrupt the course of myocardial necrosis.

A variety of thrombolytic agents are currently available that are effective in reestablishing coronary perfusion in patients with acute myocardial infarction[35-38] (see also Ch. 16). The initial agent used was streptokinase, which is produced by beta-hemolytic streptococci. Streptokinase forms a complex with plasminogen, which subsequently activates plasminogen to cleave fibrin. Streptokinase is inexpensive but causes allergic reactions and hypotension in a small percentage of patients. Urokinase is a naturally occurring thrombolytic enzyme, which has been used only sparingly in the treatment of acute myocardial infarction. Anisoylated plasminogen streptokinase activator complex (APSAC) is a formulation of streptokinase that may be given as a bolus and has a sustained duration of action. Tissue plasminogen activator (t-PA) is the newest thrombolytic agent; it has attracted considerable interest since it is the product of recombinant DNA technology. It is a naturally occurring serum protease, derived from vascular endothelium, which has a high affinity for plasminogen in the presence of fibrin and is therefore fibrin-specific. This clot specificity is relative, not absolute, and offers the theoretical benefit of concentrated efficacy in the region of the clot and less potential for hemor-

rhage. Thus far, available studies have not demonstrated a significant difference in hemorrhagic complications with any of the agents.

Numerous studies have now been performed with each of the thrombolytic agents.[35-39] Considerable data have documented the ability of each of these agents to reperfuse occluded coronary arteries and reduce mortality following acute myocardial infarction. Of interest, the ability to demonstrate myocardial salvage with thrombolytic therapy has been less consistent. Considerable debate continues about whether any of the thrombolytic agents is clearly preferable over the others. Although t-PA is fibrin-specific and has been demonstrated to achieve reperfusion in a higher percentage of patients than streptokinase, prospective comparative trials have not yet demonstrated a difference in the ability of these two agents to reduce mortality following acute myocardial infarction. All of the thrombolytic agents are associated with reocclusion, and this remains an important area for investigation.

PTCA represents an alternative approach to establishing reperfusion of occluded coronary arteries (see also Ch. 17). Several studies have demonstrated that direct PTCA may be an effective measure when applied independently of or in conjunction with thrombolytic therapy in acute myocardial infarction.[40,41] However, large prospective trials have not yet been carried out to determine the comparable benefit of direct PTCA versus thrombolytic drugs or to determine the long-term morbidity and mortality effects of such intervention. Since emergency PTCA is available at only a few medical centers, the feasibility of this approach to the treatment of acute myocardial infarction remains uncertain.

A larger issue relates to the application of PTCA following thrombolytic therapy of acute myocardial infarction. The Thrombolysis in Myocardial Infarction (TIMI-IIB) Study evaluated the potential of routine PTCA following thrombolytic reperfusion to reduce morbidity and mortality following acute myocardial infarction.[42] The results of this study suggested that routine application of PTCA at 18 to 48 hours following thrombolytic therapy was not superior to conventional medical approaches. Therefore, current strategies call for

PTCA to be used only in patients who manifest recurrent or inducible early ischemia following thrombolysis and who are appropriate for this procedure. Considerable controversy continues regarding the usefulness of salvage or rescue angioplasty, i.e., the application of PTCA to achieve reperfusion in vessels in which thrombolytic therapy has failed.

The indications for thrombolytic therapy have evolved largely from the criteria for enrollment in investigative trials. ECG evidence of ST segment elevation in two contiguous leads was required for the diagnosis of acute myocardial infarction and has largely persisted as an indication. It has generally been accepted that patients considered for thrombolytic therapy should have experienced chest pain for 6 hours or less. Exclusion criteria for thrombolytic therapy have consisted of a history of bleeding or age greater than 75 years, the latter based on the recognized increased prevalence of spontaneous intracerebral hemorrhage in this group. The potential benefit of thrombolytic therapy in patients with clinically small inferior myocardial infarctions is uncertain; however, thrombolysis appears to be useful in these patients as well.

The indications for thrombolytic therapy have come under close scrutiny because of the recognition that only a small percentage of patients with acute myocardial infarction are currently receiving this therapy, despite its proven benefit. Recent data suggest that only 20% of patients with acute myocardial infarction are currently receiving thrombolytic agents.[43] Accordingly, attempts are being made to assess the benefit of this treatment in additional subsets of patients, such as those presenting 6 to 24 hours after the onset of chest pain and those older than 75 years. The indications for thrombolytic therapy will probably be expanded in the future.

General Treatment

A number of general measures are typically recommended for the treatment of patients with acute myocardial infarction. Since hypoxemia due to ventilation-perfusion mismatch is present to some degree in nearly all patients with acute myocardial infarction, oxygen therapy is routinely administered. Similarly, the pain and accompanying anxiety secondary to myocardial infarction may have detrimental effects, and potent analgesic agents such as morphine sulfate are characteristically administered. Bed rest is typically instituted upon admission, with a gradual program of progressive ambulation thereafter. Most physicians recommend stool softeners for patients with acute myocardial infarction and mild sedation for patients who are particularly apprehensive.

Anticoagulants are used in most patients with acute myocardial infarction in whom contraindications are absent. Anticoagulation with heparin is routine for all patients who have received thrombolytic therapy. The regimen with which anticoagulants are administered varies. Patients receiving t-PA typically receive full-dose heparin therapy immediately following administration of the thrombolytic agent. Administration of heparin to patients receiving streptokinase may be given concomitantly with the drug, 4 hours after receiving the drug, or at some later period. The duration of anticoagulation with heparin varies in patients receiving thrombolytic therapy, but usually includes the first 5 to 7 days after infarction.

For the patient who has not received thrombolytic therapy, heparin is often administered for at least 48 hours to prevent deep-vein thrombosis and pulmonary emboli. In patients at high risk for systemic emboli, such as those with large transmural infarctions or congestive heart failure, heparin therapy sufficient to prolong the partial thromboplastin time (PTT) to 1.5 to 2 times control levels is administered until discharge. Some physicians elect to give these high-risk patients oral anticoagulants such as coumadin sufficient to prolong the prothrombin time to 1.3 to 1.5 times control levels (international normalized ratio [INR] 2.0 to 3.0), and to continue such therapy for at least 3 months. Analysis of data from multiple studies on the use of oral anticoagulation to reduce the long-term risk of reinfarction and death following myocardial infarction demonstrates a benefit for this therapy. However, the benefit appears comparable to that produced by aspirin, which is preferred by most physicians.

Antiplatelet drugs have been demonstrated to be of value in most patients with acute myocardial infarction. The ISIS II trial demonstrated that aspirin produced a reduction in mortality from myocardial infarction that was comparable to the reduction caused by streptokinase and that the increased survival obtained from combination therapy was additive. Therefore, aspirin at 300 mg or less daily is characteristically administered at admission to all patients with acute myocardial infarction who do not have contraindications. It should be recognized, however, that the use of aspirin and heparin together slightly increases the risk of bleeding. Most physicians continue daily aspirin therapy indefinitely.

Antiarrhythmic therapy is often indicated in patients with acute myocardial infarction. Although available studies show that prophylactic use of antiarrhythmic agents can reduce the incidence of sustained ventricular tachyarrhythmias and ventricular fibrillation,[44] most such patients are rapidly resuscitated and mortality is not reduced. Since all antiarrhythmic drugs have some side effects, most patients do not receive prophylactic antiarrhythmic agents unless they are far removed from resuscitative facilities. Antiarrhythmic agents are administered intravenously to patients with symptomatic arrhythmias or ventricular arrhythmias that are considered premonitory of ventricular tachycardia or fibrillation, i.e., those that are frequent, occur on the T wave, or are multiform.

A variety of anti-ischemic drugs may be used during and after hospitalization for acute myocardial infarction. Nitroglycerin has the ability to both reduce myocardial oxygen demand and dilate coronary vessels; it is frequently effective in eliminating chest pain. Several studies have provided evidence suggesting that intravenous nitroglycerin may reduce the infarct size and decrease mortality.[45] This agent is of particular value for this latter indication in postinfarction patients who exhibit evidence of congestive heart failure. Calcium channel blocking drugs are potent coronary artery vasodilators and may be used to treat recurrent chest pain in patients with acute myocardial infarction. Although these agents have all been evaluated for their ability to reduce infarct size and mortality following myocardial

infarction, data thus far have not demonstrated any efficacy for this indication.[46,47] The exception to this rule has been the demonstrated ability of diltiazem to reduce the rate of reinfarction in patients with non-Q wave myocardial infarctions.[48] These agents are often used in an attempt to prevent coronary spasm and reocclusion in patients who have undergone reperfusion therapy with thrombolytic agents or PTCA. However, no data are available regarding the efficacy of these agents for this purpose.

The administration of beta-blocking agents has been demonstrated to reduce both short-term and long-term mortality following acute myocardial infarction.[49,50] Beta-blocking agents administered within 12 hours of infarction can reduce short-term mortality, and long-term administration of these agents has been demonstrated to produce a salutary effect for up to 2 years. Despite these findings, many postinfarction patients should not receive beta-blocking drugs. These agents are often not administered to patients because of contraindications to the drugs (congestive heart failure, asthma, bradycardia) or because the patients are in a low-risk category and the agents have not been shown to produce significant benefit in this group. Accordingly, beta-blocking drugs are most often applied in the group of patients without contraindications who have some risk for increased mortality and in whom direct revascularization procedures are not or cannot be performed.

Test Procedures following Acute Myocardial Infarction

Test procedures following myocardial infarction are also discussed in Chapters 7 to 10, 14, and 15.

Exercise Testing

Exercise testing is performed in nearly all patients who are capable of exertion following myocardial infarction.[51] The exercise test demonstrates functional capacity and the existence of persistent ischemia and serves to identify a safe level of exertion during convalescence and later. Abnormalities during exercise testing are predictive of an increased risk of morbidity and mortality in the postinfarction period. The nature and timing of exercise testing following infarction varies. Some patients may undergo submaximal exercise testing prior to discharge. Other physicians prefer to delay the exercise test for 3 to 6 weeks, at which time a maximal symptom-limited test is performed. Although the predischarge examination may identify patients at risk, available data suggest that the incidence of complications in the first several weeks following discharge is very low in patients with uncomplicated myocardial infarction and that patients rarely experience difficulties. Although the ECG is the primary diagnostic marker monitored during exercise testing in the postinfarction period, nuclear[52] or echocardiographic[53] imaging can be added for patients with markedly abnormal ECGs or in whom additional information is desired.

Ambulatory Electrocardiographic Recording. The presence of premature ventricular contractions late during hospitalization for acute myocardial infarction is an independent risk factor for increased mortality.[54] Data from the Multicenter Postinfarction Research Group demonstrated that patients with 10 or more premature ventricular contractions per hour prior to discharge had a three- to fivefold increased risk of mortality during the ensuing 2-year period. Greater degrees of complexity of ventricular arrhythmias have also been associated with diminished survival. Although there is a good correlation between impaired left ventricular function and the presence of ventricular arrhythmias in the postinfarction period, the increased risk of mortality conveyed by the arrhythmias has been demonstrated to be independent of ventricular performance. Computer averaging of multiple ECG complexes (the signal-averaged ECG) has detected abnormalities that have also identified patients at higher risk of mortality.[55] Finally, invasive electrophysiologic testing, with attempts to provoke sustained ventricular arrhythmias by premature extrasystoles, has also been used to identify patients with an adverse prognosis following acute myocardial infarction.[56] Patients in whom sustained ventricular arrhythmias can be provoked have been shown to have a 1-year mortality rate of 30%

versus 2% in patients in whom such disturbances cannot be induced.

Unfortunately, although the presence of ventricular arrhythmias clearly is predictive of increased mortality following myocardial infarction, no data are available to establish that therapy of such arrhythmias can reverse this risk. Systematic studies assessing the efficacy of therapy in patients identified as having diminished survival by signal-averaged ECGs or invasive electrophysiologic studies have not been performed. A multicenter study (Cardiac Arrhythmia Suppression Trial) that evaluated the ability of several antiarrhythmic drugs to prolong life in postinfarction patients with frequent premature ventricular contractions demonstrated an increase in mortality following treatment with encainide and flecainide.[57] Thus, the usefulness of performing procedures to detect ventricular arrhythmias in the predischarge period, for which treatment is ineffective, is unclear. Therefore, there is no clear indication for performing signal-averaged ECGs or invasive electrophysiologic testing in most patients after myocardial infarction. Ambulatory ECG recording is usually applied in patients judged to be at high risk in the postinfarction period because of evidence of left ventricular dysfunction, recurrent ischemia, or frequent arrhythmias on telemetry. Ambulatory ECG recording with calibrated instrumentation can also be used to screen for the presence of ST segment depression during usual activities. Such ST segment abnormalities, whether accompanied or unaccompanied (silent) by chest pain, indicate an increased risk of mortality in patients after infarction. Again, however, no data are available to determine whether therapeutic interventions directed at these abnormalities will successfully increase survival.

Echocardiography and Nuclear Angiography. Left ventricular dysfunction is an important prognosticator of adverse outcome in patients after myocardial infarction. Left ventricular function can be noninvasively assessed by a variety of techniques, among which radionuclide ventriculography and echocardiography are the most common. Either procedure can be performed at rest or with exercise. Radionuclide ventriculography provides useful quantitative measurements of left ventricular ejection fraction and can yield information regarding regional left ventricular contractile abnormalities. Echocardiography can provide similar information and also is of value in detecting associated abnormalities such as mitral regurgitation and left ventricular thrombi. Echocardiography or radionuclide angiography is typically performed in patients suspected of having complications of acute myocardial infarction or as part of the process of risk stratification.

Complications

Although the period of highest mortality in patients with acute myocardial infarction occurs in the earliest hours following the onset, a number of complications may occur in the subsequent course. These complications may occur in the coronary care unit or after discharge to the medical ward. They include recurrence or extension of the ischemic process (postinfarction angina or reinfarction), mechanical abnormalities of cardiac function (ruptured papillary muscle, ventricular septal defect, severe pump dysfunction), or associated abnormalities (pericarditis, mural thrombus). All complications can have profound consequences for the patient and should be aggressively treated.

Recurrent ischemia may be encountered in the form of postinfarction angina or extension of infarction. The extension may be symptomatic or silent; in the latter case it is detected only by elevation of cardiac serum enzymes or new ECG abnormalities. Recurrent ischemia should be aggressively treated with the antianginal agents discussed above. In most cases, coronary angiography is performed, and subsequent revascularization is undertaken if indicated on the basis of these studies. In certain patients, temporary support by means of IABP counterpulsation may be performed; however, this is often a temporary measure until definitive therapy can be undertaken.

Muscle destruction secondary to myocardial infarction may lead to left ventricular dysfunction of various degrees, from mild congestive heart failure to cardiogenic shock. Patients with evidence of severe circulatory impairment must be carefully evaluated for mechanical defects such as a ruptured papillary muscle or ventricular septal defect (septal rupture). Mild congestive heart failure manifested by basilar lung rales, with or without an S3 gallop, may occur transiently following acute infarction and is typically successfully treated with diuretic drugs, vasodilators such as nitroglycerin, or inotropic agents such as dobutamine or amrinone. Clearly, it is important not to increase myocardial oxygen demand in the process of treating the heart failure. Patients with more advanced degrees of pump dysfunction should undergo invasive hemodynamic monitoring with balloon flotation right heart catheterization to measure left ventricular filling pressure (wedge pressure), cardiac output, and systemic vascular resistance. The specific therapy administered is dictated by the hemodynamic profile of the individual patient. Patients with cardiogenic shock should be aggressively stabilized and cardiac catheterization should be performed to determine whether revascularization is possible. The prognosis of cardiogenic shock remains poor, despite the availability of PTCA and CABG surgery.

A variety of mechanical defects related to rupture of the myocardium may be encountered in patients after infarction (see also Ch. 18). If some portion of the papillary muscle ruptures, a severe degree of mitral regurgitation can ensue. Such patients will typically have profound degrees of congestive heart failure. Cardiac catheterization and cardiac surgery should be rapidly performed whenever feasible. Rupture of the ventricular septum results in an acute left-to-right shunt and increased pulmonary flow. Surgery is again indicated when feasible. Acute ventricular rupture is typically fatal secondary to pericardial tamponade.

Left ventricular aneurysm formation often occurs following acute myocardial infarction. Although opinions differ as to whether aneurysm is an anatomic or a functional abnormality, most individuals agree that an aneurysm involves both diastolic and systolic deformity of the left ventricle, a localized area of the myocardium that is discretely demarcated and in which dyskinesis is present. Potential complications of left ventricular aneurysm include ventricular arrhythmias, thrombi, congestive failure, and rupture. Therapy for each of these problems should be directed as discussed above.

Right ventricular infarction is another recognized complication of acute myocardial infarction. It is typically manifested by right-sided heart failure, atrioventricular block, or hypotension. Volume administration and vasodilator drugs are typically used in the treatment of this disorder. In most cases, the symptoms resolve over a period of days.

Mural thrombi are a common complication of acute myocardial infarction and can be recorded in more than one-third of patients with transmural anterior wall infarctions.[58] Echocardiography is the best technique to diagnose thrombi and has been shown to have good sensitivity and specificity. Unfortunately, it is equivocal in many cases, and definitive recognition of the presence or absence of a clot is not possible. Although mural thrombi may be frequently seen at echocardiography after infarction, the incidence of systemic embolism continues to be low, in the range of 3%. Accordingly, most patients with evidence of mural thrombus will not have a systemic embolus. When recognized, anticoagulation certainly is in order for mural thrombus.

Pericarditis with or without effusion is an additional complication of acute myocardial infarction. The incidence of clinically overt pericarditis is clearly lower than that found at autopsy. Chest pain is the most common symptom and may occur in the absence of other physical findings of pericarditis. In fact, the chest pain and diffuse ST segment elevation on the ECG may simulate extension of the infarct or reinfarction. The classic three-component friction rub of pericarditis may come and go; it is the most specific physical finding for the diagnosis. Typically, pericarditis does not lead to significant pericardial effusion; abnormalities are therefore rarely present on the echocardiogram. Pericarditis is usually successfully treated with aspirin or other nonsteroidal anti-inflammatory agents. Pericarditis associated with acute myocardial infarction usually resolves in several days.

SUDDEN CARDIAC DEATH

Patients in whom the clinical presentation of coronary heart disease has differed markedly have been designated as having sudden cardiac death in the past. The most widely accepted definition of this syndrome is unexpected death occurring in a patient, heralded by the abrupt loss of consciousness, within 1 hour of the onset of symptoms.[50,60] However, sudden death may often be unwitnessed, and patients who are found dead within 24 hours of last being seen alive are often counted in this category. Most patients who are seen shortly after the onset of cardiac arrest manifest ventricular fibrillation. It is therefore assumed that ventricular arrhythmias are the mechanism of sudden cardiac death in nearly all patients, whether preceded by myocardial infarction or myocardial ischemia.

Sudden cardiac death is very prevalent, comprising nearly 50% of all cardiac deaths and up to 25% of all deaths in patients without prior clinical symptoms of coronary heart disease. Most patients experiencing cardiac arrest have evidence of extensive coronary artery disease and prior myocardial infarction. The recurrence rate of sudden cardiac death is up to 30% in the first year and is higher in resuscitated patients who have not had acute myocardial infarction than in resuscitated patients who sustained an acute infarction.

The course of patients with sudden cardiac death is variable and relates to the rapidity with which resuscitation is performed. It is determined by the recurrence of arrhythmias, presence and severity of left ventricular dysfunction, and presence and severity of neurologic abnormalities. In patients undergoing prompt cardioversion, there may be a rapid return of hemodynamic function and no neurologic deficit. Conversely, patients may require hemodynamic support and endotracheal intubation for several days. The most common cause of death (59% of cases) in patients resuscitated from cardiac arrest relates to neurologic abnormalities.

For patients in whom cardiac collapse occurs concomitant with the onset of acute myocardial infarction, the treatment is identical to that for other patients with acute myocardial infarction. For patients in whom sudden cardiac death occurs without infarction or late after infarction, a more detailed evaluation is indicated. Studies should be performed to detect evidence of myocardial ischemia, as well as to study the location and severity of coronary artery disease and the presence of left ventricular aneurysm. Revascularization is indicated for coronary lesions demonstrated to be responsible for myocardial ischemia. Invasive electrophysiologic testing should be undertaken in survivors of sudden death, since induction of sustained ventricular tachycardia or ventricular fibrillation that can be successfully treated by antiarrhythmic agents is associated with a substantial reduction in the mortality rate. However, it should be recognized that antiarrhythmic agents have limited efficacy (30 to 50%) in the long-term treatment of ventricular tachyarrhythmias.

The availability of automatic implantable cardioverter defibrillators (ICDs) has significantly enhanced the treatment of survivors of sudden death.[61] The device consists of sensing leads and defibrillating patches, which are sewn directly onto the epicardium, and a pulse generator, which is inserted into a subcutaneous pocket. The ICD monitors electrical activity, identifies sustained ventricular tachyarrhythmias, and delivers a countershock that causes reversion to sinus rhythm. In patients who survive cardiac arrest and in whom revascularization is not appropriate, arrhythmias are noninducible, or inducible arrhythmias cannot be suppressed by pharmacologic agents, an ICD is indicated (see also Ch. 24).

REFERENCES

1. Sarnoff SJ, Braunwald E, Welch GH Jr et al: Hemodynamic determinants of oxygen consumption of the heart with special reference to the tension-time index. Am J Physiol 192:148, 1958
2. Hillis LD, Braunwald E: Coronary artery spasm. N Engl J Med 299:695, 1978
3. Epstein SE, Talbolt TL: Dynamic coronary tone in precipitation, exacerbation and relief of angina pectoris. Am J Cardiol 48:797, 1981
4. Heberden W: Some account of a disorder of the breast. Med Trans Coll Physicians (London), 2:59, 1772
5. Hirzel HO, Leutwyler R, Krayenbuehl HP: Silent myocardial ischemia: Hemodynamic changes during dynamic exercise in patients with proven coronary artery disease despite absence of angina pectoris. J Am Coll Cardiol 6:275, 1985
6. Tennant R, Wiggers CJ: The effect of coronary occlusion on myocardial contraction. Am J Physiol 112:351, 1935
7. Gewirtz H, Ohley W, Walsh J et al: Ischemia-induced impairment of left ventricular relaxation: Relation to reduced diastolic filling rates of the left ventricle. Am Heart J 105:72, 1983
8. McNeer JF, Margolis JR, Lee KL et al: The role of the exercise test in the evaluation of patients for ischemic heart disease. Circulation 57:64, 1978
9. Hlatky AM, Pryor DB, Harrell FE Jr et al: Factors affecting sensitivity and specificity of exercise electrocardiography. Am J Med 77:64, 1984
10. Okada RD, Boucher CA, Strauss HW, Pohost GM: Exercise radionuclide imaging approaches to coronary artery disease. Am J Cardiol 46:1188, 1980
11. Armstrong WF, O'Donnell J, Dillon JC et al: Complementary value of two-dimensional exercise echocardiography to routine treadmill exercise testing. Ann Intern Med 105:829, 1986
12. Redwood DR, Rosing DR, Epstein SE: Circulatory and symptomatic effects of physical training in patients with coronary artery disease and angina pectoris. N Engl J Med 286:959, 1972
13. Parker JO, Vankoughnett KA, Farrell B: Comparison of buccal nitroglycerin and oral isosorbide dinitrate for nitrate tolerance in stable angina pectoris. Am J Cardiol 56:724, 1985
14. Miller RR, Olson HG, Amsterdam EA, Mason DT: Propranolol withdrawal rebound phenomenon. Exacerbation of coronary events after abrupt cessation of antianginal therapy. N Engl J Med 293:416, 1975
15. American College of Cardiology/American Heart Association Task Force on Assessment of Diagnostic and Therapeutic Cardiovascular Procedures: Guidelines for coronary angiography. J Am Coll Cardiol 10:935, 1987
16. CASS Principal Investigators and their Associates: Coronary artery surgery study (CASS): A randomized trial of coronary artery bypass surgery. Survival data. Circulation 68:939, 1983
17. European Coronary Surgery Study Group: Long-term results of prospective randomised study of coronary artery bypass surgery in stable angina pectoris. Lancet ii:1173, 1982

18. American College of Cardiology/American Heart Association Task Force on Assessment of Diagnosis and Therapeutic Cardiovascular Procedures: Guidelines and indications for coronary artery bypass graft surgery. J Am Coll Cardiol 17:543, 1991

19. American College of Cardiology/American Heart Association Task Force on Assessment of Diagnostic and Therapeutic Cardiovascular Procedures: Guidelines for percutaneous transluminal coronary angioplasty. J Am Coll Cardiol 12:529, 1988

20. Sherman CT, Litvack F, Grundfest W et al: Coronary angioscopy in patients with unstable angina pectoris. N Engl J Med 315:913, 1986

21. Kaplan K, Davison R, Parker M et al: Intravenous nitroglycerin for the treatment of angina at rest unresponsive to standard nitrate therapy. Am J Cardiol 51:694, 1983

22. Lewis HD Jr, Davis JW, Archibald DG et al: Protective effects of aspirin against acute myocardial infarction and death in men with unstable angina: Results of a Veterans Administration cooperative study. N Engl J Med 309:396, 1983

23. Theroux P, Ouimet H, McCans J et al: Aspirin, heparin, or both to treat acute unstable angina. N Engl J Med 319:1105, 1988

24. Gazes PC, Mobley EM Jr, Faris HM Jr et al: Preinfarctional (unstable) angina—a prospective study—ten year follow-up. Circulation 48:331, 1973

25. Conti CR, Brawley RK, Griffith LSC et al: Unstable angina pectoris: Morbidity and mortality in 57 consecutive patients evaluated angiographically. Am J Cardiol 32:745, 1973

26. DeWood MA, Stifter WF, Simpson CS et al: Coronary arteriographic findings soon after non-Q wave myocardial infarction. N Engl J Med 315:417, 1986

27. Willerson JT, Campbell WB, Winniford MD et al: Conversion from chronic to acute coronary artery disease: Speculation regarding mechanisms. Am J Cardiol 54:1349, 1984

28. Roberts CS, Maclean D, Maroko PR, Kloner RA: Early and late remodeling of the left ventricle after acute myocardial infarction. Am J Cardiol 54:407, 1984

29. Erlebacher JA, Weiss JL, Eaton LW et al: Late effects of acute infarct dilation on heart size: A two-dimensional echocardiographic study. Am J Cardiol 49:1120, 1982

30. Wynne J, Sayres M, Maddox DE et al: Regional left ventricular function in acute myocardial infarction: Evaluation with quantitative radionuclide ventriculography. Am J Cardiol 45:203, 1980

31. Kannel WB, Abbott RD: Incidence and prognosis of unrecognized myocardial infarction: An update on the Framingham study. N Engl J Med 311:1144, 1984

32. Phibbs B: "Transmural" versus "subendocardial" myocardial infarction: An electrocardiographic myth. J Am Coll Cardiol 1:561, 1983

33. Lee TH, Goldman L: Serum enzyme assays in the diagnosis of acute myocardial infarction. Ann Intern Med 105:221, 1986

34. Oh JK, Miller FA, Shub C et al: Evaluation of acute chest pain syndromes by two-dimensional echocardiography: Its potential application in the selection of patients for acute reperfusion therapy. Mayo Clin Proc 62:59, 1987

35. Gruppo Italiano per lo Studio della Streptochinasi Nell'Infarto Miocardico (GISSI): Effectiveness of intravenous thrombolytic treatment in acute myocardial infarction. Lancet ii:349, 1988

36. ISIS (Second International Study of Infarct Survival) Collaborative Group: Randomized trial of intravenous streptokinase, oral aspirin, both or neither among 17,187 cases of suspected acute myocardial infarction: ISIS-2. Lancet ii:349, 1988

37. AIMS Trial Study Group: Effect of intravenous APSAC on mortality after acute myocardial infarction: Preliminary report of a placebo-controlled clinical trial. Lancet i:545, 1987

38. European Cooperative Study Group for Recombinant Tissue-Type Plasminogen Activator: Randomized trial of intravenous recombinant tissue-type plasminogen activator versus intravenous streptokinase in acute myocardial infarction. Lancet i:842, 1985

39. Chesebro JH, Knatterud G, Roberts R: Thrombolysis in Myocardial Infarction (TIMI) trial, phase I: A comparison between intravenous tissue plasminogen activator and intravenous streptokinase. Circulation 76:142, 1987

40. Hartzler GO, Rutherford BD, McConahay DR et al: Percutaneous transluminal coronary angioplasty with and without thrombolytic therapy for treatment of acute myocardial infarction. Am Heart J 106:965, 1983

41. O'Neill W, Timmis GC, Bourdillon PD et al: A prospective randomized clinical trial of intracoronary streptokinase versus coronary angioplasty for acute myocardial infarction. N Engl J Med 314:812, 1986

42. The TIMI Study Group: Comparison of invasive and conservative strategies after treatment with intravenous tissue plasminogen activator in acute myocardial infarction: Results of the Thrombolysis

in Myocardial Infarction (TIMI) phase II trial. N Engl J Med 320:618, 1989

43. Grines CL, Nissen SE, Booth DC et al: A new thrombolytic regimen for acute myocardial infarction using half dose tissue plasminogen activator with full dose streptokinase. J Am Coll Cardiol 14:573, 1989

44. MacMahon S, Collins R, Peto R et al: Effects of prophylactic lidocaine in suspected acute myocardial infarction: An overview of results from the randomized controlled trials. JAMA 260:1910, 1988

45. Yusuf S, MacMahon S, Collins R, Peto R: Effects of intravenous nitrates on mortality in acute myocardial infarction: An overview of the randomized trials. Lancet i:1088, 1988

46. The Multicenter Diltiazem Postinfarction Trial Research Group: The effect of diltiazem on mortality and reinfarction after myocardial infarction. N Engl J Med 385:92, 1988

47. Muller JE, Morrison J, Stone PH et al: Nifedipine therapy for patients with threatened and acute myocardial infarction: A randomized, double-blind, placebo-controlled comparison. Circulation 69:740, 1984

48. Gibson RS, Boden WE, Theroux P et al: Diltiazem and reinfarction in patients with non-Q-wave myocardial infarction: Results of a double-blind, randomized, multicenter trial. N Engl J Med 315:423, 1986

49. ISIS-1 (First International Study of Infarct Survival) Collaborative Group: Randomized trial of intravenous atenolol among 16,027 cases of suspected acute myocardial infarction: ISIS-1. Lancet ii:57, 1986

50. Yusuf S, Peto R, Lewis J et al: Beta blockade during and after myocardial infarction: An overview of the randomized trials. Prog Cardiovasc Dis 27:335, 1985

51. DeBusk RF, Haskell W: Symptom-limited vs. heart-rate-limited exercise testing soon after myocardial infarction. Circulation 61:738, 1980

52. Gibson RS, Watson DD, Craddock GB et al: Prediction of cardiac events after uncomplicated myocardial infarction: A prospective study comparing predischarge exercise thallium-201 scintigraphy and coronary angiography. Circulation 68:321, 1983

53. Applegate RJ, Dell'Italia LJ, Crawford MH: Usefulness of two-dimensional echocardiography during low-level exercise testing after uncomplicated acute myocardial infarction. Am J Cardiol 60:10, 1987

54. Bigger JT, Fleiss JL, Rolnitzky LM (for the Multicenter Postinfarction Research Group): Prevalence, characteristics and significance of ventricular tachycardia detected by 24-hour electrocardiographic recordings in the late phase of acute myocardial infarction. Am J Cardiol 58:1157, 1986

55. Gomes JA, Winters SL, Stewart D et al: A new noninvasive index to predict sustained ventricular tachycardia and sudden death in the first year after myocardial infarction: Based on signal-averaged electrocardiogram, radionuclide ejection fraction and Holter monitoring. J Am Coll Cardiol 10:349, 1987

56. Gomes JAC, Hariman RI, Kang PS et al: Programmed electrical stimulation in patients with high-grade ventricular ectopy: Electrical findings and prognosis for survival. Circulation 70:43, 1984

57. The Cardiac Arrhythmia Suppression Trial (CAST) Investigators: Preliminary report: Effect of encainide and flecainide on mortality in randomized trial of arrhythmia suppression after myocardial infarction. N Engl J Med 321:406, 1989

58. Meltzer RS, Visser CA, Fuster V: Intracardiac thrombi and systemic embolization. Ann Intern Med 104:689, 1986

59. Goldstein S: The necessity of a uniform definition of sudden coronary death: Witnessed death within 1 hour of the onset of acute symptoms. Am Heart J 103:156, 1982

60. Myerburg RJ, Conde CA, Sung RJ et al: Clinical, electrophysiologic and hemodynamic profile of patients resuscitated from prehospital cardiac arrest. Am J Med 68:568, 1980

61. Mirowski M, Reid PR, Winkle RA et al: Mortality in patients with implanted automatic defibrillators. Ann Intern Med 98:585, 1983

12

Coronary Heart Disease in the Elderly

Nanette K. Wenger, M.D.

The demographic characteristics of the U.S. population are changing dramatically and will continue to do so into the 21st century. There are currently about 26 million elderly persons (older than age 65) who live independently, about 12% of the population; their numbers are expected to increase by 20% during the next decade. The most rapidly increasing component of this group is the "oldest old," greater than age 85, now numbering 2.7 million and projected to increase six-fold by the year 2030.[1]

Cardiovascular disease is the major cause of death and disability in this population, and coronary heart disease is the most prevalent problem.[2] Indeed, the majority of U.S. patients with clinical evidence of coronary heart disease are older than 65 years.[3] In excess of 3.6 million patients age 65 and older in the United States are estimated to have coronary heart disease,[4] with this problem accounting for more than two-thirds of cardiac deaths in the elderly population. The severity, clinical manifestations, and complications of coronary heart disease increase incrementally with age; the clinical presentation, management, and prognosis differ substantially from those encountered in younger coronary patients.

AGE–CORONARY DISEASE INTERACTIONS

Elderly patients[5] are a highly heterogeneous group in regard to physical, behavioral, cognitive, emotional, and social functioning, such that chronologic age poorly predicts functional capabilities. Concomitant diseases more frequently complicate treatment and alter prognosis. These features mandate consideration of physiologic rather than chronologic age and evaluation of each elderly coronary patient individually to determine the appropriate spectrum of diagnostic and therapeutic interventions. The goal should be to ameliorate suffering and disability and to prolong the duration of active and alert life.

Because of the sedentary lifestyle of many elderly patients,[5] coronary heart disease is less likely to present as typical effort-induced angina. Often arthritis, musculoskeletal problems, or claudication limits physical activity before anginal pain occurs. Dyspnea, commonly a symptom of myocardial ischemia, may be attributed to a variety of other causes. Indeed, the initial clinical manifestation of coronary heart disease in the elderly is often acute myocardial infarction (or sudden cardiac death). Further, in elderly patients with previously asymptomatic coronary atherosclerosis, myocardial infarction may often be precipitated by a variety of medical problems characterized by acute blood loss or anemia, hypotension, hypoxemia, arrhythmia, fever, or infection; or myocardial infarction can occur intraoperatively or in the perioperative period of both cardiac and noncardiac surgery.

ACUTE MYOCARDIAL INFARCTION IN THE ELDERLY

Diagnosis

Diagnosis of acute myocardial infarction is also discussed in Chapter 11.

The spontaneous presentation of myocardial infarction among aged patients differs from that of their younger counterparts in the frequency of atypical, often painless, infarction, mandating a high degree of suspicion to make the diagnosis. It has not been ascertained whether this high incidence of painless infection reflects physiologic sensory changes, alterations of perception related to aging, or whether it is attributable to the frequent comorbid problems, particularly hypertension and diabetes mellitus. Acute dyspnea, pulmonary edema, syncope, peripheral arterial embolism, and stroke are among the more dramatic presentations. Less commonly, progressive renal failure may herald myocardial infarction. More subtle signs and symptoms such as profound weakness, faintness, worsening heart failure, agitation or restlessness, acute confusion or altered mental status, change in eating habits, or sudden change in activity or other usual behaviors may provide the only clue to myocardial infarction. Silent or unrecognized myocardial infarction is also more frequent.[2] The male preponderance of myocardial infarction decreases with advancing age, with an essentially equal gender incidence beyond age 70.

Not only are the clinical manifestations of myocardial infarction less typical in the elderly, but laboratory data used to confirm the diagnosis are also problematic. Diagnostic elevations of creatine kinase MB (CK-MB) isoenzyme fractions are often encountered with total CK levels within the normal range for younger patients; older patients are likely to have lower values for total CK related to the decrease in lean body mass with aging. Because non-Q wave infarction occurs more commonly in aged patients, the more subtle electrocardiographic abnormalities are often less helpful in the diagnosis of new infarction; this limitation is compounded by the excess of conduction abnormalities on the electrocardiogram with advancing age, as well as the abnormalities reflect-

ing prior myocardial infarction or concurrent hypertension.

Clinical Course and Management

Coronary or Intensive Care Unit Phase

Admission to a coronary or intensive care unit, with its specialized personnel and technology, remains appropriate for elderly patients with acute myocardial infarction, as they benefit as much as their younger counterparts from defibrillation when needed; further, invasive monitoring of pulmonary artery pressure is more likely to guide management in elderly patients, given their excess development of heart failure and cardiogenic shock.

In the coronary care unit, elderly patients tend to have more disorientation and cerebral dysfunction than younger ones, possibly owing to the increased occurrence of hypotension, arrhythmia, and heart failure; and increased sensitivity to medications, particularly narcotics, analgesics, tranquilizers, and sedatives. Reassurance should be substituted for sedation when feasible. Elderly patients may be more anxious than their younger counterparts; may have problems understanding the complex monitoring devices; and may become confused by the unfamiliar surroundings, the multiplicity of personnel and procedures, and so forth. Limitations of vision and hearing may contribute to these problems. Concise and repeated explanations must be part of early rehabilitation, with efforts made to ensure that the aged patient remains oriented to time and place. Other problems encountered with increased frequency include difficulty with urination, particularly in males with prostatic enlargement who receive diuretic therapy, and gastrointestinal complications, which may be averted by prescribing a stool softener and a soft diet. The use of atropine to reverse sinus bradycardia may precipitate glaucoma, urinary retention, and/or confusion; alternative therapy, such as temporary pacing, may be preferable.

Thrombolytic Therapy

In contrast to the initial suggestion that thrombolytic therapy offered no survival advantage for elderly patients,[6] more recent trials of several thrombolytic agents have documented favorable outcomes, particularly in the 65- to 75-year age group; thrombolysis effects an even greater reduction in mortality than at younger ages despite the excess of bleeding complications, particularly the occurrence of cerebrovascular hemorrhage among elderly women. For patients older than age 75, decisions must be individualized on the basis of preinfarction status, comorbidity, the apparent severity of infarction, the extent of myocardium at risk, and the risk of bleeding, among others.[7]

Clinical Course

The clinical course of myocardial infarction tends to be more severe in elderly patients and is characterized by an excess of complications,[5] as well as by increased mortality. Cardiogenic shock, pulmonary edema, and congestive heart failure, major manifestations of the severity of infarction and determinants of mortality from infarction, are more common in the elderly. Elderly patients with myocardial infarction more frequently have supraventricular arrhythmias, including atrial fibrillation and flutter; and an excess occurrence of conduction defects, including atrioventricular block; ventricular aneurysm, and myocardial rupture.[2] Cardiac rupture, most frequent in the initial week or 10 days following infarction, is heralded by recurrence of chest pain, hypotension, and, preterminally, electromechanical dissociation. Of interest and therapeutic consequence is the fact that ventricular ectopic beats, even when frequent and multiform, are less likely to progress to ventricular tachycardia and fibrillation than in a younger population; given the excess of adverse effects, particularly central nervous system toxicity, from lidocaine administration in elderly patients, the prophylactic use of lidocaine to suppress ventricular ectopy is unwise because of its unfavorable risk-to-benefit ratio. It is indicated only for high-grade or symptomatic ventricular arrhythmias; when used, the loading dose does not differ from that given to younger patients because of similar volumes of distribution, but the maintenance infusion dosage must be reduced, usually by half, because of decreased drug metabolism in the elderly.[2]

Because of the increased anatomic severity of

coronary disease in the elderly, with an excess of complications and greater comorbidity, their mortality in hospital is as high as 20 to 40% (twice that of a younger population) and the hospital stay is more prolonged for survivors (almost twice that for younger individuals); they have more extended periods at bed rest or at limited activity, including a longer stay in the coronary or intensive care unit. With this increased severity of infarction, often superimposed on prior infarction, elderly patients also tend to have more residual impairment and invalidism. Additionally, physicians often underestimate the habitual physical activity of their elderly patients and may institute excessive bed rest on the basis of age rather than disease status, in addition to overmedicating their elderly patients in an attempt to provide comfort and rest.

Pharmacotherapy

Pharmacotherapy is also discussed in Chapter 16.

With advancing age, major changes occur in drug absorption, metabolism and half-life, distribution, excretion, and receptor sensitivity. Elderly patients therefore have an increase in adverse responses to drug therapy as a result of drug interactions; comorbid problems; diminished renal, hepatic, gastrointestinal, and central nervous system function; decreased lean body mass for drug distribution; and lessened compensatory responses, among others.[8,9] For example, morphine given to control pain may cause excessive respiratory depression, bradyarrhythmias, and hypotension. Elderly patients have increased sensitivity to the effects of vasodilator therapy and beta-adrenergic blocking agents because of their predisposition to orthostatic hypotension, compromised baroreceptor function, and frequently associated conduction system disease. Particularly in the hypovolemic patient, vasodilator therapy may produce unacceptable hypotension; similarly, taking nitroglycerin while standing may cause syncope. Syncope may also develop when calcium-blocking drugs are used.

Complications of antihypertensive therapy are more frequent in elderly patients, both because the diminished renal function increases the incidence of drug toxicity and because the aged patient with less sensitive baroreceptor responses is more susceptible to the orthostatic complications of volume depletion. Also, the decreased efficacy of stretch receptors in the rigid aortic wall of the aged lessens the reflex tachycardia in response to assuming an upright position. The dosage of antihypertensive drugs should be increased gradually, and blood pressure should be checked in both the sitting and standing positions. By gradually assuming the standing posture, the elderly patient may avert dizziness and syncope.

Diuretic therapy poses a particular problem since excessive diuresis with hypovolemia is poorly tolerated by the elderly individual and may result in dehydration, hypotension, azotemia, and confusion. Even with the milder thiazide diuretics, the aged patient may incur potassium depletion in addition to orthostatic complications; this depletion is especially likely in elderly patients whose dietary potassium intake is limited. Digitalis toxicity and weakness may result from hypokalemia. In addition, the hyperglycemia secondary to thiazide therapy may aggravate preexisting diabetes mellitus or glucose intolerance.

Low-Risk Elderly Coronary Patients

Despite the general increase in postinfarction risk status, some elderly coronary patients have a favorable prognosis. These individuals, typically characterized by an uncomplicated hospital course and a normal predischarge exercise test, have a low risk of proximate coronary events and an excellent prognosis for recovery; they should be encouraged to resume or undertake a reasonably active lifestyle.

EXERCISE REHABILITATION

Exercise rehabilitation is discussed in Chapter 22.

RISK STRATIFICATION: IMPLICATIONS FOR MYOCARDIAL REVASCULARIZATION

Risk stratification for myocardial revascularization is also discussed in Chapters 17 and 18.

Because of the unfavorable long-term outcome in many elderly coronary patients, which is in part related to the frequency of multivessel coronary disease and severe or unstable angina pectoris,[10] evaluation for myocardial revascularization is often undertaken; this may have to be considered in even very elderly patients.[11] Exercise testing, when feasible, can identify high-risk patients; adenosine or dipyridamole thallium studies can be performed with safety in elderly patients unable to exercise.[12,13]

Coronary angiography entails only a minor increase in risk for elderly patients. Although fewer elderly patients appear eligible for coronary angioplasty, its high rate of success and favorable long-term benefit among suitable patients, even among octogenarians, are encouraging.[14] Despite the increased perioperative mortality, the long-term success of coronary bypass surgery is equally encouraging, with 5-year event-free survival better at age 65 or older than at younger age (47% versus 39%, respectively).[15] Excellent functional improvement and long-term survival, with higher but acceptable morbidity and mortality risks, are found among octogenarians.[16] Management in the perioperative period presents the greatest challenge because of excess complications and greater requirement for temporary pacemakers, ventilatory support, and intra-aortic balloon pump counterpulsation. These entail a longer time spent at bed rest, with more of the hospitalization spent in a surgical intensive care setting.

Ambulation and gradually progressive physical activity should be initiated as soon as feasible (see also Ch. 19) as a component of postoperative management designed to help decrease complications and improve functional capacity at the time of hospital discharge. When this is not undertaken, the excessive immobilization and protracted hospital stay often result in substantial deconditioning such that, at hospital discharge, exercise tolerance is markedly decreased, even among previously active elderly coronary patients. Particularly after coronary bypass surgery, this postoperative exercise intolerance must be explained to the elderly coronary patient as related to the deconditioning of prolonged perioperative immobilization, at times combined with the prior long-term inactivity from the illness, so that the patient will not inappropriately perceive the coronary disease as excessively severe or the coronary bypass revascularization as unsuccessful.

REFERENCES

1. Pifer A, Bronte L: Squaring the pyramid. p. 3. In Pifer A, Bronte L (eds): Our Aging Society. WW Norton, New York, 1986
2. Wenger NK, Marcus FI, O'Rourke RA (eds): 18th Bethesda Conference Report: Cardiovascular disease in the elderly. J Am Coll Cardiol 10 (suppl. A):2A, 1987
3. Wenger, NK, Furberg CD, Pitt E: Coronary Heart Disease in the Elderly. Elsevier Science Publishing, New York, 1986
4. National Center for Health Statistics, DA Dawson, PF Adams: Current estimates from the National Health Interview Survey, United States, 1986. (DHHS publication no. [PHS] 87-1592.) Vital and Health Statistics. Series 10, no. 164. p. 98. Public Health Service, Hyattsville, MD, 1987
5. Wenger NK: The elderly patient with cardiovascular disease. p. 1. In Parmley WW, Chatterjee K (eds): Cardiology. JB Lippincott, Philadelphia, 1989
6. Italian Group for the Study of Streptokinase in Myocardial Infarction (GISSI): Effectiveness of intravenous thrombolytic therapy in acute myocardial infarction. Lancet i:397, 1986
7. Tanaka T, Wenger NK: Acute myocardial infarction in the elderly: Diagnosis, management prognosis. Modern Med 59:48, 1991
8. Greenblatt DJ, Sellers EM, Shader RI: Drug disposition in old age. N Engl J Med 306:1081, 1982
9. Ouslander JG: Drug therapy in the elderly. Ann Intern Med 95:711, 1981
10. Gersh BJ, Kronmal RA, Schaff HV et al: Comparison of coronary artery bypass surgery and medical therapy in patients 65 years of age or older: A nonrandomized study from the Coronary Artery Surgery Study (CASS) registry. N Engl J Med 313:217, 1985
11. Smith SC, Jr, Gilpin E, Ahnve S et al: Outlook after acute myocardial infarction in the very elderly compared with that in patients aged 65 to 75 years. J Am Coll Cardiol 16:784, 1990
12. Saunamaki KI: Early post-myocardial infarction exercise testing in subjects 70 years or more of age: Functional and prognostic evaluation. Eur Heart J 5(suppl. E):47, 1984
13. Deckers JW, Fioretti P, Brower RW et al: Ineligibility for predischarge exercise testing after myocardial infarction in the elderly: Implications for prognosis. Eur Heart J 5 (suppl. E):97, 1984
14. Jeroudi MO, Kleiman NS, Minor ST et al: Percutaneous transluminal coronary angioplasty in octogenarians. Ann Intern Med 113:423, 1990
15. Gersh BJ, Kronmal RA, Schaff HV et al: Long-term (5 year) results of coronary bypass surgery in patients 65 years old or older: A report from the Coronary Artery Surgery Study. Circulation 68 (suppl. II):II-190, 1983
16. Naunheim KS, Kern MJ, McBride LR et al: Coronary artery bypass surgery in patients aged 80 years or older. Am J Cardiol 59:804, 1987

13

Clinical Aspects of Coronary Heart Disease in Women

Barbara Packard, M.D., Ph.D.

Coronary heart disease (CHD) is the leading cause of death in U.S. women aged 75 or older and the second most common cause of death in U.S. women between 45 and 74 years (Fig. 13-1). About 245,000 of the 510,000 individuals who die of CHD each year in the United States are women. A comparison of the CHD death rates before age 75 shows that black women have approximately 1.5-fold higher death rates than white women (Fig. 13-2). The death rate for white women rises sharply after age 75. The economic cost of heart disease in women was estimated at $20 billion in 1988.

The age-adjusted CHD death rate in white women declined 47% between 1963 and 1988 (latest year for which data are available). Over the same period, the decline in men was 50%. The decline was smaller in black women (40%). The rate of decline in women slowed to an average of 3.5% per year in the 5-year period 1983 to 1988, compared with an average of 4.1% per year in the five years from 1973 to 1978 (Fig. 13-3). Both improved medical care and reduction of risk factors play important roles in the continuing decline in the CHD death rates.

Other aspects of the problem are important. CHD manifests itself initially as angina pectoris more commonly in women and as myocardial infarction in men. Infarction is more often fatal in women than in men. Women undergoing coronary artery bypass graft surgery (CABG) have a higher operative mortality, although long-term rates of survival are similar to those in men. In the last decade, the number of cardiac catheterizations in women has nearly doubled and the number of CABG procedures has nearly tripled.

Information on the differences between women and men with regard to rehabilitation after a clinical coronary event is sparse. Most of the guidelines for the rehabilitation process come from studies of men. Although some gender differences in the specific psychosocial aspects of CHD have been reported, data on this subject are also limited. Depression, anxiety, and guilt feelings about their coronary disease and their family roles have been found with such frequency in women that they are often identified as women-specific responses to CHD. It has been suggested that women are twice as likely as men to experience depression following myocardial infarction.

Such data improve our understanding of the course of CHD in women and add to our ability to detect and manage the disease. They also provide direction for lifestyle changes needed to reduce the risk of and ultimately to prevent CHD. The early prevention of CHD in women is the most important goal because of the seriousness of the disease once it develops later in life.

This chapter addresses the clinical aspects of CHD in women and gender differences in clinical manifestations, detection, and management. Although these differences have been described in various studies, further research is needed in most cases to confirm the relationship to gender or to identify the specific mechanism(s) responsible.

217

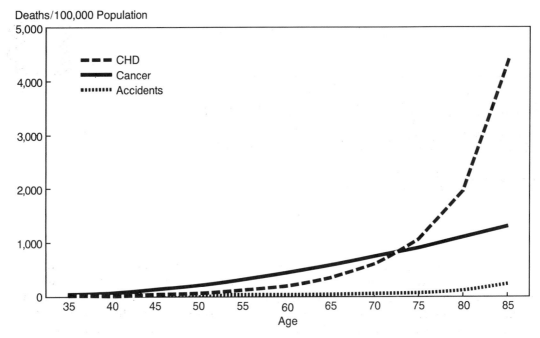

Fig. 13-1. Leading cause of death in U.S. women in 1988. (Data from the National Center for Health Statistics, Washington, D.C.)

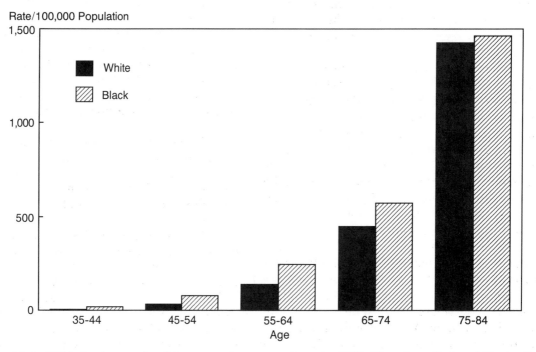

Fig. 13-2. CHD death rates for U.S. women by race and age in 1988. (Data from National Center for Health Statistics, Washington, D.C.)

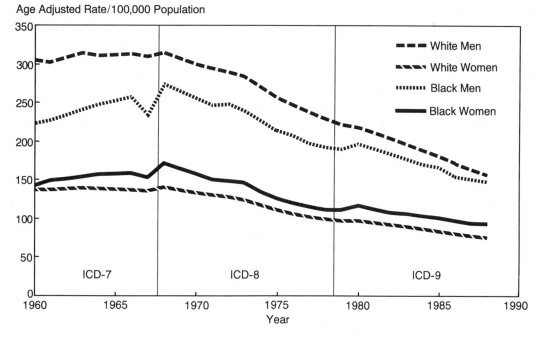

Age Adjusted Rate/100,000 Population

Fig. 13-3. CHD death rates in the United States by race and gender from 1960 to 1988. (Data from International Classification of Diseases, World Health Organization, Geneva.)

CLINICAL MANIFESTATIONS

Although the clinical features of CHD in women are the same as in men, important differences exist between the genders. Clinical manifestations of CHD increase among women after the menopause, and CHD is the leading cause of death in women beginning at age 75. Early findings of the Framingham Heart Study indicated that CHD occurs consistently at a later age among women than men. The initial clinical manifestation occurs 10 years later in women and myocardial infarction occurs 20 years later. However, 68% of coronary disease deaths in women occurred as the first clinical manifestation of CHD, compared with 49% of men.[1] Further research is needed to explain these significant differences.

Stable Angina Pectoris

The incidence of stable angina pectoris appears to be influenced by gender as well as by age and risk factor status. Angina, in the absence of myocardial infarction, is reported to be a more common clinical manifestation of CHD in women, occurring in 55% of women compared with 43% of men.[1] However, not all women presenting with precordial chest pain have angina pectoris due to CHD. In the Coronary Artery Surgery Study (CASS) Registry, 50% of women with chest pain who were referred for angiographic evaluation had little or no coronary artery narrowing compared with 17% of men.[2] In particular, young women with chest pain represent a diagnostic challenge. In women below age 45, about 56% undergoing coronary angiography for suspected CHD in one large series had normal coronary arteries or insignificant narrowing (less than 50%) of the coronary arteries.[3] It is important, therefore, to differentiate the causes of chest pain in women to avoid performing unnecessary coronary angiography in normal women.

The prognosis in women presenting with angina is unclear since many studies have not reported gender analyses. The Framingham Heart Study reported that women with angina had a better prognosis than men. At the 14-year follow-up, of those who presented with angina, 17% of women compared with 44% of men subsequently developed a more serious coronary event.[4] However, these figures may be complicated by the diagnosis of angina in women without CHD. A more recent study reported that survival free of myocardial infarction for 8 years in patients with angina was 80% in women compared with 71% in men.[5]

Lerner and Kannel reported that 86% of all angina in women is uncomplicated by myocardial infarction compared with 66% in men. In men aged 35 to 54 years, 73% of all angina occurs after myocardial infarction.[6]

Unstable Angina Pectoris

Information about unstable angina pectoris in women is available primarily from studies of surgical intervention. It appears that more women than men with a diagnosis of unstable or severe angina are referred for or undergo CABG. CASS reported that the difference in the distribution of unstable angina between women and men undergoing CABG was significant (51 and 39%, respectively).[7] Loop et al. reported that more women than men (60% versus 45%, respectively) had severe and unstable angina prior to CABG, even though the extent of coronary atherosclerosis was less and left ventricular performance was better overall in women.[8] Others demonstrated that 54% of women had unstable angina before surgery compared with 35% of men.[9] In another series of patients referred for CABG, 76.1% of women and 69.8% of men had unstable angina preoperatively.[10] Although these figures do not provide information on the prevalence and course of unstable angina in women, they do indicate that the gender distribution of clinical symptoms in patients referred for CABG may differ.

Chest Pain with Normal Coronary Arteries

Chest pain resulting from coronary artery spasm differs from typical angina pectoris. Coronary spasm in the absence of coronary atherosclerosis occurs more commonly in women than men and at a younger age than classic angina pectoris. This type of chest pain, often referred to as variant angina, generally has a good prognosis.[11,12] The so-called "variant angina" that occurs in the presence of coronary atherosclerosis is believed to be a severe form of unstable angina. Only 20% of women are affected by this type of angina, compared with 80% of men. A review by Murdaugh and O'Rourke reported that even minimal (less than 30%) coronary artery luminal narrowing adversely affected the prognosis.[13]

Growing evidence indicates that in patients with chest pain but without significant large-vessel coronary atherosclerosis, a condition known as microvascular angina may exist that cannot be detected by standard tests. Although its frequency of occurrence is unknown, in one series of patients undergoing cardiac catheterization, 20% had normal coronary arteries and two-thirds of these were women. Investigators speculated that abnormal sensory function of the nerves supplying the coronary arteries can result in an inappropriate flow response to stress and cause severe chest pain that may last longer than typical angina. The overall impact of this abnormality on the heart may be mild, but the atypical chest pain may be more difficult to manage than the typical angina of CHD.[14] Research on this interesting condition may provide additional information important to the interpretation of chest pain in women.

Myocardial Infarction

Framingham data show that myocardial infarction as the initial clinical manifestation of CHD is less common in women (34%) than in men (50%) and occurs almost 20 years later.[1] However, in women who experience a myocardial infarction, both the prognosis for survival and the subsequent clinical course are worse than in men. First episodes of infarction are more likely to be fatal within 1 year in women (39%) than in men (31%). In addition, women are twice as likely as men to die within the first few weeks following a myocardial infarction. Data from the Multicenter Investigation of the Limitation of Infarct Size

(MILIS) support the worse prognosis in women. The overall mortality rate was 36% for women and 21% for men over a 32-month mean follow-up period after myocardial infarction. The highest mortality rate was for black women (48%) followed by white women (32%), black men (23%), and white men (21%). The racial difference was not significant after adjustment of the mortality rate for baseline differences.[15] The worse prognosis in women cannot be entirely explained by the older age at which they typically have a myocardial infarction, their higher prevalence of diabetes and hypertension, or any particular characteristic of the infarction.[16]

Other features of the clinical course after myocardial infarction also appear to differ between women and men. Left ventricular ejection fraction is reported to be higher in women at hospital discharge.[15] CASS also documented this difference in women with CHD undergoing CABG, in addition to a higher wall motion score that indicated less severe ventricular dysfunction. No significant difference was reported for left ventricular end-diastolic pressure between women and men. Congestive heart failure was more frequent and severe in women.[7] One explanation for this finding of congestive heart failure in women with better ventricular systolic function may be the higher incidence in women of diabetes mellitus and hypertension with their attendant adverse influence on left ventricular diastolic function.[17] Results reported in 1974 from the Framingham Heart Study demonstrated that the relative risk of developing congestive heart failure in diabetic compared with nondiabetic subjects increased 5.3-fold in diabetic women and 2.4-fold in diabetic men.[18]

The relative risk of reinfarction is greater among women (4.9) than among men (2.2) compared to individuals of the same gender in the general population. Reinfarction occurred in 25% of the women and 22% of the men in the Framingham Heart Study within 10 years of the initial infarction.[1] Being a woman was described by Marmor as a risk factor for early recurrent infarction.[19] In addition, women who experienced a symptomatic infarction have a greater risk of recurrence than those whose infarction was silent and unrecognized.[6]

Although information about the psychosocial features of CHD in women is very limited, data from a small series of patients aged 25 to 55 years identified feelings of guilt in women during recuperation from myocardial infarction as the most striking psychosocial gender difference.[7] The study reported that women resume household activities, with associated high-energy requirements, immediately upon hospital discharge and increase their progression of activities at 3 or 4 weeks by increasing their level of household activities. Men, on the other hand, do not describe guilt feelings during convalescence after myocardial infarction and rest before progressing to walking at 3 or 4 weeks. In this small series, 71% of the women resumed sexual activity within 7 weeks compared with 88% of the men. One-third of the women returned to work, outside the home, within 3 to 6 months after myocardial infarction, compared with 90% of the men. Although the reasons for these gender differences are not known, such factors as disease severity, socioeconomic status, psychological variables, or compliance with coronary rehabilitation may be involved.[20]

Silent Ischemia

Awareness of the existence of silent or asymptomatic myocardial ischemia and its important role in myocardial infarction and sudden death has increased over the past decade. However, little information on its prevalence and significance in women is available. It has been reported that almost one-half of the cases of unrecognized myocardial infarction are completely silent.[1] The frequency of unrecognized myocardial infarction is over 25% of all infarctions in the Framingham Heart Study.[20a] Unrecognized infarctions occur more commonly among women (34%) at almost every age than among men (27%).[6] This difference remains unexplained. Since women have a higher proportion of unrecognized infarctions, there is an important need for information on silent ischemia in women.

Sudden Death

Sudden death in women occurs, on average, 20 years later than in men and is somewhat less common (37% compared with 46% of CHD deaths, respectively). However, in individuals without prior overt CHD, sudden death occurred in more women (67%) than men (55%). In individuals with prior overt CHD, over a 10-year period, sudden death occurred in 5.3% of women compared with 11.9% of men.[1] Women with diabetes who are taking antihypertensive medication appear to have an increased risk of sudden death.[21] More information is needed to understand this association.

Summary

Although the spectrum of clinical manifestations of CHD is similar between women and men, comprehensive information about specific characteristics and the course of CHD in women is not yet available. It appears that there are important gender differences that should be recognized, understood, and taken into account in the diagnosis and management of CHD in women. Although twice as many men as women who present with angina will have myocardial infarction within 4 to 8 years, the prognosis for survival after myocardial infarction is worse for women. Women also develop higher subsequent rates of congestive heart failure, postinfarction angina, and reinfarction than men. This worse course cannot be entirely explained by the older age when women typically have myocardial infarction or by the higher prevalence of hypertension and diabetes. These findings are particularly important in view of the changing demographics of the population in the United States and many other societies. CHD accounts for an increasingly larger proportion of the cause of death with age. The number of older people in the United States is increasing, and it is estimated that by the year 2050, 16% of people over age 60 will be women and about 12% will be men.[22] The burden of CHD in women can therefore be expected to increase.

DETECTION

The interpretation of chest pain and the diagnosis of CHD are more complex in women than in men. The lower prevalence of CHD in women,

particularly under age 50, and the experience that its presence is confirmed in only about one-third to two-thirds of women with typical angina and in fewer than one-fifth of women with atypical chest pain syndromes challenge the clinician. The medical history can provide valuable information about the occurrence of prior events and risk factors more frequently seen in women, such as diabetes mellitus and hypertension. It can also uncover symptoms of more advanced disease, such as congestive heart failure, reported to be twice as common in women as in men.[7] The family history is important to risk factor assessment, especially in younger women. Age and hormonal status provide further information with regard to the probability of CHD. A thorough physical examination can shed light on the possible cardiac or noncardiac origin of chest pain and elicit other signs supportive of a particular diagnosis compatible with the history.

An important objective of noninvasive diagnostic tests is to identify patients at high risk for CHD. In women with chest pain, the value of rest and exercise electrocardiography (ECG) studies in the diagnosis of CHD is controversial. In general, the lower disease prevalence in women with chest pain limits the interpretation of many of the noninvasive tests in the detection of CHD, the selection and effectiveness of interventions, and the prognosis of CHD. However, when the prevalence of disease is taken into account, similar efficacy of noninvasive testing for the detection of CHD has been established in both genders.[23] Gender, age, and the characteristics of chest pain are important in the selection and use of noninvasive studies. Current diagnostic tests for detecting CHD in women include ECG, cardiac fluoroscopy, exercise thallium scintigraphy, exercise radionuclide ventriculography, exercise echocardiography, and coronary angiography.

Electrocardiography

The resting ECG is important to the diagnosis of CHD in women, particularly because of the higher proportion of women with unrecognized infarctions.[1] In addition, the presence or absence of abnormal Q waves in the resting ECG may be influenced in women older than 50 years by the use of estrogen replacement therapy (ERT). Barrett-Connor et al. reported that the only significant difference in the resting ECG between estrogen users and nonusers in the Lipid Research Clinics Program was the lower occurrence of abnormal Q waves in postmenopausal women on ERT.[24]

The exercise ECG, despite its common use and low cost, has limited usefulness in the detection of CHD in women because of its moderate sensitivity (73 to 79%) and low specificity (59 to 66%).[25] Several studies provide data that appear to be different from those for men. Cumming et al. reported that 25% of normal women aged 20 to 39, 50% aged 40 to 59, and 66% aged 60 or more had exercise-induced ECG abnormalities compatible with ischemia.[26] The high false-positive rate in normal women limits the value of this test in the detection of CHD in women. Manca et al. found that although 18.3% of men with atypical angina and positive exercise ECG tests developed clinically overt CHD in 3 to 7 years, only 4.6% of women subsequently were diagnosed with CHD.[27] In patients with typical angina, a sensitivity of 98% in men and only 75% in women has been reported for the exercise ECG.[28] Therefore, even in women with CHD, the effectiveness of the procedure in detecting disease is poor. Better diagnostic results were seen in women with multivessel coronary involvement, of whom 93% had an abnormal exercise ECG compared with only 43% with single-vessel or no disease. This study used the sum of the 14 leads as the best independent prediction of multivessel disease.[29]

The diagnostic effectiveness of the exercise ECG is related to the characteristics of the population tested by using Bayesian factors; when the prevalence of CHD is low, the ability of the exercise ECG to detect disease is low. Diagnostic accuracy can be expected to increase in proportion to the extent (severity) of disease. However, the usefulness of the exercise ECG in diagnosing the presence or absence of CHD in women remains limited.[30] Some investigators have suggested that non-Bayesian factors may be operating, such as hemodynamic response to exercise or level of estrogen, which has digitalislike actions.[31] Until better criteria are established to select subjects or interpret results obtained in women, this test will remain of limited value in the detection of CHD in women.

Cardiac Fluoroscopy

Cardiac fluoroscopy is easy to perform. Hamby et al.[32] report that when coronary calcification is present at fluoroscopy its sensitivity and specificity in women with at least 50% coronary narrowing are 84 and 81%, respectively; and Hung et al.[29] report that these values in women with at least 70% narrowing are 79 and 83%, respectively. Since symptomatic CHD may be more common among patients with coronary calcification, this test may be useful in confirming the diagnosis in women with typical angina, especially younger women, in whom coronary artery calcification is more likely to indicate CHD.[32,33] In addition, Chaitman et al. reported that more than 80% of women with multivessel coronary artery disease had coronary calcification involving both right and left vessels.[25] Cardiac fluoroscopy for detecting calcium in the coronary arteries is cost-effective and can contribute to the detection of CHD in women.

Exercise Thallium Scintigraphy

Exercise thallium scintigraphy is more effective than exercise ECG alone for detecting CHD in women, as a result of its higher specificity. Values of 75% sensitivity and 91 to 97% specificity have been reported.[29,34] However, its diagnostic accuracy may be reduced by the attenuation of signals due to breast artifact in the anterior cardiac wall. This fixed defect in the anterolateral or anteroapical segment may result in a false-positive study. Other aspects of thallium scintigraphy, including cost, exposure of the patient to radiation, and the need for nuclear facilities, although not gender-specific, can limit its use. Therefore, careful selection of patients is necessary, especially for women in whom the prevalence of chest pain without CHD is higher than in men. Melin et al. report that the test is as accurate in women as in men when disease prevalence is taken into account.[35] Little further information is available on differences between women and men in the use of this test to diagnose CHD.

Exercise Radionuclide Ventriculography

Technetium-labeled radionuclide ventriculography, now limited in use, has reasonable sensitivity and specificity for the diagnosis of CHD in men. Since one of the abnormal responses is failure to increase the left ventricular ejection fraction at peak exercise, the test is of little value in women because of their different physiologic pattern of left ventricular function. Buonanno et al. describe a hyperdynamic condition of the left ventricle, present in women but not in men, that may account for the failure of the ejection fraction to increase with exercise in women and may result in more false-positive studies.[36] Smaller ventricular volumes and increased contractility in women have also been reported in several other studies. This condition may be a cause of transient myocardial ischemia as a result of the potential imbalance of metabolic needs and autoregulatory adaptability of the coronary vasculature. Nevertheless, for radionuclide ventriculography to be effective in the detection of CHD in women, new parameters for interpretation of the ejection fraction response in women should be developed.

Exercise Echocardiography

Although little research has been performed to study exercise echocardiography in women, available data indicate that the values for sensitivity and specificity are moderate (86%) and are similar in women and in men. An important aspect of these data is the maintenance of sensitivity in the presence of single-vessel disease.[37] Since single-vessel disease involving 50% or more narrowing occurs more frequently in women with CHD (18%) than in men with CHD (9%), exercise echocardiography may be clinically useful for the detection of CHD in women.

Because of the difficulty of diagnosing CHD by noninvasive tests involving exercise, investigators have evaluated high-dose dipyridamole echocardiography. A sensitivity of 79% and a specificity of 93% make the test more reliable in women than exercise ECG and more attractive from the point of view of safety, cost, and feasibility than exercise thallium scintigraphy. Results obtained from the dipyridamole echocardiography test do not appear to differ between women and men.[38]

Coronary Angiography

Coronary angiography is considered the definitive test to detect CHD in patients. Its main limitations are its invasiveness, cost, and potential complications, admittedly infrequent. A normal test does not necessarily eliminate other potential coronary artery abnormalities, such as spasm or small-vessel disease. As with other tests, patient selection influences diagnostic accuracy. Gender differences in the extent of atherosclerosis have been reported from angiographic studies alone or in conjunction with CABG.

Results from two large angiographic series in young women suspected of having CHD indicate that the left anterior descending coronary artery is the most common site (43 to 54%) of single-vessel disease in young women[3,39] compared with young men (36%).[40] In women under age 45 with significant CHD, 50% had only one vessel narrowed by 50% or more, 25% had two vessels involved, and 25% had three-vessel disease.

Since angiographically normal coronary arteries are frequently seen in young women with chest pain, it is important that better indicators for invasive evaluation become available. Disease is not often present in younger women with fewer than two coronary risk factors; therefore, diagnostic angiography may rarely be needed in this group of subjects.[3]

The CASS Registry offers the largest series of angiographic data in women with chronic stable chest pain and without myocardial infarction. The CASS Registry reported a prevalence of 56 to 96% for ≥70% coronary artery narrowing in women with definite angina. Moreover, left main coronary artery or three-vessel disease occurred in 40% of women older than 60 years compared with 50% of men over 50 years of age. The prevalence of left main coronary artery disease was 8 to 9% in women over a wide age range but 24% in men 70 years of age or older.[41] Similar findings for the left main and the left circumflex coronary arteries in patients 65 years of age or older with angina were reported by Boucek et al.[42] The frequency of poorer left ventricular perfusion (by scintigraphy) was 8% higher in men than in women. In this study of 100 patients of each gender, right coronary dominance was seen in 90% of women compared with 80% of men and left coronary dominance occurred in 8% of women and 19% of men. However, 55% of three-vessel disease was found in right-coronary-dominant patients and 42% in left-coronary-dominant patients. The reasons for such apparent gender-related differences in the extent of disease are unexplained.[42]

Summary

Noninvasive testing to detect CHD in women is not as useful as in men for several reasons. Chief among these is the lower prevalence of CHD in women with chest pain referred for evaluation. However, when statistical analysis of multiple clinical and diagnostic variables is performed, the accuracy of detecting CHD can be improved. Melin et al. suggested that probability analysis can assist clinical judgment in making a better prediction of the presence of disease. They found that a history of typical angina, an abnormal exercise ECG, and an exercise defect on a thallium scan combined to be the best predictor of CHD in women.[35] Other investigators have also assessed the close correlation between variables in predicting CHD by using a stepwise multiple discriminant analysis. The most predictive variable for CHD was a reversible thallium defect followed by coronary calcification and the characteristics of the chest pain.[29] If women presenting with chest pain could be classified into risk categories for CHD, better selection of diagnostic tests might be possible.

MANAGEMENT

Approaches to the management of CHD for women are the same as for men. Prevention is the most important management strategy: primary prevention through adoption and maintenance of a healthy lifestyle and secondary prevention through early and accurate diagnosis, rehabilitation with risk factor modification, and appropriate and timely intervention. The goals of management are also the same for both genders: relief of symptoms, reduction of morbidity and mortality, and maintenance of an acceptable quality of life. Owing to the diagnostic complexity of interpreting chest pain in women, it has become increasingly apparent that management of CHD in women has not been as vigorous as may be warranted. Differences in the presentation characteristics and course of CHD in women may necessitate specific considerations in its management.

Pharmacologic Therapy

The indications for pharmacologic therapy do not appear to differ between women and men, although further studies are needed to determine whether differences exist in such areas as efficacy and safety. Three major classes of drugs are effective in the management of ischemia: nitrates, beta-blocking drugs, and calcium channel-blocking agents. Gender-specific uses and side effects have been described for these agents. It is known that women have smaller coronary arteries than men, mainly as a result of differences in body size. One mechanism that may be important in women with angina may be changes in vascular tone in the area of fixed stenoses. Nitrate and calcium channel-blocking drugs may be of particular benefit, therefore, since they dilate coronary arteries. These agents are also indicated for treatment of coronary artery spasm. Another consideration in the choice of antianginal agents is the increased likelihood of Raynaud's phenomenon in women and the worsening effect of beta-blocking drugs, especially nonselective agents, on peripheral vasospasm associated with this disease.

In these women, the use of beta-blocking drugs that are cardioselective may be indicated.[43] Other than these few indications for specific antianginal agents, little information is available on gender differences in the therapeutic efficacy of vasodilator drugs for the treatment of various anginal syndromes. Because of gender differences in the severity of angina at baseline described in several studies, more intensive antianginal therapy may be warranted in selected women.[13] In general, antianginal agents may be overprescribed in women because of the low prevalence of CHD in women with chest pain.

More information exists regarding the effects of drug treatment after myocardial infarction in women. The Timolol Myocardial Infarction Study demonstrated that a beta-blocking drug prevented nonfatal reinfarction in both genders after myocardial infarction.[44–46] The Beta Blocker Heart Attack Trial reported a lower mortality rate in the treatment group for both women and men who survived the acute phase of myocardial infarction, but the difference was significant only among men.[46] Although the frequency of side effects was similar, the form of the side effects differed between women and men. The symptoms were bronchospasm, nausea, and tiredness among women and were tiredness, insomnia, and cold extremities among men.[47] Results from the Second International Study of Infarct Survival demonstrated significant therapeutic benefit of low-dose aspirin in preventing subsequent clinical manifestations of CHD in women after myocardial infarction.[48] Further studies of the role of antiplatelet agents in women with CHD are needed, and primary prevention trials of the effects of aspirin in women have not been conducted.

Thrombolytic therapy administered early after myocardial infarction has proved beneficial in restoring vessel patency and improving outcome. The GISSI trial demonstrated a significant reduction in 21-day mortality in women receiving intravenous streptokinase early after myocardial infarction.[49]

Information is unavailable on gender differences of routine therapy after myocardial infarction, although dosage considerations based on body size may be more important in women. The Multicenter Postinfarction Research Group reported on the mortality risk associated with ventricular arrhythmias in women and men. Although the distribution of frequent and repetitive runs of ventricular premature beats were similar in both genders, they were not independent risk factors in women, in contrast to their significant independent risk association with mortality in men.[50] This finding, if confirmed, may have an important influence on the treatment of postinfarction arrhythmias in women.

The role of hormone replacement therapy in the primary and secondary prevention of CHD in women is likely to have an important impact on future management strategy.

Percutaneous Transluminal Coronary Angioplasty

Important gender differences have been described by the National Heart, Lung, and Blood Institute PTCA Registry for percutaneous transluminal coronary angioplasty (PTCA). Short-term results were unfavorable in women and showed a significantly reduced clinical success rate for single-vessel disease PTCA and a similar trend for reduced rates of success for multivessel disease. The complication rate was higher, chiefly owing to the greater incidence of bradycardia, hypotension, and coronary dissection. Hospital mortality was significantly higher among women, as were the PTCA mortality rate and that associated with emergency CABG. Multivariate analysis identified being a women as an independent risk factor for PTCA. If PTCA is successful in women, long-term survival is improved compared with men. Women also experience a lower incidence of additional revascularization and restenosis.[51]

Coronary Artery Bypass Graft Surgery

CABG is an important management consideration in women. Gender differences have been reported for CABG surgery in terms of preoperative status, operative success, and postoperative outcome. Preoperative differences include both clinical and anatomic characteristics. Women undergoing CABG were older; more likely to have a history of hypertension and diabetes mellitus; and more frequently reported symptoms of severe or unstable angina, postinfarction angina, and congestive heart failure.[7,9] Women had more frequent cardiac enlargement on chest x-ray and more frequent and severe mitral regurgitation than men.[7] On the other hand, women had a lower incidence of prior myocardial infarction and better ventricular function than men. Anatomically, they also had less coronary artery disease as evidenced by less left main coronary artery stenosis and three-vessel disease.[7,8] Although the difference in age at the time of CABG in women may be related to the later onset of CHD, women appear to be at higher risk than men in terms of clinical manifestations of disease, despite having a better anatomic and functional profile.

Significant differences in operative mortality exist between the genders. CASS reported a 4.5% operative mortality in women compared with 1.9% in men.[7] Results from a large series of women undergoing CABG at the Cleveland Clinic also demonstrated the higher operative mortality rate of women (2.9 and 1.3%, respectively).[8] Findings from a more recent study are consistent with these results (4.6 and 2.6%, respectively).[10] Although the reasons for this difference in operative mortality may be related to age, preoperative clinical status, or other risk factors, at least two studies found correlations to physical size[7,8] applicable to both genders. Therefore, the higher operative mortality seen in women may be due to their smaller physical size and smaller-diameter coronary arteries and not to gender per se. Recognition of this finding and continued improvements in operative procedures and management may have a beneficial impact on operative risk in smaller patients, most of whom are women.

Postoperative outcome differs in certain aspects between women and men. Graft patency rates for women appear to be less favorable than for men, although these data come from those patients selected for repeat angiography mostly for reasons related to patient care, and therefore the

gender data may not be comparable. Long-term survival after CABG is similar between women and men. Survival for women at 5 years is 87 to 91% compared with 90 to 94% for men.[52] The 10-year survival was 78.6% for women and 78.2% for men in the Cleveland Clinic series.[8] After CABG, however, women report less improvement than men, with more days of restricted activity and more days in bed as a result of severe recurring chest pain or dyspnea.[53] Women consistently report less relief of angina than men after CABG.[52] In addition, fewer women than men return to work after CABG.[54]

Rehabilitation

Other than the short- and long-term CHD morbidity and mortality differences described throughout this chapter, few studies have been conducted related to recovery and rehabilitation in women, and therefore only limited information about gender differences is available. The beneficial effects of physical conditioning and exercise rehabilitation appear to be similar for women and men. Women develop an increased physical work capacity and lower their myocardial oxygen demand as a result of exercise training. These findings indicate that exercise training plays an important role in the rehabilitation of women, as it does in men. However, although such improvements occur, women do not remain in rehabilitation programs as men do. One study found that 19% of women left the program compared with 8% of men and that attendance rates for women were lower than for men.[55] The lack of rehabilitation programs structured to the needs of women may be responsible for this behavior. Despite the limited information available about rehabilitation in women, counseling and follow-up of psychosocial and physical outcomes should be an integral part of the management regimen for women with CHD.

Summary

In general, the same guidelines for pharmacotherapy of CHD are applied to women as are used for men. Whether the indications and dosages should be gender-specific has not been determined, although different dose effects may be seen in women because of their smaller body size and smaller coronary arteries. In addition, the efficacy of various pharmacologic agents may be influenced by the endocrine status of women at the time of administration. Information on this issue is unavailable. Women referred for PTCA and CABG appear to be older and have more severe and unstable angina. For each procedure, the outcome reflected their status, i.e., higher early mortality. Although little is known about the reasons for these differences, several characteristics have been implicated, such as age, more advanced disease, and smaller body size.

The rehabilitation aspects of the management of CHD in women should be clarified. The facts that after myocardial infarction women experience more psychosocial abnormalities and sexual dysfunction, do not return to work at the same rate as men, and have less symptomatic improvement after CABG suggest that gender differences exist. The effects of age, socioeconomic status, CHD knowledge, and health-care-seeking behavior also have yet to be evaluated.

REFERENCES

1. Kannel WB, Abbott RD: Incidence and prognosis of myocardial infarction in women: The Framingham Study. p. 208. In Eaker ED, Packard B, Wenger NK et al (eds): Coronary Heart Disease in Women. Haymarket Doyma, New York, 1987
2. Kennedy JW, Killip T, Fisher LB et al: The clinical spectrum of coronary artery disease and its surgical and medical management, 1974–1979. Circulation 66:16, 1982
3. Waters DD, Halphen C, Theroux P et al: Coronary artery disease in young women: Clinical and angiographic features and correlation with risk factors. Am J Cardiol 42:41, 1978
4. Kannel WB, Feinleib M: Natural history of angina pectoris in the Framingham Study. Prognosis and survival. Am J Cardiol 29:154, 1972
5. Elveback LR, Connolly DC: Coronary heart disease in residents of Rochester, Minnesota. V. Prognosis of patients with coronary heart disease based on initial manifestation. Mayo Clin Proc 60:305, 1985
6. Lerner DJ, Kannel WB: Patterns of coronary heart disease morbidity and mortality in the sexes: A 26-year follow-up of the Framingham population. Am Heart J 111:383, 1986
7. Fisher LD, Kennedy JW, Davis KB et al: Association of sex, physical size, and operative mortality after coronary artery bypass in the Coronary Artery Surgery Study (CASS). J Thorac Cardiovasc Surg 84:334, 1982
8. Loop FD, Golding LR, MacMillan JP et al: Coronary artery surgery in women compared with men: Analysis of risks and long-term results. J Am Coll Cardiol 1:383, 1983
9. Gardner TJ, Horneffer PJ, Gott VL et al: Coronary artery bypass grafting in women. Ann Surg 201:780, 1985
10. Khan SS, Nessin S, Gray R et al: Increased mortality of women in coronary artery bypass surgery: Evidence for referral bias. Ann Intern Med 112:561, 1990
11. Selzer A, Langston M, Ruggeroli C et al: Clinical syndrome of variant angina with normal coronary arteriogram. N Engl J Med 295:1343, 1976
12. Scholl J-M, Veau P, Benecerraf A et al: Long-term prognosis of medically treated patients with vasospastic angina and no fixed significant coronary atherosclerosis. Am Heart J 115:559, 1988
13. Murdaugh CL, O'Rourke RA: Coronary heart disease in women: Special considerations. p. 73. In O'Rourke RA (ed): Current Problems in Cardiology. Vol. 13. Year Book Medical Publishers, Chicago, 1988
14. Cannon RO, Watson RM, Rosing DR et al: Angina caused by reduced vasodilator reserve of the small coronary arteries. J Am Coll Cardiol 1:1359, 1983
15. Tofler GH, Stone PH, Muller JE et al: Effects of gender and race on prognosis after myocardial infarction: Adverse prognosis for women, particularly black women. J Am Coll Cardiol 9:473, 1987
16. Puletti M, Sunseri L, Curione M et al: Acute myocardial infarction: Sex-related differences in prognosis. Am Heart J 108:63, 1984
17. Tofler GH, Stone PH, Muller JE et al: Clinical manifestations of coronary heart disease in women. p. 215. In Eaker ED, Packard B, Wenger NK et al (eds): Coronary Heart Disease in Women. Haymarket Doyma, New York, 1987
18. Kannel WB, Hjortland M, Castelli WP: Role of diabetes in congestive heart failure: The Framingham Study. Am J Cardiol 34:29, 1974
19. Marmor A, Geltman EM, Schechtman K et al: Recurrent myocardial infarction: Clinical predictors and prognostic implications. Circulation 66:415, 1982

20. Boogaard MAK, Briody ME: Comparison of the rehabilitation of men and women post-myocardial infarction. J Cardiopulmonary Rehabil 5:379, 1985

20a. Kannel WB, Abbott RD: Incidence and prognosis of unrecognized myocardial infarction: An update on the Framingham Study. N Engl J Med 311:1144, 1984

21. Kannel WB, Cupples LA, D'Agostino RB et al: Hypertension, antihypertensive treatment, and sudden coronary death: The Framingham Study. Hypertension 11(suppl.):II-45, 1988

22. U.S. Bureau of the Census: Decennial Censuses of Population, 1900–1980, the Projections of the Population of the United States: 1982 to 2050. Current Population Reports, Series P-25, No. 922, October 1982. U.S. Bureau of the Census, Suitland, Maryland, 1982

23. Weiner DA, Ryan TJ, McCabe CH et al: Exercise stress testing: Correlations among history of angina, ST-segment response and prevalence of coronary-artery disease in the Coronary Artery Surgery Study (CASS). N Engl J Med 301:230, 1979

24. Barrett-Connor E, Wilcosky T, Wallace RB et al: Resting and exercise electrocardiographic abnormalities associated with sex hormone use in women. Am J Epidemiol 123:81, 1986

25. Chaitman BR, Bourassa MG, Lam J: Noninvasive diagnosis of coronary heart disease in women. p. 222. In Eaker ED, Packard B, Wenger NK et al (eds): Coronary Heart Disease in Women. Haymarket Doyma, New York, 1987

26. Cumming GR, Dufresne C, Kich L et al: Exercise electrocardiogram patterns in normal women. Br Heart J 35:1055, 1973

27. Manca C, Dei Cas L, Albertini D et al: Different prognostic value of exercise electrocardiogram in men and women. Cardiology 63:312, 1978

28. Detry J-MR, Kapita BM, Cosyns J et al: Diagnostic value of history and maximal exercise electrocardiography in men and women suspected of coronary heart disease. Circulation 56:756, 1977

29. Hung J, Chaitman BR, Lam J et al: Noninvasive diagnostic test choices for the evaluation of coronary artery disease in women: A multivariate comparison of cardiac fluoroscopy, exercise electrocardiography and exercise thallium myocardial perfusion scintigraphy. J Am Coll Cardiol 4:8, 1984

30. Osbakken MD: Exercise stress testing in women: Diagnostic dilemma. p. 187. In Douglas PS (ed): Heart Disease in Women. FA Davis, Philadelphia, 1989

31. Glazer MD, Hurst JW: Coronary atherosclerotic heart disease: Some important differences in men and women. Am J Noninvasive Cardiol 1:61, 1987

32. Hamby RI, Tabrah F, Wisoff BG et al: Coronary artery calcification: Clinical implications and angiographic correlates. Am Heart J 87:565, 1974

33. Uretsky BF, Rifkind RD, Sharma SC et al: Value of fluoroscopy in the detection of coronary stenosis: Influence of age, sex, and number of vessels calcified on diagnostic efficacy. Am Heart J 115:323, 1988

34. Friedman TD, Greene AC, Iskandrian AS et al: Exercise thallium-201 myocardial scintigraphy in women: Correlation with coronary arteriography. Am J Cardiol 49:1632, 1982

35. Melin JA, Wijns W, Vanbutsele RJ et al: Alternative diagnostic strategies for coronary artery disease in women: Demonstration of the usefulness and efficiency of probability analysis. Circulation 71:535, 1985

36. Buonanno C, Rossi AL, Dander B et al: Left ventricular function in men and women. Eur Heart J 3:525, 1982

37. Sawada SG, Ryan T, Fineberg NS et al: Exercise echocardiographic detection of coronary artery disease in women. J Am Coll Cardiol 14:1440, 1989

38. Masini M, Picano E, Lattanzi F et al: High dose dipyridamole-echocardiography test in women: Correlation with exercise-electrocardiography test and coronary arteriography. J Am Coll Cardiol 12:682, 1988

39. Welch CC, Proudfit WL, Sheldon WC: Coronary arteriographic findings in 1,000 women under age 50. Am J Cardiol 35:211, 1975

40. Welch CC, Proudfit WL, Sones FM et al: Cinecoronary arteriography in young men. Circulation 42:647, 1970

41. Chaitman BR, Bourassa MG, Davis K et al: Angiographic prevalence of high-risk coronary artery diseases in patient subsets (CASS). Circulation 64:360, 1981

42. Boucek RJ, Romanelli R, Willis WH et al: Sex differences in obstructive coronary artery disease in patients 65 years of age or older with angina pectoris. Circulation 66:926, 1982

43. Hutter AM: Coronary artery disease in women: Medical management. p. 229. In Eaker ED, Packard B, Wenger NK et al (eds): Coronary Heart Disease in Women. Haymarket Doyma, New York, 1987

44. Pederson TR: Six-year follow-up of the Norwegian Multicenter Study on timolol after acute myocardial infarction. N Engl J Med 313:1055, 1985

45. Rodda BE: The timolol myocardial infarction study: An evaluation of selected variables. Circulation 67 (suppl. I):I-101, 1983

46. β-Blocker Heart Attack Trial Research Group: A randomized trial of propranolol in patients with acute myocardial infarction. I. Mortality results. JAMA 247:1707, 1982

47. Furberg CD, Friedman LM, MacMahon SW: Women as participants in trials of the primary and secondary prevention of cardiovascular disease. Part II. Secondary prevention: The beta-blocker heart attack trial and the aspirin myocardial infarction study. p. 241. In Eaker ED, Packard B, Wenger NK et al (eds): Coronary Heart Disease in Women. Haymarket Doyma, New York, 1987

48. ISIS-2 (Second International Study of Infarct Survival) Collaborative Group: Randomised trial of intravenous streptokinase, oral aspirin, both, or neither among 17,187 cases of suspected acute myocardial infarction: ISIS-2. Lancet ii:349, 1988

49. Italian Group for the Study of Streptokinase in Myocardial Infarction (GISSI): Effectiveness of intravenous thrombolytic treatment in acute myocardial infarction. Lancet i:397, 1986

50. Moss AJ, Carleen E, and Multicenter Postinfarction Research Group: Gender differences in the mortality risk associated with ventricular arrhythmias after myocardial infarction. p. 204. In Eaker ED, Packard B, Wenger NK et al (eds): Coronary Heart Disease in Women. Haymarket Doyma, New York, 1987

51. Cowley MJ, Mullin SM, Kelsey SF et al: Sex differences in early and long-term results of coronary angioplasty in the NHLBI PTCA Registry. Circulation 71:90, 1985

52. Davis KB: Coronary artery bypass graft surgery in women. p. 247. In Eaker ED, Packard B, Wenger NK et al (eds): Coronary Heart Disease in Women. Haymarket Doyma, New York, 1987

53. Stanton BA, Zyzanski SJ, Jenkins CD et al: Recovery after major heart surgery: Medical, psychological, and work outcomes. p. 217. In Becker R (ed): Psychopathological and Neurological Dysfunctions Following Open-Heart Surgery. Springer-Verlag, Heidelberg, 1982

54. Stanton BA, Jenkins CD, Denlinger P et al: Predictors of employment status after cardiac surgery. JAMA 249:90, 1983

55. Oldridge NB, LaSalle D, Jones NL et al: Exercise rehabilitation of female patients with coronary artery disease. Am Heart J 100:75, 1980

14

Diagnostic Procedures for Patients with Coronary Heart Disease

Richard W. Lee, M.D.
Gordon A. Ewy, M.D.

This chapter provides an overview of the diagnostic procedures frequently used in patients with suspected or known coronary heart disease (CHD). The indications, values, and limitations of each procedure are emphasized. Some important diagnostic procedures, such as measurement of serum lipid values, measurements of blood pressure, etc., are not addressed.

THE RESTING ELECTROCARDIOGRAM

The standard 12-lead electrocardiogram (ECG), performed with the patient supine and relaxed, is a useful and important adjunct to the clinical history and physical examination in evaluating patients who have or are suspected of having CHD. Specifically, the ECG can show signs of myocardial ischemia or previous myocardial infarction and evidence of ventricular aneurysm or hypertrophy, conduction defects, and arrhythmias. It must be emphasized that a normal resting ECG (Fig. 14-1) does not rule out significant CHD. Most people with CHD but without myocardial ischemia have normal ECGs at rest.

Some ECG abnormalities are specific and sensitive, some are specific but not very sensitive, and many are nonspecific. For example, the presence of atrial fibrillation on the ECG is specific and is a sensitive method of detecting this atrial arrhythmia, but does not define its etiology. The ECG findings of an acute inferior myocardial infarction (Fig. 14-2) or an acute anterior myocardial infarction (Fig. 14-3) are specific and fairly sensitive. The sensitivity of the ECG for diagnosing acute posterior or lateral infarction is intermediate, since a higher percentage of patients with acute myocardial infarctions in these areas do not have acute ST segment changes. The classic true posterior infarction results in anterior ST segment depression and wider (greater than 0.04 second) and taller R waves in precordial leads V_1 and V_2. Acute high lateral infarctions typically have ST segment elevation in leads I and aVL, but true lateral infarctions may be silent on the ECG. When the ECG criteria of left ventricular hypertrophy are present, there is a high likelihood that the patient has left ventricular hypertrophy. On the other hand, many patients have anatomic left ventricular hypertrophy, documented either at postmortem examination or by echocardiogram, without ECG evidence of left

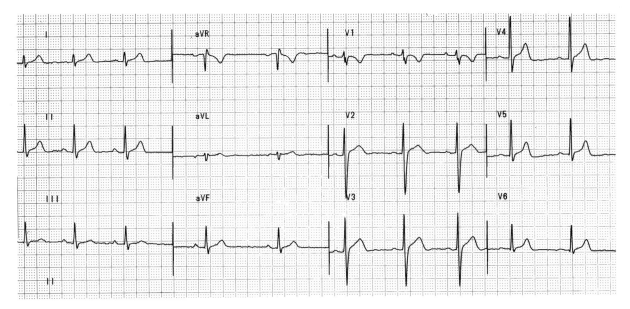

Fig. 14-1. Normal ECG.

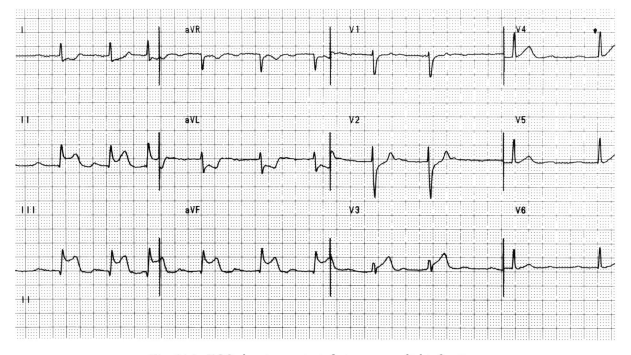

Fig. 14-2. ECG showing acute inferior myocardial infarction.

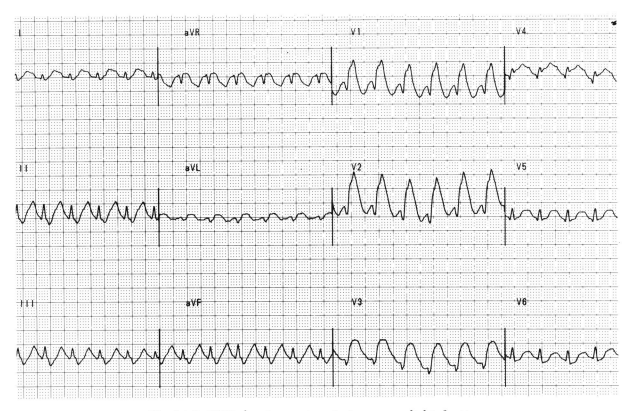

Fig. 14-3. ECG showing acute anterior myocardial infarction.

ventricular hypertrophy. This is an example of a finding that is specific but not sensitive.[1] Finally, there are so many causes of minor ST-T wave abnormalities that these changes are nonspecific.

Comparison of the patient's ECG with previous ECGs improves the diagnostic accuracy of the ECG. For example, a patient with a previously normal ECG who complains of prolonged chest pain or discomfort and has new ECG changes, such as new ST segment depression or new inverted T waves, has a high likelihood of having myocardial ischemia or an acute coronary event.

ECG ST segment elevation is not diagnostic of acute myocardial infarction. The differential diagnosis of ECG ST segment elevation includes the presence of ventricular aneurysm, pericarditis, and early repolarization.

ECG ST segment depression suggests subendocardial ischemia. Again, examining the associated clinical history and comparing the tracing with a recent but earlier ECG are most helpful. A patient without ST segment depression on the ECG who develops ST segment depression in association with chest pain has a high probability of having significant coronary obstructive disease.

Arrhythmias are common in patients with CHD. Patients with heart failure due to CHD may develop an elevation of left ventricular filling pressures that predisposes to left atrial dilatation and consequently to atrial fibrillation and flutter. Isolated ventricular premature beats are frequently present. Some are associated with complaints of palpitations; most are totally asymptomatic. A major concern in a population of patients with CHD is the development of ventricular tachycardia or ventricular fibrillation. These potentially life-threatening arrhythmias are rarely found on the routine ECG. Special recording techniques such as 24-hour ambulatory

(Holter) ECG recording, ECG event recording, or exercise testing are necessary to document most paroxysmal arrhythmias.

THE EXERCISE TEST

Exercise testing is also discussed in Chapters 7 and 8.

Exercise testing in the United States is most often performed on a treadmill (Fig. 14-4) and less frequently on a bicycle ergometer. In some patients, orthopedic or other problems preclude treadmill exercise testing, and the use of a bicycle ergometer, preferably using both arm and leg exercise testing, is necessary (Fig. 14-5). A variety of protocols have been established with the aim of gradually increasing the work load so that there is a gradual increase in heart rate and systolic blood pressure and therefore a gradual increase in oxygen uptake. Most exercise test protocols

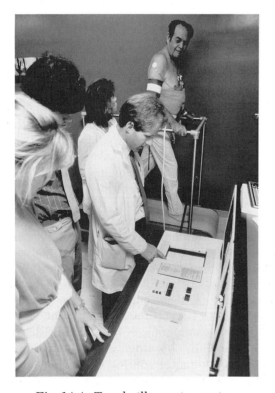

Fig. 14-4. Treadmill exercise testing.

were initially developed for testing active healthy young individuals or endurance athletes. These protocols had to be modified by the addition of lower work levels for patients with heart disease. It is not necessary to routinely measure oxygen uptake for clinical purposes, as there is a relatively good correlation between heart rate and oxygen uptake.

It is important to use multiple ECG leads when testing for CHD (Fig. 14-5), as increasing the number of leads from 1 to 12 increases the sensitivity of the test.[2] In addition to the ECG, it is important to monitor not only the blood pressure, but the patient's appearance and symptoms as well.

Various degrees of ECG ST segment depression (Fig. 14-6) have been advocated as criteria for "positive" or "negative" exercise tests, more properly designated as abnormal and within normal limits, respectively. The sensitivity of the treadmill exercise test is increased when the criteria for a positive or abnormal test are less rigid, but such criteria have a lower specificity. When more rigid criteria, such as 0.2 mV (2 mm) of flat or downsloping ST segment depression 80 msec after the end of the QRS complex are used, the criteria become very specific but less sensitive.[3] However, it is not only the depth of the ST segment depression but also the heart rate and work load at which these changes occur and the duration of the ST segment depression after the cessation of exercise that most closely correlate with the presence or absence of CHD (Fig. 14-7). ST segment depression that quickly normalizes is more likely to be a false-positive result than ST segment depression that slowly returns to baseline levels over several minutes (Fig. 14-7). The development of classic angina pectoris with exercise with ST segment changes is more predictive than ST segment changes alone.[4]

Caution must be used in patients receiving cardiac pharmacotherapy, as a variety of drugs result in false-positive ECG changes with exercise. These include digitalis, diuretic drugs, tricyclic antidepressant drugs, phenothiazines, and lithium.[5] False-positive ECG changes can also be found in the presence of hypokalemia, carbohydrate loading, alkalosis, and hyperventilation.[6] Ischemic responses can be masked by treatment

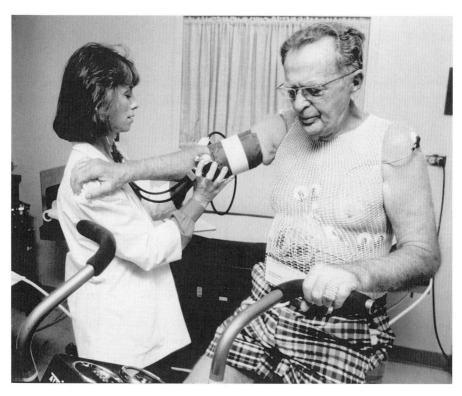

Fig. 14-5. Preparation for bicycle exercise testing. A special net is used to help stabilize the ECG electrodes.

with nitrate drugs, beta-blocking drugs, and calcium channel-blocking drugs.[7,8] Hypertensive heart disease or ventricular hypertrophy of any cause may produce a positive (abnormal) exercise test.[9] The presence of bundle branch block interferes with the interpretation of the standard ECG treadmill test. In the presence of left bundle branch block, the ECG ST segment changes cannot be interpreted. In the presence of right bundle branch block, changes confined to leads V_1, V_2, and V_3 are unreliable, but changes in the lateral or inferior leads are still predictive.[10] False-positive ECG abnormalities occur in patients with abnormal left ventricular depolarization (i.e., Wolff-Parkinson-White syndrome) and repolarization (i.e., resting ST-T wave changes). Finally, valvular heart disease, even in the absence of ventricular hypertrophy, can produce false-positive treadmill exercise tests.

The indications for exercise testing in patients with suspected or known heart disease are (1) to

determine the likelihood of disease, (2) to estimate the prognosis, (3) to determine functional capacity, (4) to evaluate the effects of therapy, and (5) to evaluate symptoms consistent with exercise-induced arrhythmias.

Determination of the Likelihood of Coronary Heart Disease

The problem with using exercise testing to identify patients with CHD is its relatively low sensitivity and specificity. Exercise testing in asymptomatic men results in an average sensitivity of 61% and a specificity of 91%. The test is much less sensitive in women. In patients with CHD, the sensitivity for detecting patients with single-vessel coronary disease is 43%, that for double-vessel disease is 67%, and that for triple-vessel disease is 86%. Another important determinant of the sensitivity and specificity of the test

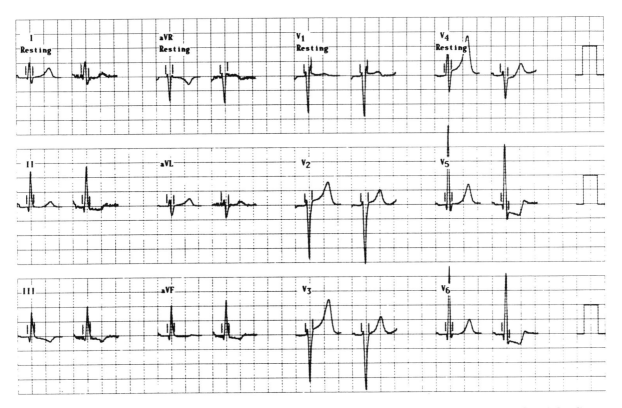

Fig. 14-6. Summary of ECG changes at rest (left of each lead) and at peak exercise (right of each lead). Note the significant downsloping ST segment depression in leads V_5 and V_6 at peak exercise that was not present at rest.

is the criterion for an abnormal test. If 0.2 mV (2 mm) of ST segment depression is necessary before the test is deemed positive (abnormal), the sensitivity decreases but the test is more specific. Yet another determinant of the sensitivity and specificity of the test is the population studied. Exercise testing has a poor sensitivity in populations of patients with a low incidence of disease. ST segment depression is most specific when not only is it marked—i.e., greater than 0.2 mV or 2 mm—but also it appears at low levels of exercise and heart rate and persists for several minutes after cessation of exercise.[11]

The specificity of exercise testing for myocardial ischemia in women is lower than that in men, and exercise testing is not generally recommended as a screening method for CHD in asymptomatic young patients of either sex without known risk factors. The prevalence of false-positive exercise ST segment responses is 4.5

times greater in women than in men.[12] Because of these problems, it is generally agreed that exercise test screening in an apparently healthy individual is indicated only for men over 40 years of age who are in high-risk occupations such as pilots or firemen and for men over 40 years of age who have two or more coronary risk factors, e.g., cholesterol greater than 240 mg/dL, blood pressure of 160/90 mmHg or greater, cigarette smoking, diabetes, relatives under 55 years with known CHD, and men or women under 40 years of age with a family history of premature coronary disease or with severe familial hyperlipoproteinemia; it may be useful for sedentary men over age 40 who plan to enter vigorous exercise programs.

The wisdom of these commonly used indications for treadmill exercise testing was recently questioned.[13] More than 3,600 asymptomatic hypercholesterolemic men (age range, 35 to 59

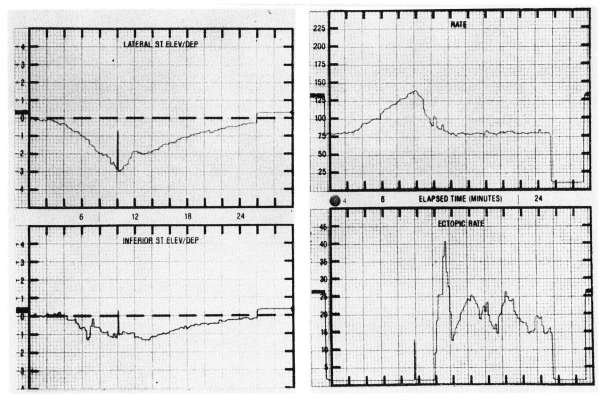

Fig. 14-7. (**Left**): Complete summary of lateral (top) and inferior (bottom) ST segment changes. Vertical line at 10 minutes indicates end of exercise. (**Right**): Heart rate (top) and ectopic rate (bottom). Vertical line at 10 minutes indicates end of exercise.

years) who were monitored in the Lipid Research Clinics Coronary Primary Prevention Trial underwent treadmill exercise testing to 90% of predicted heart rate on entry and yearly thereafter. Although this study suggested that the presence of clinically silent, exercise-induced ST segment changes was associated with an increased risk of activity-related acute coronary events, ST segment changes were not sensitive indicators of the occurrence of activity-related events.[13] For this reason, the authors concluded that the utility of the exercise test to assess the safety of physical activity among asymptomatic men who are at risk of CHD is likely to be limited.[13]

Estimation of Prognosis

The second indication for exercise testing in patients with known or suspected CHD is to determine the prognosis, i.e., to forecast the probable course of disease. This is known as risk stratification (see also Chs. 7, 8, and 11). However, prognostic variables are based on patient populations and provide only guidelines for the individual patient.

The maximal heart rate achieved is one predictor of prognosis. The inability to achieve a high heart rate with exercise while off medications such as beta-blocking drugs is a poor prognostic sign. However, patients with known CHD who achieve a heart rate of 160 beats/min or greater have only a 1 to 2% annual mortality rate.[14,15] The greater the degree of ST segment depression at lower heart rates, the worse the prognosis of the population. In general, ST segment depression of more than 0.2 mV (2 mm) in a patient with a heart rate below 120 beats/min or an exercise capacity below 6.5 METs, together with exercise ST segment depression lasting more than 6 minutes and ST segment depression in multiple leads, indicates a poor prognosis.[12]

The duration of exercise is a major determinant of prognosis.[16]

Low-level exercise testing is useful in the post-myocardial infarction patient to assess the presence of residual myocardial ischemia, to stratify for risk, and to provide guidelines for exercise rehabilitation. Several studies have confirmed the importance of a positive (abnormal) test. A 20 to 25% first-year mortality has been reported in patients with abnormal ST segment responses to low-level predischarge treadmill exercise testing after myocardial infarction.[17] Patients with positive low-level exercise tests postinfarction are candidates for more intensive evaluation and management, i.e., coronary angiography to evaluate for CABG surgery or PTCA. Symptom-limited exercise testing is frequently performed several weeks after myocardial infarction to help determine whether the patient should return to work, to determine the safety of so doing, to determine the effectiveness of therapy, or all of these features.

Determination of Functional Capacity

Another indication for exercise testing in patients with known or suspected CHD is to determine the functional capacity. Information about functional capacity is helpful in the determination of the degree of disability or degree of limitation of exercise capability.

Determination of the Effects of Therapy

In patients with known or suspected CHD, exercise testing is also performed to determine the effect of therapy. Exercise testing is most helpful when performed before and after a therapeutic intervention, such as the initiation of beta-adrenergic blocking therapy, PTCA, or CABG surgery. Exercise-induced hypertension should be reevaluated after antihypertensive therapy is given, to determine its effectiveness.

Evaluation of Arrhythmias

Finally, exercise testing is performed to evaluate exercise-induced symptomatic arrhythmia. Some patients have exercise-induced ventricular arrhythmias, including ventricular tachycardia. Repeated exercise testing is invaluable in determining the effectiveness of antiarrhythmic therapy in these patients.

The frequency or severity of ventricular ectopic beats is not diagnostic of CHD, and the appearance or disappearance of ventricular ectopic beats during exercise is also a nonspecific finding.[18,19]

Decrease in Blood Pressure

A decrease in blood pressure with exercise testing has classically been ascribed to severe CHD. Our recent study (G. Watson, G. Mechling, and G. A. Ewy, personal communication) indicates that three types of decrease in blood pressure with exercise each have different clinical implications. The first type is found in the patient who is anxious about the test and has a slightly higher blood pressure when standing before the test than he or she usually has at rest. As this individual relaxes during the first stage of exercise, blood pressure falls slightly; the patient is asymptomatic, and there are no ECG changes. The blood pressure then increases appropriately with continued exercise. This type of blood pressure response to exercise is a normal variant. The second type of fall in systolic blood pressure with treadmill exercise is characterized by a dramatic fall, i.e., 10 to 20 mmHg, during the first stage of exercise, associated with ST segment depression and symptoms of angina, dyspnea, or severe fatigue. This type of response suggests severe three-vessel or left main coronary artery disease. The third type of exercise-induced hypotension is characterized by an increasing blood pressure during the initial stages of exercise, followed by a fall in systolic blood pressure with continued exercise. In this type, only half of the patients have significant CHD. The others have a variety of etiologies for their exercise-induced hypotension. These nonischemic causes are listed in Table 14-1.

The usefulness of exercise tests, like all diagnostic tests, depends on the sensitivity, specificity, and predictive accuracy of the test. Sensitivity is defined as a true-positive (abnormal) response in a patient with CHD, while specificity is a negative (within normal limits) response in a patient without CHD. The predictive accuracy of a test is dependent not only on the sensitivity and specificity of the test, but also on the prevalence of disease in the population studied. Using ECG criteria, the sensitivity of the exercise test varies from 60 to 70% and the specificity and predictive accuracy from 85 to 90%. Sensitivity for the diagnosis of single-vessel disease ranges from 25 to 50%.

In summary, exercise testing is useful in the diagnosis and risk stratification of CHD. ECG and non-ECG variables are important in the overall interpretation of an exercise test. ECG exercise testing alone is not helpful in certain patients, such as those with left bundle branch block or other baseline ECG abnormalities that preclude accurate interpretation of the ST segment changes. Alternative studies, such as radionuclide-based exercise testing (see Ch. 9) or stress exercise echocardiography (see Ch. 10) may be indicated.

Table 14-1. Causes of Exercise-Induced Hypotension in Patients Without Severe Coronary Heart Disease

Drugs
　　Vasodilators
　　Negative inotropic agents
　　Diuretics
Orthostatic Causes
　　Idiopathic
　　Diabetes mellitus
　　Advanced age
Valvular Heart Disease
　　Aortic stenosis
　　Mitral stenosis
Cardiomyopathy
Miscellaneous
　　Left ventricular aneurysm
　　Sick-sinus syndrome
No Significant Heart Disease

THALLIUM EXERCISE TEST AND OTHER EXERCISE RADIONUCLIDE STUDIES

Exercise radionuclide studies are also discussed in Chapter 9.

Myocardial perfusion studies utilizing thallium-201 in conjunction with exercise testing are also useful techniques to detect myocardial ischemia. Thallium-201 is a metallic element with physiologic characteristics similar to those of potassium. Accordingly, thallium-201 is actively taken up by myocardial cells via the sodium-potassium adenosine triphosphatase (ATPase) pump. The principle of its usefulness is based on the fact that thallium-201 is not taken up by infarcted or ischemic myocardium, but is taken up by normal and nonischemic myocardium. Therefore, ischemic or infarcted myocardium will appear as a filling defect in the radionuclide image of the heart. A filling defect that is present immediately following peak exercise but is not present subsequently at rest denotes an area of ischemia. This phenomenon is referred to as redistribution. A filling defect both at rest and immediately after exercise indicates an area of infarct and is referred to as a fixed defect.

In practice, thallium-201 is injected intravenously near peak exercise, but at least 1 minute before the patient stops exercising. The patient is immediately placed under a large camera that is used for radioactive imaging. In most patients, the thallium will redistribute so that resting images are obtained by reimaging the patient 4 hours after exercise. In patients with very high-grade coronary arterial obstruction, redistribution images have to be taken at 24 hours and additional thallium-201 must be injected with the patient at rest.

Thallium-201 improves the sensitivity and specificity of exercise testing in the detection of CHD, with the best results obtained by using either quantitative planar or single photon emission tomography (SPECT) imaging. At present, SPECT imaging appears to be gaining acceptance as the procedure of choice for thallium exercise imaging. Within the next few years, thallium may be replaced by other agents that have better photon-imaging energy.

The major advantage of thallium imaging is that it can help in evaluating patients for CHD who have ECG abnormalities or cardiac conditions that make the routine treadmill exercise test unreliable (e.g., left ventricular hypertrophy, left bundle branch block, abnormal resting ECG, valvular heart disease, Wolff-Parkinson-White syndrome). The major disadvantage of thallium imaging is the occurrence of false-negative studies in the presence of severe triple-vessel disease. Since a filling defect depends on the difference in the amount of "filling" in one area of the heart compared with another, a diffuse but symmetric decrease in thallium-201 uptake will result in a false-negative test.

Like the routine exercise test, thallium-201 postexercise imaging is useful as a predictor of future coronary events in patients with known or suspected CHD. The number of reversible thallium defects is the best predictor of future coronary events, independent of coronary anatomy. Thallium-201 exercise testing has also been used as a prognostic indicator in predischarge risk stratification after myocardial infarction.

Radionuclide studies of cardiac function are well-accepted techniques for evaluating left and right ventricular ejection fraction and valvular regurgitation and for quantifying left-to-right shunts. Measurements of cardiac output and ventricular volumes can also be obtained with somewhat less accuracy. The measurements are independent of geometric assumptions and can be quite accurate in the presence of segmental cardiac disease. Multigated (MUGA) studies are presently the most reliable noninvasive method of determining the left ventricular ejection fraction, which is the value most commonly used to assess left ventricular systolic function. Relaxation parameters may be used to evaluate left ventricular diastolic dysfunction. The detection of segmental contraction abnormalities is important in the evaluation of patients with CHD. Another advantage of radionuclide studies of left ventricular function is the ability to obtain function measurements during exercise. The exercise ejection fraction is considered an excellent predictor of prognosis in patients with CHD.

CARDIAC CATHETERIZATION AND CORONARY ANGIOGRAPHY

Cardiac catheterization, with coronary angiography, is presently the gold standard for the evaluation of the coronary anatomy in patients with suspected or documented CHD. Specific morphologic abnormalities can be evaluated and the extent of coronary artery disease assessed by selective coronary angiography. The technique of percutaneous, retrograde cardiac catheterization via the femoral arteries, using state-of-the-art equipment, is safe when performed by well-trained and experienced personnel and is widely accepted. Another technique, the Sones technique, involves surgical cutdown over the right brachial artery and retrograde cardiac catheterization.

Minor variability in interpreting the coronary angiograms and in determining the physiologic significance of an anatomic stenosis is a minor shortcoming of the procedure. Variability in interpretation may be due to injection of inadequate amounts of contrast material or to other technical problems that result in inadequate opacification or visualization of the coronary vessel, an inadequate number of different projections, superselective injections, coronary spasm, or total occlusions. Some centers have suggested that the final cardiac catheterization report include the consensus of at least two angiographers.

Currently, only lesions obstructing more than 50% of the luminal diameter (75% of the cross-sectional area) are considered hemodynamically significant. This has been challenged by some investigators. Harrison et al.[20] concluded that the physiologic significance of some coronary obstructions cannot be determined by visual estimates of coronary artery stenosis and that computer-guided edge detection techniques are needed. Nevertheless, most clinical decisions are based on visual interpretation of the coronary angiograms.

Autopsy studies have also shown that clinical coronary angiograms tend to underestimate the severity of coronary lesions (see Ch. 2). This is because many patients have diffuse coronary atherosclerosis with one or more lesions superim-

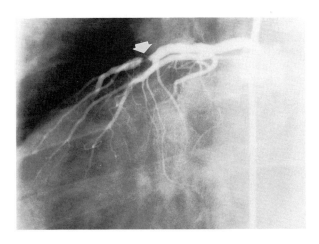

Fig. 14-8. Coronary artery stenosis (arrow).

posed. The availability of intravascular ultrasonography for intracoronary imaging may help solve this problem.

The prognosis of patients with CHD can be stratified on the basis of their coronary anatomy and ventricular function. Patients with left main coronary artery disease have a very poor prognosis. Prior to the advent of beta-adrenergic blocking drugs and other currently used forms of therapy, the 5-year survival rate of patients with single-, double-, and triple-vessel coronary artery disease was 60, 40, and 20%, respectively.[21]

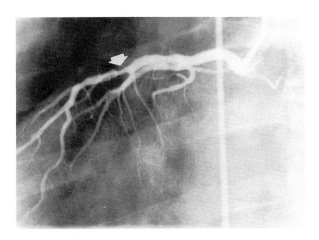

Fig. 14-9. Same coronary artery as in Figure 14-8 after successful percutaneous transluminal coronary angioplasty (PTCA).

Within each subcategory of coronary artery disease, the prognosis is worse when it is associated with poor ventricular function. CABG surgery or PTCA and medical therapy may improve prognosis (Figs. 14-8 and 14-9).

The majority of patients referred to the cardiac catheterization laboratory are referred to determine the presence and/or severity of coronary arterial disease.

RESTING ECHOCARDIOGRAPHY

Resting echocardiography is also discussed in Chapter 10.

Echocardiography (Fig. 14-10) is an examination technique that provides images of the anatomy, structural abnormalities, and blood flow of the heart and great vessels by ultrasonography.[21] Although ultrasonography may be applied in different forms (M-mode, two-dimensional [2D], spectral, and color-flow Doppler imaging) and by different techniques (transthoracic and transesophageal), all forms and techniques are encompassed by the term "echocardiography".[22] When applied by the transthoracic approach, the examination involves little patient discomfort and has not been associated with risk to the patient. The ability of echocardiography to provide unique information regarding cardiac structure and function, its lack of ionizing radiation, the portability of the instrument, and the potential for repeated studies has led to its widespread use for virtually all categories of known and suspected cardiovascular disease.[22]

In the patient with CHD, echocardiography can assess overall ventricular function or segmental ventricular wall motion abnormalities. Additional information can be obtained by two-dimensional echo-Doppler studies during or immediately after exercise testing (see Ch. 10). Laboratory and clinical studies confirm the ability of echocardiography to qualitate and detect regional myocardial ischemia. With normal systolic function, there is thickening of the ventricular wall. In the presence of ischemia, there may be lack of wall thickening, no change, or even wall thinning. Each identified ventricular segment is as-

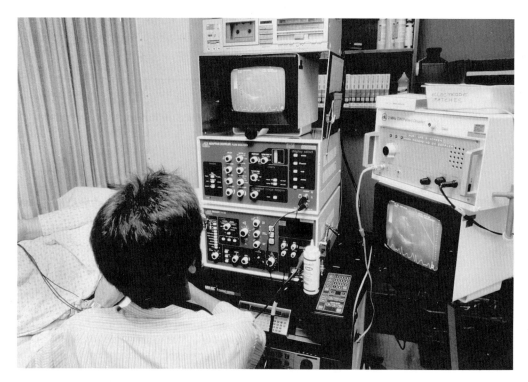

Fig. 14-10. Technician performing an echocardiogram.

sessed for its systolic wall thickening (normal, none, or decreased) and for the type of systolic wall motion (normal, hyperkinetic, hypokinetic, or dyskinetic). Despite recent advances in technology and resolution, errors in assessment are most commonly due to inadequate visualization of the segment of interest as a result of technical problems. For example, it is difficult to determine ventricular function in a patient with hyperexpanded lung fields by the transthoracic approach.

Echocardiography is not only a useful diagnostic technique for the assessment of complications of CHD, but it is also useful in the diagnosis and assessment of the complications of acute myocardial infarction. Echo-Doppler techniques can detect left ventricular aneurysm, ventricular thrombi, pericardial effusion, papillary muscle dysfunction, rupture of the interventricular septum, and mitral regurgitation. The detection of mural thrombi depends on the size and location of the thrombi. Echocardiography for detecting intracardiac thrombi has been confirmed

by numerous studies to be superior to left ventriculography.

Echocardiography is used in conjunction with exercise testing to detect myocardial ischemia, i.e., to detect areas of the myocardium at risk. Ventricular wall motion abnormalities are early markers of myocardial ischemia. These abnormalities may be detected by echocardiography. Although exercise electrocardiography remains the standard for determining myocardial ischemia with exercise, some studies have shown that regional wall motion abnormalities occur at a lower ischemic threshold than ST segment changes do. Echocardiography may allow better spatial resolution than other imaging techniques for determining wall thickness. Accordingly, an increasing number of centers use exercise echocardiography in patients with suspected or known CHD. Because of the inability of some patients to exercise, pharmacologic echocardiographic stress, such as dobutamine or persantine infusion, has also been used.

AMBULATORY ECG (HOLTER) RECORDING

The indications for ambulatory ECG recording in patients are threefold: evaluating arrhythmias, assessing the responses of arrhythmias to antiarrhythmic therapy, and monitoring the ST segment for the detection of myocardial ischemia.

Because of the sporadic occurrence of most arrhythmias, prolonged recording is required for their detection and quantification. The development of a portable monitoring system by Holter in 1961 made ambulatory ECG recording feasible. Ventricular arrhythmias are present in many patients with CHD. In many studies in which the presence of CHD was documented by the history of a previous myocardial infarction, 24-hour ambulatory ECG recording has shown ventricular ectopy in 61 to 96% of patients after a myocardial infarction.[23–28] Since there is an association between the presence and severity of ventricular arrhythmias after myocardial infarction (or other heart disease) and the occurrence of sudden cardiac death, studies have attempted to evaluate the effectiveness of antiarrhythmic therapy in these patients.

The most important of these studies is the Cardiac Arrhythmia Suppression Trial (CAST).[29] CAST was designed to test the hypothesis that suppression of asymptomatic complex ventricular arrhythmias after myocardial infarction would decrease subsequent mortality.[29] The quite unexpected results showed that patients treated with the antiarrhythmic drugs encainide or flecainide had a higher incidence of sudden death, even though the drugs were effective in decreasing the frequency of ventricular arrhythmias as judged by 24-hour ambulatory ECG.

Ambulatory ECG is useful to document the presence and type of paroxysmal arrhythmia if the patient's palpitations, or other symptoms thought to be related to arrhythmia, occur with a reasonable frequency. If the problem occurs less frequently, e.g., every week or so, use of an ECG event recorder may be more appropriate than repeating 24-hour ECG recordings for several days. ECG event recorders continuously record and erase the patient's ECG on magnetic tape. When palpitations or other symptoms occur, the event recorder is activated by the patient to store and save a variable amount of the ECG rhythm strip.

Some commercial ambulatory ECG units and analyzers are altered to meet diagnostic specifications and to accurately record ST segments. These units are used not only to detect arrhythmias, but also to monitor ST segment changes. ST segment monitoring can be used to detect the presence and frequency of ST segment changes associated with symptomatic (angina) or asymptomatic (silent) ischemia.

SIGNAL-AVERAGED ECG

A signal-averaged electrocardiogram (SAECG) is a computer-processed and -averaged, high-resolution ECG that differs from the conventional ECG by its ability to record low-amplitude signals from the heart. These low-amplitude signals, arising after ventricular depolarization (activation), are called late potentials. Late potentials are derived from areas of slow conduction in the ventricular muscle. These areas of slow conduction serve as substrates for reentrant ventricular tachyarrhythmias.[30] Experimental and clinical evidence suggests that late potentials arise from abnormal myocardium.

A conventional surface ECG records a QRS complex that reflects the net electrical activity arising from depolarization of the ventricular myocardium. It is not sensitive enough to record after-repolarization potentials. In the past, late potentials could be recorded only via intracardiac catheter electrodes. Recent technological advances have allowed the surface recording of low-amplitude late potentials. This method, SAECG, refers to a computerized processing technique that measures signals in the microvolt amplitude range while simultaneously minimizing and removing extraneous noise signals by signal averaging. Several hundred QRS complexes are filtered, amplified, and digitized to produce a high-resolution signal with an improved signal-to-noise ratio. The signal-averaged QRS complex is then filtered, removing the ultra-low-frequency signals of the ST segment and T wave. The fre-

Table 14-2.   Criteria for SAECG Analysis[a]

1. QRS duration on 12-lead ECG less than 110 msec. An SAECG is considered abnormal if one or more of the following conditions exists:
   QRS is greater than 120 msec
   RMS 40 is less than 20 μV
   LAS 40 is greater than 38 msec

2. QRS duration on 12-lead ECG greater than 110 msec (IVCD/BBB); a signal-averaged ECG is considered abnormal if RMS 40 is less than 10 μV

3. A study is nondiagnostic if the RMS 40 is greater than or equal to 10 μV

[a] Abbreviations: RMS, root mean square; LAS, low amplitude signals.

quency of high-pass filtering determines the normal values used in a laboratory.

The SAECG is obtained by attaching electrodes to the patient to obtain an orthogonal x, y, and z lead set. The electrodes are attached to the right and left midaxillary lines at the fourth intercostal space (x axis), the left subclavicular and lower thoracic areas (y axis), and the intercostal spaces anteriorly and posteriorly (z axis). A reference electrode is placed on the eighth rib, at the right midaxillary line.

A commercial SAECG unit records and processes approximately 200 beats of QRS complexes derived from each of the three leads by using vector analysis. A computerized algorithm retrogradely scans the ST segment. A 5-msec segment yielding a root mean square voltage greater than 2.5 times the noise level represents the end of the QRS complex. The following parameters are measured: (1) the root mean square (RMS) voltage of the final 40 msec of the QRS complex, (2) the duration of low amplitude signals (LAS) of less than 40 μV, and (3) the duration of the entire SAECG complex. The criteria for a positive SAECG at the University of Arizona are shown in Table 14-2.

At present the clinical utility of the SAECG has not been clearly defined. Potential applications include the risk stratification of postinfarction patients, the prediction of inducible (by electrophysiologic testing) ventricular tachycardia in patients with nonsustained ventricular tachycardia, and the evaluation of selected patients with syncope of undetermined origin.

Sudden cardiac death occurs in 10 to 12% of patients after myocardial infarction. Patients at high risk include those with residual high-grade blockage of the coronary arteries, poor ventricular function, and a substrate for ventricular arrhythmias. As noted above, current noninvasive methods for risk stratification include the use of exercise testing to determine myocardium at risk, radionuclide ventriculography or echocardiography to determine ventricular function, and ambulatory ECG monitoring to determine the presence or absence of ventricular arrhythmias. Studies have explored the use of the SAECG to enhance the ability to detect the presence or absence of areas of slow conduction, i.e., the substrate for lethal arrhythmias. Gomes et al.[31,32] prospectively observed 102 patients after myocardial infarction and showed that SAECG was an independent predictor of arrhythmic events. The event rate was 50% in patients with an abnormal SAECG, an ejection fraction of less than 40%, and an abnormal 24-hour ECG recording (more than

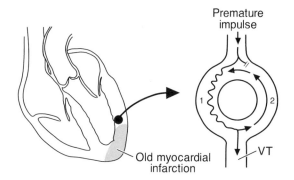

Fig. 14-11. Conditions of reentrant ventricular tachycardia. The availability of two pathways with a final common route of impulse conduction is the substrate for reentrant tachycardia. These conditions are most often present in the peri-infarction area. The two pathways must possess different properties of conduction and refractoriness. The difference in refractoriness allows for critically timed premature impulses to be blocked in one pathway but conducted down the other. If conduction proceeds sufficiently slowly through the unblocked pathway, not only does it depolarize the ventricle but, if the previously blocked pathway is no longer refractory, the impulse also conducts retrograde in the previously blocked pathway, initiating an echo beat or a reentrant tachycardia.

10 premature ventricular contractions per hour, couplets or triplets). Denniss et al.[33] showed that the presence of late potentials in patients after myocardial infarction was associated with inducibility (by invasive electrophysiologic studies) of sustained ventricular tachycardia in the electrophysiologic laboratory. Therefore, preliminary studies suggest that SAECG has potential utility as a noninvasive technique to improve the risk stratification of patients after myocardial infarction.

SAECG also promises to be of use in the diagnosis of syncope of undetermined origin. Patients with CHD may present with unexplained syncope. In some patients a diagnosis cannot be made despite extensive noninvasive studies (ambulatory ECG monitoring, electroencephalography, and echocardiography). Invasive electrophysiologic studies have induced sustained ventricular tachycardia in 30 to 40% of these pa-tients. The SAECG has been reported to predict the inducibility of sustained ventricular tachycardia. The long-term clinical implications of this finding are not known. However, if confirmed, SAECG may become an important noninvasive technique to help predict which subgroup of patients are at high risk for the development of potentially malignant arrhythmias after myocardial infarction and may accordingly identify those who should undergo electrophysiologic testing.

ELECTROPHYSIOLOGIC STUDIES

Most ventricular arrhythmias, particularly ventricular tachycardia, are due to reentry of the depolarizing impulse through an area of slowed conduction in the ventricle (Fig. 14-11). These areas of slowed conduction are almost invariably

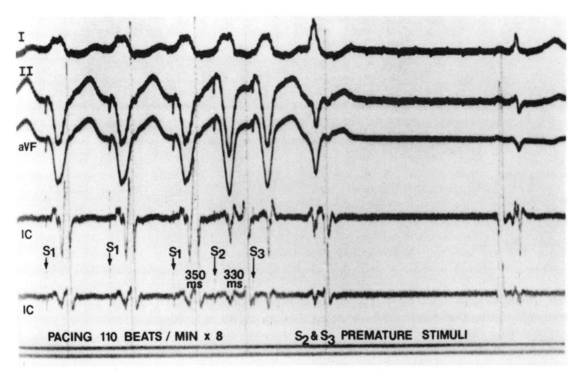

Fig. 14-12. Simultaneous frontal plane leads I, II, and aVF, and two intracardiac leads (1C). Ventricular pacing stimuli (S1 arrows) at a cycle length (S1 to S1) of 545 msec, followed by two premature stimuli at 350 msec (S2) and 330 msec (S3). The programmed stimulation is followed by a single ventricular ectopic depolarization and then resumption of sinus rhythm.

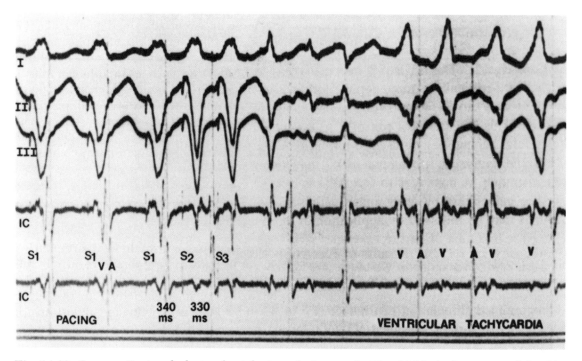

Fig. 14-13. Same patient and electrophysiologic technique as in Fig. 14-12. A shortening of the S1–S2 interval by 10 msec results in the induction of ventricular tachycardia. The intracardiac leads (1C) show 1:1 retrograde conduction from the ventricle (V) to the atrium (A).

located in the peri-infarction area. Therefore, ventricular arrhythmias are a common complication of CHD.

A clinical electrophysiologic study (EPS) is commonly performed in patients with symptomatic ventricular tachycardia and in patients with asymptomatic ventricular tachycardia associated with poor ventricular function. EPS may be performed to confirm the diagnosis of ventricular tachycardia, but most often is used to guide therapy. The electrode tip of the catheter(s) is placed in different sites within the right ventricle and at times within both ventricles. The heart is paced at a fixed rate (but above the intrinsic rate) for about eight beats, and then one to four premature stimuli are introduced. The premature stimuli are initially delivered late in diastole. The coupling interval between the last paced beat and the premature stimulus is progressively decreased until refractoriness is reached or an arrhythmia results

(Figs. 14-12 and 14-13). If a single premature stimulus fails to elicit the arrhythmia, additional premature stimuli are used.

If sustained monomorphic ventricular tachycardia is produced, the patient is said to be "inducible."[37] The patient is then given an antiarrhythmic drug, and the procedure is repeated. Only one antiarrhythmic drug is given per invasive EPS unless combination drug therapy is being tested. When groups of patients with symptomatic ventricular tachycardia are studied, those discharged on antiarrhythmic therapy that rendered them noninducible have a better prognosis than patients in whom a reasonable number of antiarrhythmic drugs were tried, all of which failed to prevent induction of sustained ventricular tachycardia during EPS. In fact, the latter group have such a poor prognosis that they are considered candidates for implantation of an automatic implantable cardioverter defibrillator.

SUMMARY

Diagnostic procedures, both invasive and non-invasive, help in the recognition and management of patients with CHD. Those engaged in coronary rehabilitation should be familiar with the indications for, value of, and limitations of such procedures.

REFERENCES

1. Devereux RB, Alonso DR, Latas EM et al: Sensitivity of echocardiography for detection of left ventricular hypertrophy. p. 16. In ter Keurs HEDJ, Schipperheyn JJ (eds): Cardiac Left Ventricular Hypertrophy. Martinus Nijhoff, Boston, 1983
2. Chaitman BR, Bourassa MG, Wagniart P et al: Improved efficiency of treadmill exercise testing using a multiple lead ECG system and basic hemodynamic exercise response. Circulation 57:71, 1978
3. Dagenais GR, Rouleau JR, Christen A et al: Survival of patients with a strongly positive electrocardiogram. Circulation 65:452, 1982
4. Cole JP, Ellestad MH: Significance of chest pain during treadmill exercise: Correlation with coronary events. Am J Cardiol 41:227, 1978
5. Dhingra RC, Wyndham C, Amat-Y-Leon F et al: Significance of A–H interval in patients with chronic bundle branch block: Clinical, electrophysiologic and follow-up observations. Am J Cardiol 37:231, 1976
6. Riley CP, Oberman A, Sheffield LT: Electrocardiographic effects of glucose ingestion. Arch Intern Med 130:703, 1972
7. Mukharji J, Kremers M, Lipscomb K et al: Early positive exercise test and extensive coronary disease: Effect of antianginal therapy. Am J Cardiol 55:267, 1985
8. Ho SWC, McComish MJ, Taylor RR: Effect of beta-adrenergic blockade on the results of exercise testing related to the extent of coronary artery disease. Am J Cardiol 55:258, 1985
9. Wroblewski EM, Pearl FJ, Hammer WJ et al: False positive stress tests due to undetected left ventricular hypertrophy. Am J Epidemiol 115:412, 1982
10. Tanaka T, Friedman MJ, Okada RD et al: Diagnostic value of exercise-induced ST-segment depression in patients with right bundle branch block. Am J Cardiol 41:670, 1978
11. Weiner DA, McCabe CH, Ryan TJ: Identification of patients with left main and three vessel coronary disease with clinical and exercise test variables. Am J Cardiol 46:21, 1980
12. Weiner DA, Ryan TJ, McCabe CH et al: Exercise stress testing: correlations among history of angina, ST-segment response and prevalence of coronary-artery disease in the coronary artery surgery study (CASS). N Engl J Med 301:230, 1979
13. Siscovick DS, Ekelund LG, Johnson JL et al: Sensitivity of exercise electrocardiography for acute cardiac events during moderate and strenuous physical activity. Arch Intern Med 151:325, 1991
14. Podrid PJ, Graboys TB, Lown B: Prognosis of medically treated patients with coronary artery disease with profound ST-segment depression during exercise testing. N Engl J Med 305:1111, 1981
15. McNeer JF, Margolis JR, Lee KL et al: The role of exercise in the evaluation of patients for ischemic heart disease. Circulation 57:64, 1978
16. Gohlke H, Samek, Betz P et al: Exercising testing provides additional prognostic information in angiographically defined subgroups of patients with coronary artery disease. Circulation 68:979, 1983
17. Theroux P, Waters DD, Halphen C et al: Prognostic value of exercise testing soon after myocardial infarction. N Engl J Med 301:341, 1979
18. Califf RM, McKinnis RA, McNeer JF et al: Prognostic value of ventricular arrhythmias associated with treadmill exercise testing in patients studied with cardiac catheterization for suspected ischemic heart disease. J Am Coll Cardiol 2:1060, 1983
19. McHenry PL, Morris SN, Kavalier M et al: Comparative study of exercise-induced ventricular arrhythmias in normal subjects and patients with documented coronary artery disease. Am J Cardiol 37:609, 1976
20. Harrison DG, White CW, Hiratzka LH et al: The value of lesion cross-sectional area determined by quantitative coronary angiography in assessing the physiologic significance of proximal left anterior descending coronary artery stenosis. Circulation 69:1111, 1984
21. Proudfit WL, Bruschke AVG, Sones FM: Natural history of obstructional coronary artery disease: 10 year study of 601 nonsurgical cases. Prog Cardiovasc Dis 21:53, 1978
22. Ewy GA, Appleton CP, DeMaria AN et al: ACC/AHA guidelines for the clinical application of echocardiography. Circulation 82:2323, 1990

23. Ruberman W, Weinblatt E, Goldberg JD et al: Ventricular premature beats and mortality after myocardial infarction. N Engl J Med 297:750, 1977

24. Califf RM, Burks JM, Behar VS et al: Relationships among ventricular arrhythmias, coronary artery disease, and angiographic and electrocardiographic indicators of myocardial fibrosis. Circulation 57:725, 1978

25. De Soyza N, Bennett FA, Murphy ML et al: The relationship of paroxysmal ventricular tachycardia complicating the acute phase and ventricular arrhythmia during the late hospital phase of myocardial infarction to long-term survival. Am J Med 64:377, 1978

26. Rehnqvist N, Lundman T, Sjorgren A: Prognostic implications of ventricular arrhythmias registered before discharge and one year after acute myocardial infarction. Acta Med Scand 204:203, 1978

27. Schulze RA, Strauss HW, Pitt B: Sudden death in the year following myocardial infarction: Relation to ventricular premature contractions in the late hospital phase and left ventricular ejection fraction. Am J Med 62:192, 1977

28. Olson HG, Lyons KP, Troop P et al: Prognostic implications of complicated ventricular arrhythmias early after hospital discharge in acute myocardial infarction: A serial ambulatory electrocardiography study. Am Heart J 108:1221, 1984

29. The Cardiac Arrhythmia Suppression Trial (CAST) Investigators: Preliminary report. Effect of encainide and flecainide on mortality in a randomized trial of arrhythmia suppression after myocardial infarction. N Engl J Med 321:406, 1989

30. Josephson ME, Horowitz LN, Farshidi A: Continuous local electrical activity. A mechanism of recurrent ventricular tachycardia. Circulation 57:659, 1978

31. Gomes JAC, Mehra R, Barreca P et al: Quantitative analysis of the high frequency components of the signal averaged QRS complex in patients with acute myocardial infarction: A prospective study. Circulation 72:105, 1985

32. Gomes JA, Winters SL, Martinson M et al: The prognostic significance of quantitative signal-averaged variable relative to clinical variables, site of myocardial infarction, ejection fraction and ventricular premature beats: A prospective study. J Am Coll Cardiol 13:377, 1978

33. Denniss AR, Richards DA, Cody DV et al: Prognostic significance of ventricular tachycardia and fibrillation induced at programmed stimulation and delayed potentials detected on the signal averaged electrocardiograms of survivors of acute myocardial infarction. Circulation 74:731, 1986

34. Mason JW, Winkle RA: Electrode-catheter arrhythmia induction in the selection and assessment of antiarrhythmic drug therapy for recurrent ventricular tachycardia. Circulation 58:971, 1978

35. Horowitz LN, Josephson ME, Farshidi A et al: Recurrent sustained ventricular tachycardia. 3. Role of the electrophysiologic study in the selection of antiarrhythmic regimens. Circulation 58:986, 1978

36. Swerdlow CD, Winkle RA, Mason JW: Determinants of survival in patients with ventricular tachyarrhythmia. N Engl J Med 308:1436, 1983

37. Rae AP, Kay HR, Horowitz LN et al: Proarrhythmic effects of antiarrhythmic drugs in patients with malignant ventricular arrhythmias evaluated by electrophysiologic testing. J Am Coll Cardiol 12:131, 1988

15

Imaging Techniques: Radionuclide Testing, PET, MRI

Byron R. Williams, Jr., M.D.

Coronary heart disease (CHD) remains a leading cause of death in the United States. Despite tremendous technologic advances, the ability to detect CHD remains a challenge to the clinician. Symptoms alone, or in combination with coronary risk factor analysis, are not adequate to detect CHD in most patients. Most patients are asymptomatic; over one-half of individuals with acute myocardial infarction or sudden cardiac death have reported no prior symptoms.[1-3] Advanced CHD is typically seen when such patients are studied by coronary angiography or at autopsy. Silent myocardial ischemic episodes appear to be more common than painful events. Asymptomatic individuals may have a less favorable prognosis when silent ischemia is present as opposed to asymptomatic individuals without evidence of silent myocardial ischemia.[4] The absence of symptoms does not assure a favorable outcome in CHD. Prognosis in individuals with CHD appears related to several factors including left ventricular function, number of coronary arteries involved, ventricular arrhythmias, and severity of ischemia. Non-invasive tests that accurately document the presence of CHD, the number of vessels involved, and, perhaps more importantly, the physiologic significance of anatomic disease could be extremely helpful in managing patients with CHD. Contemporary surgical and non-surgical techniques can restore normal or improved coronary bloodflow to previously ischemic myocardium. If we assume that most premature deaths from CHD are due to ischemic-related events (i.e., acute myocardial infarction, chronic left ventricular dysfunction, ventricular arrhythmias), the prevention or reduction of ischemic episodes might favorably influence prognosis. Efforts to accomplish this will be multifactorial but will mandate accurate assessment of myocardial ischemia and the benefits of interventions such as PTCA, CABG, and dietary or drug therapies. Ideally, this would be done with non-invasive test procedures.

THE USE OF RADIOACTIVE TRACERS FOR CARDIAC IMAGING AT REST

Nuclear cardiology has been characterized by rapid growth over the last 15 years. The primary indications for cardiac imaging at rest are (1) assessment of ventricular function, (2) intra-cardiac shunt detection, and (3) evaluation for myocardial infarction.

Although other modalities such as echocardiography (see Ch. 14), magnetic resonance imaging (MRI), and fast computed tomography can be used to assess ventricular function, radionuclide imaging remains an important technique for the non-invasive evaluation of ventricular performance. Two types of radionuclide studies are used for this purpose, the gated equilibrium study (MUGA scan) and first-pass radionuclide angiography. These techniques differ in methodology but provide similar information. In the former, red blood cells are labeled with technetium, allowing a radioactive "blood pool" for approximately 4 to 6 hours after intravenous injection of the radioactive tracer. By employing ECG gating and sophisticated computer techniques, this scan can image the patient in multiple projections. Each image is actually a summation of 150 to 300 cardiac cycles that can be played back in a continuous loop. The radioactivity counts in the ventricle are analyzed at end diastole and end systole, enabling the determination of ejection fraction and ventricular volumes. These studies compare favorably with the ejection fraction as determined at cardiac catheterization. Both visual and quantitative assessment of regional wall motion is possible with the gated blood pool technique, which is probably more accurate than the first-pass technique for this purpose. First-pass nuclear angiography involves a bolus injection of a radioactive tracer (usually technetium); it enables temporal separation of activity between right ventricle and left ventricle. This technique requires a very high count rate capability from the nuclear camera, but provides a very accurate measure of the ejection fraction. The first-pass technique probably assesses right ventricular function more reliably than the MUGA study.

Intracardiac shunts (as with septal rupture in myocardial infarction) can be identified and accurately quantitated by the first-pass technique. However, echocardiography with color flow Doppler has replaced radionuclide imaging as the non-invasive test of choice in assessing shunt lesions.

Valvular regurgitation can be assessed only indirectly by radionuclide angiography. The estimation of ventricular volume and regurgitant fraction are helpful measures for evaluating patients with regurgitant valvular lesions. In CHD, this is primarily either papillary muscle rupture secondary to acute myocardial infarction or chronic mitral regurgitation due to chronic papillary muscle dysfunction. However, again, color flow Doppler echocardiography has replaced radionuclide imaging for the non-invasive evaluation of this problem.

The clinical uses for MUGA studies remain important in the prognostic assessment following myocardial infarction and in evaluating for ventricular aneurysm in the patient with CHD and congestive heart failure.

Infarct imaging with radioactive tracers is primarily of historic interest. The technetium pyrophosphate ("hot pyp") scans are sensitive detectors of myocardial necrosis. The pyrophosphate binds to macromolecules in the infarct zone, but this requires some residual blood flow (approximately 40% of normal) into the infarcted region. These scans become positive approximately 24 to 48 hours after infarction and remain positive for approximately 7 days. By the time these scans become positive, most patients have ECG changes and enzymatic evidence of acute myocardial infarction, so that the occasional patient who is hospitalized 3 to 7 days after a presumed coronary event, whose ECG is nondiagnostic, may benefit from an avid infarct scan such as technetium pyrophosphate. In general, avid infarct imaging has limited value in clinical practice today.

Rest imaging with thallium as well as with the new technetium perfusion agents (Tc-99m Sestamibi and Tc-99m Teboroxime) is very sensitive in detecting acute myocardial infarction. When imaged as early as 6 to 12 hours into infarction, thallium images are very sensitive in detecting a perfusion defect or "cold spot"—approaching 100% accuracy in some studies. However, the logistics and expense of accomplishing this limit its usefulness.

There may be a role for Tc-99m Sestamibi imaging in patients receiving thrombolytic therapy. Because this agent does not redistribute, it can be injected in the emergency room before thrombolytic therapy is given, and the patient can be imaged later in the coronary care unit. The image obtained defines the zone of myocardium at risk for infarction when the patient presented. A follow-up study several days later may allow detection of salvaged myocardium. More clinical trials are needed to determine how practical and useful this imaging strategy will be.

Radionuclide-based ventricular function studies and myocardial perfusion studies with exercise are discussed in Chapter 9.

POSITRON EMISSION TOMOGRAPHY

The role for positron emission tomography (PET) imaging is evolving, without clear consensus by the "experts" at this time. However, clinical PET studies are being performed in about 57 medical centers in the United States and about 126 centers worldwide. The two major categories of use for clinical cardiac PET studies are (1) evaluation of myocardial perfusion, primarily for the detection of CHD and physiologic assessment of patients with known CHD, and (2) assessment of myocardial viability.

PET is a three-dimensional tomographic imaging modality that employs radioactive tracers to evaluate biochemical events and tissue perfusion. PET uses positron emitting isotopes such as oxygen-15-labeled water, rubidium-82, carbon-11, nitrogen-13-labeled ammonia, and fluorine-18-labeled deoxyglucose (FDG) for these purposes.

Clinical interest in PET has increased since the 1950s, when early research at Brookhaven National Laboratory and the University of California at Berkeley determined that positron radiopharmaceuticals could be used for medical purposes. PET pioneers at Washington University in St. Louis performed clinical tomographic imaging with positron emitting isotopes in the 1970s. Although PET can provide valuable clinical information, the expense of the equipment and the need for an on-site cyclotron had relegated the technique to research institutions. Several factors are responsible for the recent emergence of PET as a clinical technique: (1) increased medical interest in biochemical imaging, (2) improvements in PET cameras resulting in dramatic improvement in resolution and image presentation, and (3) emergence of the rubidium-82 generator that provides cardiac PET with an agent that can be used as an alternative flow tracer and does not require an on-site cyclotron. PET can provide a quantitative, high-resolution, three-dimensional image of myocardial perfusion that surpasses information obtained from conventional gamma cameras.

Sensitivity and Specificity

Current non-invasive diagnostic techniques have limitations. The sensitivity and specificity of exercise treadmill testing and exercise thallium imaging are approximately 75%/80% and 85%/90%, respectively, in symptomatic populations with CHD. These tests are of less diagnostic value in asymptomatic populations, where their diagnostic accuracy drops to much lower levels. The sensitivity of PET for diagnosing CHD approximates 90 to 95%, and its specificity is similarly high, even in asymptomatic individuals. Table 15-1 compares more than 700 patients with suspected CHD who had PET studies and coronary angiograms.[5–13] Even with single photon emission computed tomography (SPECT) thallium studies, sensitivities range from 85 to 95%; specificity is in the 75 to 85% range compared with a much higher specificity for PET imaging. The low-energy photons produced by thallium or technetium in the myocardium or cardiac blood-pool are subject to tissue attentuation. Tissue attenuation is one of the main limitations of single photon emission scans. In contrast, when a positron emitter decays, two high-energy photons are produced simultaneously through an annihilation reaction between the positron and a nearby

Table 15-1. Detection of CHD with PET

Study	No. of Patients	Sensitivity/Specificity (%)
Schelbert et al. (UCLA)[5–6]	32	97/100
Tamaki et al. (Tokyo)[7]	32	95/100
Gould et al. (Univ. of Texas–Houston)[8–9] plus personal communication	400	95/98
Yonekura et al. (Tokyo)[10]	49	97/100
Williams et al. (Atlanta)[11]	208	96/95
Go R et al. (Cleveland Clinic)[12]	202	95/82
Stewart et al. (Univ. of Michigan)[13]	60	88/90
TOTALS (Average)	983	95/94

orbital electron. These travel away from each other at approximately 180° from the site of annihilation. Each photon has approximately six times the energy of a single thallium photon. Because of this high energy, tissue attenuation losses are substantially less with PET imaging than with single photon imaging. Furthermore, a transmission image can be constructed with PET imaging by using an external positron source placed in a ring around the patient, producing a map of tissue densities of the patient's chest cavity. This image can be used to correct the final image for attenuation losses. No such attenuation correction can be performed with single photon emission studies, including SPECT imaging.

In addition, PET has the potential for metabolic imaging of the heart. Various positron emitters, including flourine-18 and carbon-11, produced in a cyclotron, can be incorporated into organic molecules to study myocardial metabolism. Flourine-18 (FDG) studies appear to be the most accurate method currently available for assessing viable myocardium. Brunken et al. reported that PET revealed residual metabolic activity in 68% of ECG-determined Q-wave myocardial regions.[14] This confirmed earlier investigations that had questioned the specificity of ECG Q-waves as indicators of transmural myocardial infarction. Several authors have demonstrated a significant advantage of PET for identifying viable myocardium compared to SPECT thallium imaging.[15,16] Based on both animal studies and clinical investigation, PET appears to be most useful for identifying both acutely infarcted myocardial regions and chronic myocardial ischemia. PET is likely, therefore, to be of great value in helping decide whether acutely damaged myocardium can be salvaged and will likely influence the management of patients immediately following myocardial infarction, especially those who have received thrombolytic therapy. PET represents significant progress in the evolution of nuclear cardiac imaging, having the ability to measure myocardial perfusion and cellular viability non-invasively and quantitatively, with a high degree of accuracy. The next decade holds great promise for advances in the clinical application of PET.

COMPUTED TOMOGRAPHY

Fast computed tomography (cine-CT) provides real time images with tomographic display in a closed-loop cine format. This is not truly a non-invasive imaging technique, since iodinizing radiation is used, with the blood pool identified by the intravenous injection of iodinated contrast medium.

Many uses for fast cine-CT have been identified; however, there is much overlap between this technique and other non-invasive modalities. The most valuable and perhaps unique indications for fast cine-CT of the heart are

1. Evaluation of coronary artery bypass graft patency: This has a 90% diagnostic accuracy but cannot define the severity of stenosis when present or adequately assess coronary flow physiologically.[17]
2. Evaluation for the complications of myocardial infarction:
   (a) thrombus formation
   (b) aneurysm formation
   (c) ventricular function.
3. Analysis of left ventricular function. Since cine-CT is a three-dimensional imaging modality, precise measurement of left and right ventricular volumes is possible. This is in contrast to the estimated volumes at cardiac catheterization, using assumed geometric models in a two-dimensional system.[18]

The use of fast cine-CT is limited in the evaluation of CHD primarily because competing techniques may be equally accurate and less invasive (e.g., echocardiography, magnetic resonance imaging, and nuclear imaging).

MAGNETIC RESONANCE IMAGING

Magnetic resonance imaging (MRI) is a non-invasive diagnostic technique with demonstrated usefulness in many cardiovascular diagnostic problems.[19] The subject being imaged is placed in the center of a higher field magnet and the sensitive nuclei respond by reorienting themselves. Radiowaves are then generated and excite or perturb the magnetized nuclei. This causes the nuclei to rotate in a different direction than their initial alignment direction in the field. Once the radio frequency is turned off, the stored energy due to displacement of the nuclei is released, as those nuclei return to their original positions. The radiowaves emit energy that identifies the type of nucleus present. Thus, images are based upon the radiofrequency signal emitted by hydrogen nuclei of tissues in the presence of a strong magnetic field. There is generally a high contrast between blood and myocardial or vessel wall, since the blood pool is a signal void. The cardiac images generated can be viewed as static or dynamic.

Although MRI can be quite useful in pediatric heart disease,[20] the primary uses in adults with heart disease appear to be related to CHD with its complications and to valvular heart disease. The current uses of MRI in CHD are to demonstrate the complications of acute myocardial infarction, such as thrombus or aneurysm formation.[21-22] There is hope that the use of MRI in CHD will be expanded to demonstrating myocardial viability, regional perfusion (with the use of magnetic resonance contrast media) and patency of coronary bypass grafts. The use of contrast agents to evaluate myocardial perfusion is a fertile area for research and involves the use of paramagnetic agents, such as gadolinium, that are attached to chelating agents; the hope is that these agents will be attached to metabolically active substances, thus developing a system that is specific for myocardium and provides a potential strategy for the evaluation of myocardial perfusion as well as myocardial metabolism.

MRI has been very effective in documenting intracardiac masses, especially in identifying mural thrombi and tumor.[23] When conventional echocardiography raises the question of an intracardiac mass but is not definitive, MRI can be a very helpful diagnostic technique. This may be the most common clinical indication for MRI cardiac studies at present.

Valvular regurgitation can be appreciated with cine-MR. Mitral regurgitation is the most common regurgitant lesion with CHD. Regurgitation through the atrioventricular valves is associated with a high velocity jet resulting in a signal void. The severity of regurgitation can be estimated from the volume of the signal void itself or in-

directly by estimating regurgitant fraction or volume after calculation of right and left ventricular stroke volumes. However, color flow Doppler echocardiography generally is used to assess mitral regurgitation because it is a more widely available and less expensive technique.

Magnetic resonance (MR) spectroscopy deserves mention as a promising new modality for the in vivo evaluation of myocardial metabolism. MR spectroscopy provides a map of the sites where an atom exists in a compound. The atoms or isotopes most commonly used for biologic studies with MR spectroscopy include hydrogen, sodium (Na-23), phosphorus (P-31), and carbon (C-13). The spectra generated by these isotopes depend on the chemical environment in which the isotope is found, as well as the properties of each isotope. The relative amplitude of the spectral peaks, as well as their location within the field, reveals much about myocardial metabolism. For example, five peaks are generated with phosphorus spectroscopy, which include inorganic phosphate and several types of organic phosphates. Each resonates in a different position in the spectral pattern, and their amplitude and position provide information about the concentration or content in the tissue being evaluated. Experimental occlusion of a coronary artery in canine hearts for approximately 15 minutes resulted in the demonstration of lipid accumulation detected by electron micrographs. Reeves et al. demonstrated increased myocardial lipid accumulation with post-ischemic dysfunction by proton MRI.[24] Tissue characterization by T1 and T2 relaxation times is another area of active research. The constants, T1 and T2, control the rate of decay of various components of the net magnetization factor. They are independent of each other and are a fundamental property of tissue. Large values of T1 and T2 indicate a slow and gradual decay. For example, T1 for fat is 180 msec, for muscle is approximately 600 msec, and for water approximates 2,500 msec. In general, T1 of diseased and damaged tissue is longer than for corresponding healthy tissue. Thus, areas of infarction can be characterized by their relaxation times and contrasted to normal adjacent myocardium.

The enormous potential for this non-invasive diagnostic technique has generated considerable interest and hope for future use. However, clinical application of most of the techniques described in this section remain to be refined and defined as to their routine clinical use.

REFERENCES

1. Midwall J, Ambrose J, Pichard A et al: Angina pectoris before and after myocardial infarction. Chest 81:681, 1982
2. Kannel WB, Abbott RD: Incidence and prognosis of unrecognized myocardial infarction. An update on the Framingham Study. N Engl J Med 311:1114, 1984
3. Lown B: Sudden cardiac death: The major challenge confronting contemporary cardiology. Am J Cardiol 43:313, 1979
4. Gottlieb SO, Weisfeldt ML, Ouyang P et al: Silent ischemia as a marker for early unfavorable outcomes in patients with unstable angina. N Engl J Med 314:1214, 1986
5. Schelbert HR, Henze E, Phelphs ME, Kuhl DE: Assessment of regional myocardial ischemia by positron emission computed tomography. Am Heart J 103:588, 1982
6. Schelbert HR, Wisenberg G, Phelps ME et al: Noninvasive assessment of coronary stenoses by myocardial imaging during pharmacologic coronary vasodilation. VI. Detection of coronary artery disease in man with intravenous N-13 ammonia and positron computer tomography. Am J Cardiol 49:1197, 1982
7. Tamaki N, Yonekura Y, Senda M et al: Myocardial positron computer tomography with ^{13}N-ammonia at rest and during exercise. Eur J Nucl Med 11:246, 1985
8. Goldstein RA, Kirkeeide RL, Demer LL et al: Relation between geometric dimensions of coronary artery stenoses and myocardial perfusion reserve in man. J Clin Invest 79:1473, 1987
9. Gould KL, Goldstein RA, Mullani NA et al: Noninvasive assessment of coronary stenoses by myocardial perfusion imaging during pharmacologic coronary vasodilation. VIII. Clinical feasibility of positron cardiac imaging without a cyclotron using generator-produced rubidium-82. J Am Coll Cardiol 7:775, 1986
10. Yonekura Y, Tamaki N, Senda M et al: Detection of coronary artery disease with ^{13}N-ammonia and high-resolution positron emission computer tomography. Am Heart J 113:645, 1987
11. Williams BR, Jansen DE, Wong LF et al: Positron emission tomography for the diagnosis of coronary artery disease: A non-university experience and correlation with coronary angiography. J Nucl Med 30:845, 1989 (abstract)
12. Go RT, Marwick TH, MacIntyre WJ et al: A prospective comparison of rubidium-82 PET and thallium-201 SPECT myocardial perfusion imaging. J Nucl Med 31:1899, 1990
13. Stewart RE, Kalus M, Moluria E et al: Rubidium-82 PET versus thallium-201. Circulation 80:204, 1989
14. Brunken R, Tillisch J, Schwaiger M et al: Regional perfusion, glucose metabolism and wall motion in patients with chronic EKG Q-wave infarctions. Circulation 73:951, 1986
15. Brunken R, Schwaiger M, Grover-McKay M et al: Positron emission tomography detects tissue metabolic activity in myocardial segments with persistent thallium perfusion defects. J Am Coll Cardiol 10:557, 1987
16. Tamaki N, Yonekura Y, Senda M et al: Value and limitation of stress Tl-201 tomography. Comparison with perfusion and metabolic imaging with positron tomography. Circulation 76 (Suppl IV):IV-4, 1987
17. Stanford W, Brundage BH, MacMillan R et al: Sensitivity and specificity of assessing coronary bypass graft patency with ultrafast computed tomography. J Am Coll Cardiol 12:1, 1988
18. Caputo GR, Lipton MJ: Evaluation of regional left ventricular function using cine CT. In Pohost GM et al (eds): New Concepts in Cardiac Imaging. Yearbook Medical, Chicago, 1988
19. Higgins CB: MR of the heart: Anatomy, physiology and metabolism. Am J Roentgenol 151:239, 1988
20. Didier D, Higgins CB, Fisher MR et al: Congenital heart disease: Gated MR imaging in 72 patients. Radiology 158:227, 1986
21. Dooms GC, Higgins CB: MR imaging of cardiac thrombi. J Comput Assist Tomogr 10:415, 1986
22. Johns JA, Leavitt MB, Newell JB et al: Quantitation of acute myocardial infarct size by nuclear magnetic resonance imaging. J Am Coll Cardiol 15:143, 1990
23. Winkler M, Higgins CB: Suspected intracardiac masses: Evaluation with MR imaging. Radiology 165:117, 1987
24. Reeves RC, Evanochko WT, Canby RC et al: Demonstration of increased myocardial lipids with post-ischemic dysfunction ("myocardial stunning") by proton nuclear magnetic resonance spectroscopy. J Am Coll Cardiol 13:739, 1989

16

Pharmacotherapy of Coronary Heart Disease and Its Complications

David Waters, M.D.
Jules Lam, M.D.
Mario Talajic, M.D.

PRINCIPLES OF CORONARY PHARMACOTHERAPY

Coronary heart disease usually presents as a chronic problem with acute, life-threatening exacerbations. Most patients with known coronary disease take one or more drugs, often over many years. These medications are potent and often costly and have the potential to induce serious side effects. On the other hand, correctly applied pharmacotherapy reduces mortality in hypertension and acute myocardial infarction, reduces complications in unstable angina, improves symptoms in stable angina and heart failure, and influences the design and conduct of rehabilitation.

The benefits of pharmacotherapy depend upon accurate diagnosis and appropriate prescription. Thrombolytic therapy can be disastrous in a patient whose chest pain is not caused by acute myocardial ischemia. An incorrect diagnosis of angina can lead to years of fruitless medical treatment. Even when the diagnosis is correct, the reflex decision to treat may be poor judgment. For example, a patient with only one or two anginal episodes per month and no limitation of ordinary physical activities probably does not require chronic antianginal therapy.

Assessing the effect of drug therapy on coronary patients is often a difficult problem. Symptoms of heart failure, myocardial ischemia, and arrhythmias exhibit wide ranges of spontaneous variability. The placebo effect enhances any intrinsic benefit from antianginal therapy. After beginning therapy with a cardiac drug, the physician should consider whether the patient's condition actually improved as a result. If not, the dose could be optimized or the drug discontinued. One of the most useful procedures in modern cardiology is stopping several unnecessary drugs for a victim of overenthusiastic polypharmacy.

The results of controlled clinical trials provide a rational basis for much of our current drug therapy in coronary patients. A benefit demonstrated in such a trial will apply with certainty only to a patient who would meet the entry criteria of the study. Furthermore, the absolute risk reduction is likely to be more relevant to the management of the individual patient than is the relative risk reduction. Thus, a drug that reduces 10-year cor-

255

onary mortality by a statistically significant 50% may not be worthwhile if the absolute mortality reduction is from 2% to 1%.

The population of patients with coronary disease is aging, and this trend will almost certainly continue. The elderly coronary patient often metabolizes and excretes drugs more slowly than the younger patient, often has a reduced body mass, and may be more sensitive to both the therapeutic effect and the adverse effects of a drug. Digitalis, verapamil, beta-adrenergic blocking drugs, nitrates, and diuretic drugs should be used with particular caution in the elderly.

Thirty years ago, digitalis, quinidine, nitrates, and the early diuretics were the most useful of the limited array of drugs available to treat coronary patients. Since then, great advances have occurred in coronary pharmacotherapy, requiring familiarity with many more drugs. The physician must also understand the limitations of drug therapy and know when to turn to other treatments, such as coronary angioplasty, coronary bypass surgery, arrhythmia surgery, and cardiac transplantation.

ANTI-ISCHEMIC DRUGS

Anti-ischemic drugs are also discussed in Chapters 11, 12, and 13.

Beta-adrenergic Blocking Drugs

The first beta-adrenergic blocking drug available in the United States was propranolol, in 1967. This drug is a competitive antagonist of both beta$_1$ and beta$_2$ stimulation and therefore results in negative chronotropic and inotropic effects in the heart, bronchoconstriction, and vasoconstriction.[1] After oral administration, propranolol improves treadmill walking time to the onset of angina and total exercise time, beginning at 1 hour and lasting for about 12 hours.[2]

Myocardial ischemia, with or without angina, occurs when coronary blood flow is decreased or when myocardial oxygen demand is increased. The three major determinants of myocardial ox-

ygen demand are systolic wall tension, heart rate, and the inotropic state of the myocardium. Propranolol and other beta-blocking drugs reduce systemic arterial pressure, heart rate, and myocardial contractility both at rest and during exercise and thus are useful in the treatment of angina. In an early uncontrolled study of patients with severe, stable angina, propranolol eliminated all episodes in 32% of patients and reduced episodes by at least one-half in 84%.[3] During a follow-up of 5 to 8 years, patients whose attacks were not reduced by at least one-half experienced a fourfold-greater mortality than the others.

Propranolol is also useful therapy for hypertension and atrial and ventricular arrhythmias. Its antihypertensive action results in part from a lowering of plasma renin activity. Common side effects include fatigue, impotence, nightmares, and cold extremities. The drug can precipitate or worsen heart failure, conduction disturbances, and bronchoconstriction in susceptible individuals. In brittle diabetic patients, propranolol can induce hypoglycemia and can also mask the premonitory symptoms of hypoglycemia. Abrupt propranolol withdrawal can induce rebound,[4] with worsening angina or myocardial infarction. Propranolol increases serum triglyceride levels and slightly lowers high-density lipoprotein (HDL) cholesterol[5]; during long-term therapy, these unfavorable metabolic effects could accelerate the progression of atherosclerosis.

The second beta-blocking drug to become available for clinical use in the United States was metoprolol, in 1978.[6] This drug preferentially antagonizes the action of sympathomimetic amines on beta$_1$ receptors and is therefore described as cardioselective. This cardioselectivity is only relative, however; at higher doses metoprolol also blocks beta$_2$ receptors. Atenolol, released in the United States in 1981, is also cardioselective and has a longer half-life so that it can be administered once per day.

Nadolol and timolol are nonselective beta-blocking drugs with longer half-lives than propranolol. They do not share the membrane-stabilizing properties of propranolol; however, this quinidinelike effect on the cardiac action potential occurs only at very high doses and is unlikely to have any clinical relevance. Pindolol and acetabulol are beta-blocking drugs with intrinsic sympathomimetic activity; that is, they not only block the beta-receptor from catecholamine stimulation but also produce low-level beta stimulation themselves. Therefore, they reduce heart rate and myocardial contractility less than other beta-blocking drugs do, potentially resulting in either fewer adverse effects or compromised efficacy, depending upon one's viewpoint.

Are cardioselectivity and intrinsic sympathomimetic activity relevant to the treatment of angina? In a study comparing five different beta-blocking drugs, including those with and without cardioselectivity and intrinsic sympathomimetic activity, no differences were seen in the degree of improvement in angina threshold.[7] In patients with peripheral vascular disease or Raynaud's phenomenon, beta-blocking drugs are often avoided entirely or cardioselective agents are used, in spite of evidence from controlled studies[8,9] that symptoms of these conditions are not worsened by either type of beta-blocking drug.

Some features of the currently available beta-blocking drugs are summarized in Table 16-1. Labetalol is a beta-blocking drug with alpha-blocking and direct vasodilating properties, making it useful for the treatment of hypertension. Esmolol is an ultra-short-acting beta-blocking drug with $beta_1$ selectivity, available only in an intravenous formulation. Its features make it ideal for the treatment of supraventricular arrhythmias or for patients at risk for serious adverse reactions to beta-blockade.[10] Sotalol, a beta-blocking drug that prolongs the action potential duration and increases the refractoriness of cardiac tissue, appears to be effective for a variety of atrial and ventricular arrhythmias. However, higher drug concentrations appear to be necessary for its antiarrhythmic efficacy than for beta-blockade.[11] Sotalol is not approved for use in the United States but is available in many other countries.

A major positive feature of beta-blocking drugs is their proven ability to reduce mortality in survivors of myocardial infarction. At least 25 randomized trials that included over 23,000 patients have evaluated the long-term use of these drugs after infarction.[12] Overall, 7.6% of eligible patients (without contraindications such as bradycardia, congestive heart failure, etc.) allocated to beta-blocking therapy and 9.4% of control subjects died, a 22% risk reduction (95% confidence

Table 16-1. Characteristics of Beta-adrenergic Blocking Drugs

Drug	Potency vs Propranolol	Cardio-selectivity	ISA	Membrane Stabilization	Elimination Half-life (hr)
Acetabulol	0.3x	+	+	+	3–4
Atenolol	1.0x	+ +	0	0	6–9
Betaxolol	1.0x	+ +	0	+	15
Carteolol	10.0x	0	+	0	5–6
Esmolol[a]	0.02x	+ +	0	0	9 min
Labetalol[b]	0.3x	0	+	0	3–4
Metoprolol	1.0x	+ +	0	0	3–4
Nadolol	1.0x	0	0	0	14–24
Oxprenolol	1.0x	0	+	+	2–3
Penbutalol	1.0x	0	+	0	27
Pindolol	6.0x	0	+ +	+	3–4
Propranolol	1.0x	0	0	+ +	3–4
Timolol	6.0x	0	0	0	4–5

[a] Available only in intravenous formulation.
[b] Also alpha-blocking activity.
Abbreviations: ISA, intrinsic sympathomimetic activity.

intervals 16 to 30%, $P < 0.001$).[12] Meta-analysis also suggests that long-term beta-blocking therapy reduces the risk of recurrent infarction by 27%, from 7.5% to 5.6%.[12] The most impressive of the long-term trials are the Norwegian Multicenter Study with timolol,[13] the β-Blocker Heart Attack Trial with propranolol,[14] and the Göteborg metoprolol study.[15] On the basis of three small trials with negative results, it has been suggested that beta-blocking drugs with intrinsic sympathomimetic activity may not reduce postinfarction mortality.[16]

Controversy exists about whether beta-blocking drugs are necessary in low-risk survivors of myocardial infarction.[17] In the β-Blocker Heart Attack Trial, the survival benefit was almost entirely restricted to patients with electrical or mechanical complications.[18] Noninvasive testing can identify a large subset of postinfarction patients with 1-year mortality risk of less than 2%.

The administration of intravenous beta-blocking drugs in the acute phase of myocardial infarction has also been shown to reduce mortality.[12] In ISIS-1, more than 16,000 patients were randomized to placebo or intravenous followed by oral atenolol; cardiovascular mortality during the first week, the primary endpoint of the study, was reduced by 15%, from 4.57% to 3.89% ($P < 0.04$).[19] Meta-analysis of early intravenous beta-blocking drug trials in acute infarction suggests that about 200 patients would have to be treated to prevent one death, one reinfarction, and one cardiac arrest during the first week,[19] (i.e., consideration of biologic versus statistical significance). In the United States, this form of therapy is not widely practiced, probably because the risk of adverse events is perceived as being greater than the potential benefit and because thrombolytic therapy is more commonly used.

Most episodes of transient myocardial ischemia in patients with coronary heart disease are unaccompanied by symptoms. The presence of silent ischemia has been reported to be an adverse prognostic factor in patients with stable[20] and unstable[21] angina and after myocardial infarction.[22] Whether treatment of silent myocardial ischemia with antianginal drugs improves the prognosis is a hotly debated question, which has not yet been definitively answered. Propranolol,[23] atenolol,[24] and metoprolol[25] all reduce the frequency and duration of silent ischemia, and one study demonstrated superiority of propranolol over nifedipine and diltiazem.[23] However, antianginal drugs usually do not eliminate all spontaneous ischemic episodes, and it is not known whether complete suppression of ischemia should be the goal of antianginal therapy.

The treatment of angina with beta-blocking drugs requires dose titration, because a favorable response may occur at any point over a wide range. Changes in heart rate are helpful in evaluating the effect of treatment. For example, if heart rate at rest remains at 70 beats/min after the institution of 160 mg/day of chronic propranolol therapy, it is reasonable to increase the dose in an attempt to increase efficacy. However, if the heart rate at the same dose is 48 beats/min with sinus rhythm, higher doses are not advisable because the risk of an adverse response outweighs the potential benefit.

In the absence of contraindications, beta-blocking drugs are the antianginal drugs of choice in patients with previous infarction, hypertension, or contraindications to alternative antianginal drugs. In most patients they are more effective than dihydropyridine calcium channel-blocking drugs or long-acting nitrate drugs. Their utility for a wide range of other cardiac conditions has been well documented over the past two decades.

Calcium Channel-Blocking Drugs

Compounds that bind to specific receptor sites associated with the voltage-dependent calcium channel and inhibit cellular uptake of calcium come from diverse chemical groups. Of the four calcium channel-blocking drugs now available in the United States, two are dihydropyridines (nifedipine and nicardipine), one is a benzodiazepine (diltiazem), and one is a phenylalkylamine (verapamil). In contrast to the beta-blocking drugs, which all have approximately similar hemodynamic effects, calcium channel-blocking drugs exhibit important differences that affect their clinical use. Some of the features of these drugs are listed in Table 16-2.

Table 16-2. Characteristics of Calcium Channel-Blocking Drugs

	Nifedipine, Nicardipine	Diltiazem	Verapamil
Hemodynamic effects			
Heart rate	↑	↓	↓
Arterial pressure	↓	↓	↓
Myocardial contractility	↓	↓	↓↓
Electrophysiologic effects	No	Yes	Yes
Oral dose range[a]	10–30 mg tid or qid	30–120 mg tid	80–160 mg bid or tid

[a] Long-acting formulations of nifedipine, diltiazem, and verapamil are available.

Each of these four drugs is approved for the treatment of angina. Because the dihydropyridines increase heart rate and occasionally worsen angina,[26] they are not the treatment of choice for stable angina. Diltiazem and verapamil do not cause reflex tachycardia and cause fewer side effects; they are therefore preferable as monotherapy for stable angina.[26,27]

Variant angina, an uncommon syndrome in which myocardial ischemia is caused by coronary spasm, is not improved by beta-blocking drugs.[28] Calcium channel-blocking drugs are extremely effective in preventing angina in this condition[29] and may also reduce the risk of myocardial infarction or sudden death.[30] In unstable angina without evidence of coronary spasm, diltiazem and propranolol are equally effective in preventing angina but rarely eliminate all attacks and probably do not reduce the risk of infarction.[31] The combination of nifedipine and propranolol for unstable angina has been shown to prevent episodes better than either of these two drugs used alone.[32,33] Indeed, most patients with unstable angina are treated with two or three antianginal drugs, often including intravenous nitroglycerin, during the acute phase.

In an attempt to duplicate the positive results with beta-adrenergic blocking drugs, at least nine controlled clinical trials have assessed the effect on mortality of calcium channel-blocking drugs after myocardial infarction.[34–42] These studies are summarized in Table 16-3. In two of the five trials with nifedipine, mortality was significantly *higher* in the group receiving active drug than in the placebo group.[34,38] The excess mortality caused by nifedipine appears to occur early, and although the exact mechanism is unknown, it may be related to drug-induced hypotension or tachycardia upsetting a tenuous balance between myocardial oxygen supply and demand in a susceptible minority of patients. These findings have generated the recommendation that nifedipine should be avoided in the acute phase of myocardial infarction unless a very compelling indication is present for its use.

Although diltiazem had no effect on overall infarction mortality in the one large trial in which it was used,[41] the investigators noted an important bidirectional effect related to left ventricular function. In patients with radiographic signs of pulmonary congestion during the acute phase of infarction, mortality was 41% higher in diltiazem-treated patients than in those taking placebo. On the other hand, patients without pulmonary congestion benefited from diltiazem; their risk reduction was 23% (confidence intervals, 2 to 39%). A similar pattern was observed when using radioisotopic left ventricular ejection fraction, dichotomized at 0.40, as an indicator of ventricular function.

In another randomized, controlled trial in which diltiazem therapy was begun from 1 to 3 days after a non-Q wave myocardial infarction and continued for up to 2 weeks, the drug significantly reduced the reinfarction rate, the primary endpoint of the study.[43] The subset of patients with non-Q wave infarction in the MDPIT study[41] showed a significant survival advantage with diltiazem. For these reasons, diltiazem is commonly used instead of beta-adrenergic blocking drug to improve the outcome after an infarction of the non-Q type.

The purpose of DAVIT-II was to determine whether the administration of verapamil, begin-

Table 16-3.   Placebo-Controlled Trials of Calcium Channel-Blocking Drugs
After Myocardial Infarction

Drug	Number of Patients	Duration of Follow-up	Mortality (%)	
			Drug	Placebo
Nifedipine				
Muller et al.[34]	171	6 months	10.1	8.5[a]
Norwegian trial[35]	227	6 weeks	8.9	8.7
SPRINT[36]	2,276	10 months	5.8	5.7
TRENT[37]	4,491	1 month	6.7	6.3
SPRINT II[38]	1,373	6 months	15.8	12.6[b]
Verapamil				
DAVIT-I[39]	1,436	6 months	12.8	13.9
DAVIT-II[40]	1,775	16 months	11.1	13.8
Diltiazem				
MDPIT[41]	2,466	25 months	13.5	13.5
Lidoflazine				
MI Study Group[42]	1,792	1–6 years	19.7	18.8

[a] At 2 weeks, mortality was 7.9 versus 0% ($P = 0.018$) in favor of placebo.
[b] Statistically significant difference in favor of placebo because of a higher early mortality in the nifedipine group.

ning 2 weeks after myocardial infarction and continuing for 12 to 18 months, might reduce total mortality or the combined endpoint of death and reinfarction, compared with placebo.[40] Although the mortality difference, 11.1% compared with 13.8%, did not attain statistical significance ($P = 0.11$), the combined endpoint was significantly less in verapamil patients, 18.0% compared to 21.6% (relative risk, 0.80; confidence intervals, 0.64 to 0.99). No benefit or adverse effect was seen in the subset of patients with heart failure. The degree of risk reduction in this trial and in the patients without pulmonary congestion in the MDPIT study is equivalent to that seen in the beta-blocking drug trials. However, a beta-adrenergic blocking drug should be the therapy of choice after myocardial infarction, particularly when left ventricular function is more compromised, on the basis of the larger number of positive studies with this class of drugs. Diltiazem or verapamil could be used if left ventricular function is well preserved and a contraindication to beta-blocking drug usage is present.

On theoretical grounds, calcium channel-blocking drugs are appealing as a choice for therapy of silent myocardial ischemia during daily life. Because most of these episodes appear at heart rates far below rates seen with ischemia induced during exercise testing, it has been assumed that reductions in coronary flow are important in their pathogenesis. Although calcium channel-blocking drugs induce coronary vasodilatation and prevent coronary spasm, they do not seem to be superior to beta-adrenergic blocking drugs in the treatment of silent ischemia.

In one uncontrolled study,[44] nifedipine reduced the number of ischemic episodes when added to baseline antianginal therapy; however, in a subsequent controlled study, the drug did not significantly decrease the number of ischemic episodes.[23] Diltiazem reduced ischemic episodes by 50% compared with placebo in a recently completed study of 60 patients with stable angina[45]; the number of episodes was reduced by at least half in 70% of patients. Whether medical treatment of silent ischemia improves the prognosis has not yet been established, and therefore routine treatment of this condition is not recommended.

Calcium channel-blocking drugs are effective vasodilators, and acute and chronic vasodilator drug therapy has become an established approach to the management of heart failure. By reducing afterload, calcium channel-blocking drugs can increase cardiac output and produce short-term amelioration of symptoms. The dihydropyridines hold an advantage over diltiazem and verapamil in these circumstances because their negative inotropic effects on the cardiac myocyte are more easily overcome by their salutory effect on afterload. However, even when these drugs induce persistent favorable hemodynamic effects, the renal and neurohumoral consequences usually induce clinical deterioration in patients with congestive heart failure.[45] Other vasodilator drugs are preferable for the treatment of heart failure; calcium channel-blocking drugs are not recommended for this problem.[46]

Calcium channel-blocking drugs inhibit the development of atherosclerosis in experimental models such as the cholesterol-fed rabbit.[47,48] The mechanism accounting for this beneficial effect is undefined but could include preservation of endothelial integrity; modulation of low-density lipoprotein (LDL) receptors to increase LDL binding, internalization and degradation by smooth muscle cells; reduction in smooth muscle cell proliferation and migration; and a reduction in the synthesis of matrix components.[47]

Two controlled clinical trials have examined the potential of calcium channel-blocking drugs to influence coronary atherosclerosis. In the INTACT study,[49] no difference in the rates of progression or regression of coronary lesions was seen at serial coronary angiography between placebo- and nifedipine-treated patients. However, new lesions appeared at a reduced rate in the nifedipine group. In another study,[50] nicardipine also had no effect on the incidence of progression and regression of established coronary lesions. However, minimal stenoses, those ≤20% in severity on the first coronary angiogram, were almost twice as likely to progress in placebo-treated controls than in nicardipine-treated patients. Further studies are under way to clarify and confirm the antiatherogenic activity of this class of drugs.

The side effects associated with calcium channel-blocking drugs are usually mild and are sometimes consequences of the therapeutic effects of these drugs. The dihydropyridines can cause dizziness, palpitations, headache, and peripheral edema. These problems are probably more common with the original formulation of nifedipine, as a result of rapid absorption and high peak serum levels, than with the longer-acting formulations or other dihydropyridines. The most common side effects of diltiazem are gastrointestinal upset, edema, and rash. Diltiazem is more likely to be tolerated than the dihydropyridines, but shares with verapamil the potential to induce or worsen conduction disturbances, particularly atrioventricular block. Verapamil and diltiazem are more likely to worsen heart failure than are the dihydropyridines and are contraindicated in patients with very low ejection fractions. The most common adverse effects of verapamil are headache and constipation.

The number of calcium channel-blocking drugs available for clinical use will increase over the next decade.[51,52] Nisoldipine, nitrendipine, nimodipine, amlodipine, isradipine, and felodipine are all dihydropyridine drugs that are nearing U.S. approval or are already available in some countries. They differ in their duration of activity and their ability to cross the blood–brain barrier, but their similarities far outweigh their differences.[52]

Nitroglycerin and Longer-Acting Nitrate Drugs

Nitroglycerin has been used to treat angina for over a century. After sublingual administration, it is absorbed within seconds and relieves anginal attacks within 2 to 5 minutes. Several mechanisms that account for its beneficial effect have been described, and the relative contribution of each of these to the clinical setting remains controversial.[53] Nitroglycerin decreases afterload and decreases preload to a greater extent, owing to venous pooling. It dilates both epicardial coronary arteries and collateral vessels and both prevents and relieves coronary spasm. It is also capable of directly dilating coronary stenoses during exercise when coronary vasoconstriction has been documented to occur.[54] This latter action may be the most relevant to ordinary angina.

All patients with angina are routinely supplied with sublingual or other nitroglycerin and should be instructed in its proper use because misconceptions abound. The drug can cause headache, palpitations, dizziness, and syncope. It should not be used for symptoms other than those related to myocardial ischemia, and patients should be instructed not to take it while standing. The prophylactic use of nitroglycerin to prevent anginal attacks can greatly enhance the exercise capacity of many patients with stable, predictable angina.

Intravenous nitroglycerin is commonly used to treat patients with unstable angina, usually in association with beta-adrenergic blocking drugs and/or calcium channel-blocking drugs.[55] This route of administration permits rapid titration of dosage in response to symptoms or to adverse events. In a randomized comparison between intravenous nitroglycerin and the combination of oral isosorbide dinitrate and topical nitroglycerin ointment in 40 patients with unstable angina, both regimens were effective in reducing anginal attacks and the difference between them did not attain statistical significance.[56] Recent evidence[57] suggests that the antiplatelet activity of intravenous nitroglycerin may contribute to its beneficial effect in unstable angina.

Intravenous nitroglycerin can also be used to treat acute heart failure. By decreasing venous return, it reduces left and right ventricular filling pressures. Its afterload-reducing effect decreases cardiac work and tends to increase cardiac output, although by reducing preload, nitroglycerin tends to reduce cardiac output, even during heart failure. The anti-ischemic activity of nitroglycerin is desirable in some types of acute heart failure, such as early after myocardial infarction. The usefulness of nitroglycerin in acute heart failure is derived primarily from preload reduction, since better arterial vasodilator drugs are available.

Few drugs can be administered in as many different ways as nitroglycerin.[58] In addition to the sublingual tablet and intravenous form, a lingual spray is available. This formulation does not lose potency with time and is probably more rapidly absorbed than the sublingual tablet, particularly if the mouth is dry. Sustained-release buccal formulations of nitroglycerin have also been shown to be effective antianginal agents.[58] Isosorbide dinitrate is the most commonly used oral nitrate preparation in North America. In Europe, one of its longer-acting metabolites, isosorbide-5-mon-

onitrate, is also available. Transdermal nitroglycerin patches have proved to be a very popular method of administration since their approval for use in the United States in 1982.

The major problem with the long-term administration of nitrate drugs by any route is the development of tolerance. Tolerance to the hemodynamic effects of nitroglycerin appears within 24 to 48 hours of chronic therapy,[59] and antianginal efficacy is completely attenuated after 7 to 10 days of continuous treatment.[58] Intermittent therapy with nitrate-free intervals of 8 to 12 hr/day has been used to circumvent the problem of tolerance, with some success.[58] Isosorbide dinitrate should be prescribed in doses of two to three times per day, with a drug-free overnight interval of at least 12 hours. Nitroglycerin patches should likewise be removed for at least 8 to 12 hours at night.[58]

Unfortunately, even with intermittent dosing regimens, treatment with long-acting nitrate drugs is associated with significant problems and limitations. Nitrate headache occurs in most patients treated with doses high enough to ensure antianginal efficacy, and often the medication is abandoned.[60] Nocturnal angina may be more frequent with intermittent nitrate drug therapy than with placebo, and placebo-treated patients may have better early-morning exercise tolerance.[61]

Tolerance develops because of a reduced ability of the administered nitrate to undergo conversion to nitric oxide, the active moiety that stimulates the enzyme guanylate cyclase, so that cyclic guanosine monophosphate accumulates and induces vascular smooth muscle relaxation. Depletion of intracellular thiol groups limits the conversion of nitrates to nitric oxide in the tolerant state. One strategy to prevent tolerance that is currently under investigation involves the administration of thiol donors such as captopril or N-acetylcysteine.

As a result of the foregoing considerations, long-acting nitrate drug preparations are not recommended as the best choice for prophylactic therapy in stable angina. In patients who do not tolerate or have contraindications to beta-adrenergic blocking drugs or calcium channel-blocking drugs, such as those with heart failure, long-acting nitrate preparations are the antianginal drugs of choice. To minimize side effects, treatment should begin with low doses, which are gradually increased. Intermittent therapy is essential, and drug administration should be discontinued in the face of side effects or a lack of efficacy. Long-acting nitrate drugs can also be used in patients with angina whose symptoms persist at an unacceptable level in spite of other antianginal drugs. The combination of a long-acting nitrate drug and a beta-adrenergic blocking drug tends to act synergistically because the beta-blocking drug prevents any nitrate-induced acceleration in heart rate. Long-acting nitrate preparations reduce the frequency of silent myocardial ischemia; however, their usefulness in this condition has not been adequately investigated.[62]

Intravenous nitroglycerin has been used in the acute phase of myocardial infarction to limit infarct size. A meta-analysis of controlled clinical trials suggests that such treatment reduces mortality by one-third, from 18 to 12% (95% confidence intervals, −18% to −49%).[63] The benefit appears to be greatest in large, anterior, Q wave infarctions and may be due to the salutory influence of the drug on ventricular remodeling.[64] Subsequent treatment with an angiotensin-converting enzyme inhibitor drug is indicated to preserve left ventricular function by preventing left ventricular aneurysm formation.[64]

THROMBOLYTIC DRUGS

Thrombolytic drugs are also discussed in Chapters 11, 12, and 13.

Thrombus formation at the site of rupture of a coronary atherosclerotic plaque is the most common precipitating event in the conversion from a chronic stable coronary syndrome to an acute ischemic coronary event such as unstable angina and acute myocardial infarction.[65–67] This understanding has led to pharmacologic interventions for acute myocardial infarction aimed at lysing the thrombus, thereby restoring coronary blood flow, interrupting the infarction process, salvaging myocardium at risk, and improving survival. Besides these thrombolytic interventions, other pharmacologic therapy involving anti-

thrombotic agents is aimed at preventing acute thrombus formation and extension at the site of a ruptured atherosclerotic plaque. Because arterial occlusion by mural thrombosis represents a dynamic process of thrombus formation and thrombus lysis, it is appropriate to discuss the thrombolytic approach and the antithrombotic approach to the management of these patients. The thrombolytic drugs are reviewed first.

The results of several large randomized clinical trials are overwhelming and have unequivocally shown the benefit of intravenous thrombolytic therapy in the management of acute myocardial infarction.[67–72] This benefit, a reduction in mortality, has been shown for three currently available thrombolytic agents,[67–72] suggesting a class action of these drugs whose benefits are related to their thrombolytic effect. However, it is still not clear whether one agent is superior to the other, and this issue is now being addressed in trials directly comparing these drugs. This has practical relevance because of the up to 10-fold difference in price between agents. Nevertheless, the advent of these agents has drastically changed not only our approach to the management of patients with acute myocardial infarction, but also the natural history of the disease. Interruption of the infarction process by the reestablishment of blood flow halts the "wavefront phenomenon" of myocardial necrosis proceeding from the subendocardial layers to the subepicardial layers,[73] thereby limiting the extent of necrosis and potentially averting a myocardial infarction, or converting a transmural infarct into a nontransmural infarct.

Mechanisms of Action and Classification

Thrombolytic agents are plasminogen activators that convert inactive plasminogen of the fibrinolytic system to the active proteolytic enzyme, plasmin, a serine protease that degrades the fibrin of a blood clot.[74] Plasmin may also degrade normal components of the hemostatic system, such as fibrinogen, and factors V, VIII, and XIII.[74] Clot lysis is induced when plasmin binds to fibrin via its lysine-binding site and degrades the fibrin polymers to fibrin degradation products. Unbound or freely circulating plasmin is rapidly inactivated by alpha$_2$-antiplasmin and alpha$_2$-macroglobulin.[75] When the antiplasmin system is overwhelmed, the unbound plasmin may rapidly degrade circulating fibrinogen and noncrosslinked fibrin, resulting in a systemic lytic state with marked fibrinogen depletion.[76] Plasminogen also binds to fibrin via its lysine-binding site, and this can be selectively inactivated pharmacologically by epsilon aminocaproic acid, which binds at that lysine site.[75,76]

The three agents that have been extensively studied as therapy for acute myocardial infarction to date include the relatively fibrin-selective thrombolytic drug tissue plasminogen activator (t-PA)[71] and the nonselective drugs streptokinase[68–70] and anisoylated plasminogen streptokinase activator complex (APSAC) (Table 16-4).[72] This classification of thrombolytic drugs in terms of their fibrin selectivity refers to their propensity for activating circulating as opposed to fibrin-bound plasminogen. The nonselective agents streptokinase, APSAC, and also urokinase tend to activate circulating plasminogen more than the fibrin selective agents t-PA and single-chain urokinase plasminogen activator (scu-PA), resulting in a greater generation of free circulating plasmin that induces fibrinogenolysis and a systemic lytic state characterized by fibrinogen depletion. A goal in the development of newer thrombolytic agents has been to improve the agent's fibrin or clot selectivity to avoid free-plasmin generation and the systemic lytic state.

Another classification of thrombolytic agents is based upon their time of introduction into clinical use. Thus, streptokinase and urokinase constitute the first-generation or "classic" agents. The search for more potent and more fibrin-selective agents has led to the introduction of the second-generation agents t-PA, APSAC, and scu-PA. However, APSAC appears to be a nonselective agent. The clot selectivity of t-PA and scu-PA occurs as a result of molecular interactions that render them more effective at the fibrin surface than in the circulating blood. The third-generation agents in development include mutants of t-PA, chimeric molecules, and thrombolytic agents attached to antifibrin antibodies; their potential role is yet unclear. It is hoped that they will not only be more effective, exceeding the 75 to 85% recanalization rate achieved with currently available drugs, but also provide a persistent long-term patency with a lesser tendency for inducing a systemic lytic state. Potentially synergistic combinations of thrombolytic agents are also being tested for this purpose.

Streptokinase

Streptokinase is derived from the beta-hemolytic streptococcus, and although the fibrinolytic activity was first described in 1933, it was not until the 1950s that it was used to treat acute myocardial infarction.[77] It is currently administered as a dose of 1.5 million units over 60 minutes. Doses of less than 1.0 million units are less effective.[78] Its plasma half-life is about 18 minutes, with a beta-elimination of 83 minutes. Strepto-

Table 16-4.   Characteristics of Thrombolytic Drugs

	Streptokinase	*t-PA*	*APSAC*
Fibrin selectivity	No	Yes	No
Fibrinogen lysis	Extensive	Moderate	Extensive
Half-life	18 min	4 min	95 min
Patency			
90 min	45%	75%	56%
24 hr	85%	85%	—
Hypotension	Yes	No	Yes
Allergic reactions	Yes	No	Yes
Approximative cost/dose	$200	$2,200	$1,500

kinase combines with circulating plasminogen to form an activator complex, which then hydrolyzes additional plasminogen to plasmin.[79]

Because of its low fibrin specificity, a systemic lytic state, with fibrinogen depletion in excess of 80%, may occur by 4 to 6 hours with the current dosing regimen. The resulting extensive fibrinogenolysis and fibrinogen degradation product generation may exert a platelet inhibitory effect that may be beneficial for preventing rethrombosis.[80] However, it appears that streptokinase by itself may promote platelet aggregation[81] or thrombin formation.[82] The antigenic properties of streptokinase may also cause fever, rash, urticaria, and angioedema.[68-70] Hypotension is a more common problem, which may be related to the activation of kinins and the complement system and to the rapidity and the magnitude of the dose administered.[83]

The efficacy of thrombolytic therapy can be measured in terms of reperfusion rate or patency rate. Reperfusion rate refers to the proportion of angiographically occluded vessels that are open on subsequent angiography after drug therapy. Patency rate refers to the proportion of infarct-related arteries that are open at an arbitrary point in time after administration of therapy, regardless of the status of the arteries at baseline. In clinical studies with streptokinase, the 90- to 120-minute angiographic reperfusion rates range from 31 to 80%,[84-87] with a mean of about 40% at 4 hours from symptom onset. The patency rates range from 42 to 77%, with a mean of about 47% at 3 hours from the onset of symptoms and about 85% at 24 hours.[88-92]

This improvement in reperfusion and patency rates is associated with a 3 to 6% improvement in left ventricular ejection fraction [70,93,94] (Table 16-5) and a consistent 21% reduction in mortality from the GISSI,[68] ISIS-2,[69] and ISAM[70] studies combined (Table 16-6). In the GISSI trial,[68] the reduction in mortality is more marked the earlier the streptokinase is given, approaching 50% when treatment is begun within 1 hour from the onset of symptoms. The ISIS-2 study[69] demonstrated a marked additive effect of aspirin, 160 mg daily, in decreasing mortality and reinfarction when combined with streptokinase. Thus, despite its lack of fibrin selectivity and its low early reperfusion rate after myocardial infarction, streptokinase is still very effective in decreasing mortality and improving left ventricular function at a reasonable cost.

Tissue Plasminogen Activator

t-PA is a serine protease and a physiologic thrombolytic agent that is naturally synthesized by vascular endothelial cells. In the early 1980s it was produced in small quantities from a melanoma cell culture, but since then it has been mass-produced for clinical use by recombinant DNA technology.[95] Recombinant t-PA was initially synthesized and tested as a two-chain enzyme, but the current commercially available product is mostly a single-chain form of t-PA.[96] This newer single-chain form of t-PA has a higher selectivity for fibrin, but it is usually given at a higher dose than the original two-chain t-PA because of its more rapid clearance.[96] Because of its strong binding affinity to fibrin, plasminogen bound to fibrin is preferentially converted to plasmin on the clot surface, rather than affecting the free circulating plasminogen unbound to fibrin.[97] Despite this relative fibrin selectivity, however, some free plasmin is generated that may lead to a 30 to 40% decrease in the plasma fibrinogen level.[96,98] This is still much less than observed with the nonselective thrombolytic agents. Other theoretical advantages of t-PA include its nonantigenicity and its much smaller potential for inducing allergic reactions or hypotension.

The half-life of t-PA is short, being less than 5 minutes, and t-PA is cleared by the liver.[99] The current dose of t-PA is 100 mg given over 3 to 4 hours. The prolonged infusion was used in the hope of preventing reocclusion; however, this dosing regimen may promote the risk of bleeding.[100] A front-loaded or bolus injection of t-PA is now being tested in combination with a shorter maintenance infusion.[101,102] This accelerated dosing regimen appears to be associated with an enhanced patency rate of 90% at 90 minutes [101] compared with 62% at 90 minutes for conventional t-PA administration in the TIMI-1 trial.[90] The accelerated dosing regimen may also be

Table 16-5.   Left Ventricular Function After Intravenous Thrombolytic Drugs

Study	Drug	Number of Patients	Entry (hr)[a]	Follow-up (days)	Ejection Fraction (%) Drug	Placebo	P
ISAM[70]	SK	1,741	6	21–28	56.8	53.9	<0.005
Kennedy et al.[93]	SK	368	6	42–56	50.8	46.6	<0.02
White et al.[94]	SK	219	4	21	59.0	53.0	<0.005
Guerci et al.[111]	t-PA	138	4	10	53.2	46.4	<0.02
Australian[113]	t-PA	144	4	7	57.7	51.7	0.04
O'Rourke et al.[112]	t-PA	126	2.5	21	61.0	54.0	<0.006
Armstrong et al.[115]	t-PA	115	3.75	9	53.6	47.8	0.017
Van de Werf and Arnold[114]	t-PA	721	5	14	50.7	48.5	0.04
Bassand et al.[125]	APSAC	230	5	14	53	47	0.002
Meinertz et al.[126]	APSAC	331	4	14	56	57	NS

[a] Hours after onset of symptoms.
Abbreviations: SK, streptokinase; NS, not significant.

more selective in lysing fresh thrombus than aged thrombus.[102]

The early clinical trials have confirmed the efficacy of t-PA in recanalizing the infarct-related artery. Indeed, recanalization rates at 90 minutes appear to be superior with t-PA (62%) than with streptokinase (31%) in the TIMI-1 trial,[90] and they were 70% for t-PA and 55% for streptokinase in the European Co-operative Study Group comparison.[103] The overall results of four angiographic trials suggest that a recanalization rate between 62 and 83%,[90,96,104,105] with a mean rate of 68%, can be achieved with t-PA. The early patency rate also appears to range between 69 and 89%, with a mean of 78% at 3 hours,[89,106–110] with a dose of about 100 mg intravenously.

Subsequent clinical trials have also demonstrated a beneficial effect of t-PA on improving left ventricular ejection fraction by 2 to 7% relative to the effect of a placebo (Table 16-5).[111–115] Also, the ASSET trial has shown a 26% decrease in mortality with intravenous t-PA relative to placebo (Table 16-6).[71]

Although t-PA appears to be superior to streptokinase in establishing patency in arteries early after infarction, the two agents appear to produce the same patency rates by 24 hours owing to the longer-term effects of streptokinase.[116] With regard to the clinical endpoints of improvement in left ventricular function and decrease in mortality, the two agents appear to be equivalent, suggesting that the clinical benefits may be more re-

Table 16-6.   Mortality Trials of Intravenous Thrombolytic Drugs

Study	Drug	Number of Patients	Entry (hr)[a]	Follow-up (days)	Mortality (%) Drug	Placebo	Risk Reduction (%)
GISSI[68]	SK	11,806	12	hosp.	10.7	13.0	18
ISIS-2[69]	SK	17,187	24	35	9.1	11.8	23
ISAM[70]	SK	1,741	6	21	5.1	6.5	22
ASSET[71]	t-PA	5,011	5	30	7.2	9.8	27
AIMS[72]	APSAC	1,004	6	30	6.3	12.1	48

[a] Hours after onset of symptoms.
Abbreviations: hosp., duration of hospitalization.

lated to the delayed than to the early patency rate. Results of the large GISSI-2 trial[117] directly comparing streptokinase with t-PA suggest that the two drugs are equally effective thrombolytic agents, although there is some question regarding the usage of subcutaneous heparin 12 hours after the use of the thrombolytic agent. Results of another large multicenter trial (ISIS-3) directly comparing streptokinase, t-PA, and APSAC, with or without heparin, are anxiously being awaited. A third trial, GUSTO, is also currently comparing these thrombolytic agents, with or without concomitant heparin use.

Anisoylated Plasminogen Streptokinase Activator Complex

APSAC is an anisoylated derivative of streptokinase that is activated by deacylation.[118,119] It is not a fibrin-selective agent, and, like streptokinase, it induces extensive fibrinogenolysis. It is more potent than an equivalent dose of streptokinase and has a much longer half-life. Its advantage over streptokinase is its ease of administration as an intravenous bolus of 30 mg or 30 units over 2 to 5 minutes and its long half-life. However, it shares the same disadvantages as streptokinase in terms of its immunogenicity and potential for inducing allergic reactions and hypotension.

Recanalization rates of the infarct-related artery range from 51 to 64%, with a mean of 54% from angiographic reperfusion studies.[120-122] The 3-hour patency rate ranges from 72 to 84%.[123,124] However, it has not been studied as extensively or in such large-scale clinical trials as streptokinase or t-PA. Similar to streptokinase, its thrombolytic efficacy is less with older clots. It has been shown to improve left ventricular ejection fraction in one study[125] but not in another study (Table 16-5),[126] but it has been shown to produce about a 47% decrease in mortality relative to placebo (Table 16-6).[72]

Patient Selection for Thrombolytic Therapy

Because of the unequivocal benefits of the thrombolytic agents, ideally all patients who present with an acute myocardial infarction should routinely receive thrombolytic therapy. However, on the basis of the well-kept registry of the GISSI-1[68] and ASSET[71] trials, only about 35% of infarction patients received thrombolytic therapy. Thus, the majority of patients are excluded because of contraindications to lytic therapy, late presentation to hospital, absence of ST segment elevation on the electrocardiogram, or age greater than 75.[127,128]

Bleeding Risk

A major concern when administering thrombolytic therapy is bleeding. This may occur with all the thrombolytic agents. Although the risk of bleeding was expected to be smaller with the fibrin-selective agents such as t-PA than the nonselective agents such as streptokinase, which induce more of a systemic lytic state, studies comparing the two drugs have shown no difference in the incidence of bleeding.[84,89,129,130] Concern about the risk of bleeding has led to absolute contraindication to lytic therapy, such as active bleeding, and relative contraindications such as uncontrolled hypertension, recent stroke or transient ischemic attack (TIA), recent trauma or surgery, cardiopulmonary resuscitation with chest compression, proliferative diabetic retinopathy, or menstruation. It is still not clear whether some of these concerns are valid. With regard to hypertension, it has been suggested that a diastolic blood pressure in excess of 100 mmHg increases the risk of intracranial hemorrhage.[131] However, the elevated blood pressure of many of these patients may respond rapidly to appropriate control of their chest pain or to nitrate drugs, nifedipine, or beta-blocking drugs if not contraindicated. In the ISIS-2 trial,[69] the 5-week vascular mortality was improved with aspirin and streptokinase for all blood pressure categories, even in patients who presented with a systolic pressure exceeding 175 mmHg. Patients with truly refractory hypertension or other important contraindications to lytic therapy may perhaps benefit from reperfusion by coronary angioplasty if this alternative is available in the hospital.

Timing

The degree of benefit of thrombolysis or any reperfusion therapy is related to the time of treatment from symptom onset, with mortality being the least when treatment is started as soon as the diagnosis of acute myocardial infarction is made. In the GISSI trial,[68] there was no mortality reduction at 21 days in those receiving streptokinase 6 hours or more after the onset of symptoms. However, in those treated within 6 hours, there was a 17% reduction in mortality (from 14.1 to 11.7%) for treatment started between 3 and 6 hours after symptom onset; a 23% reduction in mortality (from 12.0 to 9.2% for treatment between 0 and 3 hours, and an impressive 47% reduction in mortality (from 15.4 to 8.2%) for treatment started within 1 hour of symptom onset. A gradient of benefit in mortality reduction at 5 weeks with respect to the time of initiation of thrombolytic therapy was also observed in the ISIS-2 study.[69] In those treated between 12 and 24 hours, there was a 19% reduction in mortality (10.8 to 8.7%); a 13% reduction in mortality (11.8% to 10.3%) between 4 and 12 hours; and a 32% reduction in mortality (12.1 to 8.2%) between 0 and 4 hours, with the greatest decrease (42%) seen in those treated within 1 hour of symptom onset. Thus, the greatest benefit occurs in patients treated less than 1 hour from symptom onset, but substantial benefit is also obtained from treatment up to 6 hours after symptom onset. Patients treated between 6 and 24 hours may still benefit, although the benefit is smaller, and in patients without recurrent or ongoing chest pain or ischemia, the benefit may potentially not outweigh the risks. Three ongoing trials (EMERA, LATE, and TAMI-6) are assessing the benefits of treating patients who present late after their infarction.

Location of Infarct

Patients with anterior myocardial infarction conventionally treated have a worse prognosis than those with inferior myocardial infarction,[132] and they derive the most benefit from thrombo-lytic therapy.[94,113,114] Mortality reduction in patients with inferior myocardial infarction has been uncertain in several trials, including the GISSI trial.[133] The GISSI investigators have subsequently shown that the extent of myocardial injury was more important in determining mortality and thrombolytic efficacy than the conventional anterior or inferior location of the infarct.[134] Nevertheless, the ISIS-2 trial[69] has conclusively shown that there was a significant 35% reduction in mortality (from 10.0 to 6.5%) with inferior ST segment elevation. The comparative reduction in mortality with anterior ST segment elevation was 53% (from 21 to 9.8%). In contrast to the inconsistent mortality reduction, improvement in left ventricular function is more consistent with inferior infarction treated with thrombolytic therapy,[70,93,111–115] although this benefit is still lower than that observed with anterior infarction.[133]

The strongest evidence of mortality reduction with thrombolytic intervention is restricted to the subgroup of patients presenting with ST segment elevation in two contiguous leads, or those with Q wave infarction. In neither the ISIS-2[69] nor the GISSI[68] trial was a mortality reduction observed in the small subgroup of patients with ST segment depression. This may be due to the small number of patients with ST segment depression entered in these trials, but, more importantly, may reflect the fact that ST segment elevation and Q wave infarction are associated with a much higher incidence of occlusive intracoronary thrombus than infarction with ST segment depression or T wave changes.[135]

The Elderly

In-hospital mortality due to acute myocardial infarction increases markedly with age, increasing up to 50% in those over the age of 75.[136] However, these elderly patients also tend to be at a much higher risk of developing a major bleeding complication following thrombolytic therapy.[137] Because of this concern, many thrombolysis trials have excluded patients over the age of 70 or 75. Nevertheless, the ISIS-2[69] and GISSI[68] trials, which had no age limits for entry into the studies, have shown that the elderly may derive substantial benefits from thrombolytic therapy. In these trials, mortality was highest in the control group of patients over the age of 75. In the ISIS-2 trial, the 5-week mortality after streptokinase and aspirin therapy was lower than with placebo at all age groups, and especially in those over the age of 80, for whom a 45% reduction in mortality was observed relative to placebo. A similar trend was noted in the GISSI trial. However, the risk of bleeding complications as a function of age in the ISIS-2 and GISSI trials was not tabulated. Thus, in the elderly patients, the administration of thrombolytic agents should not be routine, but individualized, and the benefits should be weighed against the risks of major bleeding.

ANTITHROMBOTIC DRUGS: PLATELET INHIBITORS

Angiographic,[138] angioscopic,[139] and pathologic[65–67] studies have shown that plaque rupture or fissuring, with the resultant formation of an acute mural or occlusive thrombus, is an important mechanism in the pathogenesis of the acute ischemic coronary syndromes such as unstable angina and myocardial infarction. These intracoronary arterial thrombi have a large platelet and fibrin component: thus, drugs that inhibit platelet function and fibrin formation have been used as an antithrombotic approach to the management of these coronary syndromes. The potential of these drugs depends on their ability to interfere with essential reactions associated with arterial thrombogenesis. In this section, the platelet inhibitor drugs will be reviewed first, followed by the anticoagulant drugs.

Aspirin

Many drugs have been shown to inhibit platelet function in vitro, but only a few possess beneficial antithrombotic effectiveness when tested in humans in clinical trials.[140] Aspirin, dipyrid-

amole, and sulfinpyrazone are among the more commonly available platelet inhibitors that have been evaluated for the management of cardiovascular diseases. Aspirin acetylates the platelet cyclooxygenase enzyme and thus inhibits the formation of cyclic endoperoxides and thromboxane A_2 from platelet membrane arachidonic acid.[141] Aspirin may also inhibit platelet function independent of the acetylation of cyclooxygenase.[142] Although aspirin is rapidly cleared from the circulation, its antiplatelet effects persist for the life of the platelets, because of the irreversible acetylation of the platelet cyclooxygenase at the time of exposure.[140] Thus, aspirin (300 mg) can prolong the bleeding time for up to 5 days in normal volunteers.[143] Aspirin has been evaluated as an antithrombotic drug clinically, in doses of 160 to 1500 mg/day, but there is no indication that its beneficial effect is dose-related.[69,144,145] In fact, long-term administration of aspirin at a low dose of 1 mg/kg or even less per day significantly inhibits thromboxane A_2 generation and may even inhibit vessel wall generation of prostacyclin, a platelet-inhibitory substance naturally produced by the vessel wall.[146] However, it is unclear whether consistent beneficial antithrombotic effects can be observed with these low dosages or whether inhibition of prostacyclin has important practical implications.

Whereas the beneficial antithrombotic effects of aspirin have not been shown to be dose-related, with a dose ranging from 160 to 1,500 mg/day, it has clearly been shown that the adverse side effects, mainly gastrointestinal, become more severe as the dose is increased.[147] For these reasons, the lower clinically effective and proven dose of 160 to 325 mg/day of aspirin is recommended for the management of coronary disease. Despite this beneficial antithrombotic effect, aspirin does not prolong the reduced platelet survival time that is seen in a number of thromboembolic diseases.[148] However, even a dose of aspirin of 325 mg/day prolongs the bleeding time,[143] and its use may be associated with an increased risk of bleeding at the time of surgery.[149]

By inhibiting cyclooxygenase and thromboxane A_2 formation,[140] aspirin inhibits only one pathway of platelet aggregation, which is arachidonic acid dependent. Aspirin inhibits only partially, or does not inhibit, platelet aggregation mediated by the other two pathways of platelet aggregation and caused by adenosine diphosphate (ADP), collagen and thrombin.[140] As such, its antithrombotic effect, although present, is only partial, as platelet aggregation and thrombosis can occur through the other two pathways. In addition, aspirin does not prevent the adherence of platelets to the exposed subendothelium.[140]

Dipyridamole

Dipyridamole inhibits platelet function by increasing platelet cyclic adenosine monophosphate (cAMP) through the activation of the cAMP synthetic enzyme adenylate cyclase, the inhibition of the cAMP degradation enzyme phosphodiesterase, or the inhibition of adenosine uptake by vascular endothelium and reticulocytes, resulting in an increase in adenosine enhancing the adenylate cyclase enzyme.[150] In addition, dipyridamole normalizes a shortened platelet survival time in patients with prosthetic heart valves,[151] but, when it is used alone, its antithrombotic efficacy has not been consistent.[150] The beneficial antithrombotic effects of dipyridamole have been better demonstrated in the setting of prosthetic implants, such as artificial heart valves and arteriovenous cannulas, than on biologic surfaces.[140] Thus, the combination of dipyridamole and warfarin was more effective than warfarin alone for the prevention of thromboembolism in patients with mechanical heart valves, without excessively increasing the bleeding risk.[152] The combination of aspirin and dipyridamole has been used in numerous trials in the past, since it had been demonstrated that this combination prolonged a shortened platelet survival time more than either aspirin or dipyridamole alone.[148] This combination has been shown to have beneficial antithrombotic efficacy in patients undergoing percutaneous transluminal coronary angioplasty[153,154] (by preventing the acute thrombotic occlusions), in patients undergoing coronary artery bypass surgery,[149,155–157] in patients with known coronary artery disease,[158] in

patients with cerebrovascular disease,[159,160] and also in patients with peripheral vascular disease.[161] However, in direct comparative trials, mainly in patients undergoing coronary bypass surgery, this combination of aspirin and dipyridamole has not been shown to be significantly more effective than aspirin alone,[149,157] except perhaps in subgroups of patients with bypass grafts at high risk of occlusion such as those with poor flow or anastomosed to coronary arteries less than 1.5 mm in diameter.[149,155–157] In addition, dipyridamole does not prolong the bleeding time, and its use is not associated with increased bleeding at the time of surgery[155] or when used in combination with an anticoagulant.[152] The more common side effects observed with the use of dipyridamole are headaches, epigastric discomfort, and nausea.

Sulfinpyrazone

Sulfinpyrazone is a competitive inhibitor of platelet cyclooxygenase, but its antiplatelet mode of action is incompletely understood. It prolongs a reduced platelet survival time in patients,[162] prevents chemical injury of the endothelium,[140] and inhibits thrombosis in arteriovenous cannulas in humans.[163] Its beneficial effect is less consistent on biologic surfaces, and it has not been shown to be useful in unstable angina[164] or cerebrovascular disease,[165] although it may decrease the incidence of vascular events after myocardial infarction.[166] Common side effects of sulfinpyrazone include gastrointestinal irritation and exacerbation of peptic ulcer disease; a uricosuric effect with precipitation of uric acid stones; and high protein binding with possible displacement of, and thus increased sensitivity to, warfarin.

Unstable Angina Pectoris

Results of three randomized clinical trials have unequivocally demonstrated the value of the platelet inhibitor drug aspirin in the acute, subacute, and chronic management of patients with unstable angina (Table 16-7). The Veterans Ad-

Table 16-7. Effect of Platelet Inhibitors in Unstable Angina

Study	Number of Patients	Entry	Follow-up	Dose of ASA (mg/d)	Cardiac Endpoint (%) (Death + Nonfatal MI)		Risk Reduction (%)	P
					ASA	Placebo		
Lewis et al.[167]	1,266	48 hr	3 months	325	5.0	10.1	51	0.0005
Cairns et al.[164]	555	8 days	18 months	1,300	8.6	17.0	51	0.008
Théroux et al.[168]	479	8 hr	6 ± 3 days	650	3.3	11.9	71	0.012

Abbreviations: ASA, aspirin; MI, myocardial infarction.

ministration Cooperative Study (VACS),[167] which was the first to report the benefit of aspirin in unstable angina, randomized 1,266 patients to 324 mg of buffered aspirin or to placebo daily for 3 months. It showed a 51% decrease in death or acute myocardial infarction in the aspirin group relative to the placebo group (5 versus 10.1%) at 3 months. There was no difference in bleeding or gastrointestinal symptoms between the treated and control groups. In a longer follow-up study of 18 months, the McMaster University group[164] randomized 555 patients to aspirin, 325 mg four times daily; sulfinpyrazone, 200 mg four times daily; both of these agents; or neither. Similar to the VACS study, this Canadian study showed that the incidence of cardiac death and nonfatal myocardial infarction was reduced by 51% (8.6 versus 17.0%) in the group taking aspirin. There was no observed benefit for sulfinpyrazone either by itself or in combination with aspirin. In this study, in which a higher dose of aspirin was used, the incidence of gastrointestinal side effects was 29% higher in patients given aspirin than in the other groups. The usefulness of platelet inhibitors in the more acute management of patients with unstable angina was demonstrated in a recently published study from the Montreal Heart Institute.[168] In that study 479 patients were randomized to aspirin, 325 mg twice daily; intravenous heparin; a combination of both agents; or double placebo. At a mean of 6 days after hospital admission, when definitive therapy for the individual patient was selected, aspirin was shown to reduce the incidence of fatal and nonfatal myocardial infarction by 72% relative to placebo (11.9 versus 3.3%).

Acute Myocardial Infarction

For patients with acute myocardial infarction, ISIS-2[69] conclusively demonstrated the usefulness of aspirin in reducing mortality and recurrent coronary events. In this study, 17,187 patients with suspected acute myocardial infarction presenting within 24 hours of symptom onset were randomized to aspirin, 160 mg daily; intravenous streptokinase, 1.5 million units over 1 hour; both drugs; or double placebo. The 5-week follow-up mortality was significantly decreased by 23% by aspirin alone (from 11.8 to 9.4%), by 25% by streptokinase alone (from 12.0 to 9.2%), and by 42% by the combination of streptokinase and aspirin. In patients receiving aspirin, the decrease in mortality was similar for patients treated within 4 hours (25% decrease) and between 4 and 24 hours (21% decrease) of symptom onset. Benefits were higher in those with ST segment elevation than in those with ST segment depression, and the benefits were comparable in anterior and inferior myocardial infarction. The additive beneficial effect of aspirin and streptokinase on mortality, as well as the reduction in the high rate of reinfarction with streptokinase alone from 3.8 to 1.8% with the combination therapy, raises the possibility that aspirin enhances recanalization and/or prevents coronary reocclusion after spontaneous or streptokinase-induced recanalization. Indeed, there is a 5 to 20% risk of thrombotic reocclusion of the infarct-related artery after thrombolytic recanalization, which may be diminished by aggressive antithrombotic intervention as suggested by experimental studies.[169] These beneficial effects of aspirin, streptokinase, or both remained significant after a median of 15 months of follow-up.

Chronic Myocardial Infarction

The value of aspirin in various doses, aspirin in combination with dipyridamole, and sulfinpyrazone alone for secondary prevention following a myocardial infarction was assessed in several trials.[145] No clear definitive benefit was demonstrated for any of the three platelet inhibitor regimens from any single study. However, in a meta-analysis of these randomized trials,[145] platelet inhibitors as a class of agents reduced vascular mortality by 13% and nonfatal reinfarction by 31%. No apparent significant differences were noted among the various platelet inhibitor drug regimens or dosages. Aspirin alone appeared as effective as the combination of aspirin and dipyridamole, although the benefits of sulfinpyrazone were less striking.

Chronic Coronary Heart Disease

For patients with documented coronary heart disease and a stable anginal syndrome, the preliminary results of a 5-year angiographic follow-up trial recently completed at the Mayo Clinic suggest that the combination of aspirin and dipyridamole may reduce the incidence of myocardial infarction and prevent the development of new lesions.[158] Thus, patients with chronic stable coronary heart disease may also benefit from platelet inhibitors.

Primary Prevention of Coronary Heart Disease

In patients without overt evidence of coronary heart disease, the use of platelet inhibitors for primary prevention is controversial. The results of a double-blind, placebo-controlled trial of aspirin, 325 mg every other day versus placebo, involving 22,701 physicians in the United States[170] showed a 47% reduction in the incidence of myocardial infarction over a period of 4 to 8 years.

Total cardiovascular mortality, on the other hand, was *not reduced*, because the use of aspirin was associated with a slightly increased risk of hemorrhagic stroke. In another 5-year primary prevention trial involving 5,139 British physicians,[171] the group taking aspirin, 500 mg daily, had about the same rate of myocardial infarction and total cardiovascular death as the group instructed to avoid aspirin. Again, there was a slight increase in disabling stroke among those taking aspirin. Thus, the value of aspirin for primary prevention is less clear in terms of reducing cardiovascular mortality, although myocardial infarction may be reduced, but with an associated higher risk of hemorrhagic or disabling stroke.

Coronary Angioplasty

Coronary angioplasty is also discussed in Chapter 17.

Therapeutic atherosclerotic plaque rupture during coronary angioplasty is also associated with thrombus formation with and without thrombotic vessel occlusion. Thus, platelet inhibitors are indicated for preventing these thrombotic occlusions and associated myocardial infarctions, and treatment with these drugs should preferably be started before the procedure. Two randomized, placebo-controlled trials[153,154] have convincingly shown that the combination of aspirin and dipyridamole can significantly decrease the incidence of myocardial infarction during the periprocedural period. In the study of the Montreal Heart Institute and the Toronto General Hospital involving 376 patients,[153] there was a 77% reduction in the incidence of periprocedural Q wave infarction in those treated with aspirin, 990 mg daily, and dipyridamole, 225 mg daily, as opposed to the placebo group (1.6 versus 6.9%). However, the 6-month angiographic restenosis rate was not significantly altered by the platelet inhibitors, being 39% in the treated group and 38% in the placebo group. The other North American multicenter randomized study[154] allocated patients to aspirin, 650 mg daily, combined with dipyridamole, 225 mg daily; ticlopidine, 750 mg daily; or placebo. The acute periprocedural complication rate was again reduced by 64% (14 versus 5%) by aspirin with dipyridamole, and it was reduced by 86% (14 versus 2%) by ticlopidine, a potent experimental platelet inhibitor not yet commercially available in the United States. Here again, neither the combination of aspirin with dipyridamole nor ticlopidine was effective in reducing the angiographic restenosis rate at 6 months.

Saphenous Vein Coronary Artery Bypass Grafting

Saphenous vein coronary artery bypass grafting is also discussed in Chapter 18.

In patients undergoing saphenous vein coronary artery bypass graft surgery, thrombotic occlusion of the vein graft is an important cause of early graft failure. Thrombosis of the vein graft is thought to be due to the endothelial injury that occurs during vein harvesting and preparation, anastomotic suturing, and the subsequent exposure to the pulsatile high-pressure arterial circulation. The value of using platelet inhibitors starting in the preoperative or immediately postoperative period has been documented in several trials.[149,155–157] The use of platelet inhibitors 48 hours or more after surgery is not of value. The Mayo Clinic Study[155,156] has shown that dipyridamole, 400 mg daily, for 2 days preoperatively, followed by aspirin, 975 mg daily, and dipyridamole, 225 mg daily, starting 7 hours postoperatively, was effective in reducing early and late vein graft occlusion up to 1 year after operation. These results have been confirmed by other studies, which have also shown that aspirin alone at 325 mg daily or 975 mg daily may also improve graft survival.[149,157] However, in these latter trials, the benefit to grafts at high risk of occlusion, i.e., those with a blood flow slower than 40 ml/min or those anastomosed to coronary arteries less than 1.5 mm in diameter was less obvious[172] than in the Mayo Trial. In addition, prevention of new vein graft occlusion from 1 month to 1 year after operation was better achieved with the combination of aspirin and dipyridamole.[155,156,173] The combination of high-dose dipyridamole (400 mg daily) and low-dose aspirin (50 mg daily) has recently been shown to be effective in preventing

vein graft occlusion early and late after operation and in preventing new vein graft occlusion beyond the early phase.[173] A recently published Spanish study[174] has shown that a combination of low-dose aspirin (150 mg daily) and dipyridamole (225 mg daily) is also beneficial in preventing early vein graft occlusion and that this combination appears to be better than the low dose of aspirin (150 mg daily) alone. Furthermore, in trials in which aspirin was administered preoperatively,[149] bleeding complications were more common than in trials in which dipyridamole was administered before surgery[155,156,174] followed by aspirin 7 hours after surgery. Sulfinpyrazone was less effective than aspirin or aspirin combined with dipyridamole in preventing graft occlusion, and its use was further complicated by the development of transient renal insufficiency in about 5% of patients.[149]

Late graft failure (beyond 1 year of surgery) is probably multifactorial in etiology and is related to the development of graft atherosclerosis. The presence of risk factors for atherosclerosis predisposes to these late failures, and therefore control of risk factors is an important preventive measure. There are currently no published data on the benefit of platelet inhibitors in preventing late graft failures, although thrombotic occlusion of these atheromatous grafts is an important cause of recurrent coronary events in these coronary bypass surgery patients. However, rigorous lipid-lowering measures may be beneficial in preventing late graft failures.[175] Ongoing trials are assessing the value of aspirin, lipid-lowering agents, and their combination in this condition.

ANTITHROMBOTIC DRUGS: ANTICOAGULANTS

Anticoagulants are also discussed in Chapters 11, 12, and 13; and their characteristics are listed in Table 16-8.

Anticoagulants have been successfully used for the prevention and treatment of venous thrombosis. However, their use for the management of coronary heart disease and acute myocardial infarction has been controversial, being met with

Table 16-8. Characteristics of Anticoagulants

	Heparin	*Coumarins (Warfarin)*
Action	Enhances AT-III, inhibits factors XIIa, XIa, IXa, Xa, thrombin	Decrease factors II, VII, IX, X
Route	IV or SC	PO
Onset	Immediate	3–5 days
Drug half-life	90 min	35 hr
Monitoring	aPTT (1.5–2.5 × control)	PT: low intensity (INR, 2.0–3.0), moderate intensity (INR, 3.0–4.5)
Antagonist	Protamine	Vitamin K
Idiosyncratic reactions	Skin and fat necrosis	Thrombocytopenia

Abbreviations: AT-III, antithrombin III; aPTT, activated partial thromboplastin time; PT, prothrombin time; IV, intravenous; SC, subcutaneous; PO, oral.

enthusiasm in the early 1950s[176] and skepticism in the early 1970s,[177] when the results of several randomized studies were negative. There is now a resurgence in the use of anticoagulants in the management of the acute coronary ischemic syndromes, especially with the recognition of the role of thrombin and fibrin in arterial thrombogenesis.

Heparin

The major anticoagulant action of heparin at therapeutic concentrations is to potentiate the inhibition by antithrombin III of the activated clotting factors XIIa, XIa, IXa, Xa, and thrombin.[178] Antithrombin III is a naturally occurring inhibitor whose activity is accelerated subsequent to its conformational change induced by heparin binding. Heparin has an additional inhibitory effect on thrombin by its binding, at higher concentrations, to heparin cofactor II.[179] A third and clinically minor anticoagulant effect of heparin involves the inhibition of prothrombin by factor Xa in the absence of antithrombin III and heparin cofactor II.[180]

Heparin also interacts with platelets and may induce both a platelet proaggregatory and an antiaggregatory response.[181] In addition, heparin-associated thrombocytopenia[182] may occur between 6 and 12 days in about 5% of patients treated with heparin, and it may or may not be associated with major arterial thrombosis.[183] It is

not dose-related, and it rapidly resolves following cessation of heparin therapy. This condition is characterized by the presence of an elevated level of platelet immunoglobulin G (IgG) and the presence of a platelet-aggregating factor. The platelet-inhibitory effect of heparin may account for its prolongation of bleeding time in normal volunteers and may contribute to the hemorrhagic complications of heparin treatment, independent of its anticoagulant effects.[180]

Commercially available heparin is a heterogeneous mixture of low and high molecular weight sulfated polysaccharide fragments obtained from beef lung or pork mucosa. It appears that the low molecular weight fragments may be as antithrombotic as standard heparin, but with fewer bleeding complications because of their lesser platelet-inhibitory effects and lesser platelet-dependent thrombin generation.[180] All the heparin fragments are highly negatively charged and must be given intravenously or subcutaneously. In case of toxicity, the effect of heparin can be reversed by the administration of the positively charged protamine sulfate. The rapid onset of action of heparin, combined with its half-life of about 90 minutes, makes it an attractive drug for short-term and acute use. It is cleared mainly by the liver (80%) and the kidneys (20%).

The safest and most effective method of monitoring heparin therapy is through the use of the activated partial thromboplastin time (aPTT). The degree of anticoagulation or prolongation of the aPTT aimed for is 1.5 to 2 times the preheparin control value, and this appears to correlate well with efficacy. The actual heparin levels can also be measured by protamine sulfate titration, aiming for a level of 0.3 to 0.5 units/mm.

Oral Anticoagulants (Vitamin K Antagonists)

The oral anticoagulants, or vitamin K antagonists, do not have direct action on the blood coagulation system but inhibit the hepatic synthesis of normal vitamin K-dependent clotting factors II, VII, IX, and X and also of proteins C and S.[184] These anticoagulants work by preventing the vitamin K-dependent postribosomal gamma-carboxylation of glutamic acid residues located on these coagulation factors, a process necessary for the effective participation of these factors in the coagulation process.[185] Thus, the levels of the normal procoagulants fall with therapy as a function of their half-life, which is shortest for factor VII. As a result, an anticoagulant effect occurs within 24 hours as a result of factor VII decrease, but the full anticoagulant effect may not appear until 72 to 96 hours later, when factors IX, X, and II, with longer half-lives, become depleted.[186] Although the rate of decrease of factor VII is dependent on the loading dose, this is not the case for factors IX, X, and II. A loading dose of a vitamin K antagonist should therefore be avoided, as it may prolong the prothrombin time (PT) without achieving adequate anticoagulation, which occurs by 72 to 96 hours. In addition, the concomitant depletion of protein C (which has a half-life as short as that of factor VII) during the first day of treatment may increase the thrombogenic risk, as protein C is a natural anticoagulant.

The oral anticoagulants are structurally similar to vitamin K and comprise the indanediones and the coumarins. Warfarin (coumadin) is the most commonly used coumarin because of its predictable onset and duration of action and its excellent bioavailability. The mean half-life of a single dose is 35 hours, and its metabolism and excretion are affected by concomitant drug therapy and disease processes. The drug is highly albumin bound (99%); therefore, drugs that displace its binding to albumin can markedly enhance its anticoagulant effect by increasing the level of the free and active drug. The use of a 3- to 5-day overlap of heparin and warfarin may protect the patient against thrombus extension until the levels of factors IX, X, and II are reduced acceptably.

Use of the PT is the accepted method of monitoring warfarin anticoagulation. However, because of the differential sensitivities of the thromboplastin reagents being used in North America (less sensitive rabbit brain thromboplastin) and Europe (more sensitive human brain thromboplastin), a higher dose of warfarin was generally used for anticoagulation in North America, with an unnecessarily higher bleeding risk, without higher protection. As a result, an international normalized ratio (INR) was recommended to standardize warfarin monitoring.[187] With the INR, the patient's PT is normalized to the human brain thromboplastin equivalent by a sensitivity index reflecting the thromboplastin actually utilized. A low-intensity anticoagulation now refers to an INR between 2 and 3.0 (PT 1.3 to 1.5 times control values) and moderate anticoagulation to an INR between 3.0 and 4.5 (PT 1.5 to 2.0 times control values).

Unstable Angina

Two large randomized trials have now shown the efficacy of anticoagulants in the management of patients with unstable angina (Table 16-9). Telford and Wilson[188] showed an 80% reduction in the occurrence of myocardial infarction (from 15 to 3%) in patients with unstable angina randomized to heparin therapy for 7 days. All patients were then treated with warfarin after 7 days, and at 7 weeks the beneficial effects of heparin were still maintained. However, in that study, about half of the originally randomized patients were excluded from analysis for various reasons. Nevertheless, similar beneficial effects of heparin were demonstrated in the Montreal Heart Institute study, where Théroux et al.[168] showed an 85% decrease in myocardial infarction in patients with unstable angina randomized to heparin as opposed to placebo (1.2 versus 7.5%, $P < 0.001$). As mentioned earlier, in this study aspirin alone also significantly reduced fatal and

Table 16-9. Effect of Heparin in Unstable Angina

	Telford and Wilson[188]		Théroux et al.[168]	
	Heparin	No Heparin	Heparin	No Heparin
Number of patients	100	114	240	239
Duration of heparin therapy (days)	7	—	6	—
Mortality (%)	0	1.7	0	0.8
Myocardial infarction (%)	3.0	14.9	1.2	7.5
Risk reduction (%)	80[a]		85[a]	

[a] $P < 0.05$.

nonfatal myocardial infarction, with a nonsignificant trend favoring heparin. Heparin was significantly better than aspirin for the control of refractory angina over the 6 days of the study. Surprisingly, the combination of heparin and aspirin conferred no additional benefit over heparin alone, although there was a slight excess of bleeding complications.[168]

Acute Myocardial Infarction

Of the many trials conducted in the late 1960s to assess the efficacy of anticoagulant therapy in the management of acute myocardial infarction, only three were sufficiently large to detect a true treatment effect (Table 16-10). In the Medical Research Council[189] study involving 1,427 patients, oral anticoagulation with phenindione to maintain an INR of 2.0 to 2.5 decreased mortality by 10% relative to control (16.2 versus 18%, not significant) and reinfarction by 25% (9.7 versus 13.0%, not significant). In the Bronx Municipal Hospital study[190] involving 1,136 patients, mor-

tality was 30% lower (14.9 versus 21.2%, $P < 0.05$) in those treated with initial heparin followed by oral phenindione as opposed to control patients. The reinfarction rate was similar (11.8 versus 13%, not significant) in the two groups of patients, however. The Veterans Administration Cooperative trial[191] randomized 999 patients to initial heparin followed by warfarin, to maintain an INR of 2.0 to 2.5, or to placebo. There was a nonsignificant reduction in both mortality (9.6 versus 11.2%, 14% reduction) and reinfarction (3.4 versus 4.8%, 29% reduction) in the treated group. Thus, only one of the three studies showed a significant reduction in mortality, although a trend toward reduction was seen in the other two. A trend toward a lower reinfarction rate was also observed in the three studies. However, a consistent and significant reduction in mortality of 21 to 22% (confidence interval, −8 to −35%, $P < 0.001$) was seen when the results of all randomized trials were pooled into a meta-analysis.[192]

In the recently completed Warfarin Re-Infarction Study (WARIS),[193] 1,214 patients were ran-

Table 16-10. Effect of Anticoagulants in Acute Myocardial Infarction

Study	Drug	Number of Patients	Year	Mortality			Reinfarction			Pulmonary Embolism			Systemic Embolism		
				Drug (%)	Placebo (%)	RR (%)	Drug (%)	Placebo (%)	RR (%)	Drug (%)	Placebo (%)	RR (%)	Drug (%)	Placebo (%)	RR (%)
MRC[189]	Phenindione	1,427	1967	16.2	18	10	9.7	13.0	25	2.2	5.6	61[a]	1.3	3.4	62[a]
Bronx[190]	Phenindione	1,136	1972	14.9	21.2	30[a]	11.8	13.0	9	3.8	6.1	38	1.7	2.3	26
Veterans[191]	Warfarin	999	1973	9.6	11.2	14	3.4	4.8	29	0.2	2.6	92[a]	0.8	5.4	85[a]

[a] $P < 0.05$.
Abbreviation: RR, risk reduction.

domized to warfarin to maintain an INR of 2.8 to 4.8, or to placebo. At an average follow-up of 37 months, there was a 24% reduction in mortality (15.5 versus 20.3%, $P < 0.027$) and a 34% reduction in reinfarction (13.5 versus 20.4%, $P < 0.0007$) in those receiving oral anticoagulants as opposed to those receiving placebo. In addition, there was a significant (55%) reduction in total cerebrovascular accidents in the warfarin group. These data, combined with the previous demonstration of a significant decrease in pulmonary and systemic embolism in treated patients,[184–191] would make anticoagulant therapy a valuable and effective option after myocardial infarction. However its generalized use has been tempered by its hemorrhagic risk, the need for PT monitoring, and, most importantly, the availability of alternative antithrombotic therapy with platelet-inhibitor drugs. When prophylaxis is required against both coronary events, pulmonary or systemic thromboembolism, and left ventricular thrombosis, the documented benefits of anticoagulants outweigh these inconveniences.

The value of heparin in the management of acute myocardial infarction in the thrombolytic era is unclear. There are data to suggest that the patency rate may be improved with the concomitant use of intravenous heparin[194]; however, it is unclear whether this will translate into improved mortality or ventricular function. The recently completed GISSI-2 trial[117] has not shown that subcutaneous heparin begun 12 hours after thrombolytic therapy provided any benefit in mortality reduction, although bleeding complications were increased. The results of the ISIS-3 trial, investigating the usefulness of heparin in conjunction with t-PA, streptokinase, or APSAC, may clarify this issue. The GUSTO trial is also planning to address the value of heparin in the thrombolytic era.

Coronary Angioplasty

Coronary angioplasty is also discussed in Chapter 17.

Animal studies suggest that thrombin may be an important mediator of the acute thrombotic complications in the periangioplasty period,[195]

and heparin is routinely given during coronary angioplasty. In addition, heparin has been shown to inhibit smooth muscle cell proliferation in animal models,[196] but it is unclear whether long-term heparin or low molecular weight heparin use in humans will be effective in reducing the restenosis problem after angioplasty. Heparin given for up to 24 hours after angioplasty has not influenced the restenosis rate in humans.[197]

Saphenous Vein Coronary Artery Bypass Grafting

Saphenous vein coronary artery bypass grafting is also discussed in Chapter 18.

Oral anticoagulants appear as effective as antiplatelet drug therapy for the prevention of vein graft occlusion after surgery.[173] However, they cannot be used until after surgery, and their use is associated with an increased bleeding risk as compared with platelet-inhibitor drug therapy.[173]

LIPID-LOWERING DRUGS: RATIONALE FOR LOWERING BLOOD CHOLESTEROL LEVELS

Lipid-lowering drugs are also discussed in Chapters 5, 11, 12, and 13.

Coronary heart disease mortality in the United States has decreased steadily since 1968, and more than half of this decline has been attributed to better control of hypercholesterolemia, cigarette smoking, and hypertension.[198] Although the cause of coronary atherosclerosis is multifactorial, evidence from different sources clearly implicates elevated blood cholesterol levels as playing a central role in atherogenesis. Epidemiologic studies[199] documented a close correlation between blood cholesterol levels and coronary heart disease incidences. Subsequently, clinical trials documented that interventions to ameliorate blood lipoprotein levels reduced the incidence of coronary endpoints.

Lipid Research Clinics Coronary Primary Prevention Trial

The clinical trials have been reviewed in more detail elsewhere[200] and will be mentioned only briefly here. The Lipid Research Clinics Coronary Primary Prevention Trial was a multicenter, randomized, double-blind study to test the efficacy of cholesterol lowering in reducing the coronary heart disease incidence in 3,806 asymptomatic, middle-aged men with primary hypercholesterolemia.[201] Cholestyramine, 24 g/day, reduced LDL cholesterol levels during the 7.4 years of the study by an average of 20%, 12.6% more than the reduction achieved by diet alone in the placebo group. The cumulative 7-year incidence of the primary endpoint, definite coronary death or definite nonfatal infarction, was 7% in the cholestyramine group and 8.6% in the placebo group ($P < 0.05$). This 19% reduction was accompanied by 25, 20, and 21% reductions in the incidence rates for new positive exercise tests, angina, and coronary bypass surgery, respectively. Total mortality was not significantly different in the two groups.

Helsinki Heart Study

The Helsinki Heart Study was a 5-year, randomized, double-bind trial to assess the efficacy of simultaneously elevating HDL cholesterol and lowering non-HDL cholesterol with gemfibrozil in reducing the risk of coronary heart disease.[202] Slightly more than 4,000 asymptomatic men aged 40 to 59 with non-HDL cholesterol levels greater than 200 mg/dL were allocated to placebo or 600 mg of gemfibrozil twice daily. Gemfibrozil lowered total and LDL cholesterol levels by approximately 8% and increased HDL cholesterol levels by 10 to 14% throughout the trial. The cumulative rate of coronary endpoints, cardiac death or myocardial infarction, was 2.7% in the gemfibrozil group and 4.1% in the placebo group at 5 years, a reduction of 34% (95% confidence intervals, 8 to 53%; $P < 0.02$). There was no difference in total mortality between the groups. Taken together, these two trials provide compelling evidence that pharmacologic therapy of hypercholesterolemia

reduces the incidence of coronary disease, at least for the type of person under study. The absence of a statistically significant effect upon total mortality is not surprising because this endpoint is relatively uncommon in asymptomatic middle-aged men; it is diluted with noncoronary deaths, and the duration of the intervention was relatively short compared with the entire period over which coronary atherosclerosis evolves.

Coronary Drug Project

Evidence from the Coronary Drug Project, however, suggests that effective treatment of hypercholesterolemia will eventually have a favorable impact on mortality.[203] This study, initiated in the late 1960s, enrolled 8,341 survivors of myocardial infarction in 53 clinical centers to five different drug therapies.[204] Three of these, estrogen at two doses and dextrothyroxine, were discontinued prematurely because of excessive drug-related morbidity and mortality. One of the remaining drugs, clofibrate, reduced cholesterol levels marginally at the expense of an array of serious adverse effects, including an increased incidence of angina, thromboembolism, claudication, cardiac arrhythmias, and gallstones.

The remaining medication, niacin, reduced serum cholesterol levels by 10% and significantly reduced the 5-year incidence of definite, nonfatal myocardial infarction by 27% (from 12.2 to 8.9%).[204] In spite of this benefit, total mortality rates at 5 years, and at a mean follow-up of 6.2 years when niacin treatment was discontinued, were nearly identical in the two groups. However, after a mean follow-up of 15 years, nearly 9 years after termination of the trial, mortality in the niacin-treated group was 11% lower than in the placebo group (52 versus 58.2%, $P < 0.0004$).

The clinical endpoints used in the aforementioned trials, coronary death and myocardial infarction, are the final consequences of progression of coronary atherosclerosis. In asymptomatic subjects and even in patients with known coronary disease, these events are infrequent. Thus, testing the effect of cholesterol lowering by using these endpoints is very expensive because many subjects must be followed for at least 5 years to detect a benefit from the intervention. Using coronary angiographic endpoints to assess interventions greatly reduces the number of patients required and also somewhat shortens the needed length of the observation period per patient.

NHLBI Type II Coronary Intervention Study

In the National Heart, Lung, and Blood Institute (NHLBI) Type II Coronary Intervention Study,[205] 116 hypercholesterolemic patients with coronary atherosclerosis at coronary angiography were randomized to placebo or cholestyramine treatment and underwent repeat angiography after 5 years. LDL cholesterol levels decreased by 26% in patients treated with the resin and by 5% in control subjects. During the 5 years, coronary atherosclerosis progressed in 32% of the cholestyramine-treated patients and 49% of the control subjects ($P < 0.05$). When the results were examined independently of treatment assignment, reduction in LDL cholesterol levels and increases in HDL cholesterol levels correlated inversely with the risk of athersclerotic progression.

Cholesterol-Lowering Atherosclerosis Study

The Cholesterol-Lowering Atherosclerosis Study (CLAS) was a randomized, placebo-controlled, angiographic trial testing combined colestipol and niacin treatment in 162 nonsmoking men aged 40 to 59 years who had had previous coronary bypass surgery.[206] During 2 years of therapy, impressive modifications in lipid profiles were obtained: a 26% reduction in total plasma cholesterol, a 43% reduction in LDL cholesterol, and a 37% elevation in HDL cholesterol. The average number of lesions per patient that progressed and the percentage of subjects with new atheroma in native coronary arteries were significantly smaller in the drug treatment group. Treatment also decreased the percentage of patients with new coronary bypass graft lesions or an adverse change in coronary bypass graft status.

Regression of atherosclerosis occurred in 16.2% of colestipol–niacin-treated patients versus 2.4% of placebo-treated patients ($P < 0.002$).

Of the 162 original CLAS patients, 103 continued in a 2-year extension of the trial.[207] The favorable lipid changes were maintained, and the angiographic outcomes at four years, compared with baseline, were more impressive than the 2-year results reported in the original paper. The average number of coronary lesions that progressed was 0.9 per patient in the drug treatment group compared with 2.0 per patient in control subjects. New lesions in native arteries were found in 12.5% of drug-treated patients and 40.4% of placebo-treated patients. Drug therapy also significantly reduced the percentage of subjects with new coronary bypass graft lesions. In summary, the divergence between the two groups noted at 2 years had widened at 4 years.

Familial Atherosclerosis Treatment Study

The results of the recently completed Familial Atherosclerosis Treatment Study (FATS)[208] confirm and extend the results of CLAS. Men 62 years old or younger with documented coronary disease, a family history of premature cardiovascular events, and apolipoprotein B levels of at least 125 mg/dL were studied in FATS. All underwent baseline coronary angiography and dietary counseling. In a blinded fashion, patients were randomized to niacin, 4 g/day, plus colestipol, 30 g/day; to lovastatin, 40 mg/day, plus colestipol; or to placebo with the addition of colestipol as required. Coronary angiography was repeated after 2.5 years and the angiograms were interpreted using quantitative methodology.

The results of FATS are summarized in Table 16-11. The combination of lovastatin and colestipol reduced LDL cholesterol levels by 46% and increased HDL cholesterol levels by 15%. Niacin plus colestipol reduced LDL cholesterol levels somewhat less, by 32%, but increased HDL cholesterol levels by 43%. The conventionally treated group experienced only minor improvements in their lipid profiles, and their mean percentage coronary stenosis increased.

Table 16-11.   Results of the Familial Atherosclerosis Treatment Study[208]

Treatment Group	Number of Patients	% Change in Cholesterol		Mean Change in % Stenosis	Number of Patients with Only		Number of Patients with Coronary Events
		LDL	HDL		Progression	Regression	
Placebo ± colestipol	46	−7	+5	+2.1 ± 3.9	21	5	11
Lovastatin + colestipol	38	−46[a]	+15[a]	−0.7 ± 5.3[a]	8	12[a]	3[a]
Niacin + colestipol	36	−32[a]	+43[a]	−0.9 ± 3.0[a]	9	14[a]	2[a]

[a] $P < 0.05$ versus placebo group.

In contrast, the mean changes in percentage coronary stenosis in the two intensively treated groups were in the direction of regression and were significantly different from those in the conventionally treated group. The criterion for progression or regression of individual lesions was a stenosis diameter change of at least 10%. Regression occurred in 4 of 37 conventionally treated patients, 13 of 34 patients treated with lovastatin plus colestipol, and 15 of 32 patients treated with niacin plus colestipol.

Although only 120 patients were evaluated in FATS and the study lasted only 2.5 years, the two intensively treated groups experienced significantly fewer coronary events (3 and 2, compared with 11 in the control group). Death, proven myocardial infarction, and new refractory ischemic symptoms requiring revascularization were counted as coronary events. That the groups treated with lovastatin and niacin experienced not only a better angiographic outcome but also fewer clinical events increases the impact of the study and confirms the relevance of using angiographic changes as surrogate endpoints.

DETECTION OF HYPERLIPIDEMIA AND DIETARY TREATMENT

The National Cholesterol Education Program Expert Panel has published guidelines on the detection, evaluation, and treatment of hypercholesterolemia in adults.[209] The total cholesterol level in serum should be measured in all adults every 5 years. A total cholesterol level below 200 mg/dL is ideal and requires no further attention unless the HDL cholesterol is very low, i.e., below 30 to 35 mg/dL. In the absence of definite coronary disease or two other risk factors, a total cholesterol between 200 and 239 mg/dL should be rechecked annually and the patient should be given dietary advice. A fasting lipoprotein analysis is indicated if the screening test shows a total cholesterol level of 240 mg/dL or more, or 200 mg/dL or more in a patient with known coronary disease or at least two risk factors.

An LDL cholesterol level below 130 mg/dL is ideal and an LDL cholesterol level from 130 to 160 mg/dL is borderline. Dietary treatment is indicated for coronary patients or those with two or more risk factors with a borderline LDL cholesterol level and for other subjects with an LDL cholesterol level between 150 and 190 mg/dL. Drug therapy is recommended for all individuals with an LDL cholesterol level of 190 mg/dL or more and for coronary patients and those with two or more risk factors with an LDL cholesterol level of 160 mg/dL or more. The components of step I and step II diets are listed in Table 16-12. Total cholesterol should be rechecked at 6 weeks and 3 months after starting the step I diet. The goal of therapy is to reduce the LDL cholesterol level below 130 mg/dL for patients with coronary disease or multiple risk factors and below 160 mg/dL for others. A step II diet should be instituted if the goal of therapy is not attained with a step I diet. Drug therapy should be reserved for

Table 16-12.   National Cholesterol Education
Program Diets

Dietary Component	Diet	
	Step I	Step II
Total fat (% of total calories)	<30	<30
Saturated fatty acids (% of total calories)	<10	<7
Polyunsaturated fatty acids (% of total calories)	≤10	≤10
Monounsaturated fatty acids (% of total calories)	10–15	10–15
Dietary cholesterol (mg/day)	<300	<200
Protein (% of total calories)	10–20	10–20
Carbohydrates (% of total calories)	50–60	50–60

individuals who do not attain their LDL cholesterol targets with diet, but can be introduced sooner if the LDL cholesterol level is very high (higher than 225 mg/dL).

Bile Acid-Sequestering Agents

Cholestyramine or colestipol is recommended as the initial therapy to lower LDL cholesterol levels.[209–211] These drugs are nonabsorbable anion exchange resins that bind bile acids in the intestine to prevent their reabsorption. The cholesterol synthesized by the liver is either excreted into the circulation as lipoprotein or converted to bile acids; by interfering with the recycling of bile acids, these drugs increase the number of hepatic LDL receptors and decrease the serum LDL cholesterol level.

Gastrointestinal side effects are common with bile acid sequestrants, but are dose-related. Modest doses of these agents, 4 to 12 g/day of cholestyramine or 5 to 15 g/day of colestipol, are more likely to be tolerated and still induce significant reductions in LDL cholesterol levels. Therapy should be begun at lower levels than this, however, and be gradually increased. The use of this class of drugs is particularly attractive in younger hypercholesterolemic individuals without coronary disease, for whom therapy is likely to be required for several decades, because long-term

safety is well documented and because these drugs were used in the early positive clinical trials.[201,205,206]

Nicotinic Acid

Nicotinic acid lowers total and LDL cholesterol and triglyceride levels and raises HDL cholesterol levels. Its use in the Coronary Drug Project was associated with a long-term survival benefit.[203] The major limitation of this drug is that it induces marked flushing, which tends to decrease with continuing treatment. This prostaglandin-mediated response can be attenuated with aspirin. Hyperuricemia and abnormal liver function tests are common at higher dose levels.

Nicotinic acid should be initiated at a dose of 100 mg tid and increased gradually to at least 1 g tid; doses up to 2 g tid can be used if the initial response is not adequate. Peptic ulcer, gout, and hepatic disease are contraindications to its use. The combination of a bile acid sequestrant and nicotinic acid is commonly used in patients whose response to one drug is suboptimal.

HMG CoA Reductase Inhibitors

Lovastatin is a competitive inhibitor of the rate-limiting enzyme for cholesterol synthesis, 3-hydroxy-3-methylglutaryl coenzyme A reductase (HMG CoA reductase). Simvastatin and pravastatin are newer drugs in this class that, unlike lovastatin, have not yet been approved for clinical use. These drugs not only reduce endogenous cholesterol production but also increase hepatic LDL receptor activity. This class of drugs represents a major advance in the treatment of hypercholesterolemia because it not only produces greater decreases in LDL cholesterol levels than the drugs discussed in the previous section but does so with minimal side effects.[212]

The dose of lovastatin ranges from 20 to 80 mg/day but is usually 20 to 40 mg/day. At the upper end of this dose range, it will lower LDL cholesterol levels by an average of 40% and produce mild increases in HDL cholesterol levels and some lowering of triglyceride levels. Asymptomatic elevations of levels of hepatic enzymes or creatine kinase and myositis are the commonest side effects, occurring in fewer than 4% of patients. In combination with nicotinic acid or gemfibrozil, lovastatin may induce severe rhabdomyolysis (although this is rare); however, in general, lovastatin can be used with other lipid-lowering drugs.

If the long-term safety of lovastatin were already demonstrated, HMG CoA reductase inhibitors would be the initial drug of choice for hypercholesterolemia. It has been argued that in patients with coronary events, lovastatin should be prescribed as part of the initial therapy to induce a rapid, marked fall in LDL cholesterol levels.[213]

Gemfibrozil

Gemfibrozil is a fibric acid derivative that induces only a minor decrease in LDL cholesterol levels but increases HDL cholesterol levels by 10 to 20%. In the Helsinki Heart Study,[202] the administration of this drug was associated with a significant reduction in initial coronary events. Gemfibrozil is often used to decrease triglyceride levels in patients with combined hyperlipidemia, or, as a component of multidrug therapy, to increase HDL cholesterol levels.

Clofibrate, another fibric acid derivative that is available in the United States, is not recommended because it is associated with an increased risk of cholelithiasis.

Probucol

Probucol has been available in the United States since 1977 but is unpopular because it reduces HDL cholesterol levels by up to 25%, with only mild decreases in LDL cholesterol levels. The mechanism by which probucol lowers LDL cholesterol levels is uncertain but is probably independent of LDL receptors.[210] Probucol is a potent antioxidant agent. Oxidative modification of LDL cholesterol probably enhances its atherogenicity. Probucol retards the progression of atherosclerosis in rabbits independently of its effect on serum LDL cholesterol levels; however, such a salutary effect has not yet been demonstrated in humans.

Probucol is usually well tolerated, although it can cause headache, gastrointestinal disturbances, and mild QT interval prolongation. The usual dose is 500 mg bid. This drug is not first-line therapy for hypercholesterolemia; indeed, it is infrequently used at present.

DRUGS FOR THE TREATMENT OF HEART FAILURE

Drugs for the treatment of heart failure are also discussed in Chapters 11, 12, and 13.

Digitalis

Digitalis has been used to treat heart failure for more than 200 years, but its precise role is still a subject of debate.[214] Digitalis binds to and inhibits sodium potassium adenosine triphosphatase (ATPase) in the sarcolemmal membrane of the cardiac myocyte.[215] The intracellular sodium that tends to accumulate as a result of this inhibition is exchanged for calcium. Increased intracellular calcium levels increase contractility because more calcium is available to the contractile elements, actin and myosin.

In patients with chronic congestive heart failure, digitalis improves cardiac performance.[216] There is long-term improvement, and hemodynamic deterioration is seen after digitalis withdrawal.[216] Clinical improvement in heart failure symptoms can be expected when systolic dysfunction predominates, particularly if a third heart sound is present.[217] However, the degree of improvement is generally modest for patients in sinus rhythm, and the drug is of little benefit when heart failure is secondary to cor pulmonale or acute myocardial infarction. When valvular heart disease associated with uncontrolled atrial fibrillation was the most common cause of heart failure, digitalis established its reputation; the combined benefit of positive inotropy and slowing of the rapid ventricular rate produced much more improvement than is seen in patients with sinus rhythm.

On the basis of retrospective analysis of large data bases,[218] concern has been raised that digitalis may actually increase mortality in patients with heart failure, particularly survivors of myocardial infarction. A randomized, placebo-controlled trial has been initiated to settle this question. The margin between a therapeutic and a toxic dose level is narrower for digitalis than for any other cardiovascular drug. Adverse reactions to digitalis have been reported in 5 to 15% of hospitalized patients receiving the drug.[215] Anorexia, nausea, and vomiting are the most common noncardiac side effects; heart block and triggered arrhythmias such as junctional tachycardia or ventricular tachycardia are the serious complications seen with life-threatening digitalis toxicity.

Other Inotropic Drugs

The intravenous administration of inotropic drugs such as beta-adrenergic agonists and phosphodiesterase inhibitors improves hemodynamic measurements in both acute and chronic heart failure. Both of these classes of drugs are very useful in clinical situations in which heart failure is expected to be transient, such as after cardiac surgery. However, their role in the treatment of chronic heart failure has not been definitively established.

The phosphodiesterase inhibitors, amrinone, milrinone, and enoximone, increase cAMP levels and thus increase intracellular calcium entry to improve myocardial contractility. These drugs are also potent vasodilators and thus increase cardiac output by two mechanisms. However, these beneficial effects do not appear to translate to clinical improvement with chronic therapy. Packer et al.[219] reported that long-term oral amrinone treatment appeared to accelerate the progression of left ventricular dysfunction, exacerbate myocardial ischemia, and provoke life-threatening arrhythmias. In a controlled drug withdrawal trial, DiBianco et al. found that oral amrinone added no hemodynamic benefit to standard therapy[220] and later reported that oral mil-

rinone offered no advantage over digoxin.[221] More recently, oral enoximone was shown to produce no beneficial long-term hemodynamic effect in chronic heart failure, and more ominously, the mortality rate was higher with enoximone than placebo.[222]

Theoretically beta-adrenergic stimulation probably also exerts an unfavorable influence on the long-term evolution of chronic heart failure.[223] In fact, evidence from the postinfarction beta-blocking drug trials and small uncontrolled and controlled studies suggest that long-term beta-adrenergic blockade may improve survival in chronic heart failure. Larger studies have been initiated to test this hypothesis, but, for the moment, neither beta-adrenergic stimulation nor beta-blockade is definitively indicated for chronic heart failure.

Diuretic Drugs

Diuretic drugs are the cornerstone of therapy for chronic congestive heart failure. Renal blood flow decreases in early heart failure, so the filtration fraction increases and renal tubular sodium reabsorption is enhanced. Diuretic drugs counteract this process by increasing renal sodium and water output.

A selection of the more commonly used diuretic drugs, their dose ranges, and their duration of action are listed in Table 16-13. Diuretic drugs are used in heart failure to eliminate or prevent edema and to decrease dyspnea. A mild diuretic drug such as a thiazide is appropriate for mild heart failure. Most patients with more severe heart failure are treated with loop diuretic drugs, which are more powerful but have a shorter duration of action and thus must often be administered more than once per day. Both of these classes of drugs induce potassium loss that can lead to hypokalemia, a factor that promotes digitalis toxicity. They are therefore often combined with a potassium-sparing diuretic drug in patients with moderate to severe heart failure. Secondary hyperaldosteronism may play a significant role in advanced heart failure, and the potassium-sparing aldosterone antagonist spironolactone is a useful diuretic in this circumstance.

Table 16-13.   Features of Commonly Used Diuretic Drugs

Class of Drug	Generic Name	Daily dose (mg)	Duration of Action (hr)
Thiazide drugs	Chlorothiazide	500–1,500	6–12
	Hydrochlorthiazide	50–150	12–24
	Trichlormethazide	2–4	18–24
	Chlorthalidone	50–100	24–48
Loop diuretic drugs	Ethacrynic acid	25–150	4–6
	Furosemide	20–160	4–6
	Bumetanide	0.5–3	4–6
Carbonic anhydrase inhibitors	Acetazolamide	250–500	8–12
Potassium-sparing diuretic drugs	Spironolactone	50–200	48–72
	Triamterene	100–200	6–8
	Amiloride	5–20	12–24

In acute pulmonary edema, the intravenous administration of furosemide increases venous capacitance and decreases preload within minutes, before the onset of significant diuresis. The end result is a decrease in pulmonary congestion and dyspnea.

Common complications of diuretic drug therapy include volume depletion with fatigue, orthostatic hypotension, and prerenal azotemia; hypo- and hyperkalemia; and metabolic alkalosis. Most diuretic drugs induce hyperuricemia. Thiazide diuretic drugs also increase serum cholesterol and triglyceride levels and have a tendency to provoke or aggravate diabetes. These metabolic consequences of thiazide drugs are particularly worrisome when long-term treatment is envisaged, such as for hypertension.

Angiotensin-Converting Enzyme Inhibitors

Heart failure stimulates production of renin from the juxtaglomerular apparatus of the kidney, and this enzyme cleaves four amino acids from angiotensinogen to form angiotensin I.[224] Angiotensin I is converted to angiotensin II, a potent vasoconstrictor and stimulus for aldosterone secretion. Angiotensin-converting enzyme (ACE) inhibitors thus block both the vasoconstriction and aldosterone-mediated sodium retention caused by angiotensin II.

Captopril, enalapril, and lisinopril were the first drugs of this class to be approved for clinical use in the United States. Because of differences in serum half-lives, captopril should be given three times per day, enalapril twice per day, and lisinopril once daily. Unlike other vasodilator drugs, the dosage of these drugs is relatively easy to titrate because once the converting enzyme is completely inhibited, little further benefit can be achieved by increasing the dose. To avoid side effects due to hypotension, the starting dose should be low, followed by upward titration, if tolerated, to 25 mg tid for captopril, 5 to 10 mg bid for enalapril, and 10 to 20 mg/day for lisinopril.

These drugs reduce arterial pressure, systemic vascular resistance, and left and right atrial pressures and induce a modest increase in cardiac output. Serious adverse reactions are not common with ACE inhibitors; captopril may cause neutropenia, proteinemia, reversible renal failure, cough, and symptoms secondary to hypotension.

The ACE inhibitors are the major drugs used in the treatment of chronic heart failure that have been proven to both ameliorate symptoms and prolong life. A gradual improvement in exercise tolerance can be demonstrated over several weeks.[225] This is accompanied by a reduction in symptoms and an improvement in the quality of life. In the CONSENSUS trial, the administration of enalapril to patients with class IV heart failure reduced mortality compared with the placebo group; by 6 months, 26% of the enalapril group and 44% of the placebo group had died, a reduction of 40% ($P < 0.002$).[226] Whether this benefit would accrue to patients with less severe heart failure or even asymptomatic patients with left ventricular dysfunction is being investigated in the SOLVD trial. Until further results are available, ACE inhibitors should be used to reduce mortality and to improve symptoms in all patients with class III or IV chronic heart failure, but are not routinely indicated for class I or II patients. Diuretic and ACE inhibitor drugs act synergistically in heart failure and should be used in combination in most cases.

Other Vasodilator Drugs

The combination of hydralazine and isosorbide dinitrate reduced mortality in a Veterans Administration study of patients with chronic heart failure.[227] However, dose titration with this combination of drugs cannot be as easily achieved as with ACE inhibitors. As already noted, isosorbide dinitrate induces tolerance unless it is given intermittently and often causes side effects due to vasodilation. The hemodynamically optimal dose of hydralazine in a specific patient can vary from 10 to 150 mg tid. An additional limitation of this drug is its tendency to induce lupuslike symptoms during long-term therapy.

Prazosin, an alpha-adrenergic blocking drug has been extensively investigated for the treatment of chronic heart failure. Marked hemodynamic improvement has been documented after the first dose; however, tolerance develops rapidly in most patients,[228] and long-term controlled trials were not able to document significant benefit.

Even optimal medical therapy is not a very satisfactory approach to the problem of severe heart failure because of the persistent high mortality and often poor quality of life in survivors. In selected cases, cardiac transplantation is the preferred alternative.

ANTIHYPERTENSIVE THERAPY

Antihypertensive therapy is also discussed in Chapter 5.

Rationale for Lowering Arterial Blood Pressure

Epidemiologic studies have demonstrated that cerebrovascular accident, renal insufficiency, heart failure, myocardial infarction, angina pectoris, and coronary heart disease morbidity and mortality increase progressively with each increment in systolic and diastolic blood pressure.[229–231] Long-term clinical trials involving over 50,000 patients have been performed to assess the efficacy of antihypertensive therapy with respect to these endpoints. The incidences of congestive heart failure, renal insufficiency, and, particularly, stroke are significantly reduced by effective therapy when the blood pressure is higher than 140/90 mmHg.[231,232] The effect of treatment for mild to moderate hypertension upon coronary endpoints has been much harder to demonstrate.[232] Diuretic and beta-adrenergic blocking drugs were the most commonly used treatments in these trials, and it is possible that a more substantial benefit with respect to cardiovascular endpoints would be seen with the newer classes of antihypertensive drugs, which do not elevate cholesterol levels.

Hemodynamic Patterns in Essential Hypertension

Systemic vascular resistance is inappropriately elevated in all patients with hypertension. Other hemodynamic abnormalities tend to depend upon the age group studied. In young hypertensive patients, cardiac output is increased in association with increased sympathetic activity; with exercise, cardiac output falls and the expected decrease in systemic vascular resistance is attenuated. In middle-aged hypertensive patients (ages 30 to 60), cardiac output is usually 10 to 15% decreased and systemic vascular resistance is 15 to 20% increased. These abnormalities are usually accentuated in elderly hypertensive individuals, whose cardiac output may be decreased by 25%, with systemic vascular resistances 25% above normal.

Principles of Antihypertensive Therapy

The optimal hemodynamic approach to the treatment of established hypertension is to select a drug that corrects the underlying hemodynamic abnormality, i.e., an increased systemic vascular resistance. The ideal agent would also maintain cardiac output and perfusion to vital organs. Practical issues in drug selection include side-effect profiles and cost.

Beginning in the 1960s, a step-care approach to the treatment of hypertension was recommended, with a diuretic drug as the first drug used in patients without contraindications. Diuretic drugs initially reduce intravascular volume, increase heart rate slightly, and decrease cardiac output by less than 5%. However, after 8 weeks, cardiac output returns to near normal, intravascular volume remains only minimally reduced, and systemic vascular resistance falls.[231] As noted above, diuretic drugs cause hyperuricemia, hyperglycemia, and hypokalemia and have an adverse effect on serum lipid levels. They do not induce regression of left ventricular hypertrophy, as some other antihypertensive agents do, and they may potentiate ventricular arrhythmias.

In the treatment of hypertension, low doses of diuretic drugs are usually as effective as higher doses and are associated with fewer adverse metabolic effects. For example, 95% of the antihypertensive effect of hydrochlorothiazide can be obtained from a dose of only 25 mg/day.[233] Diuretic drugs are much less expensive than other antihypertensive therapy.

Several other classes of drugs reduce systemic vascular resistance without reducing cardiac output. Prazosin, the prototype of the alpha-adrenergic blocking drugs, reduces systemic vascular resistance, with a slight increase in cardiac output and heart rate. This drug also has a favorable effect upon serum lipids, reducing LDL cholesterol levels and increasing HDL cholesterol levels, both by about 10%.[231] The central alpha-adrenergic agonist drugs clonidine, guanabenz, guanfacine, and methyldopa reduce sympathetic nervous system activity, systemic vascular resistance, and heart rate while preserving cardiac output. With the exception of methyldopa, which lowers HDL cholesterol levels, these drugs also exert a favorable effect upon serum lipid profiles. Prazosin and alpha-adrenergic agonist drugs are effective as initial monotherapy in approximately two-thirds of patients.

The direct vasodilator drugs, hydralazine and minoxidil, are not good choices as monotherapy because they increase the heart rate and intravascular volume. The ACE inhibitors preserve or increase cardiac output while reducing systemic vascular resistance. They do not alter serum lipid levels but appear to promote regression of left ventricular hypertrophy more than do many other classes of antihypertensive drugs. Calcium channel-blocking drugs reduce systemic vascular resistance and exert a variable effect upon cardiac output; verapamil produces a decrease, and nifedipine may yield an increase. These drugs have either a neutral or beneficial effect on serum lipid levels. The response rate to ACE inhibitors as monotherapy is also approximately two-thirds, which may be slightly higher than the response rate to dihydropyridine calcium channel-blocking drugs.

In contrast to all of the aforementioned drugs, beta-adrenergic blocking agents reduce blood pressure, but increase systemic vascular resistance by 15 to 20%.[231] These drugs also reduce cardiac output and adversely affect serum lipid levels by reducing HDL cholesterol levels and increasing LDL cholesterol levels. Beta-adrenergic blocking drugs with intrinsic sympathomimetic activity, such as pindolol and acetabulol, reduce systemic vascular resistance and cardiac output slightly and do not exert the same adverse influence on serum lipid levels that other beta-blocking drugs do.

Reserpine, guanethidine, and labetalol reduce both systemic vascular resistance and cardiac output. Reserpine has an adverse effect and labetalol a neutral to adverse effect on serum lipid levels. These three drugs are not ideal antihypertensive agents.

In general, antihypertensive therapy should be tailored to the individual patient, taking into consideration coronary risk factors, concomitant conditions, compliance, cost, potential side effects, drug efficacy, age, and probable underlying hemodynamic abnormality. Combination therapy is required in many patients, and a combination of two drugs at low doses is often preferable to a high dose of one agent. Certain combinations act synergistically and beneficially; for example, the low renin state induced by an ACE inhibitor may enhance the therapeutic response to a calcium channel-blocking drug. Other combinations may increase the risk of adverse effects; for example, beta-blocking drugs, verapamil, and methyldopa all cause bradycardia. In patients whose blood pressure remains controlled on treatment for longer than 6 to 12 months, drugs can often be decreased or totally discontinued with no recurrence of hypertension.[234] Such a response is obviously more likely in mild hypertension without evidence of end organ damage. Patients in whom therapy has been discontinued should be monitored closely for recurrences.

ANTIARRHYTHMIC DRUGS

Antiarrhythmic drugs are also discussed in Chapters 11, 12, and 13.

The number of antiarrhythmic drugs available for the treatment of cardiac arrhythmias has increased dramatically over the past 10 years. All known agents act by blocking cardiac ionic channels and consequently alter the electrophysiologic properties of normal and abnormal cardiac tissue. The current classification of antiarrhythmic drugs is based on the electrophysiologic effects of individual agents on isolated tissue preparations (Table 16-14).[235] Beta-blocking (class II) and calcium antagonist (class IV) drugs have already been discussed in this chapter.

Class I Agents (Sodium Channel-Blocking Drugs)

Class I antiarrhythmic drugs depress the inward sodium current occurring during phase 0 of the action potential of fast channel tissue (atrium, ventricle, accessory pathway) and, as a result, slow the atrial and ventricular conduction. Class I agents can be further subdivided according to the relative potency of each agent, their effects

Table 16-14. Vaughan Williams Classification of Antiarrhythmic Drugs

Class I: Sodium channel-blocking drugs
  IA: Quinidine, procainamide, disopyramide
    Moderate depression of inward sodium current
    Prolongation of action potential duration
    Intermediate speed of dissociation from sodium channels
  IB: Lidocaine, mexiletine, tocainide, moricizine, phenytoin
    Weak depression of inward sodium current
    Shortening of action potential duration
    Rapid dissociation from sodium channels
  IC: Flecainide, encainide, propafenone
    Potent depression of inward sodium current
    Little effect on action potential duration
    Slow dissociation from sodium channels
Class II: Beta-adrenergic blocking drugs
  Propranolol, sotalol, others
Class III: Inhibitors of repolarization
  Amiodarone, sotalol, bretylium
Class IV: Calcium channel-blocking drugs
  Verapamil, diltiazem, nifedipine

on cardiac repolarization, and the kinetics of sodium channel blockade (Table 16-14). The pharmacokinetic properties of class I agents and other antiarrhythmic drugs are listed in Table 16-15.

Class IA Agents (Quinidine, Procainamide, Disopyramide)

Quinidine has been in use for most of this century and is currently the most widely prescribed antiarrhythmic drug in North America. It is effective in suppressing both atrial and ventricular premature contractions and prevents recurrent atrial fibrillation or flutter in about 50% of treated patients.[236] It is also effective in approximately 30% of patients with severe sustained ventricular arrhythmias when assessed with serial electrophysiologic studies.[237]

The most frequent side effects of quinidine therapy are gastrointestinal (principally diarrhea).[238,239] This limits therapy in 15 to 30% of patients but can be minimized by administering the drug with meals. Other rarer but more serious side effects include arrhythmia exacerbation (1 to 3%), thrombocytopenia, fever, and hepatic dysfunction.

Table 16-15. Pharmacokinetics of Antiarrhythmic Drugs

Class	Agent	Dose	Bio-availa-bility	Therapeutic Concentration (μg/mL)	Active Metabolites	Half-life (hr)	Excretion
IA	Quinidine	PO 200–400 mg q 4–6 h	75%	2–7	Yes	6–8	Hepatic, renal
	Procainamide	PO 50 mg/kg/day	83%	4–10	Yes	2–4	Renal
		IV 12 mg/kg L					
		2–6 mg/min M					
	Disopyramide	PO 100–200 mg qid	90%	2–8	No	7	Renal
IB	Lidocaine	IV 1.0–1.5 mg/kg L	<30%	1.5–6	Yes	1–2	Hepatic
		30 μg/kg/min M					
	Mexiletine	PO 100–300 mg tid	80%	0.5–2	No	8–12	Hepatic, renal
	Tocainide	PO 200–400 mg tid	>90%	3–10	No	14	Renal
IC	Flecainide	100–300 mg bid	>90%	0.2–1	No	13–16	Hepatic, renal
	Propafenone	150–300 mg tid	Variable	0.2–3	Yes	3–6	Hepatic
	Encainide	25–50 mg tid	>90%	NA (metabolites)	Yes	2–3 (encainide)	Renal, hepatic
						>12 (metabolites)	
III	Amiodarone	PO 200–600 mg/day	20–40%	1.0–2.5	Yes	30 days	Hepatic
	Sotalol	PO 80–240 mg bid	>90%	0.4–0.9	No	14–20	Renal, hepatic
	Bretylium	IV 5 mg/kg L	<30%	0.5–1.5	No	9	Renal
		1.4 mg/min M					

Abbreviations: L, loading; M, maintenance; NA, not applicable.

Procainamide has been in clinical use for almost 40 years. Indications for its use and associated efficacy are comparable to those of quinidine.[240-242] Long-term treatment with procainamide has been limited by two major problems. Its short half-life (2 to 4 hours) makes frequent dosing necessary, although the recent introduction of longer-acting preparations makes this less of an issue. A more serious problem is the occurrence of a lupus erythematosus–like syndrome in 30% of treated patients.[243] For these reasons, procainamide is better suited for the acute treatment of sustained arrhythmias (e.g., atrial fibrillation or ventricular tachycardia) or short-term (less than 3 months) prophylactic therapy.

The antiarrhythmic effects of disopyramide are very similar to those of quinidine and procainamide, but there are fewer gastrointestinal side effects.[244-246] Its principal side effects are related to its anticholinergic actions (dry mouth, visual blurring, and urinary retention). Disopyramide is also a potent negative inotropic agent, and this contraindicates its use in patients with a history of congestive heart failure or severe compensated left ventricular dysfunction.

Class IB Agents (Lidocaine, Mexiletine, Tocainide)

Lidocaine is the most commonly used drug for the acute termination of ventricular arrhythmias. Administration is limited to parenteral routes because of its very short half-life and extensive first-pass hepatic metabolism. It is effective in suppressing premature ventricular contractions and terminates ventricular tachycardia in 30% of episodes.[247,248] It is also effective in preventing ventricular fibrillation during the first 24 hours after myocardial infarction.[249] Therapeutic concentrations are well tolerated even in patients with congestive heart failure. Supratherapeutic concentrations cause neurologic side effects including confusion, lethargy, dysarthria, and seizures.

Two orally effective analogs of lidocaine have been in clinical use over the past 10 years. Tocainide and mexiletine are both effective in suppressing symptomatic ventricular ectopy.[250,251] They are not useful for supraventricular arrhythmias and appear to be less effective than other antiarrhythmic drugs when used as monotherapy for suppression of sustained ventricular arrhythmias.[252] Neither drug significantly depresses left ventricular function. Adverse effects are usually gastrointestinal or neurologic and limit therapy in up to one-third of patients.

Class IC agents (Flecainide, Encainide, Propafenone)

Class IC agents are potent blockers of the sodium channel. Both encainide and propafenone have active metabolites; in the case of encainide, this accounts for most of its electrophysiologic effects.[253] All class IC agents are very effective in suppressing simple and complex ventricular ectopy. Comparative studies have found flecainide to be superior to quinidine, disopyramide, mexiletine, and propafenone for this indication.[238,254] Thus, these agents would appear to be ideally suited for the treatment of patients with ventricular ectopy. However, the indications for treatment remain unresolved since it is not known whether suppression reduces the risk of sudden cardiac death. This question is currently being evaluated in the Cardiac Arrhythmia Suppression Trial (CAST). Initial results from the CAST indicate that despite suppression of ventricular ectopy, flecainide or encainide therapy paradoxically increase mortality in patients with asymptomatic ventricular ectopy after myocardial infarction.[255] This, coupled with the low risk of sudden death in placebo-treated patients, should discourage clinicians from using class IC agents to suppress asymptomatic ventricular ectopy.

The efficacy of class IC drugs in treating sustained ventricular arrhythmias is less striking. These agents suppress sustained ventricular tachycardia in 15 to 60% of patients.[256-258] Patients with preserved left ventricular function have the highest response rates, whereas only 15 to 20% of patients with coexisting coronary heart disease and left ventricular dysfunction respond fully. Ventricular tachycardias that remain inducible after treatment are frequently slower, allowing better tolerance of the arrhythmia. This represents a major advantage to the use of class IC agents in otherwise refractory patients.

These agents are also effective for supraventricular arrhythmias. For example, flecainide suppresses supraventricular tachycardia in most patients with atrioventricular nodal reentry or atrioventricular reentry using an accessory pathway.[259,260] It is also valuable in reducing the ventricular response to atrial fibrillation in patients with the Wolff-Parkinson-White syndrome.[261] These drugs have also been found useful for conversion and subsequent prophylaxis of atrial fibrillation and for suppression of ectopic atrial tachycardias.[262,263]

Mild noncardiovascular side effects (principally neurologic) occur in up to 30% of patients treated with class IC agents. Cardiovascular side effects occur less often, but may be life-threatening. Aggravation of sinus node dysfunction or atrioventricular conduction disturbance occurs in 1 to 2% of patients.[264] Exacerbation of congestive heart failure is frequently observed in patients with severely depressed left ventricular function (ejection fraction of less than 30%) when treated with flecainide or propafenone. Encainide appears to have a greater margin of safety in these patients.[240]

Class IC drugs may also worsen preexisting arrhythmias.[265] Patients with previous nonsustained or paroxysmal sustained ventricular tachycardia may develop incessant ventricular tachycardia that can be very resistant to all modes of therapy, including electrical cardioversion. These proarrhythmic properties are common to all antiarrhythmic drugs, but appear to be more frequent with class IC drugs. Patients with structural heart disease and sustained ventricular tachycardia are at highest risk. Most episodes of arrhythmia aggravation occur during initial dose titration. Therefore, before starting therapy, hospitalization is advisable for patients with serious ventricular arrhythmias. Recently, several cases of proarrhythmia have been reported in patients treated with class IC drugs for atrial arrhythmia.[266] Excessive atrial conduction slowing may lead to atrial tachycardias (including flutter) with one-to-one atrioventricular conduction. As a result, simultaneous administration of an agent to slow atrioventricular conduction is advisable when treating patients with atrial fibrillation or flutter.

Class III Agents (Amiodarone, Sotalol, Bretylium)

Class III agents act by blocking outward potassium currents, which are responsible for cardiac repolarization and lead to action potential prolongation. These agents increase cardiac refractoriness, an action that may be very useful against reentrant arrhythmias. As with other antiarrhythmic drugs, class III agents may share characteristics of other classes of agents. For example, amiodarone is also an inhibitor of sodium current (class I effect)[267] and calcium current (class IV effect).[268] Sotalol also competitively blocks beta-receptors (class II effect).

Amiodarone is perhaps the most effective antiarrhythmic agent available for clinical use. It is effective for all supraventricular arrhythmias as well as for patients with otherwise refractory ventricular tachycardia or ventricular fibrillation.[269-272] Left ventricular function is relatively unaffected by chronic amiodarone therapy, making it the drug of choice in patients with life-threatening arrhythmias and severe left ventricular dysfunction.

The advantages of amiodarone must, however, be balanced against its toxicity. The most common side effects are photodermatitis, corneal microdeposits, and asymptomatic liver function abnormalities.[273-175] Symptomatic hypo- or hyperthyroidism occurs in 2 to 4% of patients. The most feared complication of amiodarone therapy is pulmonary pneumonitis and fibrosis, an irreversible condition that can be lethal. The chances of toxicity can be minimized by ensuring that serum concentrations of the drug are less than 2.5 μg/mL.[276] Amiodarone therapy is further complicated by its very long half-life (about 30 days) and the presence of active metabolites.[277] Thus, although the drug is very effective, in a high proportion of patients (about 50%) the agent is eventually discontinued.[278]

Sotalol is effective for a variety of supraventricular and ventricular arrhythmias. Its beta-blocking actions are especially beneficial in patients whose arrhythmia is related to exercise or other conditions associated with increased catecholamines. It suppresses ventricular ectopy and prevents induction of ventricular tachycardia in

30 to 40% of cases.[279,280] It is also effective in most patients with paroxysmal supraventricular tachycardia.

Sotalol is generally well tolerated, with few of the neurologic or gastrointestinal side effects that limit other antiarrhythmic drugs. It may cause severe bradycardia in patients with underlying sinus node dysfunction and can aggravate heart failure. As with other class III agents and with class IA agents, sotalol may cause excessive prolongation of the QT interval with associated torsades de pointes ventricular arrhythmia.

REFERENCES

1. Shand DG: Propranolol. N Engl J Med 293:280, 1975
2. Thadani U, Parker JO: Propranolol in angina pectoris: duration of improved exercise tolerance and circulatory effects after acute oral administration. Am J Cardiol 44:188, 1979
3. Warren SG, Brewer DL, Orgain ES: Long-term propranolol therapy for angina. Am J Cardiol 37:420, 1976
4. Nattel S, Rangno RE, Van Loon G: Mechanism of propranolol withdrawal phenomena. Circulation 59:1158, 1979
5. Shulman RS, Herbert PN, Capone RJ et al: Effects of propranolol on blood lipids and lipoproteins in myocardial infarction. Circulation 67 (suppl. I):I-19, 1983
6. Koch-Weser J: Metoprolol. N Engl J Med 301:698, 1979
7. Thadani U, Davidson C, Singleton W, Taylor SH: Comparison of the immediate effects of five β-adrenoreceptor-blocking drugs with different ancillary properties in angina pectoris. N Engl J Med 300:750, 1979
8. Hiatt WR, Stoll S, Nies AS: Effect of β-adrenergic blockers on the peripheral circulation in patients with peripheral vascular disease. Circulation 72:1226, 1985
9. Coffman JD, Rasmussen HM: Effects of β-adrenoreceptor-blocking drugs in patients with Raynaud's phenomenon. Circulation 72:466, 1985
10. Kirshenbaum JM, Kloner RF, McGowan N, Antman EM: Use of an ultrashort-acting beta-receptor blocker (esmolol) in patients with acute myocardial ischemia and relative contraindications to beta-blockade therapy. J Am Coll Cardiol 12:773, 1988
11. Nattel S, Feder-Elituv R, Matthews C et al: Concentration dependence of class III and beta-adrenergic blocking effects of sotalol in anesthetized dogs. J Am Coll Cardiol 13:1190, 1989
12. Yusuf S, Wittes J, Friedman L: Overview of results of randomized clinical trials in heart disease. JAMA 260:2088, 1988
13. The Norwegian Multicenter Study Group: Timolol-induced reduction in mortality and reinfarction in patients surviving acute myocardial infarction. N Engl J Med 304:801, 1981
14. β-Blocker Heart Attack Trial Research Group: A randomized trial of propranolol in patients with acute myocardial infarction. JAMA 247:1707, 1982
15. Hjalmarson A, Herlitz J, Malek I et al: Effect on mortality of metoprolol in acute myocardial infarction. Lancet ii:823, 1981
16. Frishman WH, Furberg CD, Friedewald WT: β-adrenergic blockade for survivors of acute myocardial infarction. N Engl J Med 310:830, 1984
17. Griggs TR, Wagner GS, Gettes LS: Beta-adrenergic blocking agents after myocardial infarction: An undocumented need in patients at lowest risk. J Am Coll Cardiol 1:1530, 1983
18. Furberg CD, Hawkins CM, Lichstein E, for the Beta-Blocker Heart Attack Trial Study Group: Effect of propranolol in postinfarction patients with mechanical or electrical complications. Circulation 69:761, 1984
19. ISIS-1 (First International Study of Infarct Survival) Collaborative Group: Randomised trial of intravenous atenolol among 16,027 cases of suspected acute myocardial infarction: ISIS-1. Lancet ii:57, 1986
20. Rocco MB, Nabel EG, Campbell S et al: Prognostic importance of myocardial ischemia detected by ambulatory monitoring in patients with stable coronary artery disease. Circulation 78:877, 1988
21. Gottlieb SO, Weisfeldt ML, Ouyand P et al: Silent ischemia as a marker for early unfavorable outcomes in patients with unstable angina. N Engl J Med 314:1214, 1986
22. Gottlieb SO, Gottlieb SH, Achuff SC et al: Silent ischemia on Holter monitoring predicts mortality in high-risk postinfarction patients. JAMA 259:1030, 1988
23. Stone PH, Gibson RS, Glasser SP et al: Comparison of diltiazem, nifedipine, and propranolol in the therapy of silent ischemia. Circulation 80 (suppl. II):II-267, 1989

24. Chierchia S, Glazier JJ, Gerosa S: A single-blind, placebo-controlled study of effects of atenolol on transient ischemia in "mixed" angina. Am J Cardiol 60:36A, 1987

25. Willich SN, Pohjola-Sintonen S, Bhatia SJS et al: Suppression of silent ischemia by metoprolol without alteration of morning increase of platelet aggregability in patients with stable coronary artery disease. Circulation 79:557, 1989

26. Subramanian VB, Bowles MJ, Khurmi NS et al: Rationale for the choice of calcium antagonists in chronic stable angina. Am J Cardiol 50:1173, 1982

27. Klinke WP, Kvill L, Dempsey EE, Grace M: A randomized double-blind comparison of diltiazem and nifedipine in stable angina. J Am Coll Cardiol 12:1562, 1988

28. Robertson RM, Wood AJJ, Vaughn WK, Robertson D: Exacerbation of vasotonic angina pectoris by propranolol. Circulation 65:281, 1982

29. Waters DD, Théroux P, Szlachcic J, Dauwe F: Provocative testing with ergonovine to assess the efficacy of treatment with nifedipine, diltiazem and verapamil in variant angina. Am J Cardiol 48:123, 1981

30. Waters DD, Miller DD, Szlachcic J et al: Factors influencing the long-term prognosis of treated patients with variant angina. Circulation 68:258, 1983

31. Théroux P, Taeymans Y, Morissette D et al: A randomized study comparing propranolol and diltiazem in the treatment of unstable angina. J Am Coll Cardiol 5:717, 1985

32. Muller JE, Turi ZG, Pearle DL et al: Nifedipine and conventional therapy for unstable angina pectoris: a randomized, double-blind comparison. Circulation 69:729, 1984

33. Gottlieb SO, Weisfeldt ML, Ouyang P et al: Effect of the addition of propranolol to therapy with nifedipine for unstable angina pectoris: A randomized, double-blind, placebo-controlled trial. Circulation 73:331, 1986

34. Muller JE, Morrison J, Stone PH et al: Nifedipine therapy for patients with threatened and acute myocardial infarction: A randomized, double-blind, placebo-controlled comparison. Circulation 69:740, 1984

35. Sirnes PA, Overskeid K, Pedersen TR et al: Evolution of infarct size during the early use of nifedipine in patients with acute myocardial infarction: the Norwegian Nifedipine Multicenter Trial. Circulation 70:638, 1984

36. The Israeli SPRINT Study Group: Secondary prevention reinfarction Israeli nifedipine trial (SPRINT). A randomized intervention trial of nifedipine in patients with acute myocardial infarction. Eur Heart J 9:354, 1988

37. Wilcox RG, Hampton JR, Banks DC et al: Trial of early nifedipine in acute myocardial infarction: The TRENT study. Br Med J 293:1204, 1986

38. The SPRINT Study Group: The secondary prevention re-infarction Israeli nifedipine trial (SPRINT). II. Results. Abstract. Eur Heart J 9 (suppl. 1):350, 1988

39. The Danish Study Group on Verapamil in Myocardial Infarction: Verapamil in acute myocardial infarction. Eur Heart J 5:516, 1984

40. The Danish Study Group on Verapamil in Myocardial Infarction: Effect of verapamil on mortality and major events after acute myocardial infarction (The Danish verapamil infarction trial II—DAVIT II). Am J Cardiol 66:779, 1990

41. The Multicenter Diltiazem Postinfarction Trial Research Group: The effect of diltiazem on mortality and reinfarction after myocardial infarction. N Engl J Med 319:385, 1988

42. The Myocardial Infarction Study Group: Secondary prevention of ischemic heart disease: A long term controlled lidoflazine study. Acta Cardiol 24 (suppl.):7, 1979

43. Gibson RS, Boden WE, Théroux P et al: Diltiazem and reinfarction in patients with non-Q-wave myocardial infarction. N Engl J Med 315:423, 1986

44. Cohn PF, Vetrovec GW, Nesto R, Gerber FR, and the Total Ischemia Awareness Program Investigators: The nifedipine-total ischemia awareness program: A national survey of painful and painless myocardial ischemia including results of antiischemic therapy. Am J Cardiol 63:534, 1989

45. Barjon JN, Rouleau JL, Bichet D et al: Chronic renal and neurohumoral effects of the calcium entry blocker nisoldipine in patients with congestive heart failure. J Am Coll Cardiol 9:622, 1987

46. Packer M, Kessler PD, Lee WH: Calcium-channel blockade in the management of severe chronic congestive heart failure: a bridge too far. Circulation 75 (suppl. V):V-56, 1987

47. Overturf M: Are calcium ion antagonists effective anti-atherogenic agents? Arteriosclerosis 10:961, 1990

48. Henry PD: Calcium antagonists as anti-atherosclerotic agents. Arteriosclerosis 10:963, 1990

49. Lichtlen PR, Hugenholtz PG, Rafflenbeul W et al: Retardation of angiographic progression of coronary artery disease by nifedipine. Lancet 335:1109, 1990

50. Waters D, Lespérance J, Francetich M et al: A controlled clinical trial to assess the effect of a calcium channel blocker upon the progression of coronary atherosclerosis. Circulation 82:1940, 1990

51. Waters D: The future of calcium channel blockade. Can J Cardiol 5:181, 1989

52. Freedman DD, Waters DD: 'Second generation' dihydropyridine calcium antagonists. Drugs 34:578, 1987

53. De Coster PM, Chierchia S, Davies GJ et al: Combined effects of nitrates on the coronary and peripheral circulation in exercise-induced ischemia. Circulation 81:1881, 1990

54. Gage JE, Hess OM, Murakami T et al: Vasoconstriction of stenotic coronary arteries during dynamic exercise in patients with classic angina pectoris: reversibility by nitroglycerin. Circulation 73:865, 1986

55. Conti CR: Use of nitrates in unstable angina pectoris. Am J Cardiol 60:31H, 1987

56. Curfman GD, Heinsimer JA, Lozner EC, Fung HL: Intravenous nitroglycerin in the treatment of spontaneous angina pectoris: a prospective, randomized trial. Circulation 67:276, 1983

57. Diodati J, Théroux P, Latour JG et al: Effects of nitroglycerin at therapeutic doses on platelet aggregation in unstable angina pectoris and acute myocardial infarction. Am J Cardiol 66:683, 1990

58. Parker JO: Nitrate therapy in stable angina pectoris. N Engl J Med 316:1635, 1987

59. Packer M: Are nitrates effective in the treatment of chronic heart failure? Antagonist's viewpoint. Am J Cardiol 66:458, 1990

60. Waters DD, Juneau M, Gossard D et al: Limited usefulness of intermittent nitroglycerin patches in stable angina. J Am Coll Cardiol 13:421, 1989

61. Abrams J: Interval therapy to avoid nitrate tolerance: paradise regained? Am J Cardiol 64:931, 1989

62. Chatterjee K: Role of nitrates in silent myocardial ischemia. Am J Cardiol 60:18H, 1987

63. Yusuf S, Sleight P, Held P, McMahon S: Routine medical management of acute myocardial infarction. Circulation 82 (supp. II):II-117, 1990

64. Pfeffer MA, Braunwald E: Ventricular remodeling after myocardial infarction. Circulation 81:1161, 1990

65. Davies MJ, Thomas AC: Plaque fissuring—the cause of acute myocardial infarction, sudden ischemic death, and crescendo angina. Br Heart J 53:363, 1985

66. Falk E: Unstable angina with fatal outcome: Dynamic coronary thrombosis leading to infarction and/or sudden death. Autopsy evidence of recurrent mural thrombosis with peripheral embolization culminating in total vascular occlusion. Circulation 71:699, 1985

67. Fuster V, Badimon L, Cohen M et al: Insights into the pathogenesis of acute ischemic syndromes. Circulation 77:1213, 1988

68. Gruppo Italiano per lo Studio della Streptochinasi nell'Infarto Miocardico (GISSI): Effectiveness of intravenous thrombolytic treatment in acute myocardial infarction. Lancet i:397, 1986

69. ISIS-2 (Second International Study of Infarct Survival) Collaborative Group: Randomized trial of intravenous streptokinase, oral aspirin, both, or neither among 17,187 cases of suspected acute myocardial infarction: ISIS-2. Lancet ii:349, 1988

70. The I.S.A.M. Study Group: A prospective trial of intravenous streptokinase in acute myocardial infarction (I.S.A.M.). N Engl J Med 314:1465, 1986

71. Wilcox RG, von der Lippe G, Olsson CG et al: Trial of tissue plasminogen activator for mortality reduction in acute myocardial infarction. Lancet ii:525, 1988

72. AIMS Trial Study Group: Effect of intravenous APSAC on mortality after acute myocardial infarction: preliminary report of placebo-controlled clinical trial. Lancet i:545, 1988

73. Reimer KA, Jennings RB: The "wavefront phenomenon" of myocardial ischemic cell death. II. Transmural progression of necrosis within the framework of ischemic bed size. (Myocardium at risk) and collateral flow. Lab Invest 40:633, 1979

74. Collen D: On the regulation and control of fibrinolysis: Edward Kowalski Memorial lecture. Thromb Haemostasis 43:77, 1980

75. Aoki N, Moroi M, Matsuda M, Tachiya K: The behavior of α_2-plasmin inhibitor in fibrinolytic states. J Clin Invest 60:361, 1977

76. Aoki N, Moroi M, Matsuda M, Tachiya K: Effects of α_2-plasmin inhibitor on fibrin clot lysis: Its comparison with α_2-macroglobulin. Thromb Haemostasis 39:22, 1978

77. Fletcher AP, Alkjaersig N, Smyrniotis FE, Sherry S: The treatment of patients suffering from early myocardial infarction with massive and prolonged streptokinase therapy. Trans Assoc Am Physicians 71:289, 1958

78. Gottlich CM, Cooper B, Schumacher JR, Hillis D: Do different doses of intravenous streptokinase alter the frequency of coronary reperfusion in acute myocardial infarction? Am J Cardiol 62:843, 1988

79. Davies MC, Englert ME, De Renzo EC: Interaction of streptokinase and human plasminogen. I. Combining of streptokinase and plasminogen observed in the ultracentrifuge under a variety of experimental conditions. J Biol Chem 239:2651, 1964

80. Buluk K, Malofiejew M: The pharmacological properties of fibrinogen degradation products. Br J Pharmacol 35:79, 1969

81. Fitzgerald DJ, Catella F, Roy L, FitzGerald GA: Marked platelet activation in vivo after intravenous streptokinase in patients with acute myocardial infarction. Circulation 77:142, 1988

82. Owen J, Friedman KD, Grossman BA et al: Thrombolytic therapy with tissue plasminogen activator or streptokinase induces transient thrombin activity. Blood 72:616, 1988

83. Lew AS, Laramee P, Cercek B et al: The hypotensive effect of intravenous streptokinase in patients with acute myocardial infarction. Circulation: 72:1321, 1985

84. The TIMI Study Group: The thrombolysis in myocardial infarction (TIMI) trial. N Engl J Med 312:932, 1985

85. Spann JF, Sherry S, Carabello BA et al: Coronary thrombolysis by intravenous streptokinase in acute myocardial infarction: Acute and follow-up studies. Am J Cardiol 53:655, 1984

86. Rogers WJ, Mantle JA, Hood WP, Jr, et al: Prospective randomized trial of intravenous and intracoronary streptokinase in acute myocardial infarction. Circulation 68:1051, 1983

87. de Marneffe M, Van Thiel E, Ewalenko M et al: High-dose intravenous thrombolytic therapy in acute myocardial infarction: Efficiency, tolerance, complications and influence on left ventricular performance. Acta Cardiol 40:183, 1985

88. Schwartz F, Hoffmann M, Schuler G et al: Thrombolysis in acute myocardial infarction: effect of intravenous followed by intracoronary streptokinase application on estimates of infarct size. Am J Cardiol 53:1505, 1984

89. Verstraete M, Bory M, Collen D et al: Randomized trial of intravenous recombinant tissue-type plasminogen activator versus intravenous streptokinase in acute myocardial infarction. Lancet i:842, 1985

90. Chesebro JH, Knatterud G, Roberts R et al: Thrombolysis in Myocardial Infarction (TIMI) trial, phase I: a comparison between intravenous tissue plasminogen activator and intravenous streptokinase. Circulation 76:142, 1987

91. Stack RS, O'Connor CM, Mark DB et al: Coronary perfusion during acute myocardial infarction with a combined therapy of coronary angioplasty and high-dose intravenous streptokinase. Circulation 77:151, 1988

92. Taylor GJ, Mikell FL, Moses HW et al: Intravenous versus intracoronary streptokinase therapy for acute myocardial infarction in community hospitals. Am J Cardiol 54:256, 1984

93. Kennedy JW, Martin GV, Davis KB et al: The Western Washington Intravenous Streptokinase in Acute Myocardial Infarction randomized trial. Circulation 77:345, 1988

94. White HD, Norris RM, Brown MA et al: Effect of intravenous streptokinase on left ventricular function and early survival after acute myocardial infarction. N Engl J Med 317:850, 1987

95. Pennica D, Holmes WE, Kohr WJ et al: Cloning and expression of human tissue-type plasminogen activator cDNA in E. coli. Nature (London) 301:214, 1983

96. Mueller HS, Rao AK, Forman SA, and the TIMI Investigators: Thrombolysis in Myocardial Infarction (TIMI): comparative studies of coronary reperfusion and systemic fibrinogenolysis with two forms of recombinant tissue-type plasminogen activator. J Am Coll Cardiol 10:479, 1987

97. Hoylaerts M, Rijken DC, Lijnen HR, Collen D: Kinetics of the activation of plasminogen by human tissue plasminogen activator: Role of fibrin. J Biol Chem 257:2912, 1982

98. Rao AK, Pratt C, Berke A et al: Thrombolysis in Myocardial Infarction (TIMI) trial—phase I: Hemorrhagic manifestations and changes in plasma fibrinogen and the fibrinolytic system in patients treated with recombinant tissue plasminogen activator and streptokinase. J Am Coll Cardiol 11:1, 1988

99. Lucore CL, Fry ETA, Nachowiak DA, Sobel BE: Biochemical determinants of clearance of tissue-type plasminogen activator from the circulation. Circulation 77:906, 1988

100. Gold HK, Johns JA, Leinbach RC et al: A randomized, blinded, placebo-controlled trial of recombinant human tissue-type plasminogen activator in patients with unstable angina pectoris. Circulation 75:1192, 1987

101. Neuhaus KL, Feuerer W, Tebbe U et al: Efficacy of a 90-minute infusion of 100 mg tissue plasminogen activator (rt-PA) in acute myocardial infarction. Eur Heart J 9 (suppl. 1):9, 1988

102. Kanamasa K, Watanabe I, Cercek B et al: Selective decrease in lysis of old thrombi following rapid administration of tissue plasminogen activator. J Am Coll Cardiol 14:1359, 1989

103. European Cooperative Study Group for Recombinant Tissue-Type Plasminogen Activator: Randomized trial of intravenous recombinant tissue-type plasminogen activator versus intravenous streptokinase in acute myocardial infarction. Lancet i:842, 1985

104. Williams DO, Borer J, Braunwald E et al: Intravenous recombinant tissue-type plasminogen activator in patients with acute myocardial infarction. A report from the NHLBI Thrombolysis in Myocardial Infarction trial. Circulation 73:338, 1986

105. Gold HK, Leinbach RC, Garabedian HD et al: Acute coronary reocclusion after thrombolysis with recombinant human tissue-type plasminogen activator: Prevention by a maintenance infusion. Circulation 73:347, 1986

106. Topol EJ, Califf RM, George BS et al: A randomized trial of immediate versus delayed elective angioplasty after intravenous tissue plasminogen activator in acute myocardial infarction. N Engl J Med 317:581, 1987

107. Topol EJ, George BS, Kereiakes DJ et al: A randomized controlled trial of intravenous tissue plasminogen activator and early intravenous heparin in acute myocardial infarction. Circulation 79:281, 1989

108. Simoons ML, Arnold AER, Betriu A et al: Thrombolysis with rt-PA in acute myocardial infarction: No beneficial effects of immediate PTCA. Lancet i:197, 1988

109. Johns JA, Gold HK, Leinbach RC et al: Prevention of coronary artery reocclusion and reduction in late coronary artery stenosis after thrombolytic therapy in patients with acute myocardial infarction. Circulation 78:546, 1988

110. Neuhaus K, Tebbe U, Gottwik M et al: Intravenous recombinant tissue plasminogen activator (rt-PA) and urokinase in acute myocardial infarction: results of the German Activator Urokinase Study (GAUS). J Am Coll Cardiol 12:581, 1988

111. Guerci AD, Gerstenblith G, Brinker JA et al: A randomized trial of intravenous tissue plasminogen activator for acute myocardial infarction with subsequent randomization to elective coronary angioplasty. N Engl J Med 317:1613, 1987

112. O'Rourke M, Baron D, Keogh A et al: Limitation of myocardial infarction by early infusion of recombinant tissue-type plasminogen activator. Circulation 77:1311, 1988

113. National Heart Foundation of Australia Coronary Thrombolysis Group: Coronary thrombolysis and myocardial salvage by tissue plasminogen activator given up to 4 hours after onset of myocardial infarction. Lancet i:203, 1988

114. Van de Werf F, Arnold AER: Intravenous tissue plasminogen activator and size of infarct, left ventricular function, and survival in acute myocardial infarction. Br Med J 297:1374, 1988

115. Armstrong PW, Baigrie RS, Daly PA et al: Tissue Plasminogen Activator Toronto (TPAT): Randomized trial in myocardial infarction. J Am Coll Cardiol 13:1469, 1989

116. White HD: GISSI-2 and the heparin controversy. Lancet 336:247, 1990

117. GISSI-2: A factorial randomised trial of alteplase versus streptokinase and heparin versus no heparin among 12,490 patients with acute myocardial infarction. Lancet 336:65, 1990

118. Smith RAG, Dupe RI, English PD, Green J: Fibrinolysis with acylenzymes: A new approach to thrombolytic therapy. Nature (London) 290:505, 1981

119. Anderson JL: Development and evaluation of anisoylated plasminogen streptokinase activator complex (APSAC) as a second generation thrombolytic agent. J Am Coll Cardiol 10:22B, 1987

120. Anderson JL, Rothbard RL, Hackworthy RA et al: Multicenter reperfusion trial of intravenous anisoylated plasminogen streptokinase activator complex (APSAC) in acute myocardial infarction: Controlled comparison with intracoronary streptokinase. J Am Coll Cardiol 11:1153, 1988

121. Timmis AD, Griffin B, Crick JCP, Sowton E: Anisoylated plasminogen streptokinase activator complex in acute myocardial infarction: A placebo-controlled arteriographic coronary recanalization study. J Am Coll Cardiol 10:205, 1987

122. Bonnier HJRM, Visser RF, Klomps HC, Hoffmann HJML, and the Dutch Invasive Reperfusion Study Group: Comparison of intravenous anisoylated plasminogen streptokinase activator complex and intracoronary streptokinase in acute myocardial infarction. Am J Cardiol 62:25, 1988

123. Brochier ML, Quillet L, Kulbertus H et al: Intravenous APSAC versus intravenous streptokinase in evolving myocardial infarction. Drugs 33 (supp. 3):140, 1987

124. Kasper W, Meinertz T, Wollschlager H et al: Early clinical evaluation of the intravenous treatment of acute myocardial infarction with anisoylated plasminogen streptokinase activator complex. Drugs 33:112, 1987

125. Bassand JP, Machecourt J, Cassagnes J et al: Multicenter trial of intravenous anisoylated plasminogen streptokinase activator complex (APSAC) in

acute myocardial infarction: Effects on infarct size and left ventricular function. J Am Coll Cardiol 13:988, 1988

126. Meinertz T, Kasper W, Schumacher M, Just H, for the APSAC Multicenter Trial Group: The German multicenter trial of anisoylated plasminogen streptokinase activator complex versus heparin for acute myocardial infarction. Am J Cardiol 62:347, 1988

127. Jagger JD, Murray RG, Davies MK et al: Eligibility for thrombolytic therapy in acute myocardial infarction. Lancet i:34, 1987

128. Murray N, Lyons J, Layton C, Balcon R: What proportion of patients with myocardial infarction are suitable for thrombolysis? Br Heart J 57:144, 1987

129. White HD, Rivers JT, Maslowski AH et al: Effect of intravenous streptokinase as compared with that of tissue plasminogen activator on left ventricular function after first myocardial infarction. N Engl J Med 320:817, 1989

130. Magnani B, for the PAIMS Investigators: Plasminogen Activator Italian Multicenter Study (PAIMS): Comparison of intravenous recombinant single-chain human tissue-type plasminogen activator (rt-PA) with intravenous streptokinase in acute myocardial infarction. J Am Coll Cardiol 13:19, 1989

131. Althouse R, Weaver WD, Kennedy JW: Transient elevation of diastolic blood pressure in acute myocardial infarction—A contraindication to thrombolytic therapy? Circulation 76 (suppl. IV):IV-306, 1987

132. Norris RM, Caughey DE, Mercer CJ et al: Prognosis after myocardial infarction: 6 year follow-up. Br Heart J 36:786, 1974

133. Bates ER, Califf RM, Stack RS et al: Thrombolysis and Angioplasty in Myocardial Infarction (TAMI-1) Trial: Influence of infarct location on arterial patency, left ventricular function and mortality. J Am Coll Cardiol 13:12, 1989

134. Mauri F, Gasparini M, Barbonaglia L et al: Effectiveness of streptokinase in acute myocardial infarction: A problem of myocardial injury extent rather than infarct site. Data from GISSI trial. Am J Cardiol 63:1291, 1989

135. DeWood MA, Stifter WF, Simpson CS et al: Coronary arteriographic findings soon after non-Q-wave myocardial infarction. N Engl J Med 315:417, 1986

136. Robinson K, Conroy RM, Mulcahy R: Risk factors and in-hospital course of first myocardial infarction in the elderly. Clin Cardiol 11:519, 1988

137. Lew AS, Hod H, Cercek B et al: Mortality and morbidity rate of patients older and younger than 75 years with acute myocardial infarction treated with intravenous streptokinase. Am J Cardiol 59:1, 1987

138. Ambrose JA, Winters SL, Stern A et al: Angiographic morphology and pathogenesis of unstable angina pectoris. J Am Coll Cardiol 5:609, 1985

139. Sherman CT, Litvack F, Grundfest W et al: Coronary angioscopy in patients with unstable angina pectoris. N Engl J Med 315:913, 1986

140. Harker LA, Fuster V: Pharmacology of platelet inhibitors. J Am Coll Cardiol 8 (supp. B):21B, 1986

141. Roth GL, Majerus PW: The mechanism of the effect of aspirin on human platelets. I. Acetylation of a particulate fraction protein. J Clin Invest 56:624, 1975

142. Buchanan MR, Riscke JA, Hirsh J: Aspirin inhibits platelet function independent of the acetylation of cyclo-oxygenase. Thromb Res 25:363, 1982

143. Mielke CH, Ramos JC, Britten AFH: Aspirin as an antiplatelet agent: template bleeding time as a monitor of therapy. Am J Clin Pathol 59:236, 1973

144. Hirsh J, Salzman EW, Harker L et al: Aspirin and other platelet active drugs. Relationship among dose, effectiveness, and side effects. Chest 95 (supp.):12S, 1989

145. Antiplatelet Trialists' Collaboration: Secondary prevention of vascular disease by prolonged antiplatelet treatment. Br Med J 296:320, 1988

146. Preston FE, Whipps S, Jackson CA et al: Inhibition of prostacyclin and platelet thromboxane A_2 after low-dose aspirin. N Engl J Med 304:76, 1981

147. Graham DY, Smith LJ: Aspirin and the stomach. Ann Intern Med 104:390, 1986

148. Harker LA, Slichter SJ: Arterial and venous thromboembolism: Kinetic characterization of evaluation of therapy. Thromb Diath Haemorrh 31:188, 1974

149. Goldman S, Copeland J, Moritz T et al: Improvement in early saphenous vein graft patency after coronary artery bypass surgery with antiplatelet therapy: Results of a Veterans Administration Cooperative Study. Circulation 77:1324, 1988

150. FitzGerald GA: Dipyridamole. N Engl J Med 316:1247, 1987

151. Harker LA, Slichter SJ: Studies of platelet and fibrinogen kinetics in patients with prosthetic heart valves. N Engl J Med 283:1302, 1970

152. Chesebro JH, Fuster V, Elveback LR et al: Trial of combined warfarin plus dipyridamole or aspirin therapy in prosthetic heart valve replacement. Danger of aspirin compared with dipyridamole. Am J Cardiol 51:1537, 1983

153. Schwartz L, Bourassa MG, Lesperance J et al: Aspirin and dypyridamole in the prevention of restenosis after percutaneous transluminal coronary angioplasty. N Engl J Med 318:1714, 1988

154. White CW, Chaitman B, Lassar TA et al: Antiplatelet agents are effective in reducing the immediate complications of PTCA: Results from the ticlopidine multicenter trial. Abstract. Circulation 76 (suppl. IV):IV-400, 1987

155. Chesebro JH, Clements IP, Fuster V et al: A platelet inhibitor-drug trial in coronary-artery bypass operations, benefit of perioperative dipyridamole and aspirin therapy on early postoperative vein-graft patency. N Engl J Med 307:73, 1982

156. Chesebro JH, Fuster V, Elveback LR et al: Effect of dipyridamole and aspirin on late vein-graft patency after coronary bypass operations. N Engl J Med 310:209, 1984

157. Brown BG, Cukingnan RA, DeRouen T et al: Improved graft patency in patients treated with platelet-inhibiting therapy after coronary bypass surgery. Circulation 72:138, 1985

158. Chesebro JH, Webster MWI, Smith HC et al: Antiplatelet therapy in coronary disease progression: Reduced infarction and new lesion formation. Circulation 80 (suppl. II):II-266, 1989

159. Bousser MG, Eschwege E, Haugenau M et al: "AICLA" controlled trial of aspirin and dipyridamole in the secondary prevention of atherothrombotic cerebral ischemia. Stroke 14:5, 1983

160. American-Canadian Cooperative Study Group: Persantine-aspirin trial in cerebral ischemia. II. Endpoint results. Stroke 16:406, 1985

161. Hess H, Mietaschk A, Deichsel G: Drug-induced inhibition of platelet function delays progression of peripheral occlusive arterial disease: a prospective double-blind arteriographically controlled trial. Lancet i:415, 1985

162. Steele PP, Rainwater J, Vogel R: Platelet suppressant therapy in patients with prosthetic cardiac valves: Relationship of clinical effectiveness to alteration of platelet survival time. Circulation 60:910, 1979

163. Kaegi A, Pineo GF, Shimizu A et al: Arteriovenous-shunt thrombosis: prevention by sulfinpyrazone. N Engl J Med 290:304, 1974

164. Cairns JA, Gent M, Singer J et al: Aspirin, sulfinpyrazone, or both in unstable angina. N Engl J Med 313:1369, 1985

165. Canadian Cooperative Study Group: A randomized trial of aspirin and sulfinpyrazone in threatened stroke. N Engl J Med 299:53, 1978

166. Report from the Anturane Reinfarction Italian Study: Sulfinpyrazone in post-myocardial infarction. Lancet i:237, 1982

167. Lewis HD, Davis JW, Archibald DG et al: Protective effects of aspirin against acute myocardial infarction and death in men with unstable angina. Results of a Veterans Administration Cooperative Study. N Engl J Med 309:396, 1983

168. Théroux P, Ouimet H, McCans J et al: Aspirin, heparin, or both to treat acute unstable angina. N Engl J Med 319:1105, 1988

169. Gold HK, Coller BS, Yasuda T et al: Rapid and sustained coronary artery recanalization with combined bolus injection of recombinant tissue-type plasminogen activator and monoclonal antiplatelet GPIIb/IIIa antibody in a canine preparation. Circulation 77:670, 1988

170. The Steering Committee of the Physicians' Health Study Research Group: Preliminary report: Findings from the aspirin component of the ongoing Physicians' Health Study. N Engl J Med 318:262, 1988

171. Peto R, Gray R, Collins R et al: A randomized trial of the effects of prophylactic daily aspirin among male British doctors. Br Med J 296:313, 1988

172. Lam JYT, Solymoss BC, Campeau L: Care of the patient with previous coronary bypass surgery. Cardiovasc Clin 21:62, 1991

173. Pfisterer M, Jockers G, Regenass S et al: Trial of low dose aspirin plus dipyridamole versus anticoagulants for prevention of aortocoronary vein graft occlusion. Lancet ii:1, 1989

174. Sanz G, Pajaron A, Alegria E et al: Prevention of early aortocoronary bypass occlusion by low dose aspirin and dipyridamole. Circulation 82:765, 1990

175. Blankenhorn DH, Nessim SA, Johnson RL et al: Beneficial effects of combined colestipol-niacin therapy on coronary atherosclerosis and coronary venous bypass grafts. JAMA 257:3233, 1987

176. Wright IS, Marple CD, Beck DF: Report of the committee for the evaluation of anticoagulants in the treatment of coronary thrombosis with myocardial infarction. Am Heart J 36:801, 1948

177. Wasserman AJ, Gutterman LA, Yoe KB et al: Anticoagulants in acute myocardial infarction: The failure of anticoagulants to alter mortality in randomized series. Am Heart J 71:43, 1966

178. Rosenberg RD, Damus PS: The purification and mechanism of action of human antithrombin-heparin cofactor. J Biol Chem 248:6490, 1973

179. Tollefsen DM, Petska CA, Monafo WJ: Activation of heparin cofactor II by dermatan sulfate. J Biol Chem 258:6713, 1983

180. Ofosu FA, Blajchman MA, Hirsh J: The inhibition of heparin of the intrinsic pathway activation of factor X in the absence of antithrombin III. Thromb Res 20:391, 1980

181. Salzman EW, Deykin D, Shapiro RM: Effect of heparin and heparin fractions on platelet aggregation. J Clin Invest 65:64, 1980

182. Kelton JG, Levine MN: Heparin-induced thrombocytopenia. Semin Thromb Hemostasis 12:59, 1986

183. Weismann RE, Tobin RW: Arterial embolism occurring during systemic heparin therapy. Arch Surg 76:219, 1958

184. Jackson CW, Suttie JW: Recent developments in understanding the mechanism of vitamin K and vitamin K antagonist drug action and the consequences of vitamin K action in blood coagulation. Prog Hematol 10:333, 1977

185. Olson RE, Suttie JW: Vitamin K and γ-carboxy-glutamate biosynthesis. Vitam Horm 35:59, 1977

186. O'Reilly RA, Aggeler PM: Determinants of the response to oral anticoagulant drug in man. Pharmacol Rev 22:35, 1970

187. Hirsh J, Deykin D, Poller L: "Therapeutic range" for oral anticoagulant therapy. Chest 89:11S, 1986

188. Telford AM, Wilson C: Trial of heparin versus atenolol in prevention of myocardial infarction in intermediate coronary syndrome. Lancet i:1225, 1981

189. Report of the Working Party on Anticoagulant Therapy in Coronary Thrombosis to the Medical Research Council: Assessment of short-term anticoagulant administration after cardiac infarction. Br Med J 1:335, 1969

190. Drapkin A, Merskey L: Anticoagulant therapy after acute myocardial infarction: relation of therapeutic benefit to patient's age, sex and severity of infarction. JAMA 222:541, 1972

191. Cooperative Clinical Trial: Anticoagulants in acute myocardial infarction: results of a Cooperative Clinical Trial. JAMA 225:724, 1973

192. Yusuf S, Wittes J, Friedman L: Overview of results of randomized clinical trials in heart disease. 1. Treatments following myocardial infarction. JAMA 260:2088, 1988

193. Smith P, Arnesen H, Holme I: The effect of warfarin on mortality and reinfarction after myocardial infarction. N Engl J Med 323:147, 1990

194. Hsia J, Hamilton WP, Kleinan N et al: A comparison between heparin and low dose aspirin as adjunctive therapy with tissue plasminogen activator for acute myocardial infarction. N Engl J Med 323:1433, 1990

195. Heras M, Chesebro JH, Webster MWI et al: Hirudin, heparin, and placebo during deep arterial injury in the pig: The in vivo role of thrombin in platelet-mediated thrombosis. Circulation 82:1476, 1990

196. Clowes AW, Karnowsky MJ: Suppression by heparin of smooth muscle cell proliferation in injured arteries. Nature (London) 265:625, 1977

197. Ellis SG, Roubin GS, Wilentz J et al: Effect of 18- to 24-hour heparin administration for prevention of restenosis after uncomplicated coronary angioplasty. Am Heart J 117:777, 1989

198. Goldman L, Cook EF: The decline in ischemic heart disease mortality rates: an analysis of the comparative effects of medical intervention and changes in lifestyle. Ann Intern Med 101:825, 1984

199. Keys A: Coronary heart disease in seven countries. Circulation 41 (suppl. I):I-1, 1970

200. Waters D, Lespérance J: Regression of coronary atherosclerosis: An achievable goal? Review of results from recent clinical trials. Am J Med (in press)

201. Lipid Research Clinics Program: The Lipid Research Clinics Coronary Primary Prevention trial results. JAMA 251:351, 1984

202. Frick MH, Elo O, Haapa K et al: Helsinki Heart Study: primary-prevention trial with gemfibrozil in middle-aged men with dyslipidemia. N Engl J Med 317:1237, 1987

203. Canner PL, Berge KG, Wenger NK et al: Fifteen year mortality in Coronary Drug Project patients: Long-term benefit with niacin. J Am Coll Cardiol 8:1245, 1986

204. The Coronary Drug Project Research Group: Clofibrate and niacin in coronary heart disease. JAMA 231:360, 1985

205. Brensike JF, Levy RI, Kelsey SF et al: Effects of therapy with cholestyramine on progression of coronary arteriosclerosis: Results of the NHLBI Type II Coronary Intervention Study. Circulation 69:313, 1984

206. Blankenhorn DH, Nessim SA, Johnson RL et al: Beneficial effects of combined colestipol-niacin therapy on coronary atherosclerosis and coronary venous bypass grafts. JAMA 257:3233, 1987

207. Cashin-Hemphill L, Sanmarco ME, Blankenhorn DH: Augmented beneficial effects of colestipol-

niacin therapy at four years in the CLAS trial. Abstract. Circulation 80 (suppl. II):II-381, 1989

208. Brown G, Albers JJ, Fisher LD et al: Regression of coronary artery disease as a result of intensive lipid-lowering therapy in men with high levels of apolipoprotein B. N Engl J Med 323:1289, 1990

209. The Expert Panel: Report of the National Cholesterol Education Program Expert Panel on detection, evaluation, and treatment of high blood cholesterol in adults. Arch Intern Med 148:36, 1988

210. Witztum JL: Current approaches to drug therapy for the hypercholesterolemic patient. Circulation 80:1101, 1989

211. Stein EA: Management of hypercholesterolemia. Am J Med 87 (suppl. 4A):4A-20S, 1989

212. Grundy SM: Drug therapy: HMG CoA reductase inhibitors for treatment of hypercholesterolemia. N Engl J Med 319:24, 1988

213. Roberts WC: Lipid-lowering therapy after an atherosclerotic event. Am J Cardiol 64:693, 1989

214. Parmley WW: Should digoxin be the drug of first choice after diuretics in chronic congestive heart failure? J Am Coll Cardiol 12:265, 1988

215. Smith TW: Digitalis. Mechanisms of action and clinical use. N Engl J Med 318:358, 1988

216. Arnold SB, Byrd RC, Meister W et al: Long-term digitalis therapy improves left ventricular function in heart failure. N Engl J Med 303:1443, 1980

217. Lee DC, Johnson RA, Bingham JB et al: Heart failure in outpatients: A randomized trial of digoxin versus placebo. N Engl J Med 306:699, 1982

218. Yusuf S, Wittes J, Bailey K, Furberg C: Digitalis—A new controversy regarding an old drug: the pitfalls of inappropriate methods. Circulation 73:14, 1986

219. Packer M, Medina N, Yushak M: Hemodynamic and clinical limitations of long-term inotropic therapy with amrinone in patients with severe chronic heart failure. Circulation 70:1038, 1984

220. DiBianco R, Shabetai R, Silverman BD et al: with the Amrinone Multicenter Study Investigators: Oral amrinone for the treatment of chronic congestive heart failure: Results of a multicenter randomized double-blind and placebo-controlled withdrawal study. J Am Coll Cardiol 4:855, 1984

221. DiBianco R, Shabetai R, Kostuk W et al: A comparison of oral milrinone, digoxin, and their combination in the treatment of patients with chronic heart failure. N Engl J Med 320:677, 1989

222. Uretsky BF, Jessup M, Konstam MA et al: Multicenter trial of oral enoximone in patients with moderate to moderately severe congestive heart failure. Circulation 82:774, 1990

223. Packer M: Pathophysiological mechanisms underlying the effects of β-adrenergic agonists and antagonists on functional capacity and survival in chronic heart failure. Circulation 82 (supp. I):I-77, 1990

224. Cody RJ: Pharmacology of angiotensin-converting enzyme inhibitors as a guide to their use in congestive heart failure. Am J Cardiol 66:7D, 1990

225. Captopril Multicenter Research Group: A placebo-controlled trial of captopril in refractory chronic congestive heart failure. J Am Coll Cardiol 2:755, 1983

226. The CONSENSUS Trial Study Group: Effects of enalapril on mortality in severe congestive heart failure. N Engl J Med 316:1429, 1987

227. Cohn JN, Archibald DG, Ziesche S et al: Effect of vasodilator therapy on mortality in chronic congestive heart failure: Results of a Veterans Administration cooperative study. N Engl J Med 314:1547, 1986

228. Packer M, Medina N, Yushak M: Role of the renin-angiotensin system in the development of hemodynamic and clinical tolerance to long-term prazosin therapy in patients with severe chronic heart failure. J Am Coll Cardiol 7:671, 1986

229. Kannel WB: Some lessons in cardiovascular epidemiology from Framingham. Am J Cardiol 37:269, 1976

230. The Pooling Project Research Group: Relationship of blood pressure, serum cholesterol, smoking habit, relative weight and ECG abnormalities to incidence of major coronary events: Final report of the pooling project. J Chronic Dis 31:201, 1978

231. Houston MC: New insights and new approaches for the treatment of essential hypertension: Selection of therapy based on coronary heart disease risk factor analysis, hemodynamic profiles, quality of life, and subsets of hypertension. Am Heart J 117:911, 1989

232. O'Kelly BF, Massie BM, Tubau JF, Szlachcic J: Coronary morbidity and mortality, pre-existing silent coronary artery disease, and mild hypertension. Ann Intern Med 110:1017, 1989

233. Carney S, Gilles AI, Morgan T: Optimal dose of a thiazide diuretic. Med J Aust 2:692, 1976

234. Finnerty FA, Jr: Stepped-down therapy versus intermittent therapy in systemic hypertension. Am J Cardiol 66:1373, 1990

235. Vaughan Williams EM: A classification of antiarrhythmic actions reassessed after a decade of new drugs. J Clin Pharmacol 24:129, 1984

236. Coplen SE, Antman EM, Berlin JA et al: Efficacy and safety of quinidine therapy for maintenance of sinus rhythm after cardioversion. Circulation 82:1106, 1990

237. Dimarco JP, Garan H, Ruskin JN: Quinidine for ventricular arrhythmias: Value of electrophysiologic testing. Am J Cardiol 51:90, 1983

238. The Flecainide-Quinidine Research Group: Flecainide vs quinidine for treatment of ventricular arrhythmias: a multicenter clinical trial. Circulation 67:1117, 1983

239. Cohen IS, Jick H, Cohen SI: Adverse reactions to quinidine in hospitalized patients: Findings based on data from the Boston Collaborative Drug Surveillance Program. Prog Cardiovasc Dis 20:151, 1977

240. Giardina EGV, Fenster PE, Bigger JT, Jr, et al: Efficacy, plasma concentrations and adverse effects of a new sustained release procainamide preparation. Am J Cardiol 46:855, 1980

241. Giardina EGV, Bigger JT, Jr: Procaine amide against re-entrant ventricular arrhythmias. Circulation 48:959, 1973

242. Waxman HL, Buxton AE, Sadowski LM et al: The response to procainamide during electrophysiological study for sustained ventricular tachyarrhythmias predicts the response to other medications. Circulation 67:30, 1983

243. Blomgren SE, Condemi JJ, Vaughan JH: Procainamide-induced lupus erythematosus: Clinical and laboratory observations. Am J Med 52:338, 1972

244. Lerman BB, Waxman HL, Buxton AE et al: Disopyramide: Evaluation of electrophysiologic effects and clinical efficacy in patients with sustained ventricular tachycardia or ventricular fibrillation. Am J Cardiol 51:759, 1983

245. Kimura E, Mashina S, Tanaka T: Clinical evaluation of antiarrhythmic effects of disopyramide by multiclinical controlled double-blind methods. Int J Clin Pharmacol Ther Toxicol 18:338, 1980

246. Morady F, Scheinman MM, Desai J: Disopyramide. Ann Intern Med 96:337, 1982

247. Griffith MJ, Linker NJ, Garratt CJ et al: Relative efficacy and safety of intravenous drugs for termination of sustained ventricular tachycardia. Lancet 336:670, 1990

248. Harrison DC, Sprouse JG, Morrow AG: The antiarrhythmic properties of lidocaine and procaine amide. Circulation 28:486, 1963

249. Lie KI, Wellens HJ, vanCapelle FJ et al: Lidocaine in the prevention of primary ventricular fibrillation. N Engl J Med 291:1324, 1974

250. Kutalek SP, Morganroth J, Horowitz LN: Tocainide: a new oral antiarrhythmic agent. Ann Intern Med 103:387, 1985

251. Mehta J, Conti CR: Mexiletine, a new antiarrhythmic agent, for treatment of premature ventricular complexes. Am J Cardiol 49:455, 1982

252. DiMarco JP, Garan H, Ruskin JN: Mexiletine for refractory ventricular arrhythmias: Results using serial electrophysiologic testing. Am J Cardiol 47:131, 1981

253. Woosley RL, Wood AJJ, Roden DM: Drug therapy: encainide. N Engl J Med 318:1107, 1988

254. Klempt HW, Nayebagha A, Fabry E: Antiarrhythmic efficacy of mexiletine, propafenone and flecainide in ventricular premature beats. A comparative study in patients with myocardial infarction. Z Kardiol 71:340, 1982

255. The Cardiac Arrhythmia Suppression Trial (CAST) Investigators: Preliminary report: Effect of encainide and flecainide on mortality in a randomized trial of arrhythmia suppression after myocardial infarction. N Engl J Med 321:406, 1989

256. Webb CR, Morganroth J, Senior S et al: Flecainide: Steady state electrophysiologic effects in patients with remote myocardial infarction and inducible sustained ventricular arrhythmia. Am J Cardiol 8:214, 1986

257. Horowitz LN: Encainide in lethal ventricular arrhythmias evaluated by electrophysiologic testing and decrease in symptoms. Am J Cardiol 58:83C, 1986

258. Heger JJ, Hubbard J, Zipes DP et al: Propafenone treatment of recurrent ventricular tachydia: comparison of continuous electrocardiographic recording and electrophysiologic study in predicting drug efficacy. Am J Cardiol 54:40D, 1984

259. Hoff PI, Tronstad A, Oie B, Ohm OJ: Electrophysiologic and clinical effects of flecainide for recurrent paroxysmal supraventricular tachycardia. Am J Cardiol 62:585, 1988

260. Zee-Cheng CS, Kim SS, Ruffy R: Flecainide acetate for treatment of bypass tract mediated reentrant tachycardia. Am J Cardiol 62:23D, 1988

261. Kim SS, Smith P, Ruffy R: Treatment of atrial tachyarrhythmias and preexcitation syndrome with flecainide acetate. Am J Cardiol 62:29D, 1988

262. Berns E, Rinkenberger RL, Jeang MK et al: Ef-

ficacy and safety of flecainide acetate for atrial tachycardia or fibrillation. Am J Cardiol 59:1337, 1987

263. Antman EM, Beamer AD, Cantillon C et al: Long-term oral propafenone therapy for suppression of refractory symptomatic atrial fibrillation and atrial flutter. J Am Coll Cardiol 12:1005, 1988

264. Morganroth J, Anderson JL, Gentzkow GD: Classification by type of ventricular arrhythmia predicts frequency of adverse cardiac events from flecainide. J Am Coll Cardiol 8:607, 1986

265. Zipes DP: Proarrhythmic events. Am J Cardiol 61:70A, 1988

266. Feld, GK, Chen PS, Nicod P et al: Possible atrial proarrhythmic effects of class IC antiarrhythmic drugs. Am J Cardiol 66:378, 1990

267. Yabek SM, Kato R, Singh BN: Acute effects of amiodarone on the electrophysiologic properties of isolated neonatal and adult cardiac fibres. J Am Coll Cardiol 5:1109, 1985

268. Nattel S, Talajic M, Quantz M, DeRoode M: Frequency-dependent effects of amiodarone on atrioventricular nodal function and slow-channel action potentials: evidence for calcium channel-blocking activity. Circulation 76:442, 1987

269. Marcus FI: Clinical pharmacology of amiodarone. Ann NY Acad Sci 427:112, 1984

270. Rosenbaum MB, Chiale PA, Halpern MS et al: Clinical efficacy of amiodarone as an antiarrhythmic agent. Am J Cardiol 38:934, 1976

271. Wellens HJJ, Lie KI, Bar FW et al: Effect of amiodarone in the Wolff-Parkinson-White syndrome. Am J Cardiol 38:189, 1976

272. Waxman HL, Groh WC, Marchlinski FE et al: Amiodarone for control of sustained ventricular tachyarrhythmias. Clinical and electrophysiologic effects in 51 patients. Am J Cardiol 50:1066, 1982

273. Harris LW, McKenna WJ, Rowland E et al: Side effects of long-term amiodarone therapy. Circulation 67:45, 1983

274. Rotmensch HH, Belhassen B, Swanson BN et al: Steady-state serum amiodarone concentration: Relationships with antiarrhythmic efficacy and toxicity. Ann Intern Med 101:462, 1984

275. Greene HL, Graham EL, Werner JA et al: Toxic and therapeutic effects of amiodarone in the treatment of cardiac arrhythmias. J Am Coll Cardiol 2:1114, 1983

276. Nattel S, Talajic M: Recent advances in understanding the pharmacology of amiodarone. Drugs 36:121, 1988

277. Talajic M, DeRoode MR, Nattel S: Comparative electrophysiologic effects of intravenous amiodarone and desethylamiodarone in dogs: evidence for clinically relevant activity of the metabolite. Circulation 75:265, 1987

278. Smith WM, Lubbe WF, Whitlock RM et al: Long-term tolerance of amiodarone treatment for cardiac arrhythmias. Am J Cardiol 57:1288, 1986

279. Senges J, Lengfelder W, Jauernig R et al: Electrophysiologic testing in assessment of therapy with sotalol for sustained ventricular tachycardia. Circulation 69:577, 1984

280. Nademanee K, Feld G, Hendrickson BS et al: Electrophysiologic and antiarrhythmic effects of sotalol in patients with life-threatening ventricular tachyarrhythmias. Circulation 72:555, 1985

MYOCARDIAL REVASCULARIZATION AND OTHER SURGICAL PROCEDURES FOR CORONARY HEART DISEASE AND ITS COMPLICATIONS

17

Coronary Angioplasty and Coronary Atherectomy

M. Nagui Sabri, M.D.
Michael J. Cowley, M.D.

The era of interventional cardiology began in 1977 with the introduction of percutaneous transluminal coronary angioplasty (PTCA) by Gruentzig et al. as a nonsurgical method of myocardial revascularization.[1] Clinical application of PTCA grew rapidly, with an increase in the number of procedures in the United States from 6,000 in 1981 to more than 250,000 in 1989. In contrast, the volume of coronary artery bypass graft surgery (CABG) has increased only slightly in recent years and is currently estimated at 280,000 operations annually. Balloon angioplasty remains the cornerstone of nonsurgical myocardial revascularization, although newer percutaneous transluminal techniques such as atherectomy, stents, and laser angioplasty are undergoing clinical evaluation. The term *interventional cardiology* refers to these various methods of nonsurgical catheter-based treatment of coronary artery obstructions. The most important of these techniques will be reviewed here.

PERCUTANEOUS TRANSLUMINAL CORONARY ANGIOPLASTY

Current Status

Clinical applications of PTCA grew rapidly because of the demonstration of immediate and long-term efficacy and of the major improvements in equipment and technology that enabled improved results and treatment of a wider spectrum of disease. PTCA was used initially only for patients with single-vessel coronary disease, with early success rates of only about 60%.[1,2] The National Heart, Lung, and Blood Institute (NHLBI) PTCA Registry, representing procedures from more than 100 centers between 1977 and 1981, reported angiographic success ($\geq 20\%$ improvement in luminal diameter) in 67% of lesions and clinical success (angiographic success, with no major inhospital complications) in 62% of patients.[3,4] Major complications (myocardial infarction, death, need for emergency CABG) occurred in about 9% of patients. Long-term follow-up after successful PTCA showed sustained improvement in the majority (60 to 80%) of patients. Several reports have confirmed this satisfactory long-term outcome at mean follow-up intervals of 5 to 9 years after PTCA[5-8] (Table 17-1). Results from the NHLBI PTCA Registry (average follow-up of 5 years) showed continued symptomatic improvement in 89% of patients. Fifty-nine percent of patients were event-free and improved, 15% had had repeat PTCA, 12% had had CABG, 8.6% had had myocardial infarction, and 5.4% had died. (Event-free is defined as no myocardial infarction, CABG, or death.) Including patients with repeat PTCA, 67% were improved without cardiac events or need for CABG surgery during follow-up.[6] Long-term results from the original cohort of patients who had had PTCA in Zurich[5] showed similar outcomes, with an actuarial survival of 93% at 6 years after successful PTCA. Similar results have also been reported by Talley et al. at Emory University[7] and by Webb et al. at the San Francisco Heart Institute[8] (Table 17-1). Most patients (72 to 88%) in these reports had single-vessel coronary disease and normal left ventricular function, representing a relatively low-risk population for follow-up events.

Factors adversely affecting long-term outcome after PTCA include age over 65 years, multivessel coronary disease, unstable clinical status, and abnormal left ventricular function.

Technique

PTCA is performed similarly to diagnostic coronary angiography, using primarily the percutaneous femoral artery approach with 8 or 9 French guiding catheters with preshaped tip configurations (Fig. 17-1). The angioplasty balloon catheters have a lumen for balloon inflation and a central lumen through which a 0.014- to 0.018-in. flexible-tip guide wire is advanced across the obstruction. The catheter is then advanced over the wire and into the stenosis, and multiple balloon inflations are performed until satisfactory luminal improvement is achieved. Inflated balloon diameters range from 1.5 to 4 mm. Current catheters have shaft diameters of 2.7 to 4 French and tip profiles of 0.027 to 0.050 in. Several lower-profile catheters have a balloon mounted on a guide wire and are useful for traversing extremely tight stenoses. Patients are sedated as for diagnostic coronary angiography and premedicated with aspirin (325 to 650 mg) for antiplatelet effect. Heparin (10,000 units intravenously) is given to prevent thrombus formation during intracoronary manipulation. Patients also receive topical or intravenous nitrate drugs for coronary vasodilatation during the procedure. PTCA is performed with cardiac surgery standby available. Following PTCA, patients are monitored overnight by electrocardiographic (ECG) telemetry and then observed and discharged home 1 to 2 days after the procedure. Patients are continued on aspirin (80 to 325 mg/day) indefinitely and usually receive a calcium blocking drug for 3 to 6 months.

Table 17-1. Long-Term Outcome After Successful PTCA

Trial	No. of Patients	Follow-up (mean yrs)	Single-Vessel Disease	Angina-Free	Myocardial Infarction	CABG	Repeat PTCA	CABG/PTCA	Total Mortality (%)	Actuarial Survival (%)	Event-Free Survival (%)
Talley et al.[7]	338	5	82	85	5.6	12	22	30	3.0	97	81.7
Gruentzig et al.[5]	133	6	58	67		14	20	35	6.8	93	79
Kent et al.[6]	1,000	5.7	72	73	12	18	20	36	6.6	94.5	70
Webb et al.[8]	140	9	87	85	9	16	27	41	7.1	93	76

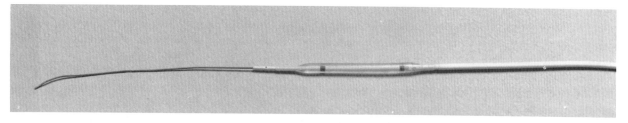

Fig. 17-1. A 3-mm angioplasty balloon catheter (inflated) and guidewire.

Early exercise testing (2 to 10 days after PTCA) is useful to assess improvement and to establish a baseline for follow-up. Repeat exercise testing with or without thallium at 3 to 6 months is often done to assess for restenosis, with periodic exercise testing at 1- to 2-year intervals to evaluate for late recurrence of stenosis or progression of coronary disease in the PTCA-dilated or other coronary arteries.

Mechanism of Effect of PTCA

The mechanism(s) of luminal widening with balloon angioplasty are multifactorial.[9] It was originally postulated to be due to plaque compression and redistribution. Later, it was demonstrated that plaque compression was only a minor component of luminal improvement and that stretching of the vessel wall with increase of the overall vessel diameter was a more important factor. The most important element of luminal improvement is plaque disruption with cracks, fractures, and dissection of the intima and occasionally the media of the vessel wall. These effects produce local vascular injury, which in most instances is "controlled" and results in a larger lumen and in improved patency. The relative contributions of each of these factors and the final angiographic result depend upon variables such as severity and composition of the lesion, size of the balloon and vessel, and technical aspects of the procedure. In most instances, PTCA effects major improvement in lumen diameter, with residual narrowing of <30%. Some degree of intimal disruption occurs in all successful dilatations; major dissection occurs in 5 to 10% and may produce acute myocardial ischemia or occlusion

for which urgent surgery may be required. Healing at the dilated site occurs over a period of weeks and involves platelet deposition and initiation of a repair response, vascular remodeling, elastic recoil, and various degrees of neointimal fibrous proliferation. The net result is persistent improvement of most lesions, although significant clinical recurrence develops in about 30% of patients.

Current and Evolving Indications for PTCA

Single-Vessel Disease
PTCA is now used in a widening spectrum of patients, depending on the extent of disease, type of ischemic syndrome, and special clinical subgroups. Single-vessel coronary disease is the most widely accepted and clearest indication for PTCA. When revascularization is warranted in these patients, angioplasty is generally the preferred approach if feasible. However, CABG may be more appropriate in some patients with single-vessel disease if unfavorable features for angioplasty are present that would cause a low success rate or a significantly increased risk; these include chronic total occlusion, extreme vessel tortuosity, heavy calcification or marked angulation, ostial or diffuse lesions, and vessels having had multiple restenoses after PTCA.

Multivessel Disease
A substantial proportion of patients undergoing PTCA nowadays have multivessel disease. An important consideration in this setting is the completeness of revascularization that can be achieved. Complete revascularization with

CABG is generally accepted to be associated with improved outcome. However, the importance of complete revascularization with PTCA is not as clear and depends on the severity and extent of the nonrevascularized segments. Incomplete revascularization in patients with multivessel disease may result from inability to dilate all attempted sites. It may also be intentional: borderline significant or noncritical lesions (50 to 70% stenosis) may not warrant intervention; similarly, small vessels and branches or lesions and segments distal to nonviable myocardial zones often do not merit dilatation. Some vessels are not technically suitable for PTCA, and dilatation is not attempted. In some situations a "culprit" vessel can be identified as a major cause of unstable or worsening symptoms, and dilatation of this vessel may result in sufficient revascularization.[10]

Numerous reports have shown high success rates and relatively low complication rates in selected cohorts undergoing multiple-vessel PTCA[11-18] (Table 17-2). Clinical and angiographic success rates in excess of 85 to 90% are common, with the incidence of major complications ranging from 3 to 7%. The incidence of Q wave myocardial infarction is 1 to 3% (4 to 5% if non Q wave infarction is included), urgent CABG rates are 1 to 3%, and in-hospital mortality ranges from 0 to 3%. These results primarily reflect patients with two-vessel disease and a smaller proportion with three-vessel disease. Long-term follow up after multiple-vessel PTCA has shown generally low coronary event rates and high rates of continued improvement during average follow-up durations of 1 to 2 years (Table 17-3).

Several reports have also shown similar initial and follow-up results with PTCA of all three major arteries,[17,18] with angiographic success in more than 95% of lesions and success of revascularization of all vessels attempted in 82% (Fig. 17-2). During a mean follow-up of 2 years, the clinical recurrence rate was approximately 40%, and repeat PTCA was successful in most of these patients. About 10% had CABG during follow up, 4% had a myocardial infarction, 4% died, and an event-free outcome was greater than 50%. Actuarial survival at 3 years was 96% and 91% in these two studies.[17,18]

PTCA after CABG

PTCA is increasingly used in patients with prior CABG who develop graft failure, stenosis of the grafts, or progression of disease in the native or the grafted vessels. Since the risk of reoperation is higher than with a first operation, PTCA represents an attractive alternative for patients who have suitable lesions. Prior CABG patients now make up about 15% of patients having PTCA. The majority have PTCA of vein graft lesions, and a smaller proportion have PTCA of native segments beyond the graft insertion or of ungrafted vessels; PTCA is rare in an internal mammary artery (IMA) graft. Primary success is reported in 80 to 90% of these patients; this rate is slightly lower than in patients without prior CABG.[19-21] The angiographic success rate for bypass grafts is higher than for the nongraft lesions. The incidence of major complications is similar to that in

Table 17-2.   Immediate Results of Multivessel PTCA

				Complications (%)		
Trial	No. of Patients	Clinical Success (%)	Angiographic Success (%)	Myocardial Infarction	CABG	Death
Cowley et al.[11]	100	95	92	4.0	4.0	0
Vandormael et al.[13]	73	87	80	3.0	4.0	0
Myler et al.[14]	494	95	88	3.0	2.8	0.4
Deligonul et al.[15]	254	85	86	2.1	6.4	1.8
Mata et al.[16]	74	100	93	1.4	0	0
MCV	860	97	94	1.4	1.7	0.6

Abbreviation: MCV, The Medical College of Virginia.

Table 17-3.   Long-Term Follow-up After Multivessel PTCA

Trial	No. of Patients	Follow-up Duration (mo)	Symptom Status (%)		Late Events (%)			
			Asympto-matic	Improved	Recurrence	Myocardial Infarction	CABG	Death
Cowley et al.[11]	44	>12	48	82	34	2	18	0
Vandormael et al.[12]	66	>6	56	80	32	3	9	2
Myler et al.[14]	286	21	68	83	35	1	3	1
Deligonul et al.[15]	373	27	—	64	30	3	13	5
Mata et al.[16]	72	5.5	40	75	34	3	1	0
MCV	337	25	51	88	30	1	7	3

Abbreviation: MCV, The Medical College of Virginia.

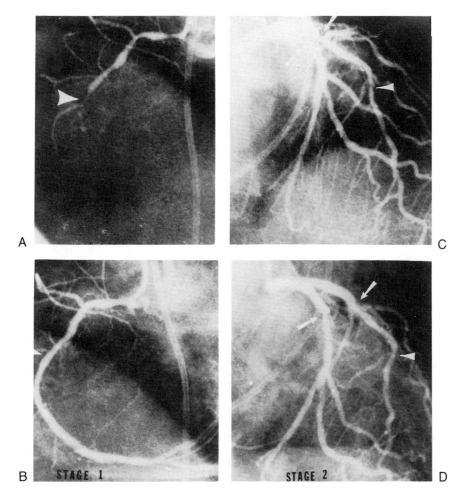

Fig. 17-2. Staged multivessel PTCA. (**A & B**) Successful stage I PTCA of a totally occluded right coronary artery (large arrowhead). (**C & D**) Successful stage II PTCA of proximal left anterior descending and circumflex arteries (arrows) and late mid-left anterior descending (small arrowhead) lesions.

patients without prior surgery: myocardial infarction in 2–6%, emergency or urgent CABG in 1 to 3%, and a hospital mortality of 0 to 2%, depending on baseline clinical risk profiles.[20] Vein graft lesions are more likely to be friable and to contain thrombus, which may embolize following PTCA. This occurs in 5 to 10% of graft dilatations and may produce myocardial infarction. Embolism is more common in older grafts (>5 years) and grafts with diffuse degenerative changes or thrombus. Diffusely diseased grafts carry a high risk of major embolization and are a contraindication to PTCA. PTCA is also feasible for IMA graft lesions. These occur most often at the distal insertion site, and success rates are in excess of 90% with current low-profile balloon dilatation equipment.[20]

Restenosis of vein grafts is more common than for native vessels, and the rate is dependent on the location of the lesion within the graft. The overall recurrence rate is 35 to 40%, with rates of about 25% at the distal insertion site, 40 to 45% for lesions in the body of the vein graft, and 50 to 60% for proximal or aorto-ostial graft lesions. After successful PTCA, prior CABG patients show similar clinical improvement. Although reports on long-term outcome are limited, available information suggests clinical recurrence rates of 20 to 25%, late CABG in fewer than 10%, and actuarial survival at 3 years of about 90%.[20,21]

PTCA in the Elderly

The elderly make up an increasing proportion of patients undergoing myocardial revascularization and represent a group in whom PTCA is an attractive alternative to CABG. Results of PTCA in patients older than 70 years show success rates ranging from 80 to 94% and relatively low complication rates: Q wave myocardial infarction in 1 to 4%, need for urgent CABG in 1 to 5%, and a hospital mortality rate of 1 to 2%.[22–24] Although the mortality rate is severalfold higher than in younger patients, it compares favorably with the operative mortality rate in elderly patients. Long-term follow-up results indicate comparable levels of clinical improvement after PTCA to those in younger patients, although the elderly have higher event rates and increased mortality rates during follow-up. Nevertheless, a high proportion of elderly patients have a satisfactory long-term outcome after PTCA.

Restenosis

Definitions

Restenosis is a major clinical and cost-related limitation of PTCA. The term "restenosis" refers to a return of luminal narrowing at a PTCA site. Restenosis is determined by angiography, using either visual or quantitative estimation. A variety of definitions have been used; each is arbitrary and has limitations.[25,26] Some definitions compare the relative degree of worsening with the original extent of improvement, some compare narrowing at follow-up with the final procedural result, and others use either absolute lumen diameter or narrowing above a certain level (50 or 70%) for restenosis. The most widely accepted definition is narrowing of >50% at follow-up evaluation. The incidence of restenosis depends on which definition is used and may not correlate with the functional importance of the residual narrowing or with clinical evidence of myocardial ischemia. For this reason, the term *clinical recurrence* is often used to describe symptomatic or important restenosis for which additional intervention may be needed. The reported occurrence of restenosis also depends on the proportion of patients who have follow-up coronary angiography and the proportion who are symptomatic. For clinical purposes, restenosis is best viewed as a discrete variable that is either present, absent, or partial. However, since most patients with restenosis have severe luminal narrowing (70 to 80%), the rates of restenosis in various reports have been similar, regardless of the definition used.

Incidence and Timing

The incidence of restenosis in most studies is in the 30 to 40% range, depending on definitions, patient population, symptom status, the time frame considered, and restudy rates. Since patients with recurrent angina are more likely to have repeat coronary angiography, this cohort is biased toward higher restenosis rates. In the NHLBI PTCA Registry report on restenosis,[25]

56% of patients with angina at follow-up had angiographic evidence of restenosis compared with only 14% of asymptomatic patients. Much of the variation in restenosis rates in reported studies reflects differences in baseline clinical and angiographic variables in the study groups.

Restenosis usually occurs within 3 to 6 months after PTCA and is generally manifested by the return of symptoms in a pattern similar to that before PTCA. Several serial angiographic studies designed to evaluate the time course of restenosis have shown that although recurrent stenosis of 50% can occur within a few days, probably as a result of elastic recoil and/or thrombosis, restenosis most often occurs gradually between 1 and 3 months.[27,28] Restenosis was less common between 3 and 6 months and was rare after 6 months. Recurrence of symptoms more than 6 to 12 months after PTCA is usually due to progression of disease in another vessel, rather than to restenosis.[29]

Mechanisms

The mechanism(s) of restenosis are multifactorial and include mechanical, viscoelastic, and hemodynamic factors, as well as the vascular healing response to injury following balloon-induced barotrauma. Elastic recoil is probably an important early factor, which occurs in response to stretching at the dilated site. Increasing evidence indicates that intimal hyperplasia and smooth muscle cell proliferation play a major role in the process of restenosis. Vascular smooth muscle cell growth and intimal hyperplasia occur in response to balloon injury of the vessel wall, with associated platelet deposition and release of platelet-derived growth factor (PDGF) and other mitogens at the site. Smooth muscle cell proliferation begins 2 to 3 days after PTCA and is complete by 7 to 14 days in experimental models.[30] Mechanical stretching of the vessel may also stimulate proliferation. Restenosis may therefore represent an exaggerated proliferative healing response.

Predictive Factors

Predictors of restenosis (Table 17-4) can be divided into clinical, angiographic, and procedural factors.

Table 17-4. Factors Predictive of Restenosis of Coronary Arteries

Clinical Factors
Male gender
Cigarette smoking
Unstable/recent-onset angina
Previous restenosis
Diabetes mellitus
Angiographic Factors
Location
Ostial LAD
Ostial RCA
Proximal vein graft
Multilesion/multivessel PTCA
PTCA of total occlusion
Severe stenosis pre-PTCA
Procedural Factors
High-grade residual stenosis and/or high translesional gradient after PTCA

Abbreviations: LAD, left anterior discending artery; RCA, right coronary artery.

Clinical Factors. In multiple studies, male gender, diabetes mellitus (particularly insulin-dependent), and unstable angina are associated with an increased restenosis rate.[25–28] Continued smoking after PTCA also has been associated with a higher restenosis rate.

Angiographic factors. Proximal left anterior descending (LAD) artery lesions, ostial stenoses, vein grafts, and vessels with total occlusion have increased restenosis rates.[25–28] In addition, more severe stenoses, lesions at bifurcations or bends, and multiple lesions have higher restenosis rates.[31]

Procedural factors. High-grade post-PTCA residual stenosis (>30%) and a higher residual translesional gradient (>15 to 20 mmHg) are associated with higher restenosis rates.[25–28] Large intimal dissections appear to have higher rates of restenosis, whereas small dissections have lower rates. Other procedural factors have not shown a consistent relationship with restenosis.

Detection

Recurrence of angina within 3 to 6 months after PTCA suggests restenosis and warrants further evaluation. Exercise testing may also detect restenosis in patients with silent myocardial ischemia or with few or atypical symptoms. The predictive value of symptoms for restenosis has ranged from 40 to 90%.[29] Exercise testing with thallium imaging improves the detection of restenosis compared with exercise testing alone. Several studies have also shown that early exercise testing after PTCA can predict future cardiac events and recurrence of angina.[32,33] Therefore, exercise testing, particularly with thallium, is useful after PTCA to detect significant residual stenosis or predict restenosis or progression of the coronary atherosclerotic disease.

Prevention

Randomized clinical trials of a variety of mechanical and pharmacologic interventions have been evaluated for the prevention of restenosis; most of these trials have shown no beneficial effects of the interventions.[28,34]

Antiplatelet Agents.   Pretreatment with aspirin (325 mg/day) before PTCA significantly reduces the rate of procedural complications (myocardial infarction, acute closure). However, several well-designed randomized trials investigating the use of aspirin alone or in combination with dipyridamole failed to show a beneficial effect on restenosis.[28,35] In a multicenter trial, ticlopidine was also ineffective in preventing restenosis.[35a] A multicenter study of ciprostene, a stable prostacycline analog administered intravenously for 48 hours after PTCA, showed a trend toward reduced restenosis and a significant reduction in combined clinical events during the study follow-up period.[28] Further studies of this agent are warranted.

Anticoagulants.   Warfarin for 6 months had no effect on restenosis compared with aspirin in one randomized trial.[35b] Heparin given for 24 hours after PTCA showed no effect on restenosis and was associated with increased bleeding complications.

Fish Oil.   Studies of N-3 omega fatty acids have shown conflicting results regarding restenosis[28]: among five published clinical trials, one showed significant reduction of the angiographic restenosis rate,[36] one showed lower recurrence rates assessed by either angiography or exercise test-

ing, and three showed no beneficial effect. In the study that showed a clear reduction in restenosis, the drug treatment was started 5 to 7 days before PTCA for maximal effect. At present, the role of N-3 fatty acids in the prevention of restenosis is uncertain.

Other Agents.   Several studies in which a large single dose of corticosteroid hormone was administered showed no effect on restenosis. Similarly, studies of the calcium-blocking drugs nifedipine and diltiazem showed no effect on restenosis rates.

Treatment

Repeat PTCA is the usual treatment for restenosis and is associated with higher success rates and lower complication rates than the initial procedures. Subsequent restenosis after repeat PTCA occurs with similar or only slightly higher frequency than following the initial procedures, so that the majority of patients have sustained improvement after repeat PTCA.

PTCA in Acute Myocardial Infarction

PTCA was initially used in acute myocardial infarction in conjunction with intracoronary streptokinase infusion (1) to achieve reperfusion in arteries that failed thrombolysis or (2) to treat severe residual stenosis after successful reperfusion in order to reduce the incidence of reocclusion.[37,38] PTCA was subsequently used as primary therapy for reperfusion as an alternative to thrombolytic therapy. The current use of PTCA for myocardial infarction has evolved considerably on the basis of accumulated experience and the results of several major clinical trials.

PTCA for acute myocardial infarction is still viewed as a method to achieve reperfusion (with or without thrombolytic therapy) and as a method to treat residual coronary artery obstruction following thrombolytic therapy for reperfusion.

Primary PTCA

The use of PTCA as the primary method to achieve reperfusion, without antecedent thrombolytic therapy, was first reported by Hartzler et al.[39] The potential advantages include avoidance of bleeding complications from thrombolytic agents and higher initial vessel patency rates than with thrombolysis. Reported success rates with primary PTCA of 83 to 95% exceed the best results with intravenous thrombolytic therapy (65 to 80% patency at 90 minutes).[39] However, the higher initial patency rate is offset by a higher reocclusion rate. In addition, primary PTCA currently is not feasible at most hospitals because of the lack of availability of immediate cardiac catheterization and/or the lack of a skilled interventional team. Trials comparing primary PTCA with intravenous thrombolysis have not been performed. Primary PTCA is most appropriate for patients who have a contraindication to thrombolytic therapy or who can be transferred or admitted to a tertiary care facility rapidly enough to warrant immediate angioplasty intervention.

Immediate PTCA

This term describes PTCA performed immediately after successful thrombolytic therapy for acute myocardial infarction. Three major randomized trials (TAMI-1, TIMI-2, and the European Cooperative Study Group) have evaluated this approach.[40–42] None of the three studies showed improvement in predischarge left ventricular exection fraction between the immediate and the "deferred" approach. In addition, hospital mortality and the need for emergency CABG were higher with immediate PTCA. Furthermore, in the TAMI-1 trial, when the 98 patients randomized to deferred (7 days) PTCA were reevaluated, only 35% actually had PTCA.[40] The others either had elective CABG or had a negative exercise test or lesion regression to <50% and no longer needed revascularization. Therefore, immediate PTCA following thrombolytic therapy is generally not warranted for patients who are clinically stable with evidence of reperfusion.

Deferred PTCA

The TIMI-2 trial compared "routine" PTCA at 18 to 48 hours after myocardial infarction (invasive strategy) with a conservative strategy of no revascularization unless recurrent or residual ischemia was present on predischarge exercise testing after infarction. The primary endpoints of death or nonfatal myocardial infarction at 6 weeks were not different between the two groups, and the predischarge left ventricular ejection fraction was also similar. These results support a conservative initial approach after thrombolytic therapy for myocardial infarction, particularly for patients who met the TIMI eligibility criteria. However, 25% of the patients in the "conservative" arm of the study required cardiac catheterization and myocardial revascularization procedures.

Salvage PTCA

Salvage PTCA refers to immediate angioplasty for reperfusion after failed thrombolytic therapy. Reported success rates range from 70 to 92%, which is lower than with primary PTCA.[38] Reocclusion rates are relatively high with salvage PTCA after tissue plasminogen activator (t-PA) therapy, but improved results have been reported with salvage PTCA in conjunction with the nonselective agents, urokinase or streptokinase.[38]

PTCA for Cardiogenic Shock

Cardiogenic shock warrants an aggressive approach and is one of the clearest indications for acute intervention in myocardial infarction. Available results from small nonrandomized series of such patients indicate that PTCA in this setting can improve reperfusion rates and provide hemodynamic stabilization. Survival rates have been higher in patients in whom PTCA is successful and in those with predominantly single-vessel coronary disease or cardiogenic shock due to right ventricular infarction. The long-term outcome has been satisfactory in those who survived their hospitalization.[43]

Complications

Incidence

Complications of PTCA include those associated with routine angiography and those related to the coronary angioplasty. Of the latter, the most important is acute vessel closure, which is responsible for most of the major complications of angioplasty: acute myocardial infarction, emergency CABG, and death. The incidence of major complications has declined with increasing experience and improvements in technology.[44] The overall incidence of major complications in the NHLBI PTCA Registry (1977 to 1982) was 9.3%, with myocardial infarction in 5%, emergency CABG in 6.3%, and a hospital mortality of 1.0%. Results from the 1985 to 1986 NHLBI PTCA Registry, which reflects a more contemporary experience in a higher-risk population, showed an overall major complication rate of 7.2%, with nonfatal myocardial infarction in 4.3%, emergency CABG in 3.4%, and a hospital mortality of 1.0%.

Predictive Factors

Baseline clinical and angiographic factors have been identified as predictors of complications with PTCA. The incidence of major complications increases with increasing extent of coronary disease, as well as with increasing age. Multivariate predictors of inhospital mortality include older age, female gender, three-vessel or left main coronary disease, as well as a history of congestive heart failure, reflecting significant left ventricular dysfunction.[44,45]

Acute Closure

Acute closure occurs in 2 to 5% of PTCA procedures.[4,44] Closure occurs more frequently in women and in patients undergoing multivessel PTCA.[44,46] Angiographic predictors include long lesions, lesions with bend angles of >45°, presence of thrombus, branch points, and total arterial occlusions.[46] Treatment of acute closure by repeat PTCA is usually successful when prolonged balloon inflations (several minutes) with standard or special perfusion catheters are used. If thrombus is present, intracoronary urokinase infusion is often effective in conjunction with repeat PTCA. Recently, newer devices such as laser-assisted balloon angioplasty,[47] directional atherectomy,[48] and intracoronary stents[49] have been used successfully to treat acute closure. However, the long-term value of stents has been discouraging.

Selection of Patients for PTCA

Selection of patients for PTCA involves integration of clinical and angiographic factors: (1) likelihood of success, (2) risk of abrupt closure,

(3) chance of restenosis, and (4) adequacy of the revascularization that can be achieved. These variables must be weighed in individual patients for each of the clinically important lesions and compared with the expected outcome of alternative therapy, either medical management or CABG. Although baseline clinical factors such as age, gender, extent of disease, and presence of left ventricular dysfunction are important, the most important determinants of suitability and outcome of PTCA are specific characteristics of the lesion. These include length, severity and location of the lesion, as well as morphologic factors such as the presence of calcification, eccentricity, tortuosity, angulation, irregularity, thrombus, branching, and total occlusion. On the basis of empiric and published experience, an American Heart Association and American College of Cardiology (AHA/ACC) Task Force on Coronary Angioplasty developed a scheme to classify lesions and to stratify the risk and likelihood of success.[50] Lesions were classified as type A (no unfavorable features), which have a high (>85%) expected success rate and low risk; type B (one or more unfavorable features), which have a moderate (60 to 85%) expected success rate and moderate risk; and type C lesions, which have either an expected low (<60%) success rate or a high risk based on very unfavorable morphology. The predictive value of this scheme has recently been validated for multivessel disease by Ellis et al.[51] Their modified classification, which further subdivided the intermediate (type B) risk group on the basis of absence (B1) or presence (B2) of multiple factors, provided significant additional predictive information on the procedural outcome compared with the standard AHA/ACC scheme.

Patients with high-success-rate, low-risk lesions are appropriate candidates for PTCA even if two or three vessels are involved, particularly when the probability of restenosis is not excessive. In contrast, high-risk features may favor CABG even in patients with single-vessel disease. Adequacy of revascularization is an important consideration, and selection of patients for PTCA should offer a reasonable probability of successful treatment of all clinically important ischemic zones compared with CABG.

PTCA and CABG are both palliative measures and should be viewed as complementary, rather than competing, strategies. Atherosclerosis is a progressive process, and many patients may require additional and possibly alternative interventions and preventive measures in the future. The obvious advantages of PTCA of simplicity, lower initial cost, and shorter recovery time are at least partly offset by the relatively high recurrence of stenosis and need for additional costly procedures. At present, only about 40 to 50% of patients who require myocardial revascularization are acceptable candidates for PTCA, whereas more than 90% are candidates for CABG. The most important limitations of PTCA are restenosis and acute vessel closure, and the most frequent exclusions are for unsuitable lesions, particularly chronic total occlusions, or for excessive risk and diffuse disease. The most important limitations of CABG are vein durability and the comorbidity associated with the operation. The most important exclusions for CABG are small vessels, distal disease, and major noncardiac medical problems. Present guidelines suggest that single-vessel disease and discrete two- (and possibly three-) vessel coronary disease with favorable lesion characteristics and good left ventricular function are acceptable situations for PTCA as well as CABG. In contrast, CABG is most appropriate in patients with extensive multivessel disease, left main coronary artery disease, or multivessel disease with significant left ventricular dysfunction.

Randomized Clinical Trials

Several major clinical trials are underway to compare PTCA with CABG in patients with multivessel coronary disease. The EAST (Emory Angioplasty Surgery Trial) has completed enrollment, with nearly 400 patients randomized[52]; the study is currently in the follow-up phase. The BARI (Bypass-Angioplasty Revascularization Intervention) Trial is an NHLBI-sponsored multicenter study, which will complete recruitment in 1991. More than 1,500 patients have been enrolled to date and will be monitored for 5 years; the BARI primary endpoint is 5-year mortality. Both studies will also assess multiple secondary clinical endpoints, as well as socioeconomic and cost factors. Several additional multicenter trials are in progress in Europe. The results of these studies should clarify the relative value of PTCA in the various heterogeneous subsets of patients with multivessel disease who require myocardial revascularization.

ALTERNATIVE INTERVENTIONAL TECHNIQUES

Although PTCA represents a major advance in nonsurgical myocardial revascularization, angioplasty has significant limitations that restrict its wider application. They include chronic occlusion, diffuse disease, acute closure, and restenosis. These limitations have led to the development of alternative devices, such as mechanical atherectomy, laser angioplasty, and cardiovascular stent systems, that offer improved safety, efficacy, and long-term artery patency. Several atherectomy systems have undergone multicenter clinical evaluation. The term *atherectomy* refers to the removal of plaque material from the vessel wall by excision or ablation. The three types of currently available systems can be considered to be directional, rotational, and extractional.

Directional Coronary Atherectomy

Device

Directional coronary atherectomy (DCA) is the most widely evaluated of the newer devices and has recently received U.S. Food & Drug Administration premarket approval for general use. The catheter system (Devices for Vascular Intervention, Inc., Redwood City, CA) is designed to cut and remove tissue.[53,54] The catheter has a cylindrical metallic housing with an open window on one side, a flexible nose cone at the distal end, a balloon support member opposite the window, and a central cup-shaped cutter which rotates at 2,000 rpm (Fig. 17-3). The catheter has a central lumen through which a guide wire can be manipulated into the distal vessel (Fig. 17-4). The device is positioned into the lesion, and the balloon is inflated to compress the open window into the plaque. The cutter is slowly advanced to shave the plaque protruding into the housing

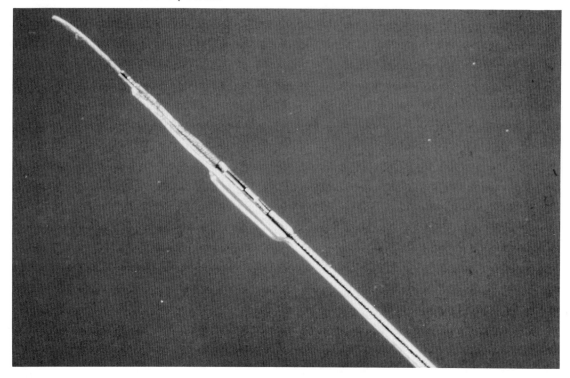

Fig. 17-3. Directional coronary atherectomy device.

window, and the atheroma is trapped in the nose cone. The window is redirected within the lesion, and cutting cycles are repeated circumferentially around the wall until the plaque has been removed. The DCA catheters are large (5, 6, and 7 French size) and require large-diameter (9.5 to 11 French size) guide catheters.

Current Experience
DCA has been performed in more than 1,500 patients through mid-1990. The U.S. experience at 12 centers through November 1989 has recently been reported, representing 958 procedures and 1,069 lesions in 873 patients.[55] Native vessels were treated in 83% and vein grafts in 17%; the left anterior descending artery was the artery most frequently treated (64%), followed by the right coronary artery (26%), the circumflex artery (7%), and the left main coronary artery (3%). Overall, the DCA success rate was 85%, and an additional 7% of patients had successful PTCA after an unsuccessful attempt at DCA. In some patients, high-grade lesions were predilated with a small balloon catheter to allow passage of the larger DCA catheter. The success rate was significantly higher for restenosis lesions (89%) than for de novo lesions (79%); it was also influenced by which vessel was treated (left anterior descending 88%, right coronary 80%, circumflex 85%, left main 61%; $P < 0.001$). Lesion calcification was associated with a lower success rate (70% versus 88%) than for noncalcified lesions ($P < 0.001$). In addition, the lesion length affected the success rate (focal 86%, tubular 86%, diffuse 75%; $P < 0.005$).

Complications
The incidence of major complications with DCA was 4.9%, with 3.7% attributable to DCA. Q wave myocardial infarction occurred in 0.8%, death occurred in 0.5%, and CABG was needed in 4.1%. Major complications were more common with right coronary artery, diffuse (>2 cm long) lesions, eccentric lesions, and de novo lesions.

Restenosis
The restenosis rate after DCA depends on the type of vessel (native or graft) and history of prior PTCA. The restenosis rate for de novo lesions

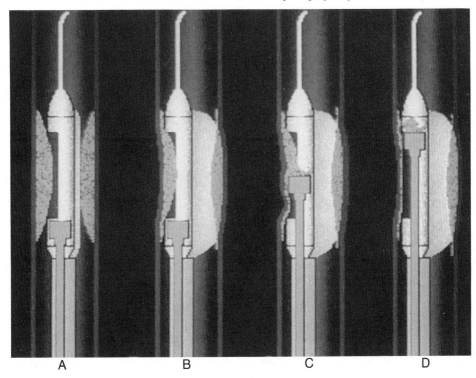

Fig. 17-4. Mechanism of directional coronary atherectomy. (**A**) Device is positioned across the stenosis. (**B**) Low pressure balloon inflation to allow protrusion of plaque into the window. (**C & D**) Rotating cup-shaped blade cuts lesion and collects tissue pieces in distal chamber.

appears to be similar to that of PTCA (about 30% for both native vessels and vein grafts). However, the restenosis rate after DCA of previously restenotic lesions appears to be considerably higher, in the range of 45% for native vessels and about 65% for vein grafts.[56]

Histopathologic analysis of DCA specimens has shown a high incidence of intimal hyperplastic changes in restenosis lesions compared with de novo atheromatous plaques. In addition to plaque elements, arterial media has been present in about 40% of specimens and adventitia in 15 to 25% of samples.[57]

Uses

The angiographic results after DCA are generally characterized by a widely patent lumen with smooth margins and almost no residual narrowing. The technique has been associated with a low incidence of dissection compared with PTCA, and late acute closure has been rare. The directional control of this technique makes it par-

ticularly well suited for highly eccentric lesions. DCA also appears useful for other lesions unfavorable for PTCA, such as ostial lesions, complex or markedly irregular stenoses, and vein grafts (Fig. 17-5). Because of the size and the rigid housing of the device, the technique is best suited for proximal segments in large vessels without prominent tortuosity.

High-Speed Rotational Atherectomy

Device

The Rotablator device (Heart Technologies, Bellevue, WA) (Fig. 17-6) contains a catheter with an elliptical burr at the tip, which is coated with tiny diamond chips. The burr is connected to a drive shaft, which is rotated by a compressed air motor at rates of 160,000 to 180,000 rpm. A central lumen allows passage of a 0.009-in. stainless steel guide wire, which is advanced across the lesion

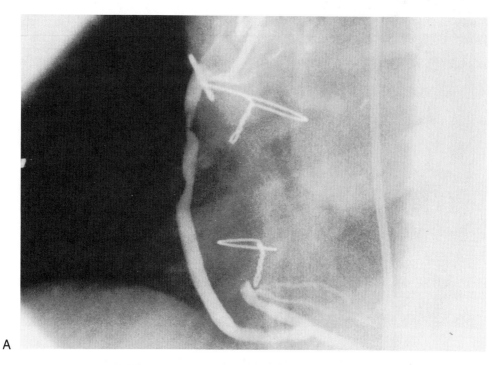

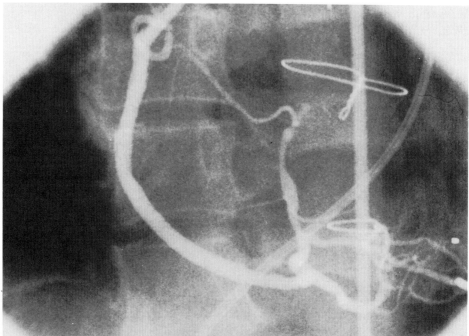

Fig. 17-5. Directional coronary atherectomy. Right coronary vein graft: (**A**) before and (**B**) after successful atherectomy.

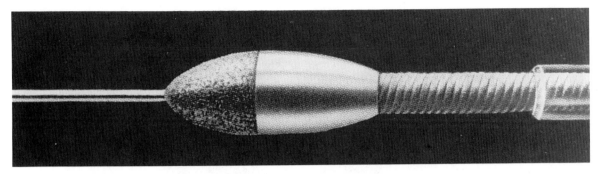

Fig. 17-6. Rotational atherectomy device (Rotablator).

and over which the catheter is advanced to the obstruction. The high-speed rotating burr abrades the plaque on contact, producing a sanding or polishing effect that releases microparticles into the distal circulation. Most of the particles are <5 μm in size and pass freely through the capillary bed without obstructing blood flow. The device appears to have a selective cutting effect, which preferentially ablates rigid noncompliant tissue (including calcified plaque) while displacing or deflecting elastic (normal) tissue. Burrs range from 1.25 to 2.75 mm in diameter.[58]

Current Experience

Following several pilot studies a multicenter study was begun, and results on 118 patients, including 140 lesions, have been reported.[59] Vessels treated were the left anterior descending arteries in 45%, right coronary artery in 36%, circumflex artery in 16%, and left main coronary artery in 3%. Most lesions (>85%) were complex (AHA/ACC type B or C). Success was achieved in 95% and adjunctive PTCA was performed for further luminal widening in 42%. Complications included non-Q wave myocardial infarction in 4.8% and emergency or urgent CABG in 0.8%. The device produces very smooth luminal margins with a low incidence of dissection; acute closure has been rare. Data on restenosis, based on angiographic 6-month follow-up in more than 150 patients, show a restenosis rate of 32%. Because of its size and flexibility, this device is well suited for distal lesions in smaller or tortuous vessels. Although it effectively ablates long lesions, flooding of the microcirculation with particulate debris

and associated transient ischemia or stunning has occurred with diffuse lesions.

Extraction Atherectomy

Device

The transluminal extraction catheter (TEC) (Interventional Technologies Inc., San Diego, CA) (Fig. 17-7) is a motor-driven rotary torque tube with an open conical cutting head and a central guide wire lumen. The catheter is attached to a vacuum pump and rotates at low speed (750 rpm) to excise the plaque material, which is removed by vacuum suction. Catheter sizes vary from 5.5 to 7 French size and require large (10 French size) guide catheters.[60]

Current Experience

Clinical experience in more than 100 patients at four centers has shown an overall primary success rate of >93% (92% in native vessels and 96% in vein grafts).[61] Mean stenosis was reduced from 74 to 35%. A significant proportion of patients had unfavorable lesions (diffuse, thrombus, or vein graft stenoses). Urgent CABG was done in 5%, mortality in patients without recent myocardial infarction was 0.7%, vessel perforation occurred in 2%, and embolization occurred in 1.5%. Adjunctive PTCA was performed in approximately two-thirds of patients. Angiographic 6-month follow-up in more than 100 patients showed restenosis in 44%. The device appears to be particularly effective for complex, thrombotic, or vein graft lesions; owing to its size and inflexibility, it

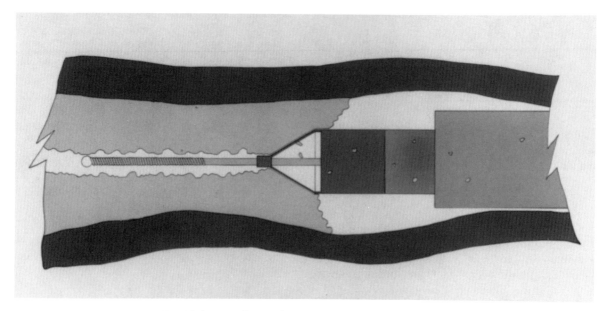

Fig. 17-7. Transluminal extraction catheter (schematic).

is best suited for proximal lesions in straight vessel segments.

Laser Angioplasty

Mechanism

Another method of nonsurgical plaque removal involves the use of laser energy. The most important medical lasers are CO_2, Nd:YAG, argon, and excimer. The first three of these are continuous-wave systems, whereas the excimer is a pulsed system. Continuous-wave lasers ablate by heat absorption (photothermal effect), causing vaporization, thermal necrosis, and acoustic shock trauma. Pulsed lasers, which use high energy, have a nonthermal or photochemical mechanism, which breaks molecular bonds and vaporizes without thermal damage. Initial vascular application was limited, owing to difficulties with the safety and control of bare laser fibers. Laser thermal angioplasty involving a catheter with a metallic cap at the tip ("hot tip") was developed to apply controlled thermal energy by heating the tip with argon or Nd:YAG lasers. The system was effective in large peripheral arteries, but the intense heat produced a significant incidence of

thrombosis and spasm in coronary arteries, and clinical use has since been limited. Continuous-wave lasers are generally not well suited for direct coronary application because of the undesirable thermal effects. Of the available pulsed-wave systems, the excimer has the most favorable energy characteristics and has been most widely used.[62]

Excimer Laser Angioplasty

Excimer refers to *excited-state dimer* lasers in which an inert gas (argon, xenon, or krypton) is associated with a halogen (fluorine or chlorine). These ultraviolet lasers have minimal tissue penetration and ablate on contact; of these, the XeCl 308-nm laser is the most reliable. The Dimer excimer laser (Advanced Interventional Systems, Irvine, CA) has been the most widely used. This system involves a multifiber catheter with a concentric array of 200-μm optical fibers around a central lumen for a 0.018-in. guide wire. Catheter sizes include 1.3, 1.6, and 2.0-mm diameter.[63] Results of excimer laser coronary angioplasty (ELCA) have been reported in 685 patients from 13 centers; 823 lesions were treated, with 9% total occlusions and 12% vein grafts.[64] Laser success, defined as >20% reduction of stenosis or creation of a lumen diameter near the catheter diameter by laser alone, was achieved in 83% of patients, and the success rate of the procedure (including adjunctive balloon dilatation) was 93%. Stand-alone laser angioplasty was done in 43% of patients. With the use of the newer 2.0-mm catheter, the laser success rate was 89% and the stand-alone laser rate was 56%. Procedural success exceeded 90% for both short lesions and stenoses >20 mm in length. Complications included acute occlusion in 5.2%, dissection in 13%, perforation in 1%, myocardial infarction in 0.4%, urgent CABG in 2%, and death in 0.2%. Additional experience with XeCl ELCA has been reported from Germany: a high clinical success rate was achieved, although a significant incidence of complications was encountered in patients with unstable angina or recent infarction.[65] Limited data are available on restenosis after ELCA. Preliminary results from Haase et al. indicate restenosis in 43% (42 of 107), with a rate of 35% (18 of 57) in patients who had stand-alone laser treatment and 56% (28 of 50) in patients who had adjunctive PTCA after an inadequate stand-alone result.[66] ELCA appears to be effective for a broad spectrum of coronary stenoses, including lesions unfavorable for balloon angioplasty, such as long, calcified, or diffuse lesions and ostial lesions. The technique is still limited by the ability to create a lumen only as large as the catheter diameter and an apparent higher incidence of complications in unstable ischemic syndromes. However, catheter technology is evolving, and this technique remains a promising new intervention whose role remains to be defined.

Endovascular Stents

Mechanical stents are an adjunct to PTCA and provide intraluminal scaffolding at the dilated site. They are designed to maintain a widely patent lumen by splinting dissection flaps against the vessel wall and by preventing elastic recoil.[67] Stents in current use are made of inert metal and are self-expanding or balloon-expandable. They are permanently implanted by using a balloon catheter delivery system and are slightly oversized for the lumen diameter to prevent migration and maintain maximum lumen size. Experimental studies indicate that endothelialization occurs within 2 to 3 weeks. Stents are foreign bodies that are thrombogenic. Thrombotic occlusion was a significant problem in early clinical use; however, aggressive anticoagulation following stent implantation has reduced the incidence of stent thrombosis. Stents are currently under evaluation for the treatment of acute vessel closure and for prevention of restenosis following PTCA. They are effective for the correction of PTCA-induced occlusive dissections and may reduce the need for urgent CABG; they are less effective when acute closure is secondary to thrombus formation. They have also been useful in improving immediate angiographic results when suboptimal results are obtained with PTCA owing to nonocclusive intimal tears or dissections or to elastic recoil of the dilated site. This application may also be promising in the prevention of restenosis. Preliminary experience suggests that implantation of a single stent for a discrete lesion in large arteries (≥3.2 mm in diameter) is associated with a restenosis rate as low as 15%. In contrast, arteries smaller than 3.0 mm in diameter and lesions longer than 15 mm, requiring multiple overlapping stents, have had prohibitively high restenosis rates of 55 to 100%.[68] Recent evidence also suggests that stenting of saphenous vein grafts is associated with a low restenosis rate. Randomized clinical trials to evaluate stenting for prevention of restenosis are currently under way.

SUMMARY

Interventional cardiology includes an increasing array of techniques for nonsurgical myocardial revascularization. PTCA is highly effective for patients with favorable angiographic anatomy. Its relative role in comparison with CABG in the heterogeneous subgroups of patients with multivessel coronary disease will be clarified by the results of ongoing clinical trials. Newer interventional devices promise to improve on some of the current limitations of PTCA and may further expand the clinical indications for PTCA.

REFERENCES

1. Gruentzig AR, Senning A, Siegenthaler WE: Nonoperative dilatation of coronary artery stenosis: Percutaneous transluminal coronary angioplasty. N Engl J Med 301:61, 1979
2. Kent KM, Bentivoglio LG, Block PC et al: Percutaneous transluminal coronary angioplasty: Report from the Registry of the National Heart, Lung and Blood Institute. Am J Cardiol 49:2011, 1982
3. Cowley MJ, Dorros G, Kelsey SF et al: Acute coronary events associated with percutaneous transluminal coronary angioplasty. Am J Cardiol 53:12C, 1983
4. Detre K, Holubkov R, Kelsey S et al: Percutaneous transluminal coronary angioplasty in 1985–1986 and 1977–1981. The National Heart, Lung and Blood Institute Registry. N Engl J Med 318:265, 1988
5. Gruentzig AR, King SB, Schlumpf M et al: Long-term follow-up after PTCA: The early Zurich experience. N Engl J Med 316:1127, 1987
6. Kent KM, Cowley MJ, Kelsey SF et al: Long term follow up of the NHLBI Registry. Circulation 74 (suppl. II):II-280, 1986
7. Talley JD, Hurst JW, King SB et al: Clinical outcome 5 years after attempted percutaneous transluminal coronary angioplasty in 427 patients. Circulation 77:820, 1988
8. Webb JG, Myler RK, Shaw RE et al: Bidirectional cross over and late outcome after coronary angioplasty and bypass surgery: 8 to 11 year follow-up. J Am Coll Cardiol 16:57, 1990
9. Waller BF, Garfinkel HJ, Rogers FJ et al: Early and late morphologic changes in major epicardial coronary arteries after percutaneous transluminal coronary angioplasty. Am J Cardiol 53:42C, 1984
10. Wohlgelernter D, Cleman M, Highman HA et al: Percutaneous transluminal coronary angioplasty of the "culprit" lesion for management of unstable angina pectoris in patients with multivessel coronary artery disease. Am J Cardiol 58:460, 1985
11. Cowley MJ, Vetrovec GW, DiSciascio G et al: Coronary angioplasty of multiple vessels: Short-term outcome and long-term results. Circulation 72:1314, 1985
12. Vandormael MG, Deligonul U, Kern MJ et al: Multilesion coronary angioplasty: Clinical and angiographic follow up. J Am Coll Cardiol 10:246, 1987
13. Vandormael MG, Chaitman BR, Ischinger T et al: Immediate and short-term benefit of multilesion coronary angioplasty: Influence of degree of revascularization. J Am Coll Cardiol 6:983, 1985
14. Myler RK, Topol EJ, Shaw RE et al: Multiple vessel coronary angioplasty: Classification, results and patterns of restenosis in 494 consecutive patients. Cathet Cardiovasc Diagn 13:1, 1987
15. Deligonul U, Vandormael MG, Kern MJ et al: Coronary angioplasty: A therapeutic option for symptomatic patients with two and three vessel coronary disease. J Am Coll Cardiol 11:1173, 1988
16. Mata LA, Bosch X, David PR et al: Clinical and angiographic assessment 6 months after double-vessel PTCA. J Am Coll Cardiol 6:1239, 1985
17. Hartzler GO, Rutherford BD, McConahay DR et al: "High risk" percutaneous transluminal coronary angioplasty. Am J Cardiol 61:33G, 1988
18. DiSciascio G, Cowley MJ, Vetrovec GW et al: Triple vessel coronary angioplasty: Acute outcome and long-term results. J Am Coll Cardiol 12:42, 1988
19. Douglas JS, Jr: Angioplasty of saphenous vein and internal mammary artery bypass grafts. p. 327. In Topol EJ (ed): Textbook of Interventional Cardiology. WB Saunders, Philadelphia, 1990
20. Dorros G, Lewin RF, Mathiak LM: Coronary angioplasty in patients with prior coronary artery bypass surgery. p. 791. In Dorros G (ed): Cardiology Clinics: Coronary Angioplasty. Vol. 7. WB Saunders, Philadelphia, 1989
21. Webb JG, Myler RK, Shaw RE et al: Coronary angioplasty after coronary bypass surgery: Initial results and late outcome in 422 patients. J Am Coll Cardiol 16:812, 1990
22. Simpfendorfer C, Raymond R, Schraider J et al: Early and long-term results of percutaneous transluminal coronary angioplasty in patients 70 years of age and older with angina pectoris. Am J Cardiol 62:959, 1988
23. Holt GW, Sugrue DD, Bresnahan JF et al: Results of percutaneous transluminal coronary angioplasty for unstable angina pectoris in patients 70 years of age and older with angina pectoris. Am J Cardiol 61:994, 1988
24. Dorros G, Janke L: Percutaneous transluminal coronary angioplasty in patients over the age of 70 years. Cathet Cardiovasc Diagn 12:223, 1986
25. Holmes DR, Vlietstra RE, Smith HC et al: Restenosis after PTCA: A report from the PTCA registry of the NHLBI. Am J Cardiol 53:77C, 1984
26. Califf RM, Ohman EM, Frid DJ et al: Restenosis: The clinical issues. p. 363. In Topol EJ (ed): Textbook of Interventional Cardiology. WB Saunders, Philadelphia, 1990
27. Serruys PW, Luitjen HE, Beatt KJ et al: Incidence of restenosis after successful coronary angioplasty:

A time-related phenomenon. A quantitative angiographic study in 342 consecutive patients at 1, 2, 3 and 4 months. Circulation 77:361, 1988

28. Nobuyoshi M, Kimura T, Nosaka H et al: Restenosis after successful percutaneous coronary angioplasty: Serial angiographic follow-up of 229 patients. J Am Coll Cardiol 12:616, 1988

29. Joelson JM, Most AS, Williams DO: Angiographic findings when chest pain recurs after successful PTCA. Am J Cardiol 60:792, 1987

30. Liu MW, Roubin GS, King SB: Restenosis after coronary angioplasty: Potential biologic determinants and role of intimal hyperplasia. Circulation 79:1374, 1989

31. Ellis SG, Roubin GS, King SB et al: Importance of stenosis morphology in the estimation of restenosis risk after elective percutaneous coronary angioplasty. Am J Cardiol 60:30, 1989

32. Deligonul U, Vandormael MG, Younis LT, Chaitman BR: Prognostic significance of silent ischemia detected by early treadmill exercise after coronary angioplasty. Am J Cardiol 64:1, 1989

33. Stuckey TD, Burwell LR, Nygaard TW et al: Quantitative exercise thallium-201 scintigraphy for predicting angina recurrence after percutaneous transluminal coronary angioplasty. Am J Cardiol 63:517, 1989

34. McBride W, Lange RA, Hillis LD: Restenosis after successful coronary angioplasty: Pathophysiology and prevention. N Engl J Med 318:1734, 1988

35. Schwartz L, Bourassa MG, Lesperance J et al: Aspirin and dipyidamole in the prevention of restenosis after PTCA. N Engl J Med 318:1714, 1988

35a. White CW, Knudson M, Schmidt D et al: Neither ticlopidine nor aspirin-dipyridamole prevents restenosis post-PTCA: Results of a randomized placebo-controlled multicenter trial (abstract). Circulation 76 (suppl. IV): IV-213, 1987

35b. Thornton MA, Gruentzig AR, Hollman J et al: Coumadin and aspirin in prevention of recurrence after transluminal coronary angioplasty: A randomized study. Circulation 69:721, 1984

36. Dehmer GJ, Popma JJ, Vanden Berg EK et al: Reduction in the rate of early restenosis after coronary angioplasty by a diet supplemented with n-3 fatty acids. N Engl J Med 319:733, 1988

37. Topol EJ: Coronary angioplasty for acute myocardial infarction. Ann Intern Med 109:970, 1988

38. Topol EJ: Mechanical interventions for acute myocardial infarction. p. 269. In Topol EJ (ed): Textbook of Interventional Cardiology. WB Saunders, Philadelphia, 1990

39. Hartzler GO, Rutherford BD, McConahay DR: Percutaneous transluminal coronary angioplasty: Application for acute myocardial infarction. Am J Cardiol 53:17C, 1984

40. Topol EJ, Califf RM, George BS et al: A randomized trial of immediate vs delayed elective angioplasty after intravenous tissue plasminogen activator in acute myocardial infarction. N Engl J Med 317:581, 1987

41. The TIMI Study Group: Comparison of invasive and conservative strategies following intravenous tissue plasminogen activator in acute myocardial infarction: Results of the Thrombolysis in Myocardial Infarction (TIMI) II trial. N Engl J Med 320:618, 1989

42. Simoons ML, Arnold AR, Betriu A et al: Thrombolysis with rt-PA in acute myocardial infarction: No beneficial effects of immediate PTCA. Lancet i:197, 1988

43. O'Neill W, Erbel R, Laufer N et al: Coronary angioplasty therapy of cardiogenic shock complicating acute myocardial infarction. Circulation 72 (suppl. III):III-309, 1985

44. Holmes DR, Holubkov R, Vlietstra RE et al: Comparison of complications during percutaneous transluminal coronary angioplasty from 1977 to 1981 and from 1985 to 1986: the NHLBI PTCA Registry. J Am Coll Cardiol 12:1149, 1988

45. Cowley MJ, Kelsey SF, Holubkov R et al: Factors influencing outcome with coronary angioplasty: The 1985–1986 NHLBI PTCA Registry (abstract). J Am Coll Cardiol 11 (suppl. II):II-148A, 1989

46. Ellis SG, Roubin GS, King SB et al: Angiographic and clinical predictors of acute closure after native vessel coronary angioplasty. Circulation 77:372, 1988

47. Spears JR, Reyes VP, Wynne J et al: Percutaneous coronary laser balloon angioplasty: Initial results of a multicenter experience. J Am Coll Cardiol 16:293, 1990

48. Whitlow PL, Robertson GC, Rowe MH et al: Directional coronary atherectomy for failed percutaneous transluminal coronary angioplasty (abstract). Circulation 82 (suppl. III):III-1, 1990

49. Sigwart U, Urban P, Golf S et al: Emergency stenting for acute occlusion after coronary balloon angioplasty. Circulation 78:1121, 1988

50. Ryan TJ, Faxon DP, Gunnar RM et al: Guidelines for percutaneous transluminal coronary angioplasty: A report of the American College of Cardiology/American Heart Association Task Force on Assessment of Diagnostic and Therapeutic Cardiovascular Procedures. J Am Coll Cardiol 12:529, 1988

51. Ellis SG, Vandormael MG, Cowley MJ et al: Coronary morphologic and clinical determinants of procedural outcome with angioplasty for multivessel coronary disease. Circulation 82:1193, 1990

52. King SB III, Lembo NJ, Hale EC et al: The Emory angioplasty vs surgery trial (EAST): Analysis of baseline patient characteristics (abstract). Circulation 82 (suppl. III):III–508, 1990

53. Simpson JB, Johnson DE, Thapliyal HV: Transluminal atherectomy: A new approach to the treatment of atherosclerotic vascular disease. Circulation 72 (suppl. III):III–146, 1985

54. Robertson GC, Hinohara T, Selmon HR et al: Directional coronary atherectomy. p. 563. In Topol EJ (ed): Textbook of Interventional Cardiology. WB Saunders, Philadelphia, 1990

55. DCA Investigators: Directional coronary atherectomy: Multicenter experience (abstract). Circulation 82 (suppl. III):III–71, 1990

56. DCA Investigators: Restenosis following directional coronary atherectomy in a multicenter experience (abstract). Circulation 82 (suppl. III):III–679, 1990

57. Safian RD, Gelbfich JS, Erny RE et al: Coronary atherectomy: Clinical, angiographic and histological findings and observations regarding potential mechanisms. Circulation 82:69, 1990

58. Bertrand ME, Fourrier JL, Auth DC et al: Percutaneous coronary rotational atherectomy. p. 580. In Topol EJ (ed): Textbook of Interventional Cardiology. WB Saunders, Philadelphia, 1990

59. Buchbinder M, O'Neill W, Warth D et al: Percutaneous coronary rotational ablation using the rotablator: Results of a multicenter study (abstract). Circulation 82 (suppl. III):III–309, 1990

60. Stack R, Quigley PJ, Sketch MH et al: Extraction atherectomy. p. 590. In Topol EJ (ed): Textbook of Interventional Cardiology. WB Saunders, Philadelphia, 1990

61. Sketch MH, O'Neill W, Tcheng JE et al: Early and late outcome following coronary transluminal extraction-endarterectomy: A multi-center experience (abstract). Circulation 82 (suppl. III):III–310, 1990

62. Forrester JS: Laser angioplasty: current and future prospects. p. 738. In Topol EJ (ed): Textbook of Interventional Cardiology. WB Saunders, Philadelphia, 1990

63. Litvack F, Grundfest WS, Goldenberg T et al: Excimer laser angioplasty. p. 682. In Topol EJ (ed): Textbook of Interventional Cardiology. WB Saunders, Philadelphia, 1990

64. Litvack F, Margolis J, Rothbaum D et al: Excimer laser coronary angioplasty: Acute results of the first 685 consecutive patients (abstract). Circulation 82 (suppl. III):III–71, 1990

65. Karsch KR, Haase KK, Voelker W et al: Percutaneous coronary excimer laser angioplasty in patients with stable and unstable angina pectoris. Circulation 81:1849, 1990

66. Haase KK, Mauser M, Baumbach A et al: Restenosis after excimer laser coronary angioplasty (abstract). Circulation 82 (suppl. III):III–672, 1990

67. Sigwart U, Puel J, Mirkovitch V et al: Intravascular stents to prevent occlusion and restenosis after transluminal angioplasty. N Engl J Med 316:701, 1987

68. Muller DWM, Ellis SG: Advances in coronary angioplasty: Endovascular stents. Coronary Artery Dis 1:438, 1990

MYOCARDIAL REVASCULARIZATION AND OTHER SURGICAL PROCEDURES FOR CORONARY HEART DISEASE AND ITS COMPLICATIONS

18

Surgical Intervention in Coronary Heart Disease

Mark W. Connolly, M.D.
Robert A. Guyton, M.D.

Since the initiation of surgical revascularization for coronary heart disease over 30 years ago, coronary artery bypass grafting (coronary bypass) has been and continues to be a proven, effective therapy for relieving symptomatic angina pectoris, prolonging survival, and improving the quality of life. The efficacy of this procedure is represented by the fact that more than 230,000 coronary bypass operations are performed annually in the United States.[1] The treatment of coronary heart disease has progressed from nonoperative management with nitrate drugs and beta-blocking agents in the 1950s to an aggressive multimodality approach using coronary risk factor control, blood pressure control, calcium channel-blocking drugs, new antiarrhythmic and lipid-lowering drugs, thrombolytic enzymes, angioplasty, and surgical interventions. The exact roles of these modalities in the diverse subsets of patients afflicted with coronary heart disease are uncertain today. Although treatment regimens have changed drastically over the last four decades and will continue to change well into the future, surgical revascularization, particularly with the internal mammary artery, remains the mainstay end therapy for severe symptomatic coronary heart disease when other therapies are unsuccessful or contraindicated. This chapter provides an overview of state-of-the-art surgical interventions in coronary heart disease in the 1990s.

HISTORICAL NOTE

Surgical attempts to achieve palliative relief from angina pectoris began well before stenotic coronary artery lesions were defined anatomically by coronary angiography.[2] Left cervical sympathectomy in the 1920s,[3] scarification of the epicardium to stimulate new vessel growth in 1930s,[4] and direct implantation of the internal mammary artery into a myocardial tunnel by Vineberg and Miller[5] preceded the development of coronary bypass. During the 1950s several small series reported results with blind,[6] direct,[7] and carbon dioxide gas[8] coronary endarterectomy without cardiopulmonary bypass. The development of coronary cineangiography by Sones and Shirey[9] at the Cleveland Clinic in 1958 to anatomically define coronary stenotic lesions formed the foundation for coronary bypass. As the technique of cardiopulmonary bypass pioneered by

323

Gibbon came into clinical use, Favaloro[10] at the Cleveland Clinic began performing reversed aortocoronary saphenous vein bypass grafting in 1967. In 1968 Green et al.[11] and Bailey and Hirose[12] reported the direct anastomosis of the left internal mammary artery to the anterior descending coronary artery.

In the early 1970s numerous reports described the advantages of coronary bypass, leading to its rapidly increasing use in the treatment of coronary heart disease. By 1980, the number of coronary bypass operations performed annually in the United States approached 200,000. Because of the substantial impact on the health and financial resources of the United States and the questioned uncertainty of long-term survival and quality-of-life results from coronary bypass surgery, large randomized prospective clinical trials were begun in the late 1970s.

PROSPECTIVE RANDOMIZED CLINICAL TRIALS

As operative mortality for coronary bypass decreased throughout the 1970s, the limits of the indications for coronary bypass were extended to include almost all patients with symptomatic coronary heart disease. The medical community questioned the benefit and possible overuse of coronary bypass in patients with stable angina pectoris. Three large randomized prospective trials comparing medical and surgical therapy in patients with chronic, stable angina were undertaken to give clinicians a better understanding of what types of patients could benefit from coronary bypass. Many reports, interpretations, and critiques have been written about each of these trials. Physician bias before and after randomization, medical-to-surgical crossover, biostatistical methods, treatment received versus treatment prescribed, and inappropriate conclusions based on small subgroup numbers cloud the results of these trials.[13] The relevance of these trials is further brought into question by the continuing changes in therapeutic methods: new treatments including thrombolytic agents, calcium channel-blocking drugs, coronary angioplasty, and ex-

panded use of the internal mammary artery conduit. Despite deficiencies in the trials and changes in treatment methods, much was learned and worthwhile inferences can be made about the benefits of surgery in subsets of coronary patients. The entry criteria and patient characteristics of each of the three major trials (the Veterans Administration [VA] Trial, the European Coronary Surgery Study [ECSS], and the Coronary Artery Surgery Study [CASS]) have been previously described in detail in the literature.

Veterans Administration Trial

In the VA Trial significant surgical benefit over medical therapy was shown in (1) patients with greater than 50% left main coronary artery stenosis (80 versus 64% survival at 30 months; $P < 0.02$),[14] (2) patients with triple-vessel disease with an ejection fraction less than 50%,[15] and (3) high-risk patients with two or more of the following clinical characteristics: resting ST segment depression, prior myocardial infarction, hypertension, or impaired left ventricular function.[16] At 11.2 years, for all patients, no significant difference was found between medical and surgical therapy; and the surgical benefits observed at 7 years diminished to nonsignificance at 11 years. The 5-year nonfatal myocardial infarction rates were similar for both groups (14% medical versus 15% surgical).[15]

Criticisms of the study included an overall high operative mortality rate (5.8%), a high perioperative infarction rate (18%), a low vein graft patency rate (70% at 1 year), and a small number of bypass grafts placed (1.9 per patient), suggesting incomplete revascularization. A 38% crossover from medical to surgical therapy took place.

European Coronary Surgery Study

Unlike the VA study, the ECCS showed a significant improvement in survival after surgery compared with medical therapy at 5 years (93 versus 83%; $P < 0.0001$), at 8 years (89 versus 80%; $P < 0.0022$), and at 12 years (71 versus 68%; $P < 0.04$).[17] The lower surgical mortality in the ECSS than in the VA Trial reflected, at least in part, improvements in surgical techniques during the several years between the two studies. Subgroups of patients with triple-vessel disease and with double-vessel disease that included stenosis of the proximal left anterior descending coronary artery also showed significantly improved survival with surgery. Other independent prognostic variables associated with surgical benefit included abnormal resting electrocardiogram (ECG), ST segment depression on the exercise ECG, peripheral vascular disease, and increased age. The overall operative mortality was 3.3%, with a better graft patency rate (74 to 81%, ranging from 1 to 5 years) than in the VA study. The incidence of myocardial infarction, as in the VA study, was not significantly different at 5 years (11% medical versus 15% surgical).[18] Surgery did not appear to influence the annual rate of retirement from work.[17,18] Surgery further provided a decrease in anginal status, a decrease in medication requirement, and an increase in exercise tolerance.[19]

Again, a high crossover rate (36%) occurred from medical to surgical therapy,[1] and only 63% of the patients randomized to surgical therapy were operated on within 3 months. Furthermore, 6 of the 21 surgical deaths occurred in patients who died awaiting surgery.

Coronary Artery Surgery Study

This large clinical trial registered 24,959 patients who underwent cardiac catheterization, but only 780 of these patients were actually randomized. No statistically significant difference in 5-year survival was found between the randomized groups (90% medical versus 92% surgical).[20] Operative mortality was low at 1.4% (range, 0.6 to 11%), and the perioperative infarction rate was 6.4%.[21] Medical survival was also excellent, with an annual mortality rate of 1.6%. Randomized patients with an abnormal ejection fraction (between 35 and 50%) and triple-vessel disease showed an improved 7-year surgical survival (88%) compared with those randomized to medical therapy (65%).[22] Improvement in angina, exercise tolerance, and medication requirements

were demonstrated after coronary bypass. Similar to the VA trial and the ECSS, 5-year freedom from myocardial infarction was not different between the groups (82% medical versus 83% surgical); nor did employment and recreational endpoints differ.[23]

Analysis of the nonrandomized patients in the CASS registry produced valuable data. Operative mortality in the 6,630 nonrandomized patients was 2.3% (range, 0.3 to 6.4%).[21] Increased age, female sex, congestive heart failure, left main coronary artery stenosis, impaired left ventricular function, and emergent operation were determined to be significant predictors of increased operative mortality.[21] Various preoperative patient characteristics then became available for assessing the relative risk and benefit of operation. Improved 5-year surgical survival was demonstrated for patients who were randomizable (but not entered because of severity of angina [class III and IV]) and who had triple-vessel disease and severe angina with or without abnormal left ventricular function.[24] Early operation was a strong predictor of survival.[25] Patients 65 years of age and older had greater 5-year surgical survival (79% versus 64% with medical therapy; $P < 0.0001$) and greater absence of angina (67% versus 26%); surgery was an independent beneficial predictor of survival.[26] Lastly, patients with abnormal exercise test results (>1-mm ST segment depression or low exercise tolerance) demonstrated better 7-year survival with surgery than medical therapy.[27]

As in the VA trial and the ECSS, medical crossover to surgery was high at 23.5% (4.7%/yr). More importantly, a strong selection bias of the randomized patients favoring medical therapy may have occurred. Of the 2,099 patients "eligible" for randomization, only 780 were actually randomized. The other 1,319 patients were not randomized mainly because of clinical judgment and physician bias.[22] Of the four groups in the CASS, randomized-medical (390 patients), randomized-surgical (390 patients), nonrandomized-medical (745 patients), and nonrandomized-surgical (570 patients) groups, the nonrandomized-surgical group had a significantly higher incidence of left main, proximal left anterior descending, and triple-vessel coronary artery disease.[24] Clearly, the higher-risk patients were directed toward and received surgery without randomization. With the higher-risk patients excluded, the differences between medical and surgical therapy were minimized, since both groups contained only low-risk patients with a favorable prognosis. Thus, physician bias and exclusion of high-risk patients must be taken into consideration when interpreting the conclusion of the CASS investigators that medical and surgical therapy provide equal survival benefit. Furthermore, the significantly better results for both medical and surgical therapy in the CASS compared with the VA Trial and the ECSS could be explained by this biased randomization of patients with favorable medical outcomes.[28]

None of the trials indicated efforts at or results from intensive coronary risk factor modification (see Ch. 5).

Conclusions

Although deficiencies existed in each of the randomized trials, a tremendous amount of information became available; clinicians were given a data base for referring patients to surgery who have chronic, stable angina or who are asymptomatic after acute myocardial infarction. The following conclusions are relevant:

1. Results of both medical and surgical therapies have improved dramatically since the 1960s.
2. Operative mortality was low, suggesting improved surgical methods.
3. Compared with medical therapy, surgery offered better relief of angina, increased exercise capacity, and decreased medication requirements.
4. Surgery improved survival in patients with left main coronary artery disease, triple-vessel disease (especially with impaired left ventricular function), double-vessel disease that included proximal left anterior descending artery stenosis, or a positive exercise test.
5. Surgery did not decrease the incidence of nonfatal myocardial infarction over that for medical therapy.
6. Left ventricular function (strongest predictor),

age, extent of coronary artery disease, female gender, and associated medical diseases were important risk factors for operative mortality.

In conclusion, medical therapy should be recommended for low-risk patients with documented moderate coronary artery obstruction, until symptoms cannot be controlled with medical treatment and revascularization becomes necessary.

Furthermore, the clinical trials delineated subgroups of patients in whom surgical intervention offers significant benefit, primarily on the basis of angiographic coronary obstruction and ventricular function. Operative benefits and risks can be predicted from angiographic data. Hence, coronary cineangiography continues to be essential in evaluating the coronary patient and determining optimal therapy.

CORONARY ANGIOPLASTY

The rapid growth of coronary angioplasty in the 1980s was as prominent as the growth of coronary bypass in the 1970s. It is estimated that more than 400,000 angioplasties were performed in 1991. Indications for coronary angioplasty quickly expanded from single-vessel to triple-vessel disease and from severe to moderate stenoses. Methods, indications, and results for angioplasty are discussed in detail in Chapter 17.

Restenosis

Despite improvement in techniques, the restenosis rate following coronary angioplasty remains 25 to 30%.[29,30] Patients with multivessel disease are especially susceptible to restenosis, with approximately 50% sustaining restenosis of at least one vessel site. Angioplasty of restenotic sites has about the same success rate as the initial procedure.

Survival Data

The hospital mortality rate for coronary angioplasty at Emory University Hospitals is less than 0.1% for single-vessel disease and 0.5% for multivessel disease. Myocardial infarction occurs in approximately 2% of patients.[31] Emergency surgery is necessary in 2 to 3%. Comparable results have been reported from other major cardiac centers.

Abrupt closure during angioplasty is the most life-threatening event. Predictors of abrupt closure are high lesional gradients and intimal tear or dissection of the dilated site.[32] Thirty percent of these patients require emergency coronary bypass, and the mortality rate ranges from 2 to 12%. Myocardial damage, determined by cardiac enzyme elevation, occurs in 25 to 50% of failed-angioplasty patients who require emergency coronary bypass. The 1-year mortality rate is 1% if myocardial infarction does not occur compared with 7% if myocardial infarction does occur.

Long-term survival after coronary angioplasty has been excellent. The early experience of Gruentzig et al. in Zürich for 133 patients revealed a 96% 5-year survival, with 97% free of death, myocardial infarction, or need for coronary bypass.[33] Emory University reported an excellent 97% 3-year survival for 966 patients who underwent multivessel angioplasty. Event-free survival was 80% at 3 years.[34]

Similar to surgery patients, approximately 85% of coronary angioplasty patients have symptomatic relief of angina and excellent (>95%) survival. Thirty percent of patients require repeat angioplasty, and 15 to 20% eventually require coronary bypass.

Surgical Back-up

Surgical back-up for angioplasty requires a concerted effort among the medical, surgical, and anesthesia teams. High-risk angioplasty patients, in whom acute closure could result in hemodynamic compromise, should be discussed with the surgical team prior to the procedure. A high-risk angioplasty involves potential cumulative loss of 40 to 45% of left ventricular muscle mass (angio-

plasty plus previous infarction). In our recent experience at Crawford Long Hospital of Emory University, emergency surgery occurred in 3% of angioplasty patients, and coronary bypass during the same hospitalization was required for another 6%. Hospital mortality was 0 in 47 emergency operations for failed angioplasty. The perioperative complication rate was high, at 68%. The perioperative myocardial infarction rate was 21%, which was markedly lower than the 71% perioperative rate previously reported from Emory University in 1982. This decreased perioperative infarction rate after failed angioplasty has occurred despite a decrease in the use of the intra-aortic balloon pump (IABP). More rapid revascularization and modification of myocardial protection techniques during coronary bypass most probably account for these improved results. Acceptance by the angioplasty operator of the need for emergency surgery leads to greater myocardial salvage and lower perioperative myocardial infarction rates.

A relative contraindication to angioplasty is coronary anatomy such that abrupt closure could cause left ventricular pump failure and consequent mortality. Patients with left main coronary artery stenosis or multivessel disease with left ventricular dysfunction fall into this high-risk category. A patient with a 30% left ventricular ejection fraction and a stenotic coronary vessel supplying 20% of the remaining viable myocardium should not undergo angioplasty.

Comparison of Coronary Angioplasty and Coronary Bypass Surgery

The explosive use of coronary angioplasty has led to dramatic changes in the coronary patient cohorts undergoing specific therapies. At Emory, between 1981 and 1988, 14,078 patients underwent diagnostic cardiac catheterization.[35] Of the 1,704 patients found to have significant disease in 1981, 52% were treated medically, 44% surgically, and 4% by angioplasty. In 1988, of 1,719 such patients, 41% were treated with medical therapy, 29% by coronary bypass, and 30% by angioplasty. The coronary bypass population was older in 1988 than in 1981 (45% older than 65 years in 1988 versus 26% in 1981) and had poorer ventricular function (30% with ejection fraction of <50% in 1988 versus 24% in 1981). The angioplasty group was significantly younger, had less severe disease, and had better ventricular function. Hence, a marked increase in angioplasty for one- and two-vessel disease has occurred, while the recent coronary bypass patients are older, have poorer ventricular function, and have more triple-vessel coronary disease.

To further examine these patient trends in therapy, three Emory patient cohorts with one- and two-vessel disease were retrospectively studied: 100 coronary bypass patients in 1979, 100 coronary bypass patients in 1984, and 100 coronary angioplasty patients in 1984.[36] The 1984 patients (coronary bypass and angioplasty) had identical preoperative characteristics to the 1979 patients, but the 1984 angioplasty patients were significantly younger and had higher ejection fractions than the 1984 coronary bypass patients. This study also revealed a continuing trend toward angioplasty for one- and two-vessel disease, as one-third of the 1984 coronary bypass cohort would have undergone angioplasty according to the more current angioplasty angiographic criteria. The indications for coronary bypass are becoming more restrictive, while those for coronary angioplasty are becoming less restrictive.

Surgical methods have changed greatly since the early days of coronary bypass. Advances in anesthetic management, cardiopulmonary bypass, myocardial protection, hemodynamic monitoring, critical-care medicine, and antibiotic drugs have all contributed to an operative mortality approaching zero in elective low-risk coronary bypass patients. To compare the results for one- and two-vessel disease between angioplasty and coronary bypass, a group of 1,376 Emory University patients were selected retrospectively by using three CASS criteria (age younger than 66 years, ejection fraction greater than 35%, no congestive heart failure).[36] The hospital mortality for coronary bypass in this CASS-equivalent low-risk group was excellent at 0.07% (1 of 1,376 patients). This compared favorably with a 0.1% mortality for angioplasty.

At the Cleveland Clinic, 781 patients with isolated left anterior descending coronary disease treated between 1980 and 1984 by either coronary bypass or coronary angioplasty were retrospectively analyzed.[37] Five-year survival was slightly better for coronary bypass (98 versus 95%; $P < 0.02$), but coronary bypass patients had a much higher event-free survival from myocardial infarction, repeat bypass grafting, angioplasty, and death (93 versus 62%; $P < 0.0001$). This type of event-free survival analysis, expanded to include overall hospital stay and costs, should be the focus of future prospective, randomized trials.

Results of prospective, randomized trials are needed, and five studies are presently in progress: the Emory Angioplasty Surgery Trial (EAST), the Bypass Angioplasty Revascularization Investigation (BARI), Coronary Angioplasty versus Bypass Revascularization Investigation (CABRI), German Angioplasty Bypass Investigation (GABI), and the Randomized Intervention Treatment of Angina (RITA). A large prospective, randomized trial comparing medical therapy and coronary angioplasty appears unlikely to be done. Angioplasty and coronary bypass both offer excellent invasive therapeutic benefits for patients with coronary heart disease. Since excellent proven results are obtained from surgery, overutilization of angioplasty should be cautiously avoided until the results of the randomized trials are known. Coronary bypass with use of the internal mammary artery (IMA) is the gold standard of invasive therapy against which the long-term results of angioplasty should be tested.

CORONARY ARTERY BYPASS SURGERY

Indications

Considering the results of the randomized trials and the present state of coronary angioplasty, the current indications (Table 18-1) for coronary bypass in symptomatic patients, after defining coronary anatomy and left ventricular function by cardiac catheterization, are as follows:

Table 18-1. Current Indications for Coronary Bypass

To relieve anginal symptoms
    Refractory to medical therapy
    Poor patient compliance with medical therapy
    Angioplasty contraindicated
To improve quality of life
    Medical therapy limits lifestyle
    Angioplasty contraindicated
To prolong life
    Left main coronary artery disease
    Triple-vessel disease
    Double-vessel disease and poor left ventricular
        function and/or proximal left anterior descend-
        ing artery disease
To preserve left ventricular function
    Compelling coronary anatomy present
    Large area of left ventricle at risk
    Previous myocardial infarctions

1. To relieve anginal symptoms in patients when medical therapy and/or angioplasty has failed or is contraindicated
2. To improve the quality of life in patients when medical therapy limits lifestyle and work ability and when angioplasty is contraindicated
3. To prolong life in patients with left main coronary artery disease, triple-vessel disease, and double-vessel disease with proximal left anterior descending stenosis with or without left ventricular dysfunction
4. To preserve left ventricular function in asymptomatic patients with compelling coronary anatomy (left main equivalent or proximal dominant-vessel stenosis) and significant left ventricular mass at risk, particularly when previous myocardial infarction has already compromised left ventricular function

As the results of the prospective angioplasty-coronary bypass trials become known, as more pharmacologic and invasive therapies become available, and as surgical techniques improve, these indications for coronary bypass will continued to be refined.

Operative Technique

Although each patient's operative management is individualized, an overview of the surgical technique for elective coronary bypass at Emory University Hospitals will be summarized. Variations of this method for specific patient subsets, such as those with acute myocardial infarction or mitral regurgitation, will be discussed subsequently.

After insertion of hemodynamic monitoring lines (Swan–Ganz catheter, radial arterial pressure, large-bore intravenous access), patients undergo induction with combination benzodiazapene, fentanyl, and enflurane anesthetics. Antibiotic prophylaxis with a second- or third-generation cephalosporin is given. After positioning, placement of a Foley catheter, and skin preparation with topical Betadine, a sternotomy incision is performed. The internal mammary artery(s) (IMA) is dissected from the chest wall, while the saphenous vein(s) is harvested from the lower leg(s). After heparinization, an aortic and a single, double-stage right atrial cannula are placed through pursestring sutures. Cardiopulmonary bypass is instituted through a membrane oxygenator to achieve blood flows of 2.5 L/min/m^2 and a mean arterial perfusion pressure of approximately 60 mmHg. Hematocrit is maintained above 18% with homologous blood transfusions if necessary. The patient is cooled to a body temperature of 25 to 28°C depending on the severity of disease, left ventricular function, and expected aortic crossclamp time. Venting of the left ventricle is not routinely performed. The coronary vessels to be bypassed are examined and dissected free from surrounding epicardium where suitable for bypass. The aorta is then crossclamped after manual inspection for atherosclerotic disease. Cold (4°C) crystalloid or blood, potassium (18 mEq/L) oxygenated cardioplegic solution is injected antegrade through the aortic root while topical iced saline is placed on the heart. Retrograde cardioplegic techniques through the coronary sinus may be used if the antegrade technique is not adequate, such as with left main or equivalent coronary disease. Myocardial termperatures are not routinely obtained, but are usually lower than 15°C when measured. Reversed saphenous-vein-to-coronary-artery anastomoses are performed with a continuous Prolene suture beginning with the vessel supplying the most viable myocardial area at risk. Cardioplegic solution is infused down the completed vein graft for further myocardial protection and estimation of graft flows. Cardioplegic solution is also reinfused into the aortic root at 20- to 30-minute intervals. The in situ internal mammary anastomosis is usually performed last while the patient is being rewarmed. The aortic clamp is removed, and vein grafts are measured for length and anastomosed to the ascending aorta with a side-biting J clamp. The heart is defibrillated if spontaneous sinus rhythm has not occurred. The vein grafts and aorta are de-aired, and all anastomoses are checked for hemostasis. The patient is weaned from cardiopulmonary bypass with pharmacologic assistance (inotropic agents, vasoconstrictor drugs, and vasodilator drugs), if necessary, to maintain a cardiac index greater than 2.2 L/min/m^2. Cannulas are removed, protamine is given to reverse the effect of the heparin, and mediastinal and pleural drainage tubes and pacing wires are placed. After adequate hemostasis is obtained, the chest is closed. The patient is then transferred to an intensive care unit for careful hemodynamic monitoring. Patients are weaned off pharmacologic support as tolerated and extubated 12 to 24 hours later, usually the morning after operation.

Perioperative Mortality and Morbidity

In approximately 9,000 nonrandomized patients entered into the CASS between 1974 and 1979, the overall 30-day operative mortality was 2.3%.[38] Increased age, female sex, severity of angina, presence of congestive heart failure, triple-vessel disease, left ventricular dysfunction, left main coronary disease, and diabetes mellitus[39] were all significant predictors of increased operative mortality.

Between 1976 and 1979, 3,040 patients at Emory University Hospitals underwent coronary bypass, with an overall mortality of 0.8%.[40] This low operative mortality (<2%) was also reported by other groups.[41] The presence of a low ejection fraction (<35%) doubled the mortality compared with that in patients with ejection fractions greater than 35%. The severity of left ventricular

function has been and continues to be the most significant predictor of operative mortality.

Age also plays an extremely important role in determining operative risk. Older patients have more severe coronary artery disease, more peripheral vascular disease, a higher incidence of unstable angina and previous myocardial infarction, and lower ejection fractions and include more females.[42] Operative mortality for patients older than 70 years is increased (3 to 11% in various series), but long-term survival is not impaired compared with that in younger patients.[43–45]

Several studies have reported operative mortalities two to three times higher for women than men. Women tend to be older and to have more severe angina and a higher incidence of congestive heart failure.[46–48] When height is considered in the analysis, female sex may not be a significant variable.[46] This increased risk is believed to be attributable to smaller-diameter coronary vessels in patients with smaller body habitus.

Perioperative complications of coronary bypass include myocardial infarction (5 to 12%), cerebrovascular accident (1 to 3%), requirement for postoperative inotropic (10 to 50%) and intra-aortic (2 to 6%) balloon pump support, sternal infection (1 to 2%), diaphragm paralysis (5 to 20%), pneumonia (1 to 2%), prolonged ventilatory dependence (1 to 2%), significant pleural effusion (1 to 2%), symptomatic pericarditis (4 to 8%), gastrointestinal ileus (2 to 4%), and ulnar nerve palsy (0 to 1%).

Long-Term Results

As documented by the randomized trials, long-term actuarial survival of coronary bypass patients with chronic, stable angina pectoris can be expected to be greater than 90% at 5 years and 80% at 10 years. Similar results have been obtained for patients with unstable angina undergoing surgical revascularization.[49–51] At 10 years, approximately 70% of patients show improvement over their preoperative anginal status, with 35 to 45% completely free of angina. As reported by Kirklin et al.,[52] 70% of coronary bypass patients at 5 years and 50% at 10 years can be expected to be free of ischemic events (return of angina, myocardial infarction, or sudden death).

Long-term survival after coronary bypass is adversely affected by certain risk factors.[53] The number and severity of obstruction of diseased coronary arteries, impairment of left ventricular function, incomplete revascularization, and nonuse of the IMA are the most significant predictive long-term risk factors. As in early mortality, left ventricular dysfunction is the most significant predictor.

Complete Revascularization

Complete revascularization is usually defined as bypass grafting performed to at least one vessel supplying the myocardial regions of significantly stenotic left anterior descending, circumflex, and/or right coronary arteries. Several studies[54,55] have shown improvement in survival and anginal symptoms with complete revascularization compared with incomplete revascularization (one or more regions not bypassed). Jones et al.[55] at Emory University reported improved 5-year survival (88.5 versus 83.5%; $P < 0.001$) and freedom from angina (70 versus 58%) in patients who were

completely revascularized (Fig. 18-1). Every effort is made to bypass regions compromised by significantly diseased coronary arteries in order to preserve as much viable myocardium as possible. Since left ventricular dysfunction is the strongest predictor of both short- and long-term survival, complete revascularization to preserve myocardium is necessary to enhance survival benefit.

Internal Mammary Artery

The long-term efficacy of coronary bypass is directly related to the patency of the bypass conduit. Occlusion of grafts correlates with increased angina, left ventricular dysfunction, and decreased survival.[56] Between 10 and 20% of saphenous vein grafts are occluded at 1 year. After 1 year, the vein graft occlusion rate is 2 to 4% per year up to 5 years and then 4 to 8% per year, with 50 to 60% of vein grafts occluded at 10 years. Antiplatelet drugs such as dipyridamole and aspirin may improve patency rates.[57]

The IMA appears to be relatively immune to the accelerated atherosclerotic process compared with vein grafts, and patency at 10 years is greater

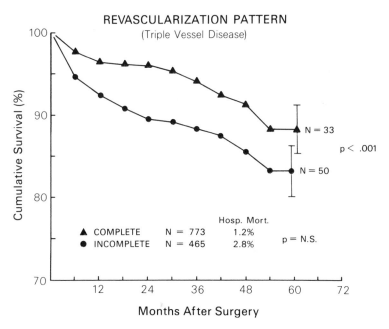

Fig. 18-1. Actuarial survival curve for patients with complete and incomplete surgical revascularization. (From Jones et al.[55] with permission.)

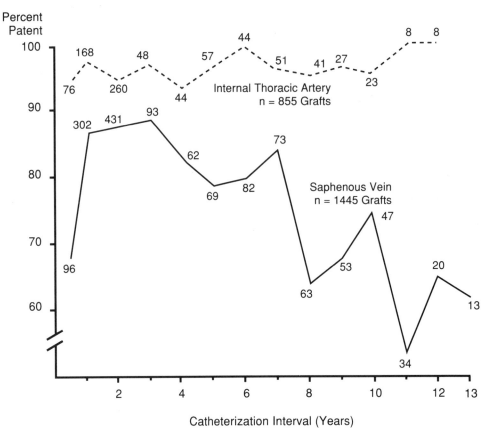

Fig. 18-2. Patency rates for IMA and saphenous vein grafts to the left anterior descending coronary artery. (From Loop et al.[60] with permission.)

than 90% (Fig. 18-2). This increased long-term patency has correlated with improved patient survival, even in the presence of poor left ventricular function (Fig. 18-3). Several studies have demonstrated greater than 90% 10-year survival in patients with an IMA graft compared with 60 to 70% 10-year survival in patients with vein grafts only.[58–60] Analysis of all the CASS patients who underwent coronary bypass showed that the use of the IMA as a bypass graft was an independent predictor of improved survival.[61] Surgical therapy has changed since these clinical trials. Saphenous vein grafts were almost exclusively used in the clinical trials, whereas today more than 80% of operations include the use of the internal mammary artery as a bypass conduit.

Proudfit et al. from the Cleveland Clinic retrospectively selected patients according to CASS criteria during the time period of the CASS and showed a significantly improved 10-year survival in patients who had IMA grafting (91%; $P <$ 0.0001), compared with medical patients (77%) and coronary bypass patients with saphenous vein grafting only (76%).[62] Fifteen-year follow-up has shown improved survival, less angina, lower rate of myocardial infarction, and fewer reoperations in patients receiving at least one IMA graft.[59]

Because of these markedly improved results, the use of the in situ IMA conduits has been expanded to free (aortocoronary), sequential, and bilateral right and left IMA grafts. Patency rates

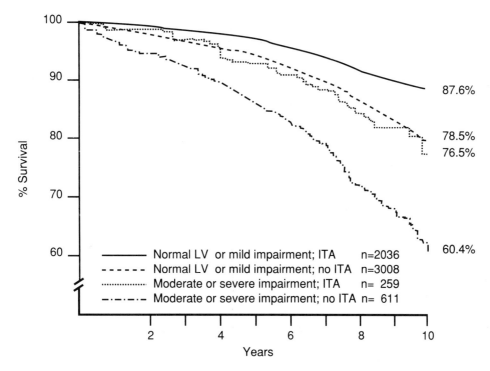

Fig. 18-3. Long-term survival rates comparing IMA and vein graft-only patients with normal or mild left ventricular dysfunction ($P < 0.0001$) and moderate or severe left ventricular dysfunction ($P < 0.0002$). (From Loop et al.[60] with permission.)

and survival data are similar to the in situ left IMA.[63–65] The use of bilateral IMAs may improve survival and freedom from angina even more than single-IMA grafting.[64]

This increased use of arterial conduits has expanded to the use of the right gastroepiploic artery; preliminary reports of its use have been promising.[66]

Complications attributed to the use of IMAs include increased sternal infections, particularly with bilateral IMAs (1 to 4%), brachial plexus injury of the ulnar and median nerves, and chest wall costochondral disarticulations. Increased sternal infections appear to be related to increased age and insulin-dependent diabetes mellitus, as well as to use of bilateral IMAs.[67]

Reoperations

Because of prolonged survival, progression of native-vessel coronary disease, occlusion of vein grafts, and failure to undertake efforts to prevent progression of atherosclerosis, an increased number of patients are returning for reoperation. Although these patients have an increased risk for operative mortality and perioperative myocardial infarction compared with patients undergoing primary revascularization,[68] long-term survival approaches that of primary operations. Lytle et al.[69] at the Cleveland Clinic reviewed 1,500 reoperations from 1967 to 1984, reporting a 3 to 4% operative mortality, with 5-year and 10-year survival at 90 and 75%, respectively. Advanced age and left ventricular dysfunction were predictors of decreased late survival. Since these patients have more severe coronary disease, improved operative and myocardial protection techniques (perhaps with retrograde cardioplegia) may further decrease operative mortality and perioperative myocardial infarction rates.

Coronary patients referred to surgery are divided into diverse subsets with different physiologic and mechanical presentations requiring individualized preoperative evaluation, surgical techniques, and postoperative care to produce favorable results. In particular, the various sequelae of myocardial infarction separate coronary patients into these surgical groups. Mechanical complications such as acute mitral regurgitation, ventricular septal defect and ventricular aneurysm, and physiologic complications such as acutely infarcting myocardium, chronic poor ventricular function, cardiogenic shock, and ischemic cardiomyopathy all require specific individual attention by the cardiac surgeon. In the past, surgical mortality has been extremely high for these high-risk patients. New developments in myocardial protection, surgical techniques, ventricular assist devices, and pharmacologic inotropic and immunosuppressive therapies have produced favorable short- and long-term surgical results. Surgical intervention for each of these subsets will be individually discussed.

ACUTE MYOCARDIAL INFARCTION: SURGICAL INTERVENTION

Unstable postinfarction angina has been reported to occur in 12 to 60% of patients, with late in-hospital mortality as high as 70% without intervention.[70] This high-risk group has been particularly difficult for the cardiac surgeon. High operative mortalities reported in the early 1970s ranged up to 50% for surgical revascularization after acute myocardial infarction. Conservative treatment was recommended, and surgery was delayed for at least 6 weeks after infarction.[71–73] In the late 1970s, improved methods of myocardial protection, anesthetic management, and surgical technique led to markedly improved sur-

gical results with early revascularization.[74–76] Jones et al. at Emory University reported no hospital mortality in 35 patients operated on within 30 days of infarction; 10 patients had surgery within 24 hours.[76] Interest in early surgical intervention was rekindled, and attempts at early coronary bypass after acute myocardial infarction were begun.

In Spokane, Dewood et al.[77] reported operation on 701 patients within 24 hours of onset of infarction. Mortality was 5% for the patients with transmural infarction and 3% for those with nontransmural infarction. Comparison with results of nonoperative medical treatment was not done. Emergency surgical revascularization could be performed in these high-risk patients with an operative mortality similar to that in patients undergoing elective coronary bypass. Increased age, transmural infarction, and cardiogenic shock were the most significant predictive risk factors for increased operative mortality in these patients.[78,79] Acceptable long-term results, with 80 to 90% 5-year and 70 to 80% 10-year survival in patients operated on less than 30 days following infarction have also been documented.[80]

In patients with acute myocardial infarction, early revascularization to salvage infarcting myocardium and preserve ventricular function is the primary goal of therapy. Thrombolytic agents and angioplasty are other effective methods of early reperfusion. Still to be addressed are (1) the period after total occlusion of a coronary artery within which reperfusion can salvage ischemic myocardium and improve early and late ventricular function and (2) the method of reperfusion that provides maximum salvage of the myocardium at risk.

Experimental studies in dogs have demonstrated that 2 hours of left anterior descending coronary artery occlusion followed by 4 hours of reperfusion (snare release) produced a 27% loss of myocardium at risk and a 39% return of normal function at 2 weeks.[81] Since the human heart develops collateral flow to chronically compromised regions, the period available for reperfusion to preserve human myocardium is unknown. Rogers et al.[82] reported improvement in ejection fraction and regional wall function in 43 patients, with an average time to surgical reperfusion of 8 hours. Although clinical studies are not completely conclusive, surgical reperfusion up to 8 hours may effectively salvage myocardium and preserve function. Others have also demonstrated enhancement of global ejection fraction with early coronary bypass after acute myocardial infarction.[83,84]

Reperfusion with thrombolytic agents such as streptokinase and recombinant tissue-type plasminogen activator (rt-PA) have also been shown to reduce mortality and to preserve left ventricular function.[85,86] A high risk of reocclusion after thrombolysis has led to interventional revascularization with angioplasty and coronary bypass. The cooperative Thrombolysis and Angioplasty in Myocardial Infarction (TAMI) study reported a low mortality, with significant preservation of regional and global left ventricular function, in patients undergoing emergency coronary bypass after thrombolytic therapy and unsuccessful or contraindicated angioplasty.[87] Coronary bypass after thrombolytic therapy is a safe and effective means of ensuring reperfusion. Bleeding complications and the need for blood transfusion are potential complications when surgery is performed after thrombolytic therapy.

Another interesting subgroup of patients with acute ischemia includes those experiencing failed coronary angioplasty. Although acute occlusion of a coronary artery is a rare complication, excellent surgical results have been reported after failed angioplasty.[88,89] These patients are usually hemodynamically stable, and quick surgical revascularization can be achieved.

Experimental laboratory data have shown that controlled, modified surgical reperfusion of ischemic myocardium may be superior to medical reperfusion such as thrombolysis and/or angioplasty. Axelrod et al.[90] demonstrated that when 4 hours of reperfusion followed a 2-hour anterior descending artery occlusion in a dog model, surgical reperfusion, initially with cold-blood, low-Ca^{2+} cardioplegia or with warm-blood, amino-acid-induction cardioplegia and left ventricle venting, produced significant reductions in infarct size (48 versus 18 to 19%; $P < 0.05$) compared with uncontrolled, unmodified, unvented medical reperfusion. Decompression of the left ventricle during reperfusion and use of a modi-

Table 18-2. Contents of Substrate-Enriched Blood Cardioplegia

Components	Crystalloid Content	Concentration Delivered
Blood	—	20–30% Hct
KCl	50 mEq/L	12–16 mEq/L
THAM (0.3 M)	260 mL	—
Glucose	16.2 g/L	>400 mg/dL
Aspartate	10.1 g/L	12 mmol/L
Glutamate	11.0 g/L	12 mmol/L
CPD	65 mL	500–600 mmol/L
Allopurinol	0.68 g/L	1 mmol/L
pH	—	7.8 at 37°C
Osm	—	370–400 mOsm/L

fied substrate-rich reperfusate before revascularization appear to be important methods for increasing myocardial salvage and improving ventricular function.[91,92] These techniques may limit the so-called reperfusion injury that may occur with medical revascularization of acutely ischemic muscle. Cheung et al.[93] at Emory University extended these concepts to a chronic dog model and demonstrated a significant benefit with controlled surgical reperfusion. In a 2-hour anterior descending artery ischemic dog model, surgical reperfusion with a substrate-enriched blood cardioplegia (Table 18-2) with left ventricular decompression was compared with "medical" (unmodified blood) reperfusion. At 1 week, myocardial necrosis of the ischemic area at risk was significantly less (19 versus 38%; $P < 0.5$) (Fig. 18-4) and recovery of regional wall function was greater (52 versus 19% of control systolic shortening; $P < 0.05$) (Fig. 18-5) in the surgical group. Although clinical randomized trials have not been performed, the experimental evidence is compelling, and variations of these modified reperfusion techniques are used today in patients with ongoing ischemia who are undergoing surgical revascularization.

Our clinical operative technique in patients with acute myocardial infarction is modified from the methods used in elective procedures. Since rapid revascularization of ischemic muscle is the overwhelming goal, expeditious transport to the

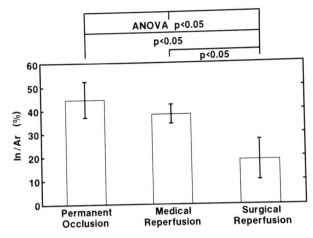

Fig. 18-4. Comparison of infarct size, determined by the area of necrosis divided by the area at risk, with surgical reperfusion vs. medical reperfusion and permanent left anterior descending artery occlusion. Abbreviations: In, infarct size; Ar, area of necrosis. (From Cheung et al.,[93] with permission.)

operating suite, insertion of hemodynamic monitoring lines, and anesthesic induction are performed. Patients are quickly placed on cardiopulmonary bypass and cooled to a core temperature of 25 to 28°C. The left ventricle is vented for decompression to decrease the work load. Myocardial arrest and protection are performed with antegrade cold (4°C) potassium (18 mEq/L), oxygenated crystalloid, or blood cardioplegia. Retrograde coronary sinus cardioplegic methods may be used next to ensure protection of the ischemic myocardium that is not reached by the antegrade technique. The distal anastomosis is performed with a reversed saphenous vein. Oxygenated cardioplegic solution is then infused through the completed anastomosis into the ischemic area. Because of time constraints and inability to infuse cardioplegic solution before grafting into the infarcting area, the IMA is not ordinarily used unless the patient is hemodynamically stable without chest pain before anesthetic induction. The remaining distal anastomoses are completed and aortic proximal anastomoses are usually performed with the aorta still completely crossclamped. Next, a warm oxygenated blood cardioplegia dose is adminis-

tered antegrade for 3 minutes. The aortic crossclamp is removed, and reperfusion is continued with the left ventricle decompressed, to limit myocardial work and reperfusion injury, for 20 to 30 minutes before weaning from cardiopulmonary bypass is attempted. Spontaneous sinus rhythm usually occurs 3 to 5 minutes after the aortic crossclamp is removed. Catecholamines and/or intra-aortic balloon pump assistance are used only if necessary.

At Crawford Long Hospital of Emory University, 69 patients underwent emergency coronary bypass between 1983 and 1986.[94] The indications for operation were continued acute myocardial infarction (19 patients), failed angioplasty (28 patients), and unstable angina pectoris refractory to medical therapy (22 patients). The time from the initial ischemic event to surgical reperfusion varied considerably, from an average of 144 minutes in the angioplasty group to 460 minutes in the myocardial infarction group. Operative mortality was 4.3% (3 of 69 patients, 2 patients in the myocardial infarction group and 1 patient in the unstable angina group). Two of the three deaths occurred in patients older than 75 years with severe preoperative pump failure. The overall complication rate was low, and the average postoperative hospital stay was 9 days. This retrospective study demonstrated not only that surgical revascularization can be safe and effective but also that acutely ischemic coronary patients are a heterogeneous group, requiring patient-by-patient decisions regarding therapy.

Our current strategy for early reperfusion of acute myocardial infarction entails early (less than 6 hours) thrombolytic therapy with streptokinase or rt-PA. If the infarction is large or hemodynamic compromise is present, immediate cardiac catheterization is undertaken and angioplasty of the infarct-related artery may be performed. If hemodynamic pump failure is present, immediate surgical intervention is considered. Early operative intervention is usually reserved for acutely ischemic patients with threatened left ventricular power failure or extension of the original infarct. If surgical revascularization can be performed within 3 hours, such as in patients with failed angioplasty or in-hospital myocardial

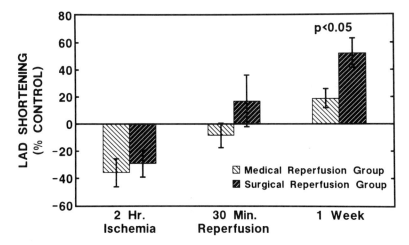

Fig. 18-5. Comparison of regional wall shortening, 1 week after reperfusion, in surgical treatment group (significantly improved recovery of regional wall shortening [52% of control]) vs. group undergoing medical reperfusion (19% of control; $P < 0.05$). Abbreviations: LAD, left anterior descending (regional wall). (From Cheung et al.,[93] with permission.)

infarction, emergency surgery may salvage myocardium, and we do not hesitate to proceed immediately.

CARDIOGENIC SHOCK: SURGICAL INTERVENTION

Cardiogenic shock secondary to left ventricular pump failure is a devastating complication of acute myocardial infarction. The incidence of cardiogenic shock in patients experiencing acute myocardial ischemia is 10 to 15%, occurring most frequently in patients with previous infarctions. Shock is defined as a systolic blood pressure less than 90 mmHg, poor peripheral perfusion, oliguria, and a cardiac index less than 2.0 L/min/m^2 or a pulmonary capillary wedge pressure acutely elevated to greater than 25 mmHg. Extensive transmural infarction involving greater than 40% of the left ventricle (including damage from prior infarction) is generally required for pump failure. Conservative medical therapy has resulted in an 80 to 90% hospital mortality for these desperately ill patients. In the 1970s, surgical revascularization improved survival, but results were still dis-

couraging, with 30 to 50% hospital mortality. Recently, with an organized, concerted medical-surgical effort directed toward early surgical revascularization of patients with cardiogenic shock, survival is significantly better.

Cheung et al.[95] reviewed 121 patients at Crawford Long Hospital of Emory University who underwent emergency coronary bypass. Twenty-eight patients (23%) had pump failure, with six of these patients requiring external cardiopulmonary resuscitation. Rapid surgical revascularization was performed after expeditous attempts at stabilization with catecholamines and/or IABP, and after defining the coronary anatomy with cardiac catheterization. The average time from the beginning of myocardial ischemia to the first distal anastomosis was 277 minutes. The operative technique was similar to that discussed in the previous section. There were 4 hospital deaths (14%) in the 28 patients with pump failure. Postoperative complications requiring additional therapy or prolonged hospital stay occurred in half of the patients. Three-year survival, including hospital deaths, was 88% by life table analysis. All patients who worked preoperatively returned to work postoperatively. Age greater than 70 years and preoperative requirement for IABP were significant independent risk factors for hospital mortality.

Laks et al.[96] from the University of California, Los Angeles, using controlled modified reperfusion, reported a 70% hospital survival with a 48% late survival in patients with cardiogenic shock. Most patients were operated on an average of 4 days after infarction. Earlier surgical intervention may have improved their survival results.

More recently, portable ventricular assist devices (VADs) that are used as adjuncts may improve survival. Pennington[97] in St. Louis reported on the use of portable extracorporeal membrane oxygenation (ECMO) in 20 patients with shock. Philips[98] has used percutaneous cardiopulmonary bypass, and Rose et al.[99] have used percutaneous transseptal left atrial-femoral bypass; all these modalities support the failing ventricle until more definitive therapy (angioplasty, coronary bypass, implantable long-term VADs, transplantation) can be performed.

Emory University presently uses a portable Cardio-Pulmonary System (CPS; Bard) with a BioMedicus centrifugal pump head. This system can be quickly primed and easily set up for emergency use. Specially developed percutaneous femoral artery and vein cannulas are inserted in the cardiac catheterization laboratory, intensive care unit, or emergency room.

Cardiogenic shock after acute myocardial infarction is a surgical emergency, demanding rapid intervention. Mechanical support with VADs may be used to stabilize the patient until revascularization or to support the failing heart until cardiac recovery or transplantation. Rapid surgical intervention can be very successful in these high-risk patients.

ISCHEMIC MITRAL REGURGITATION: SURGICAL INTERVENTION

Mitral valve incompetence of various degrees, secondary to myocardial infarction, is present in approximately 3 to 15% of coronary patients undergoing cardiac catheterization. These patients represent a heterogeneous group ranging from those with acute papillary muscle rupture and cardiogenic shock to those with chronic mild to moderate mitral regurgitation with minimal congestive heart failure symptoms. The mechanical morphologic etiology of mitral valve regurgitation encompasses papillary muscle elongation, papillary muscle rupture, and/or ventricular and mitral annular dilatation. The presence of ischemic mitral regurgitation adversely affects long-term survival in coronary patients.[100]

Surgery with and without valve replacement for ischemic mitral regurgitation carries an operative mortality up to 50%, with an average of numerous reported series at 21%.[101] Because of this increased mortality, much controversy exists over whether to repair or replace the mitral valve and the ultimate effect on left ventricular function and long-term survival.

Acute papillary muscle rupture resulting in severe mitral regurgitation is best treated by early combined coronary bypass and mitral valve replacement or repair. Only 25% of patients with complete papillary muscle rupture and 70% of those with partial rupture survive the first 24 hours with nonsurgical treatment.[102,103] These acutely ill patients may require pharmacologic and IABP support until surgery. Associated risk factors are low ejection fraction, severe congestive heart failure, acute renal and pulmonary failure, increased age, and increased severity of coronary artery disease. Operative mortality ranges between 10 and 30% if intervention occurs before multisystem failure ensues. Long-term survival is dependent on the severity of postoperative ventricular dysfunction.

The operative technique is similar to that described above. Primarily, revascularization with saphenous veins to significantly diseased vessels is accomplished first for cardioplegic solution graft infusion during the mitral part of the operation. Retrograde cardioplegic solution infusion may also be used to protect viable and ischemic myocardium during repair or replacement of the mitral valve.

Mitral valve replacement is usually performed in these acutely ill patients to ensure a completely competent functioning valve. During mitral valve replacement, preservation of the subvalvular mitral leaflet apparatus has been shown experimentally to provide supportive chordal integrity of left ventricular contour, enhancing ventricular function postoperatively.[104] Clinically, this technique has improved postoperative ventricular function and survival rates, even in patients with low ejection fractions.[105,106] Complete coronary revascularization of all threatened areas is equally important for improved results.

Mitral valve repair may be performed in acutely ill patients who are not in multisystem failure, who are younger than 70 years and have an ejection fraction greater than 35%; or in patients presenting with severe mitral regurgitation in stable condition after recovery from the acute infarction period. Kay et al.[107] in Los Angeles reported excellent short- and long-term results using valve repair for ischemic mitral regurgitation. Significantly fewer thromboembolic events, endocarditis, and anticoagulant complications occurred with repair than with prosthetic valve replacement.

Patients with mild to moderate ischemic mitral regurgitation pose a different problem for the cardiac surgeon. What effect does moderate mitral regurgitation have on perioperative and long-term ventricular function and, ultimately, on long-term survival if the mitral valve is left uncorrected? The long-term survival factor must be weighed against the increased operative mortality for combined coronary bypass and mitral valve replacement or repair.

Arcidi et al.[108] at Emory University retrospectively analyzed 58 patients operated on between 1977 and 1983 who had moderate mitral regurgitation and coronary heart disease and who underwent only coronary bypass. Hospital mortality was excellent at 3.4% (2 of 58 patients). Long-term 5-year survival was 77%, with 66% in functional class I and II, and 84% returned to work. This compared with a 25% hospital mortality and 31% 5-year survival in 20 unmatched patients who received combined valve replacement and coronary bypass during the same period.

Because of these results of coronary bypass alone in patients with moderate ischemic mitral regurgitation, we take a conservative approach. The recent use of intraoperative transesophageal echocardiography is a useful adjunct for decision-making about the mitral valve. Long-term ventricular deterioration and congestive heart failure occur infrequently, and survival rates are excellent when complete revascularization is accomplished.

LEFT VENTRICULAR ANEURYSM: SURGICAL INTERVENTION

The incidence of left ventricular aneurysm after acute transmural myocardial infarction ranges from 5 to 30%.[109,110] Most aneurysms occur in the anteroapical segments of the left ventricle (70 to 80%) with left anterior descending coronary artery disease (90%), concomitant multivessel disease (75%), and poor collateral circulation. Nonsurgical treatment has resulted in 3-year survival as low as 25% and 5-year survival as low as 10%.[110,111]

Grossly, the aneurysm often consists of a thin, white, easily demarcated fibrous scar with a smooth endocardial surface. Mural thrombi are present in 20 to 50% of aneurysms, but the risk of thromboembolism is less than 10%. An enlarged ventricular cavity results in increased ventricular volume, increased wall tension on viable myocardium according to Laplace's law, distortion of ventricular fiber geometry, and paradoxical movement of the aneurysm reducing forward-stroke volume.[112,113] All these produce various degrees of hemodynamic ventricular dysfunction.

Indications for surgery have been angina only (52%), angina and congestive heart failure (25%), congestive heart failure only (10%), intractable ventricular arrhythmias (10%), and thromboembolic events (3%).[114–116] Left ventricular aneurysm resection has had a 2 to 20% operative mortality. Better results have been achieved in the last 5 years secondary to improved myocardial protection, complete revascularization, and tachyarrhythmia surgery. Operative risk factors are the presence of ventricular arrhythmias, severe congestive heart failure, acute myocardial infarction, and severe coronary artery disease.[114,116–118] Late survival among hospital survivors is 70 to 75% at 5 years and 38 to 45% at 8 years.[115,117,118] Significant improvement in congestive heart failure symptoms and functional status occurs after surgery. Postoperative studies have demonstrated improved hemodynamic function of the left ventricle as represented by an increased cardiac index, exercise ejection fraction and decreased left ventricular end-diastolic volume.[114,119]

At Emory University, patients with left ventricular aneurysms are rarely operated on for symptoms of congestive heart failure only. Medical management is encouraged. Thromboembolism from mural thrombi is infrequent. Refractory angina, with or without heart failure, requiring coronary bypass is the most common indication for surgery, followed by ventricular tachyarrhythmia. For small aneurysms without symptoms of heart failure, only coronary bypass is performed. Moderate-sized aneurysms are usually resected or plicated if symptoms of heart failure are present. Mural thrombi are removed at this time if the ventricle is opened. Large aneurysms are usually present with heart failure symptoms. Ventricular reconstruction, according to the ventricular patching techniques described by Jantene,[120] is performed. Plication or linear resection and primary repair of large aneurysms compromises left ventricular volume and geometry and causes postoperative low-output states. Ventricular patching with Teflon-supported Dacron or pericardium is performed to recreate normal ventricular geometry as much as possible. An aneurysmal ventricular septum is plicated or is included in the patch repair to further prevent ventricular dyskinesis and failure.

The presence of left ventricular aneurysm after myocardial infarction is a significant adverse risk factor for survival. Although operative mortality is increased with aneurysmectomy compared with that of coronary bypass alone, surgical repair when indicated markedly improves symptoms and late survival over medical therapy. Complete revascularization is necessary for these improved results.

VENTRICULAR SEPTAL DEFECT: SURGICAL INTERVENTION

Ventricular septal rupture occurs in 1 to 2% of patients with acute infarction, 2 to 14 days after the initial ischemic event. Cardiogenic shock ensues, resulting in only 50% survival at 1 week and only 20% at 1 month.[121,122] The majority of postinfarction ventricular septal defects are located in the anterior or apical septum.

Patients are stabilized with inotropic drugs and IABP to maintain peripheral perfusion and kidney function. Since medical management alone results in a high mortality, surgery is almost always necessary. Operative survival ranges from 30 to 70%, with a 57% average from several reports.[123] Patients older than 70 years have an extremely high mortality. The timing of surgery remains controversial. Since earlier series[124] reported an extremely high mortality with immediate surgery, delayed operation until friable myocardium becomes more suitable for repair has been advocated by some. We generally undertake surgical repair promptly after the diagnosis is made, before the patient succumbs to multisystem failure from a low-output state. Immediate surgical intervention after initial attempts at stabilization clearly salvages some patients who would otherwise die. Rarely, patients present without cardiogenic shock; they can be managed medically while surgery is delayed. Depending on the location of the defect, the repair is performed through a right or left ventriculotomy. The defect is patched with Teflon-pledgetted sutures and Dacron, Gore-tex material, or pericardium. Concomitant mitral valve repair for papillary muscle rupture, left ventricular infarctectomy, and coronary bypass are performed when indicated.

Late survival, excluding operative mortality, is 75 to 90% at 5 years with good functional status.[125,126] Residual ventricular septal defects can occur early or late after repair (5 to 10%), and patients should be monitored closely postoperatively.

CHRONIC POOR LEFT VENTRICULAR FUNCTION: SURGICAL INTERVENTION

As other forms of nonsurgical therapy for coronary heart disease have become effective palliative procedures, the patient population referred to surgery is becoming increasingly older, with a greater prevalence of severe coronary artery disease and poor left ventricular function. Many patients are returning to surgery for the second and third time.

Left ventricular function is the most important risk factor for survival in medically and surgically treated groups. The randomized trials demonstrated significantly improved late survival in patients with depressed ejection fraction (25 to 50%) and triple-vessel disease surgically revascularized for stable angina compared with survival in medically treated cohorts.[22] Subsequent studies[127,128] have supported the CASS trial results, and, if operative mortality for these patients is less than 7 to 10%, there may be significant long-term advantages from surgery.[128,129] With present anesthetic techniques and methods of myocardial protection, operative mortality rates lower than 5% can be achieved, even in patients with ejection fractions less than 25%.

The history or presence of congestive heart failure symptoms in coronary patients being evaluated for coronary bypass is a great concern to the surgeon. The presence of heart failure signifies severe ventricular dysfunction, categorizing these patients as poor early and late survival risks. Interestingly, as noted in the review by Wechsler and Jarod,[130] the severity of congestive heart failure (class III or IV) does not necessarily correlate with measured cineangiographic parameters such as ejection fraction and wall motion score. Hence, the real incidence of congestive heart failure (class III or IV) in patients undergoing coronary bypass is approximately 3 to 5%. The dilemma exists in differentiating between failure secondary to nonviable myocardium and that from chronically ischemic myocardium with reversible dysfunction after revascularization.

At Emory University, patients presenting with angina, significant coronary artery disease, and low ejection fraction (less than 20%) with or without the clinical presence of heart failure are offered surgical revascularization. With current methods, even though operative mortality is increased, long-term benefits from surgery far outweigh those from medical therapy. Left ventricular aneurysmectomy is performed if indicated. Frequently these patients require minimal to moderate postoperative inotropic and/or IABP support and have only slightly increased hospital

stays (1 or 2 days). Symptoms of heart failure may or may not improve. Almost all patients receive anginal palliation.

Even in patients with ejection fractions less than 15% and significant heart failure, if angina and significant coronary lesions supplying functioning myocardium are present, revascularization is offered. The increased surgical risk is thoroughly discussed with the patient and family. Evaluation for transplantation may take place preoperatively, and the placement of an intraoperative ventricular assist device (VAD) may be an option if the patient cannot be weaned from cardiopulmonary bypass.

HEART TRANSPLANTATION

End-stage heart failure secondary to ischemic cardiomyopathy is treated today by heart transplantation, the only effective form of therapy for these terminally ill patients. Survival after heart transplantation has improved significantly over the last decade. The 1989 report of the Registry of the International Society for Heart Transplantation[131] noted an 80% 3-year survival and a 73% 10-year survival. Over 2,500 heart transplant procedures are performed annually worldwide, the majority in the United States.

Ischemic cardiomyopathy is the indication for approximately 40% of heart transplantations. Patients present with severe congestive heart failure without angina secondary to multiple myocardial infarctions and often have had one or more bypass operations. Life expectancy of less than 1 year is characteristic. The severity of heart failure ranges from home care with diuretics and afterload-reducing drugs to cardiogenic shock requiring admission to the intensive care unit for IABP and inotropic support. Some patients may require an implantable VAD. Approximately 30% of recipient-listed patients die befort transplantation.

Thorough psychosocial evaluations for patient compliance and family support, right and left heart catheterization, endomyocardial biopsy, and histocompatibility blood testing are done preoperatively. The only absolute contraindication is active infection. Relative contraindications are pulmonary hypertension (>7 Wood units after pharmacologic afterload reduction), insulin-dependent diabetes mellitus, renal insufficiency, poor compliance attributes, drug or alcohol abuse, active peptic ulcer disease, and age greater than 65 years.

Suitable candidates undergo orthotopic transplantation, and rejection is suppressed with triple-drug (steroid, azothiaprine, cyclosporin A) immunotherapy. In patients with elevated pulmonary vascular resistance, heterotopic "piggyback" transplantation is considered. Frequent endomyocardial biopsies are performed early, and rejection episodes are treated initially with bolus steroids. If necessary, monoclonal antilymphocytic immunoglobin therapy with OKT3 is used to suppress severe rejection. Infection and rejection are the most common modes of death. The presence of pulmonary hypertension adversely affects early and late survival, and the use of cyclosporin A has significantly increased survival.

Since January 1988, 60 adult transplants (50% for ischemic cardiomyopathy) have been performed at Emory University, with one early and three late deaths (personal communication, K. Kanter, 1990). Ninety-three percent of patients are alive and well with class I and II functional class. Four were heterotopic recipients.

VENTRICULAR ASSIST DEVICES

In patients who cannot be weaned from cardiopulmonary bypass, patients who experience sudden cardiogenic shock in the intensive care unit or cardiac catheterization laboratory, and transplant recipients refractory to pharmacologic and IABP support, a VAD may be lifesaving.

At Emory University the Cardiopulmonary Support System (Bard, Inc., with Biomedicus pump), the Nimbus Hemopump, and Abiomed ventricular bypass system are used to support the left and/or right ventricle until native ventricular function recovers. The Novacor left ventricular assist device is approved for bridge to transplantation. Farrar et al.[132] reported on a multi-institutional study using the heterotopic Pierce-Donachy (Thoratec, Berkeley, CA) prosthetic ventricular pump in 29 candidates for transplantation. Eight patients initially died, and 21 were successfully transplanted; 19 of the 21 were alive at 7 to 39 months. Complications of thromboembolism and infection are still prominent with VAD use.

SUMMARY

The prospective clinical trials of the 1970s demonstrated that many coronary patients could benefit significantly from coronary bypass. With newer methods of myocardial protection, operative mortality remains low even in high-risk patients who are older and/or have more severe coronary artery disease and poorer ventricular function. Long-term survival is often significantly prolonged, and the functional class is improved. Myocardial infarction produces subsets of high-risk surgical patients with acute and chronic mechanical dysfunction. Even these severely ill patients may benefit significantly from appropriate surgical intervention.

Coronary patients make up a heterogenous group; each patient requires specific therapies or combinations of therapies throughout his or her individual coronary history. The 1990s will be an aggressive, invasive decade. Defining coronary artery anatomy by cardiac catheterization is paramount for choosing therapy. Cooperation between the cardiologist and cardiac surgeon on a per-patient basis will determine which medical and surgical interventions are appropriate to optimize survival and quality of life.

REFERENCES

1. Vital and Health Statistics. 13:47, 1985
2. Connolly JE: The history of coronary artery disease. J Thorac Cardiovasc Surg 76:733, 1978
3. Coffee WB, Brown PK: The surgical treatment of angina pectoris. Arch Intern Med 31:200, 1923
4. Beck CS, Tietry VL, Moritz AR: Production of collateral circulation to the heart. Proc Soc Exp Biol Med 32:759, 1935

5. Vineberg AM, Miller WD: An experimental study of the physiological role of the anastomosis between the left coronary circulation and left internal mammary artery into the left ventricular myocardium. Surg Forum 5:294, 1950

6. Bailey CP, May A, Lemon WM: Survival after coronary endarterectomy in man. JAMA 164:641, 1957

7. Longmire WP, Jr, Cannon JA, Kattus AA: Direct-vision coronary endarterectomy for angina pectoris. N Engl J Med 259:993, 1958

8. Sawyer PN, Koplitt M, Sobel S et al: Experimental and clinical experience with coronary gas endarterectomy. Arch Surg 95:736, 1967

9. Sones FM, Jr, Shirey EK: Cine coronary arteriography. Mod Concepts Cardiovasc Dis 31:735, 1962

10. Favaloro RG: Saphenous vein graft in the surgical treatment of coronary artery disease: Operative technique. J Thorac Cardiovasc Surg 58:178, 1969

11. Green GE, Stertzer SH, Reppert EH: Coronary arterial bypass grafts. Ann Thorac Surg 5:433, 1968

12. Bailey CP, Hirose T: Successful internal mammary-coronary arterial anastomosis using a "minivascular" suturing technique. Int Surg 49:416, 1968

13. Landolt CL, Guyton RA: Lessons learned from randomized trials of coronary bypass surgery: Viewpoint of the surgeon. Cardiology 73:212, 1986

14. Takaro T, Hultgren HN, Lipton MJ et al: The VA Cooperative Randomized Study for Coronary Arterial Occlusive Disease. II. Subgroup with significant left main lesions. Circulation 54(suppl. III):III-107, 1976

15. The Veterans Administration Coronary Artery Bypass Surgery Cooperative Study Group: Eleven-year survival in the Veterans Administration randomized trial of coronary bypass surgery for stable angina. N Engl J Med 311:1333, 1984

16. Detre KM, Takaro T, Hultgren H et al: Long-term mortality and morbidity results of the Veterans Administration randomized trial of coronary bypass surgery. Circulation 72(suppl. V):V-84, 1985

17. Varnauskas E and European Coronary Surgery Study Group: Twelve-year followup of survival in the randomized European Coronary Surgery Study. N Engl J Med 319:332, 1988

18. Varnauskas E and European Coronary Surgery Study Group: Survival, myocardial infarction, and employment in a prospective randomized study of coronary bypass surgery. Circulation 72(suppl. V):V-90, 1985

19. European Coronary Surgery Study Group: Long-term results of prospective randomized study of coronary bypass surgery in stable angina pectoris. Lancet ii:1173, 1982

20. CASS Principal Investigators and Their Associates: Coronary artery surgery study (CASS): A randomized trial of coronary artery bypass surgery. Survival data. Circulation 68:939, 1983

21. Kennedy JW, Kaiser GC, Fisher LD et al: Multivariant discriminant analysis of the clinical and angiographic predictors of operative mortality from the Collaborative Study in Coronary Artery Surgery (CASS). J Thorac Cardiovasc Surg 80:876, 1980

22. Passamani E and CASS Principal Investigators: A randomized trial of coronary artery bypass surgery: Survival of patients with low ejection fraction. N Engl J Med 342:1665, 1985

23. CASS Principal Investigators and Their Associates. Coronary Artery Surgery Study (CASS): A randomized trial of coronary artery bypass. Quality of life in patients randomly assigned to treatment groups. Circulation 68:951, 1983

24. Kaiser GC, Davis KB, Fisher LD et al: Survival following coronary artery bypass grafting in patients with severe angina pectoris (CASS): An observational study. J Thorac Cardiovasc Surg 89:513, 1985

25. Myers WO, Schaff HV, Gersh BJ et al: Improved survival of surgically treated patients with triple vessel coronary artery disease and severe angina pectoris: A report from the Coronary Artery Surgery Study (CASS) Registry. J Thorac Cardiovasc Surg 97:487, 1989

26. Gersh BJ, Kronmal RA, Schaff HV et al: Comparison of coronary artery bypass surgery and medical therapy in patients 65 years of age and older: A randomized study from the Coronary Artery Surgery Study (CASS) Registry. N Engl J Med 313:317, 1985

27. Wiener DA, Ryan TJ, McCabe CH et al: Value of exercise testing in determining the risk classification and the response to coronary artery grafting in three-vessel coronary artery disease: A report from the Coronary Artery Surgery Study (CASS) Registry. Am J Cardiol 60:262, 1987

28. Gunnar RM, Loeb HS: An alternative interpretation of the results of Coronary Artery Surgery Study. Circulation 71:193, 1985

29. Leimgruber PP, Roubin GS, Hallman J et al: Restenosis after successful coronary angioplasty in

patients with single vessel disease. Circulation 73:710, 1986

30. Roubin GS, King SB III, Douglas JS: Restenosis after percutaneous transluminal coronary angioplasty: The Emory University Hospital Experience. Am J Cardiol 60:39B, 1987

31. Bredlau CE, Roubin GS, Leimgruber PP et al: In-hospital morbidity and mortality in patients undergoing elective coronary angioplasty. Circulation 72:1044, 1985

32. Ellis SA, Roubin GS, King SB III, et al: Angiographic and clinical predictors of acute closure after native vessel coronary angioplasty. Circulation 77:372, 1988

33. Gruentzig AR, King SB III, Schlumpf M et al: Long-term follow-up of 428 consecutive patients after percutaneous coronary angioplasty. The early Zurich experience. N Engl J Med 316:1127, 1987

34. Roubin GS, Sutor C, Lembo NJ et al: Prognosis after multivessel angioplasty (PTCA) in patients with coronary artery disease. Circulation 76(suppl. IV):IV-465, 1987

35. Weintraub WS, Jones EL, King SB III et al: Changing use of coronary angioplasty and coronary bypass surgery in the treatment of chronic coronary artery disease. Am J Cardiol 65:183, 1990

36. Arcidi JM, Powelson SW, King SB III et al: Trends in invasive treatment of single-vessel and double-vessel coronary disease. J Thorac Cardiovasc Surg 95:773, 1988

37. Kramer JR, Proudfitt WL, Loop FD et al: Late follow-up of 781 patients undergoing percutaneous transluminal angioplasty or coronary artery bypass grafting for an isolated obstruction in the left anterior descending coronary artery. Am Heart J 118:1144, 1989

38. Myers WO, Marshfield WI, Davis K et al: Surgical survival in the Coronary Artery Surgery Study (CASS) Registry. Ann Thorac Surg 40:245, 1985

39. Solomon NW, Page US, Okies JE et al: Diabetes mellitus and coronary artery bypass. J Thorac Cardiovasc Surg 85:264, 1983

40. Jones EL, Craver JM, King SB III et al: Clinical, anatomic, and function descriptors influencing morbidity, survival and adequacy of revascularization following coronary bypass. Ann Surg 192:390, 1980

41. Daly PO: Early and late five-year results for coronary artery bypass grafting. J Thorac Cardiovasc Surg 97:67, 1989

42. Horneffer PJ, Gardner TJ, Manolio TA et al: The effects of age on outcome after coronary bypass surgery. Circulation 76(suppl. V):V-6, 1987

43. Horvath KA, Disesa VJ, Pugh PS et al: Favorable results of coronary artery bypass grafting in patients older than 75 years. J Thorac Cardiovasc Surg 99:92, 1990

44. Rose DM, Gelbfish J, Jacobowitz JJ et al: Analysis of morbidity and mortality in patients 70 years of age and over undergoing isolated coronary bypass surgery. Am Heart J 110:341, 1985

45. Acinapura AJ, Rose DM, Cunningham JN, Jr et al: Coronary artery bypass in septuagenarians. Circulation 78(suppl. I):I-79, 1988

46. Fisher LD, Kennedy JW, Davis KB et al: Association of sex, physical size, and operative mortality after coronary artery bypass in the Coronary Artery Surgery Study (CASS). J Thorac Cardiovasc Surg 84:334, 1982

47. Gardner JS, Horneffer PJ, Gott VL et al: Coronary artery bypass grafting in women. Ann Surg 201:780, 1985

48. Richardson JV, Cyrus RJ: Reduced efficacy of coronary artery bypass grafting in women. Ann Thorac Surg 42:516, 1986

49. Kamer GC, Schaff HV, Killip T: Myocardial revascularization for unstable angina. Circulation 79(suppl. I):I-60, 1989

50. McCormick JR, Schick EC, McCabe CH et al: Determinants of operative mortality and long-term survival in patients with unstable angina. J Thorac Cardiovasc Surg 89:683, 1985

51. Rahimtoola SN, Nunley D, Grunkemeier G et al: Ten-year survival after coronary bypass surgery for unstable angina. N Engl J Med 308:676, 1983

52. Kirklin JW, Naftel DC, Blackstone EH et al: Summary of a consensus concerning death and ischemic events after coronary artery bypass surgery. Circulation 79(suppl. I):I-81, 1989

53. Hall RJ, Elayda MA, Gray A et al: Coronary artery bypass: long-term follow-up of 22,284 consecutive patients. Circulation 68(suppl. II):II-20, 1983

54. Buda AJ, MacDonald IL, Anderson MJ et al: Long-term results following coronary bypass operations, importance of preoperative factors and complete revascularization. J Thorac Cardiovasc Surg 82:383, 1981

55. Jones EL, Craver JM, Guyton RA et al: Importance of complete revascularization in performance of the coronary bypass operation. Am J Cardiol 51:7, 1983

56. Grodin CM, Campeau L, Thorton J et al: Coronary artery bypass grafting with saphenous vein. Circulation 79(suppl. I):I-24, 1979

57. Chesebro JH, Fuster V: Platelet-inhibitor drugs before and after coronary artery bypass surgery and coronary angioplasty: The basis of their use, data from animal studies, clinical trial data, and current recommendations. Circulation 73:297, 1986

58. Loop FD, Lytle BW, Cosgrove DM: New arteries for old. Circulation 79(suppl. I):I-40, 1984

59. Cameron P, Kemp HG, Jr, Green GE: Bypass surgery with the internal mammary artery graft: 15 year follow-up. Circulation 74(suppl. III):III-30, 1986

60. Loop FD, Lytle BW, Cosgrove DM et al: Influence of the internal-mammary-artery graft on 10-year survival and other cardiac events. N Engl J Med 314:1, 1986

61. Cameron A, Davis KB, Green CE et al: Clinical implications of the internal mammary artery bypass grafts: The Coronary Artery Surgery Study experience. Circulation 77:815, 1988

62. Proudfit WL, Kramer JR, Gormastic M et al: Ten-year survival of patients with mild angina or myocardial infarction without angina: A comparison of medical and surgical treatment. Am Heart J 119:942, 1990

63. Loop FD, Lytle BW, Cosgrove DM et al: Free (aorto-coronary) internal mammary artery graft. J Thorac Cardiovasc Surg 92:827, 1986

64. Galbut DL, Troad EA, Dorman MJ et al: Twelve-year experience with bilateral internal mammary artery grafts. Ann Thorac Surg 40:264, 1985

65. Fiore AC, Naunham KS, Dean P et al: Results of internal thoracic artery grafting over 15 years: Single versus double grafts. Ann Thorac Surg 49:202, 1990

66. Kusukawa J, Kirota Y, Kawanura K et al: Efficacy of coronary artery bypass surgery with gastroepiploic artery. Circulation 80(suppl. I):I-135, 1989

67. Cosgrove DM, Lytle BW, Loop FD et al: Does bilateral internal mammary artery grafting increase surgical risk? J Thorac Cardiovasc Surg 95:850, 1988

68. Foster ED, Fisher LD, Kaiser CL et al: Comparison of operative mortality and morbidity for initial and repeat coronary artery bypass grafting: The Coronary Artery Surgery Study (CASS) Registry. Ann Thorac Surg 38:563, 1984

69. Lytle BW, Loop FD, Cosgrove DM et al: Fifteen hundred coronary reoperations. J Thorac Cardiovasc Surg 93:847, 1987

70. Norris RM, Sammel NL: Predictors of late hospital death in acute myocardial infarction. Prog Cardiovasc Dis 23:179, 1980

71. Fraker TD, Wagner GS, Rosati RA: Extension of myocardial infarction: incidence and prognosis. Circulation 60:1126, 1980

72. Dawson JT, Hall RJ, Hallman GL et al: Mortality in patients undergoing coronary artery bypass surgery after myocardial infarction. Am J Cardiol 33:483, 1974

73. Mundth ED, Buckley MJ, Leinbach RC et al: Surgical intervention for the complications of acute myocardial ischemia. Ann Surg 178:379, 1973

74. Levine FH, Gold HK, Leinbach RC et al: Safe early revascularization for continuing ischemia after acute myocardial infarction. Circulation 60(suppl. I):I-5, 1979

75. Nunley EL, Grunkemeier GL, Teply JF et al: Coronary bypass operation following acute complicated myocardial infarction. J Thorac Cardiovasc Surg 85:485, 1983

76. Jones EL, Waites TF, Craver JM et al: Coronary bypass operation for relief of persistent pain following acute myocardial infarction. Ann Thorac Surg 32:33, 1981

77. Dewood MA, Spores J, Berg B, Jr et al: Acute myocardial infarction: A decade of experience with surgical reperfusion in 701 patients. Circulation 68(suppl. II):II-8, 1983

78. Naunheim KS, Kesler KA, Kanter KR et al: Coronary artery bypass for recent infarction. Circulation 78(suppl. I):I-122, 1988

79. Gardner TJ, Stuart RS, Greene PS et al: The risk of coronary bypass surgery for patients with postinfarction angina. Circulation 79(suppl. I):I-79, 1989

80. Floten HS, Ahmad A, Swanson JS et al: Long-term survival after postinfarction bypass operation: Early versus late operation. Ann Thorac Surg 48:757, 1989

81. Kloner RA, Ellis SC, Lange R et al: Studies of experimental coronary artery reperfusion: Effects on infarct size, myocardial function, biochemistry, and ultrastructure and microvascular damage. Circulation 68(suppl. I):I-8, 1983

82. Rogers WJ, Hood WP, Jr, Mantle JA et al: Return of left ventricular function after reperfusion in patients with myocardial infarction: Importance of subtotal stenosis or intact collaterals. Circulation 69:338, 1984

83. Phillips SJ, Kongtahworn C, Zeff RH et al: Emergency coronary artery revascularization: A possible therapy for acute myocardial infarction. Circulation 60:241, 1979

84. Flameng W, Sargeanit P, Vanhaecke J et al: Emergency coronary bypass grafting for evolving

myocardial infarction: Effects on infarct size and left ventricular function. J Thorac Cardiovasc Surg 94:124, 1987

85. Simoons M, Serruys P, Brand M et al: Early thrombolysis in acute myocardial infarction: Limitation of infarct size and improved survival. J Am Coll Cardiol 7:717, 1986

86. Williams PO, Borer J, Braunwald E et al: Intravenous recombinant tissue-type plasminogen activator in patients with acute myocardial infarction: A report from the NHLBI thrombolysis in myocardial infarction trial. Circulation 73:338, 1986

87. Kereiakes DJ, Topol EJ, George BS et al: Emergency coronary artery bypass surgery preserves global and regional left ventricular function after intravenous tissue plasminogen activator therapy for acute myocardial infarction. J Am Coll Cardiol 11:899, 1988

88. Murphy DA, Craver JM, Jones EL et al: Surgical revascularization following unsuccessful percutaneous transluminal coronary angioplasty. J Thorac Cardiovasc Surg 84:342, 1982

89. Cowley MJ, Dorros A, Kelsey SF et al: Emergency coronary bypass surgery after coronary angioplasty: The National Heart, Lung, and Blood Institute's percutaneous transluminal coronary angioplasty registry experience. Am J Cardiol 53:226, 1984

90. Axelrod HL, Galloway AC, Murphy MS et al: A comparison of methods for limiting myocardial infarct expansion during the acute reperfusion—primary role of unloading. Circulation 76(suppl. V):V-28, 1987

91. Laschinger JC, Grossi EA, Cunningham JN, Jr et al: Adjunctive left ventricular unloading during myocardial reperfusion plays a major role in minimizing myocardial infarct size. J Thorac Cardiovasc Surg 90:80, 1985

92. Allen BS, Okamoto F, Buckberg GD et al: Studies of controlled reperfusion after ischemia. XV. Immediate functional recovery after six hours of regional ischemia by careful control of conditions of reperfusion and composition of reperfusate. J Thorac Cardiovasc Surg 92:621, 1986

93. Cheung EH, Arcidi JM, Dorsey LM et al: Reperfusion of infarcting myocardium: Benefit of surgical reperfusion in a chronic model. Ann Thorac Surg 48:331, 1989

94. Guyton RA, Langford DA, Arcidi JM et al: Intervention in acute myocardial infarction: The role of surgical managment. p. 65. In Reves JG (ed): Acute Revascularization of the Infarcted Heart. Grune & Stratton, Orlando, FL, 1987

95. Cheung EH, Morris DC, Liberman HA et al: Emergency coronary bypass for left ventricular pump failure. Emory Univ J Med 3:276, 1988

96. Laks H, Rosenkranz E, Buckberg GD: Surgical treatment of cardiogenic shock after myocardial infarction. Circulation 74(suppl. II):II-11, 1986

97. Pennington DG: Emergency management of cardiogenic shock. Circulation 79(suppl. I):I-149, 1989

98. Phillips SJ: Percutaneous cardiopulmonary bypass and innovations in clinical counterpulsation. Crit Care Cardiol II:149A, 1988

99. Rose DM, Grossi EA, Laschinger JC et al: Strategy for treatment of acute evolving myocardial infarction with pulsatile left heart assist device—can this modality increase survival and enhance myocardial salvage? Crit Care Clin 2:251, 1986

100. Rankin JS, Hickey MJ, Smith LR et al: Ischemic mitral regurgitation. Circulation 79(suppl. I):I-116, 1989

101. Replogle RL, Campbell CD: Surgery for mitral regurgitation with ischemic heart disease: Results and strategies. Circulation 79(suppl. I):I-122, 1989

102. Sanders RJ, Neubuerger KT, Ravin A: Rupture of papillary muscles: occurrence of rupture of the posterior muscle in posterior myocardial function. Dis Chest 36:316, 1957

103. Vlodaver Z, Edwards JE: Rupture of ventricular septum or papillary muscle complicating myocardial infarction. Circulation 55:815, 1977

104. Sarris GE, Miller DC: Role of the mitral subvalvular apparatus in left ventricular systolic mechanics. Semin Thorac Cardiovasc Surg 1:133, 1989

105. David TE, Ho WC: The effect of preservation of chordae tendinae on mitral valve replacement for postinfarction mitral regurgitation. Circulation 74(suppl. I):I-116, 1986

106. Goor DA, Mohr R, Lavee J et al: Preservation of the posterior leaflet during mechanical valve replacement for ischemic mitral regurgitation and complete myocardial revascularization. J Thorac Cardiovasc Surg 96:253, 1988

107. Kay GL, Kay JH, Zubiate P et al: Mitral valve repair for mitral regurgitation secondary to coronary artery disease. Circulation 74(suppl. I):I-88, 1986

108. Arcidi JM, Jr, Hebeler RF, Craver JM et al: Treatment of moderate mitral regurgitation and coronary disease by coronary bypass alone. J Thorac Cardiovasc Surg 95:951, 1988

109. Gorlin R, Klein MD, Sullivan JM: Prospective

correlative study of ventricular aneurysm. Mechanistic concept and clinical recognition. Am J Med 42:512, 1967

110. Cheng TO: Incidence of ventricular aneurysm in coronary artery disease. Am J Med 50:340, 1971

111. Cabin HS, Roberts WC: True left ventricular aneurysm and healed myocardial infarction: Clinical and necropsy observations including quantification of degrees of coronary arterial narrowing. Am J Cardiol 46:754, 1980

112. Austen WG, Tsurekawa T, Bender HW et al: The acute hemodynamic effects of left ventricular aneurysm. J Surg Res 2:161, 1962

113. Klein MD, Herman MV, Gorlin R: A hemodynamic study of left ventricular aneurysm. Circulation 35:614, 1967

114. Cosgrove DM, Lytle BW, Taylor PC et al: Ventricular aneurysm resection: Trends in surgical risk. Circulation 79(suppl. I):I-97, 1984

115. Olearchyk AS, Lemole GM, Spagna PM: Left ventricular aneurysm: Ten years experience in surgical treatment of 244 cases. J Thorac Cardiovasc Surg 88:544, 1984

116. Stephenson LW, Hargrove WC, Ratcliff MB et al: Surgery for left ventricular aneurysm: Early survival with and without endocardial resection. Circulation 79(suppl. I):I-108, 1989

117. Magovern GJ, Sakert T, Simpson K et al: Surgical therapy for left ventricular aneurysms: A ten-year experience. Circulation 79(suppl. I):I-102, 1989

118. Barratt-Boyes BG, White HG, Agnew TM et al: The results of surgical treatment of left ventricular aneurysms. J Thorac Cardiovasc Surg 87:87, 1984

119. Taylor NC, Barsher R, Crossland P et al: Does left ventricular aneurysmectomy improve ventricular function in patients undergoing coronary bypass surgery? Br Heart J 54:145, 1985

120. Jantene AD: Left ventricular aneurysmectomy. J Thorac Cardiovasc Surg 89:321, 1985

121. Dellborg M, Held P, Swedberg K et al: Rupture of the myocardium: Occurrence and risk factors. Br Heart J 54:11, 1985

122. Shapira I, Isakor A, Burke M et al: Cardiac rupture in patients with acute myocardial infarction. Chest 92:219, 1987

123. Hill DJ, Stiles QR: Acute ischemic ventricular septal defect. Circulation 79(suppl. I):I-112, 1989

124. Campion BC, Harrison CE, Jr, Giuliani ER et al: Ventricular septal defect after myocardial infarction. Ann Intern Med 70:251, 1967

125. Daggett WM, Buckley MJ, Akins CW et al: Improved results of surgical management of postinfarction ventricular septal rupture. Ann Surg 196:269, 1982

126. Daggett WM, Guyton RA, Mundth ED et al: Surgery for post-myocardial infarct ventricular septal defect. Ann Surg 186:260, 1977

127. Pigott JD, Kouchoukos NT, Oberman A et al: Late results of surgical and medical therapy for patients with coronary artery disease and depressed left ventricular function. J Am Coll Cardiol 5:1036, 1985

128. Beunous EP, Mark DB, Pollack BG et al: Surgical survival benefits for coronary disease patients with left ventricular dysfunction. Circulation 78:I151, 1988

129. Alderman EL, Fisher LD, Litwin P et al: Results of coronary artery surgery in patient with poor left ventricular function (CASS). Circulation 68:785, 1983

130. Wechsler AS, Junod FL: Coronary bypass grafting in patients with chronic congestive heart failure. Circulation 79(supp. I):I-92, 1989

131. Heck CF, Shumway SJ, Kay MP: The Registry of the International Society for Heart Transplantation: Sixth Official Report—1989. J Heart Transplant 8:271, 1989

132. Farrar DJ, Hill JD, Laman AG et al: Heterotopic prosthetic ventricles as a bridge to cardiac transplantation—multicenter study. N Engl J Med 318:333, 1988

IV

Rehabilitative Care

19

In-hospital Exercise Rehabilitation After Myocardial Infarction and Myocardial Revascularization: Physiologic Basis, Methodology, and Results

Nanette K. Wenger, M.D.

Current management of the patient with myocardial infarction is characterized by earlier ambulation after the acute episode, significant decrease in the restriction of physical activity and imposed invalidism, and earlier discharge from the hospital for appropriately selected patients.[1,2]

During the past decade there has been a dramatic change in the pathophysiologic severity of acute myocardial infarction, related predominantly to earlier and more intensive interventions during the acute phase of myocardial infarction, particularly the application of coronary thrombolysis with and without subsequent coronary angioplasty or coronary bypass surgery. In contrast to the lessened myocardial necrosis, residual ischemia, and resultant myocardial dysfunction in this population, there are likely to be increasing numbers of seriously ill, often elderly patients who have previously survived myocardial infarction, coronary angioplasty, and coronary bypass surgery and who now have severe and disabling myocardial ischemia, myocardial dysfunction, or combinations of these. This changing spectrum of coronary disease requires individualization of the approach to acute coronary care.

HISTORICAL PERSPECTIVE

More than 200 years ago Heberden advocated physical activity for patients with angina pectoris and described its beneficial effect, but this wisdom was forgotten following the clinical description of myocardial infarction by Herrick in 1912.[3] In the early 1900s, patients were kept at absolute bed rest for a minimum of 6 to 8 weeks; virtually all voluntary movements were restricted, and patients were fed, bathed, and dressed by nursing personnel; protracted hospitalization and bed rest for 3 to 4 months were the mainstays of treatment. It was believed that even minimal physical exertion would predispose to ventricular aneurysm and ventricular rupture and that the increased arterial hypoxemia with activity would result in arrhythmia, recurrent myocardial infarction, and sudden cardiac death. Even after dismissal from the hospital, modestly strenuous activities such as climbing stairs were deferred for at least a year, and a return to productive work or to normal living was unusual.

Morphologic studies of the healing of myocardial infarction by Mallory et al.[4] reinforced this empiric custom of the 1920s and 1930s; they reported that at least 6 weeks of prolonged bed rest were required for the transformation of necrotic myocardium into firm scar tissue: "To advise less than three weeks in bed is unwise, even for patients with the smallest myocardial infarcts." Lewis[5] also recommended a minimum of 6 to 8 weeks of strict bed rest for patients with coronary occlusion, "during the whole of this period the patient is to be guarded by day and night nursing and helped in every way to avoid voluntary movement or effort." Patients were cautioned to lie as still as possible to avert arrhythmia, asystole, or myocardial aneurysm formation or rupture. The applicability of the data of Mallory et al.[4] to patients with myocardial infarction in the 1990s has been called into question. Criteria for the diagnosis of infarction in their series required development of new Q waves on the electrocardiogram (ECG); massive left ventricular infarction was common in their autopsy series, and, even today, such patients are unlikely to survive. Contemporary patients often have less extensive non-Q wave infarction or limited infarction secondary to treatment with coronary thrombolysis.

Jetter and White[6] described a higher incidence of myocardial rupture among postinfarction patients in mental hospitals than among patients in private hospitals; they postulated that this was attributable to the increased activity of mentally deranged patients compared with the enforced bed rest of patients hospitalized for routine private medical care.

In the 1940s, Samuel Levine of Boston began the "chair treatment of acute coronary thrombosis," initiating "the present trend in coronary care ... liberalization of the rigid restrictions of activity hitherto practiced."[7,8] Levine emphasized that "long continued bed rest saps morale, provokes desperation, unleashes anxiety and ushers in hopelessness of the capacity of resuming a normal life." Although he did not advocate physical activity, Levine and Lown's regimen allowed the patient to sit in a chair for 1 to 2 hours, beginning the first day after myocardial infarction.[8] The sitting position was believed beneficial because it increased peripheral venous pooling, decreased venous return, and reduced cardiac work. Although no randomized study was undertaken, no complications attributable to this management appeared among the 81 patients initially reported. Levine further theorized that this therapeutic approach would reduce thromboembolic and respiratory complications, a thesis that subsequently has been well documented and accepted. An enhanced sense of well-being and easier resumption of activity were also described.[8]

Dock[9] also decried the extended period at bed rest and emphasized the excessive risk of thromboembolism, bone demineralization, muscular wasting, gastrointestinal and urologic problems, and vasomotor instability with prolonged immobilization; he favored the use of a bedside commode (rather than a bedpan) as a means of avoiding the Valsalva maneuver. It has subsequently been documented that these activities do not entail an increase in myocardial oxygen demand; for example, less energy is required to use a bedside commode than to use a bedpan,[10,11] and cardiac output and myocardial work are less in the sitting than in the recumbent position.[12] Harrison[13] cited the "abuse" of bed rest as a therapeutic measure for patients with cardiovascular disease and warned that excessive physician caution would result in incapacitating cardiac neuroses among postinfarction patients. He emphasized that both John Hunter and Sir William McKenzie had lived active lives after apparent myocardial infarctions that had not been treated with bed rest.

The cardiac catheterization studies of Stead et al. in the 1940s[14] demonstrated that fear and anxiety markedly increased cardiac output and cardiac work. It was suggested that enforced bed rest might exert a paradoxic effect, with the patient's fear of impending death or disability or the concern about prolonged invalidism resulting in an increase in myocardial oxygen demand as a response to emotional stress. In 1950, Irvin and Burgess[15] further criticized the customary lengthy immobilization at bed rest; they noted that few data supported the advocacy of prolonged immobilization and that there was mounting evidence of its deleterious effects. They emphasized that bed rest could be "advantageously and safely shortened."

As recently as the early 1970s, clinical practice in the United States varied considerably, with the duration of enforced bed rest varying from 1 day to 4 weeks after uncomplicated myocardial infarction and the duration of hospitalization encompassing from 2 to 6 weeks or more.[16,17] Many physicians continued to perpetuate the misconception that optimal care for the patient with an uncomplicated myocardial infarction was prolonged bed rest and hospitalization. The advent of the coronary care unit, in addition to enabling ECG surveillance and the recognition, prevention, and treatment of life-threatening arrhythmias, enabled physiologic monitoring of patients with recent myocardial infarction and compilation of information regarding their clinical course, natural history, and prognosis. Most of the serious complications of myocardial infarction were found to occur during the first days of hospitalization, and the majority of patients with initially uncomplicated myocardial infarction had little or no in-hospital mortality and few significant late hospital complications.[18] Most patients without continued or recurrent cardiac pain, serious rhythm disorders, cardiac decompensation, or other major complications appeared able to safely leave the hospital by the end of the first week if the home circumstances were appropriate. These safety data and the information that prolonged restriction of activity may adversely affect recovery encouraged early ambulation, in-hospital physical activity programs, and early discharge from the hospital for most patients after myocardial infarction. Indeed, Rose[19] suggested that the burden of proof now lies with the physician who advocates extensive activity restriction as beneficial for the patient with uncomplicated acute myocardial infarction. On the other hand, patients with recurrent ischemia after myocardial infarction are at increased risk for late complications[20]; early coronary angiography is typically undertaken to determine their suitability for myocardial revascularization procedures. Their ambulation should be more gradual and more carefully supervised. Major changes in the pattern of care have occurred since Newman et al.[21] characterized as "early ambulation" 3 to 5 minutes of walking twice daily during the fourth week after infarction. These advances have been extended to the care of patients after myocardial revascularization procedures.

PHYSIOLOGIC BASIS FOR EARLY AMBULATION

The decrease in physical work capacity after hospitalization for myocardial infarction, coronary angioplasty, or coronary bypass surgery typically reflects both the severity of the underlying coronary disease and the deconditioning from bed rest. Information about the deleterious effects of prolonged immobilization at bed rest provided the impetus for recommending early ambulation for most patients after acute myocardial infarction and myocardial revascularization procedures.[22,23] Comparable regimens are equally appropriate and necessary for patients who have undergone coronary angioplasty or coronary bypass surgery. Not only can appropriately selected patients be mobilized with safety in the initial days after myocardial infarction, but this approach affords significant advantages.

The most marked alteration after prolonged bed rest is a decrease in physical work capacity, as a result of a diminution in stroke volume and maximal cardiac output. A study[22] of healthy young college students placed at strict bed rest for 21 days (at that time the traditional management for myocardial infarction), showed that their physical work capacity decreased 20 to 25%; at least 3 weeks of physical training were required to restore their pre-bed rest status (Fig. 19-1). The postillness fatigue, weakness, and tiredness of the patient who has been at prolonged bed rest for myocardial infarction (or for any other medical problem) often are caused less by the disease than by the activity restriction imposed for the illness. The higher the level of physical fitness before the period at bed rest, the longer the retraining needed to restore the former functional level after resumption of activity.[22] Extrapolation of these data to the patient with myocardial infarction indicates that the previously highly fit individual or the patient who regularly performs heavy manual labor rapidly incurs a more severe decrease in function and requires more pro-

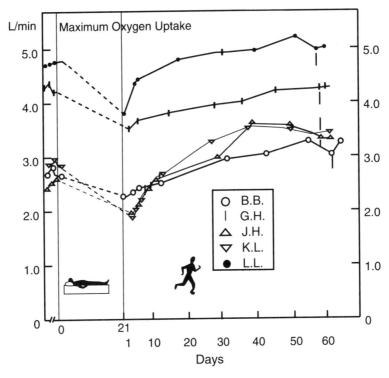

Fig. 19-1. Changes in maximal oxygen uptake with bed rest and training. Individual data before and after bed rest and at various intervals during training. Arrows indicate circulatory studies. Heavy bars mark the time during the training period at which the maximal oxygen uptake had returned to the control value before bed rest. (From Saltin et al.[22] with permission.)

longed rehabilitative physical activity to resume the former lifestyle. The data of Saltin et al.[22] additionally demonstrated that after training, the physical work capacity of their previously sedentary college students could be increased to a level greater than that prior to the 3 weeks of bed rest. Extrapolation to the patient with myocardial infarction explains the otherwise paradoxic observation that many previously sedentary patients who undertake rehabilitative exercise training after myocardial infarction and who have no major residual myocardial dysfunction can perform at higher levels of activity than before their illness.

When ambulation is begun after prolonged bed rest, orthostatic hypotension and reflex tachycardia are often encountered; neither of these responses are desirable in the patient with recent myocardial infarction.[24] Although loss of normal postural vasomotor reflexes plays a role, these adverse responses are due in large part to the hypovolemia that occurs with bed rest. Circulating blood volume begins to decrease within 24 hours and intravascular volume may decrease by 700 to 800 mL within 7 to 10 days at strict bed rest.[25] Patients with congestive heart failure, who do not incur a decrease in circulating blood volume, do not manifest tachycardia and postural hypotension when initially mobilized after bed rest.[24] An orthostatically induced decrease in ventricular filling accounted for most of the decrease in exercise tolerance after bed rest in middle-aged subjects[26]; a significantly greater decline in peak oxygen uptake occurred with upright exercise than during supine exercise in normal middle-aged men after 10 days at bed rest. Deterioration in control of the venous capacitance vessels may magnify the effects of orthostatic stress with upright exercise; pooling of 300 to 800 mL of blood in the leg veins on standing further decreases left ventricular volume and filling pressure, limiting the oxygen transport capacity; thus, the decrease in physical work capacity reflects hypovolemia, not left ventricular dysfunction. Subsequent submaximal effort is characterized by an increase in heart rate and rate–pressure product, increasing myocardial oxygen demand.[26] Intermittent exposure of the patient to gravitational stress by sitting or standing may limit the exercise intolerance resulting from bed rest. Cardiac work is less in the seated than in the supine position; nonetheless, activity as light as sitting in a chair two or three times daily seems adequate to limit the hypovolemia attendant on prolonged immobilization and the resultant orthostatic hypotension, deterioration of oxygen transport capacity, and effort intolerance.[26] Importantly, this intensity of activity is within the capability of most coronary patients. The exposure to gravitational stress seems more important than the intensity of the activity in preventing the deterioration of exercise tolerance after protracted bed rest. Even minimal regular gravitational effect on the cardiovascular system appears to preserve the ability of cardiovascular mechanisms to adequately compensate during the orthostatic stress of resuming the upright posture following prolonged periods at bed rest. An additional undesirable consequence of the bed rest-induced hypovolemia is an increase in blood viscosity, because plasma volume contracts disproportionately to the decrease in red blood cell mass.[27] Increased blood viscosity predisposes to thromboembolic complications; venous circulatory stasis, due to limited use of the leg muscle pump, augments the thromboembolic risk. Radioactive fibrinogen studies have documented forming clot in the leg veins of about one-third of patients at bed rest after myocardial infarction.[28–30]

There is a modest diminution in pulmonary ventilation as a result of a decrease in lung volume and vital capacity at bed rest; this appears important in patients with associated chronic pulmonary disease, which is not an unusual combination. Negative nitrogen and protein balances occur[31] that may adversely affect healing of necrotic myocardium.

Finally, immobilization results in a decrease in skeletal muscle mass and muscular contractile strength and efficiency; contractile strength may diminish by 10 to 15% within the first week at bed rest.[32] Inefficiently functioning muscle requires more oxygen for the performance of comparable work than does trained muscle, and this increased demand is imposed on an impaired oxygen transport system and potentially ischemic myocardium in the patient with recent infarction.

These adverse cardiovascular changes due to bed rest begin within a few days, with elderly patients especially susceptible to these adverse effects of immobilization. Early ambulation is designed to avert or lessen the detrimental physiologic effects of prolonged bed rest and to prepare the patient for activities needed for convalescence at home, a limited but important goal. Additionally, this approach lessens the deleterious psychological responses, anxiety and depression, that accompany with varying severity many episodes of acute myocardial infarction.[33–35] The gradual and progressive increases in activity allowed each day provide tangible reinforcement of the physician's statement that the patient is improving and can expect to return to a normal or near-normal lifestyle.

SELECTION OF PATIENTS FOR AND METHODOLOGY OF EARLY AMBULATION

Appropriate selection of patients for early ambulation is important, as is surveillance of their activity. Ambulation may begin as early as the first day in the coronary care unit for the patient with uncomplicated myocardial infarction with a favorable prognosis—the patient without significant arrhythmia, heart failure, hypotension or clinical shock, or persistent or recurrent chest pain. Patients whose hospital course is characterized by these complications require appropriate care at bed rest; gradually progressive ambulation should be initiated once these complications have been controlled and stabilized; these patients often require a more prolonged hospitalization and more gradual increases in physical activity. Patients with uncomplicated myocardial infarction make up more than half of all patients admitted to coronary care units in the United States[36]; in general, they tend to be younger and to have an initial episode of myocardial infarction. In recent years, early intervention procedures for acute myocardial infarction, coronary thrombolysis and acute coronary angioplasty, have transiently delayed ambulation to limit the risk of bleeding.

General guidelines for initial physical activity in the coronary care unit are that it should be primarily dynamic and of low intensity, 1 to 2 METs, i.e., one to two times the resting metabolic rate (1 MET = approximately 3.5 mL O_2/kg body w/min). Activities should be gradually progressive in work demand and should be supervised by an individual capable of assessing the patient's response. Self-care activities meet these specifications; patients may feed themselves, bathe and perform personal care, use a bedside commode, and perform selected arm and leg flexibility and range-of-motion exercises to maintain muscle tone and joint mobility. Patients should be encouraged to sit on the side of the bed or in a bedside chair to minimize intravascular volume depletion. Incentive spirometry is important for postoperative patients. No significant increase in cardiac work (as measured by the rate–pressure product) was evident[37] with postural change or with selected passive and active exercises performed by patients in the coronary care unit.

A wide variety of early ambulation protocols, defining steps or stages of activity progression, are used in many community hospitals, medical centers, and university complexes. Although most formats are comparable, there is benefit to a predefined activity regimen, as it is unrealistic to expect busy clinicians to write detailed daily physical activity orders for each patient. At Grady Memorial Hospital in Atlanta, GA, under the supervision of the Emory University School of Medicine, a prototype early ambulation program has been operative since the early 1960s (Table 19-1).[38] It delineates prescribed exercises, hospital "daily-living" activities, and recreational and educational activities of parallel intensity for each of a series of steps. The protocol is incorporated in the patient's record, which enables the

physician to indicate daily approval for progression of the patient from one activity level to the next; the nurse or therapist who supervises the activity documents the patient's daily clinical response (heart rate, blood pressure, and symptoms if appropriate). In addition to providing a structure for and documentation of care, the protocol facilitates communication among the health professionals caring for the patient. The original 14-step program was designed to meet the needs of patients hospitalized for 2 to 3 weeks for acute myocardial infarction. The current version has been curtailed and now entails seven steps or stages of gradually progressive activity; the first two are designated as coronary care unit activities, and the next five are performed in a general medical care area. Advantages of a predefined rehabilitation activity format include more efficient implementation by the hospital staff, ensuring that consistent information about activity is provided for the patient, and permitting the staff to describe for the patient and family the planned progression of activities.

ECG monitoring facilitates surveillance of the response to early ambulation in the coronary care unit. Generally accepted guidelines[39,40] for an appropriate response to low-intensity early ambulation (1 to 2 METs) in the coronary care unit or surgical intensive care unit include (1) a heart rate response less than 120 beats/min or 15 to 20 beats/min above the resting heart rate in patients receiving beta-adrenergic blocking drugs; (2) no chest discomfort, dyspnea, palpitations, or exercise fatigue; (3) no appearance of arrhythmias; (4) no increase in ST segment displacement on the ECG suggestive of myocardial ischemia; and (5) no decrease in systolic blood pressure of more than 10 to 15 mmHg. The usual response to exercise is a slight increase in systolic blood pressure; in this clinical setting, a fall in systolic blood pressure usually indicates activity-induced ischemic ventricular dysfunction, with inadequacy of the cardiac output to meet the demand. Excessive effect of vasodilator drugs such as nitrate preparations and calcium-blocking drugs may also engender this postural hypotension. An increase in excess of 180 mmHg in systolic blood pressure or a diastolic blood pressure greater than

Table 19-1.   In-Patient Rehabilitation: 7-Step Myocardial Infarction Program[a]

Step	Date	M.D. Initials	Nurse/PT Notes	Supervised Exercise	CCU/Ward Activity	Educational-Recreational Activity
				CCU		
1	—			Active and passive ROM all extremities, in bed Teach patients ankle plantar and dorsiflexion—repeat hourly when awake	Partial self-care Feed self Dangle legs on side of bed Use bedside commode Sit in chair 15 min 1–2 times/day	Orientation to CCU Personal emergencies, social service aid as needed
2	—			Active ROM all extremities, sitting on side of bed	Sit in chair 15–30 min 2–3 times/day Complete self-care in bed	Orientation to rehabilitation team, program Smoking cessation Educational literature if requested Planning transfer from CCU
				Ward		
3	—			Warm-up exercises, 2 METs: stretching, calisthenics Walk 50 ft and back at slow pace	Sit in chair ad lib To ward class in wheelchair Walk in room	Normal cardiac anatomy and function Development of atherosclerosis What happens with myocardial infarction
4	—			ROM and calisthenics, 2.5 METs Walk length of hall (75 ft) and back, average pace Teach pulse counting	Out of bed as tolerated Walk to bathroom Walk to ward class, with supervision	Coronary risk factors and their control
5	—			ROM and calisthenics, 3 METs Check pulse counting Practice walking few stairsteps Walk 300 ft bid	Walk to waiting room or telephone Walk in ward corridor prn	Diet Energy conservation Work simplification techniques (as needed)
6	—			Continue above activities Walk down flight of steps (return by elevator) Walk 500 ft bid Instruct on home exercise	Tepid shower or tub bath with supervision To occupational therapy, cardiac clinic teaching room, with supervision	Heart attack management: Medications Exercise Surgery Response to symptoms Family, community adjustments on return home
7	—			Continue above activities Walk up flight of steps Walk 500 ft bid Continue home exercise instruction; present information regarding outpatient exercise program	Continue all previous ward activities	Discharge planning: Medicions, diet, activity Return appointments Scheduled tests Return to work Community resources Educational literature Medication cards

[a] Grady Memorial Hospital and Emory University School of Medicine (revised, 1980). (From Wenger,[75] with permission.)

110 mmHg with low levels of activity suggests that antihypertensive therapy may be needed.

An inappropriate physiologic response to any level of activity signifies that the work load is excessive and requires that the patient's activity plan be revised, with return to a less demanding activity level, and that the clinical status be reevaluated to determine the need for diagnostic and therapeutic interventions. When the response is appropriate, the patient may progress to an activity level of greater intensity. Advantages of structured and supervised early ambulation include (1) detection of inappropriate physiologic responses to low-level activity, (2) avoidance of excessive levels of activity early in the clinical course, and (3) encouragement of the timid patient who is fearful of performing physical activity without supervision and direction.

After successful coronary angioplasty, patients typically have few or no symptoms and often have good ventricular function. When angioplasty is unrelated to an episode of infarction, the appropriate emphasis is on prevention of deconditioning and disability during the characteristically brief hospital stay.[41]

Mobilization of the patient after coronary bypass surgery is often begun in the surgical intensive care unit. Local discomfort at the sternotomy site or the site of saphenous vein removal is often the factor that limits mobility. Postoperative pericarditis may be associated with both chest discomfort and tachycardia and may delay ambulation.[42,43] Hypovolemia often occurs from excessive diuresis in the postoperative period after coronary bypass surgery; early ambulation may be associated with both hypotension and reflex tachycardia in this setting.[42]

After transfer from the coronary care unit to a progressive care or general medical area, the goal of rehabilitative physical activity is to continue to limit the deleterious physiologic and psychological effects of bed rest and to help patients increase their functional status to a level that enables the performance of customary self-care and homebound activities at the time of discharge from the hospital. The current duration of hospital stay in the United States is about 1 week for the patient with an uncomplicated clinical course.[1,18] This requires gradual progression from bed rest to the work intensity required to perform household tasks, an energy expenditure of 2 to 3 METs. Also, predischarge exercise testing (see Ch. 7 and 8) is inappropriate for a patient who has remained at bed rest or at a bed-and-bathroom-privileges activity level throughout the hospitalization; progressive ambulation permits an assessment of both risk status and exercise capacity to be derived from this test.

A variety of physical activities may be undertaken[38]; basic requirements are that they be of low intensity (2 to 3 METs) and be supervised by a trained individual who can monitor the physiologic responses cited above. Patients continue to perform personal care and to sit in a chair for increasing periods. They perform, with supervision, selected low-intensity dynamic rhythmic exercises involving the arms, legs, and trunk. After these "warm-up" exercises, the major prescriptive component of in-hospital physical activity is walking, with gradually progressive increases in pace and distance, based on the patient's tolerance. Ideally, these activities are performed several times each day, interspersed with rest periods. Elastic support stockings help decrease leg pain and edema at saphenous vein incision sites in the legs in postoperative patients. The emphasis is on dynamic exercise, with initial limitation of isometric exercise. Isometric exercise does not elicit (as does dynamic exercise) a heart rate response proportional to the intensity of the activity. It is associated with little heart rate change but may evoke a significant increase in blood pressure,[44] which appears related to the percentage of maximal voluntary contraction of the involved muscle group. Isometric activities involving less than 20% of the maximal voluntary contraction elicit only a minimal increase in blood pressure, whereas activities characterized by more than 20% of the maximal voluntary contraction of the muscle group may exert a profound hypertensive effect (Fig. 19-2). This sudden increase in afterload may be poorly tolerated by a potentially ischemic left ventricle and may precipitate chest pain or arrhythmia. This feature explains why low-level isometric activities are well tolerated by most coronary patients. It also emphasizes the importance of exercise training in

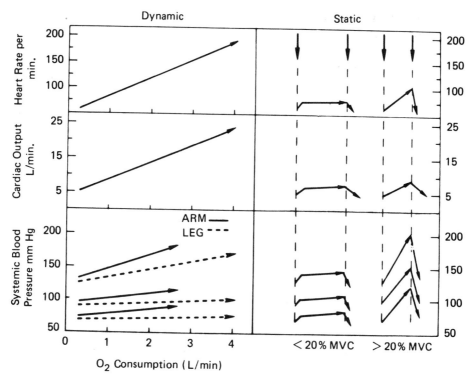

Fig. 19-2. Hemodynamic responses to dynamic exercise (running, solid line); cranking arm ergometer (dotted line); and to static exercise (handgrip). Abbreviation: MCV, maximal voluntary contraction. (From Nutter[38a] with permission.)

that 20% of the maximal voluntary contraction of trained muscle allows an absolute increase in work.

An appropriate response to physical activity is gauged by criteria comparable to those used during the coronary care unit stay. ECG monitoring or telemetry is required only for selected patients, particularly those with prior serious ventricular arrhythmias or evidence of asymptomatic myocardial ischemia.

Increments in the intensity of in-hospital daily activities should parallel the serial progression of prescribed daily exercise; recreational, diversional, and educational activities of a comparable work level should be offered (Table 19-1). More impaired patients are taught energy-conserving techniques for the performance of activities of daily living. Patients who must climb steps at home should practice this before dismissal from the hospital, walking down a flight of stairs one

day and returning by elevator, and walking slowly up a flight of steps the next day. Accomplishing this task safely under supervision in the hospital minimizes the anxiety of the patient and family often associated with initial stair-climbing at home.

RESULTS: SAFETY AND BENEFITS OF EARLY AMBULATION AND EARLY HOSPITAL DISCHARGE

Early experience with nonrandomized, early mobilization in the hospital uniformly suggested favorable results in enabling self-care, improved attitude and emotional status of the patient, earlier discharge from the hospital, and earlier and more complete return to work.[45] The 10-year follow-up data of Brummer et al.[46] showed no significant differences in outcome as bed rest was progressively decreased from 16.2 to 10.3 days and hospitalization was abbreviated from 22.6 to 18.9 days. No apparent detrimental effects of early mobilization and shortened hospital stay for patients with uncomplicated myocardial infarction were found in other studies in which earlier hospital discharge was progressively undertaken. The feasibility of early mobilization and early discharge from hospital has been repeatedly demonstrated, as has its cost-effectiveness and safety.[36,47,48]

Several well-designed controlled studies have further documented the safety of early ambulation and early discharge from the hospital for appropriately selected patients after myocardial infarction. There was no increase in either short- or long-term morbidity or mortality rates or in the incidence of complications[49]; indeed, some studies suggested a more favorable outcome among these patients. Early mobilization and earlier discharge from the hospital commonly go hand in hand, the former facilitating the latter.[45]

Groden and Brown[50] compared the effects of early and late mobilization after myocardial infarction on the results of psychological tests administered at discharge from the hospital and 1 year later. Patients mobilized earlier had lower neuroticism scores at the time of discharge from the hospital, but these scores did not persist at 1 year; this suggests that the initial advantages of early mobilization may be lost when patients return home without continued rehabilitative care. In a subsequent study, Groden[51] again found no adverse effects of early mobilization; benefits included a reduction in psychological complications and earlier return to work.

No medical disadvantages (increases in morbidity or mortality rates) were associated with early ambulation in a randomized British study coordinated by Harpur et al.,[52] with no differences in incidence of coronary death, recurrent myocardial infarction, congestive heart failure, significant arrhythmias, or ventricular aneurysm. However, patients in the early-mobilization group returned to work earlier.

In a prospective study at the Massachusetts General Hospital,[53] no differences were evident in morbidity and mortality, subsequent therapy, anxiety and depression, or return to work in pa-

tients discharged at 2 and 3 weeks after uncomplicated myocardial infarction. The additional week of hospitalization did not appear to provide benefit; the shorter hospital stay enabled substantial reductions in hospital expenses and better use of hospital beds,[54] without compromising the health of the patients.

The study of Bloch et al.[55] in Geneva revealed no difference in mortality or morbidity rates or in the results of an exercise test at 1 year in patients randomized to early mobilization or a traditional hospital regimen; however, the early-mobilization group resumed work earlier and had a significantly lower incidence of disability (psychological factors were the primary contributors to the disability).

Early-mobilization trials in recent years have been characterized by progressively earlier and more intensive ambulation. The difficulties in pooling or comparing the results of many of these studies are that the early-mobilization groups of the earlier studies correspond to the late-mobilization (control) groups of the later reports and that low-level earlier ambulation is often compared with activities of only slightly greater intensity or supervised ambulation is compared with informal and unsupervised activity.[56] In one such study, although neither beneficial nor deleterious effects were identified from a structured early-ambulation dynamic-activity program compared with informal early ambulation; the supervised program may have helped identify earlier a subset of patients who needed coronary bypass surgery,[56] suggesting benefit from observation of the patient during activity for adverse responses to exercise.

Thus, in addition to the general acceptance and adoption of early ambulation, numerous controlled studies worldwide have unequivocally confirmed the safety of supervised early mobilization for appropriately selected patients. Correctly designed and supervised early ambulation has not increased the hospital or follow-up complications of myocardial infarction (angina pectoris, reinfarction, arrhythmias, congestive heart failure, ventricular aneurysm, cardiac rupture, sudden cardiac death, and so forth).[57,58] The complications of prolonged immobilization at bed rest (decreased physical work capacity, hypovolemic orthostatic intolerance, predisposition to thromboembolism, pulmonary atelectasis, decrease in muscle mass and muscular contractile strength, and anxiety and depression)[30] have been effectively reduced. Emotional complications are common with myocardial infarction, with depression occurring in response to anticipated invalidism and future restrictions of lifestyle. Depression may also follow coronary bypass surgery. The reassurance offered by the performance of progressive physical activity improves the patient's self-confidence and self-image. In addition, many psychotropic drugs are inadvisable for patients with recent infarction because of their adverse effects on heart rate, blood pressure, and cardiac rhythm; early ambulation thus assumes greater importance in helping to limit psychological complications. Significantly greater disability has been demonstrated at follow-up examination with the traditional hospital regimen than with early ambulation,[55] and in some studies early ambulation has facilitated return to work. It should be reemphasized, however, that the home situation and access to medical care must be appropriate when early discharge from the hospital is contemplated; for example, someone must be available to prepare meals, shop for groceries, help with household tasks, obtain prompt medical aid if needed, and so forth.

There are, however, patients with multiple serious complications of myocardial infarction or coronary bypass surgery for whom in-hospital exercise, even at low intensity, is inappropriate. Intermittent dobutamine infusions, given to healthy men placed at enforced bed rest, appeared able to maintain exercise tolerance, at least in part by maintaining or increasing the activity of some aerobic enzymes in human skeletal muscle.[59] The safety and applicability of this intervention for subgroups of seriously ill coronary patients has not been assessed.

PREDISCHARGE EXERCISE TESTING

Predischarge exercise testing is also discussed in Chapters 7 and 8.

Exercise testing is the cornerstone of risk strat-

ification procedures[60] performed before discharge from the hospital after myocardial infarction[61] or other coronary events. The exercise test begins at low intensity and is often designed to evoke a heart rate response below 120 to 130 beats/min or 70% of the predicted heart rate for age; in many medical centers, patients are tested to a sign- or symptom-limited endpoint, or, alternatively, a 5-MET level is used as an endpoint in the absence of limiting symptoms.[62] Predischarge exercise testing requires prior progressive ambulation to be able to ascertain reliably the patient's functional capacity. With appropriate selection of patients, early exercise tests performed in experienced exercise laboratories have not been associated with appreciable complications and have provided valuable prognostic information to guide patient care.

Exercise testing before hospital discharge after myocardial infarction and other coronary events offers several potential clinical benefits[63–65] (see also Chs. 7 and 8). It allows more precise definition of safely tolerated activity levels and, for the relatively unimpaired patient, can identify the readiness to more rapidly resume normal out-of-hospital activity levels and return to work. It aids in identification of activity-precipitated treatable mechanisms of impairment: chest pain, arrhythmias, ventricular dysfunction, and ST-T ECG changes of myocardial ischemia. Thus, it may identify the high-risk patient who requires additional early diagnostic and therapeutic interventions[40,66] because of an increased risk of proximate coronary events, and more gradual and supervised increases in activity level during convalescence.

Low exercise capacity, with ECG or symptomatic evidence of myocardial ischemia at low levels of exercise, suggests severe and typically multivessel coronary obstruction and characterizes the patient at high risk who may benefit from additional diagnostic studies, especially coronary angiography, and additional medical or earlier surgical intervention.[67–69] Poor exercise capacity, often due to ischemic left ventricular dysfunction, is commonly associated with the development of angina pectoris and ST segment changes and ventricular arrhythmias on the exercise ECG. Further, the decision that early exercise testing is deemed unwise identifies the patient at greatest risk.

Finally, the performance of a predischarge exercise test often decreases the fear, common in patients after myocardial infarction, that activity may result in recurrent infarction or sudden cardiac death; it may therefore have a positive psychological impact[70] (see Chs. 26 and 28) by demonstrating the level of activity that can be performed without adverse effects; it may also increase motivation for subsequent participation in exercise training.

CONVALESCENT PHYSICAL ACTIVITY

Although they are not, in the strictest sense, components of early ambulation, recommendations for physical activity during the initial weeks of convalescence at home deserve mention. More than 85% of patients with uncomplicated myocardial infarction, employed at the time of infarction, can and do return to work by 8 to 12 weeks after infarction, typically returning to their former jobs.[1,16] For low-risk patients identified at predischarge exercise testing who do not require surveillance of rehabilitative exercise training, posthospital activities should be designed to gradually and progressively increase endurance. During the initial days at home, patients should continue at the activity level of the last days in the hospital; the amount of rest should also be specified. They may perform customary household tasks; dynamic "warm-up" exercises should precede walking, and the distance and pace of walking should gradually be increased. Patients who have had significant limitation of activity during hospitalization commonly initially describe a lack of energy on return home; this reflects their increase in perceived exertion required to perform a given task because it entails a greater proportion of their diminished physical work capacity. Continued activity will increase their stamina and endurance. Indeed the "spontaneous" improvement in function described during convalescence[71] probably reflects the change in medical and community attitudes to-

ward activity for patients after myocardial infarction, enabling and encouraging nonstructured "exercise training."

Walking is a major activity during convalescence, with progressive increases in the pace and distance advised. Because patients are taught during the hospitalization to monitor their pulse rate response to exercise or to use a rating of perceived exertion,[72] they can ascertain whether walking elicits an appropriate response. Predischarge exercise testing can precisely guide activity recommendations. Patients initially walk in and around their homes, walking outdoors when they can avoid extremes of temperature and humidity. In larger communities, enclosed shopping malls offer temperature- and humidity-controlled sites for walking. Other low-risk patients may prefer home exercise, guided by videotapes, that are available on physician recommendations.[73] These specific activity recommendations help structure the patient's day during convalescence, which otherwise contrasts unfavorably with the highly scheduled hospital stay or the pre-illness occupation.

Patients who can walk at a speed of 3.5 miles/h without difficulty have an activity level of 4 to 5 METs. Such patients can be expected to return to most relatively sedentary occupations in today's society, which generally require an energy expenditure of 3 to 4 METs. Patients whose occupations require higher levels of physical activity may require more intense and more prolonged exercise training before resuming work (see Chs. 29 and 30).

SUMMARY

Early ambulation of the patient after myocardial infarction and myocardial revascularization procedures is the accepted standard of care,[74] designed to minimize or avert the detrimental physiologic effects and resultant functional impairment from prolonged bed rest and to prevent or limit anxiety and depression. It facilitates the current, shorter hospital stay and an improved use of hospital beds, with saving in medical care costs[36]; it also permits the appropriate perform-

ance of a predischarge exercise test. The increased physical work capability and the improved self-image of the patient at the time of discharge from the hospital have been associated with an earlier and more complete return to work. The approach is desirable, feasible, simple, cost-effective, and safe.

REFERENCES

1. Wenger NK, Hellerstein HK, Blackburn H, Castranova SJ: Physician practice in the management of patients with uncomplicated myocardial infarction—changes in the past decade. Circulation 65:421, 1982
2. Topol EJ, Burek K, O'Neill WW et al: A randomized controlled trial of hospital discharge three days after myocardial infarction in the era of reperfusion. N Engl J Med 318:1083, 1988
3. Herrick JB: Clinical features of sudden obstruction of the coronary arteries. JAMA 59:2015, 1912
4. Mallory GK, White PD, Salcedo-Salgar J: The speed of healing of myocardial infarction: A study of the pathologic anatomy in seventy-two cases. Am Heart J 18:647, 1939
5. Lewis T: Diseases of the Heart. p. 49. Macmillan, New York, 1933
6. Jetter WW, White PD: Rupture of the heart in patients in mental institutions. Ann Intern Med 21:783, 1944
7. Levine SA: Some harmful effects of recumbency in the treatment of heart disease. JAMA 126:80, 1944
8. Levine SA, Lown B: The "chair" treatment of acute coronary thrombosis. Trans Assoc Am Physicians 64:316, 1951
9. Dock W: The evil sequelae of complete bed rest. JAMA 125:1083, 1944
10. Wanka J: Bedpan vs. commode in patients with myocardial infarction. Cardiac Rehabil 1:7, 1970
11. Winslow EH, Lane LD, Gaffney FA: Oxygen uptake and cardiovascular response in patients and normal adults during in-bed and out-of-bed toileting. J Cardiac Rehabil 4:348, 1984
12. Coe WS: Cardiac work and the chair treatment of acute coronary thrombosis. Ann Intern Med 40:42, 1954
13. Harrison TR: Abuse of rest as a therapeutic measure for patients with cardiovascular disease. JAMA 125:1075, 1944
14. Stead EA Jr, Warren JV, Merrill AJ et al: The cardiac output in male subjects as measured by the technique of right atrial catheterization. Normal values with observations on the effect of anxiety and tilting. J Clin Invest 24:326, 1944
15. Irvin CW Jr, Burgess AM Jr: The abuse of bed rest in the treatment of myocardial infarction. N Engl J Med 243:486, 1950
16. Wenger NK, Hellerstein HK, Blackburn HW, Castranova SJ: Uncomplicated myocardial infarction: Current physician practice in patient management. JAMA 224:511, 1973
17. Duke M: Bed rest in acute myocardial infarction. A study of physician practices. Am Heart J 82:486, 1971
18. Swan HJC, Blackburn HW, DeSanctis R et al: Duration of hospitalization in "uncomplicated completed acute myocardial infarction." An ad hoc committee review. Am J Cardiol 37:413, 1976
19. Rose G: Early mobilization and discharge after myocardial infarction. Mod Concepts Cardiovasc Dis 41:59, 1972
20. Singer DE, Mulley AG, Thilbault GE, Barnett GO: Unexpected readmissions to the coronary-care unit during recovery from acute myocardial infarction. N Engl J Med 304:626, 1981
21. Newman LB, Andrews MF, Koblish MO, Baker LA: Physical medicine and rehabilitation in acute myocardial infarction. Arch Intern Med 89:552, 1952
22. Saltin B, Blomqvist G, Mitchell JH et al: Response to exercise after bed rest and after training. Circulation 37–38 (suppl. VII):VII-1, 1968
23. Chobanian AV, Lille RD, Tercyak A, Blevins P: The metabolic and hemodynamic effects of prolonged bed rest in normal subjects. Circulation 49:551, 1974
24. Fareeduddin K, Abelmann WH: Impaired orthostatic tolerance after bed rest in patients with myocardial infarction. N Engl J Med 280:345, 1969
25. Hyatt KH, Kamenetsky LG, Smith WM: Extravascular dehydration as an etiologic factor in postrecumbency orthostatism. Aerosp Med 40:644, 1969
26. Hung J, Goldwater D, Convertino VA, et al: Mechanisms for decreased exercise capacity after bed rest in normal middle-aged men. Am J Cardiol 51:344, 1983
27. Miller PB, Johnson RL, Lamb LE: Effects of moderate physical exercise during four weeks of bed rest on circulatory functions in man. Aerosp Med 36:1077, 1965

28. Nicolaides AN, Kakkar VV, Renney JTG et al: Myocardial infarction and deep-vein thrombosis. Br Med J 1:432, 1971

29. Maurer BJ, Wray R, Shillingford JP: Frequency of venous thrombosis after myocardial infarction. Lancet ii:1385, 1971

30. Lies JL, Carretta RF, Amsterdam EA et al: Lower extremity venous thrombosis in coronary-care unit patients: Prevention by early ambulation and confirmation by I^{125} fibrinogen and venography. Circulation 50 (suppl 3):298, 1974

31. Lynch TN, Jensen RL, Stevens PM et al: Metabolic effects of prolonged bed rest: Their modification by simulated altitude. Aerosp Med 38:10, 1967

32. Bonner CD: Rehabilitation instead of bed rest? Geriatrics 24:109, 1969

33. McPherson BD, Paivio A, Yuhasz MS et al: Psychological effects of an exercise program for post-infarct and normal adult men. J Sports Med Phys Fitness 7:95, 1967

34. Cassem NH, Hackett TP: Psychiatric consultation in a coronary care unit. Ann Intern Med 75:9, 1971

35. Hackett TP, Cassem NH: Psychological adaptation to convalescence in myocardial infarction patients. p. 253. In Naughton JP, Hellerstein HK, Mohler IC (eds): Exercise Testing and Exercise Training in Coronary Heart Disease. Academic Press, San Diego, 1973

36. Pryor DB, Hindman MC, Wagner GS et al: Early discharge after acute myocardial infarction. Ann Intern Med 99:528, 1983

37. DeBusk RF, Spivack AP, van Kessel A et al: The coronary care unit activities program: Its role in post-infarction rehabilitation. J Chronic Dis 24:373, 1971

38. Wenger NK: Coronary Care—Rehabilitation of the Patient with Symptomatic Coronary Atherosclerotic Heart Disease. Publication 70-002-F. Prepared for the Coronary Care Committee, Council on Clinical Cardiology, and the Committee on Medical Education. American Heart Association, Dallas, TX, 1981

38a. Nutter DO: Exercise and the heart. p. 235. In Hurst JW (ed): The Heart, Update I. McGraw-Hill, New York, 1979

39. Report of the Inter-Society Commission for Heart Disease Resources: Optimal resources for the care of patients with acute myocardial infarction and chronic coronary heart disease. Circulation 65:654B, 1982

40. Council on Scientific Affairs: Physician-supervised exercise programs in rehabilitation of patients with coronary heart disease. JAMA 245:1463, 1981

41. Cragg DR, Friedman HZ, Almany SL et al: Early hospital discharge after percutaneous transluminal coronary angioplasty. Am J Cardiol 64:1270, 1989

42. Dion WF, Grevenow P, Pollock ML et al: Medical problems and physiologic responses during supervised inpatient cardiac rehabilitation: The patient after coronary artery bypass grafting. Heart Lung 11:248, 1982

43. Silvidi GE, Squires RW, Pollock ML, Foster C: Hemodynamic responses and medical problems associated with early exercise and ambulation in coronary artery bypass graft surgery patients. J Cardiac Rehabil 2:355, 1982

44. Nutter DO, Schlant RC, Hurst JW: Isometric exercise and the cardiovascular system. Mod Concepts Cardiovasc Dis 41:11, 1972

45. Wenger NK: Early ambulation after myocardial infarction: Rationale, program components and results. p. 53. In Wenger NK, Hellerstein HK (eds): Rehabilitation of the Coronary Patient. John Wiley & Sons, New York, 1978

46. Brummer P, Kallio V, Tala E: Early ambulation in the treatment of myocardial infarction. Acta Med Scand 180:231, 1966

47. McNeer JF, Wallace AG, Wagner GS et al: The course of acute myocardial infarction. Feasibility of early discharge of the uncomplicated patient. Circulation 51:410, 1969

48. McNeer JF, Wagner GS, Ginsburg PB et al: Hospital discharge one week after acute myocardial infarction. N Engl J Med 298:229, 1978

49. Rowe MH, Jelinek MV, Liddell N, Hugens M: Effect of rapid mobilization on ejection fractions and ventricular volumes after acute myocardial infarction. Am J Cardiol 63:1037, 1989

50. Groden BM, Brown RIF: Differential psychological effects of early and late mobilisation after myocardial infarction. Scand J Rehabil Med 2:60, 1970

51. Groden BM: The management of myocardial infarction. A controlled study of the effects of early mobilization. Cardiac Rehabil 1:13, 1971

52. Harpur JE, Kellett RJ, Conner WT et al: Controlled trial of early mobilization and discharge from hospital in uncomplicated myocardial infarction. Lancet ii:1331, 1971

53. Hutter AM Jr, Sidel VW, Shine KI, DeSanctis RW: Early hospital discharge after myocardial infarction. N Engl J Med 288:1141, 1973

54. Baughman KL, Hutter AM Jr, DeSanctis RW, Kallman CH: Early discharge following acute myocardial infarction. Long-term follow-up of randomized patients. Arch Intern Med 142:875, 1982

55. Bloch A, Maeder JP, Haissly JC et al: Early mobilization after myocardial infarction. A controlled study. Am J Cardiol 34:152, 1974

56. Sivarajan ES, Bruce RA, Almes MJ et al: In-hospital exercise after myocardial infarction does not improve treadmill performance. N Engl J Med 305:357, 1981

57. Boyle JA, Lorimer AR: Early mobilisation after uncomplicated myocardial infarction. Prospective study of 538 patients. Lancet II:346, 1973

58. Hayes MJ, Morris GK, Hampton JR: Comparison of mobilization after two and nine days in uncomplicated myocardial infarction. Br Med J 3:10, 1974

59. Sullivan MJ, Merola AJ, Timmerman AP et al: Drug-induced aerobic-enzyme activity of human skeletal muscle during bedrest deconditioning. J Cardiopulmonary Rehabil 6:232, 1986

60. Gunnar RM, Bourdillon PDV, Dixon DW et al: Guidelines for the early management of patients with acute myocardial infarction. A report of the American College of Cardiology/American Heart Association Task Force on Assessment of Diagnostic and Therapeutic Cardiovascular Procedures (Subcommittee to Develop Guidelines for the Early Management of Patients with Acute Myocardial Infarction). J Am Coll Cardiol 16:249, 1990

61. Hamm LF, Stull GA, Crow RS: Exercise testing early after myocardial infarction: Historic perspective and current uses. Prog Cardiovasc Dis 28:463, 1986

62. Guidelines for exercise testing. A report of the American College of Cardiology/American Heart Association Task Force on Assessment of Diagnostic and Therapeutic Cardiovascular Procedures (Subcommittee on Exercise Testing). J Am Coll Cardiol 8:725, 1986

63. Jelinek MV, Ziffer RW, McDonald JG, Hale GS: Shortened cardiac rehabilitation: A three year experience. Aust NZ J Med 10:171, 1980

64. DeBusk RF, Houston N, Haskell W et al: Exercise training soon after myocardial infarction. Am J Cardiol 44:1223, 1979

65. Lindvall K, Erhardt LR, Lundman T et al: Early mobilization and discharge of patients with acute myocardial infarction. A prospective study using risk indicators and early exercise tests. Acta Med Scand 206:169, 1979

66. DeBusk RF, Blomqvist CG, Kouchoukos NT et al: Identification and treatment of low-risk patients after acute myocardial infarction and coronary-artery bypass graft surgery. N Engl J Med 314:161, 1986

67. Theroux P, Waters DD, Halphen C et al: Prognostic value of exercise testing soon after myocardial infarction. N Engl J Med 301:341, 1979

68. Weld FM, Chu KL, Bigger JT Jr, Rolnitzky LM: Risk stratification with low-level exercise testing 2 weeks after acute myocardial infarction. Circulation 64:306, 1981

69. Starling MR, Crawford MH, Richards KL, O'Rourke RA: Predictive value of early postmyocardial infarction modified treadmill exercise testing in multivessel coronary artery disease detection. Am Heart J 102:169, 1981

70. Ewart CK, Taylor CB, Reese LB et al: Effects of early postmyocardial infarction exercise testing on self-perception and subsequent physical activity. Am J Cardiol 51:1076, 1983

71. Savin WM, Haskell WL, Houston-Miller N, DeBusk R: Improvement in aerobic capacity soon after myocardial infarction. J Cardiac Rehabil 1:337, 1981

72. Borg GA: Psychophysical bases of perceived exertion. Med Sci Sports Exercise 14:377, 1982

73. Wenger NK: Review: Cardiac Rehabilitation Exercise Video Series, by Videocare. JAMA 260:271, 1988

74. American Association of Cardiovascular and Pulmonary Rehabilitation: Guidelines for Cardiac Rehabilitiation Programs. Human Kinetics Books, Champaign, IL, 1991

75. Wenger NK: Rehabilitation of the patient with atherosclerotic coronary heart disease. p. 1110. In Hurst JW (ed): The Heart. 7th ed. McGraw-Hill, New York, 1990.

20

Exercise Training for the Coronary Patient

Larry F. Hamm, Ph.D.
Arthur S. Leon, M.D.

GOALS OF CORONARY REHABILITATION

The ultimate goal of coronary rehabilitative services is to help patients with coronary heart disease (CHD) resume active and productive lives for as long as possible, within the limitations imposed by their disease process.[1] Objectives for accomplishing this include (1) attainment of optimal physiologic, psychosocial, vocational, and recreational status; (2) prevention of progression or reversal of the underlying atherosclerotic process; and (3) reduction of risk of reinfarction and sudden death and alleviation of angina pectoris.[1–6]

Medically supervised exercise training is the focal point of a coronary rehabilitation program[6–8]; other essential elements of outpatient comprehensive coronary rehabilitation are addressed in Chapters 25 to 31. This chapter focuses on the exercise training component of coronary rehabilitation. This includes discussion of the potential benefits of exercise training, potential candidates among coronary patients for rehabilitative exercise programs, preexercise evaluation and exercise prescription, special concerns during exercise for patients taking various cardiovascular drugs, and potential hazards associated with exercise training. Basic principles, methods, and protocols of exercise testing before undertaking exercise training have been discussed in Chapters 7 and 8.

BENEFITS ATTRIBUTED TO EXERCISE TRAINING

The potential benefits of exercise training for patients recovered from myocardial infarction or following percutaneous transluminal coronary angioplasty (PTCA) or coronary surgical procedures are summarized in Table 20-1 and discussed below.[6]

Counteracting of the Deleterious Effects of Physical Inactivity

Limitation of the deleterious effects of physical inactivity is also discussed in Chapter 19.

Deleterious effects of physical inactivity, and particularly of bed rest, include reduced physical work capacity and maximal oxygen uptake ($\dot{V}o_2max$); skeletal muscle wasting; bone demineralization; increased resting heart rate; decreased blood volume; loss of postural vasomotor reflexes, resulting in orthostatic hypotension; re-

Table 20-1. Potential Benefits of Exercise Training for the Coronary Patient

1. Counteracts the deleterious effects of physical inactivity
2. Improves functional capacity
3. Improves cardiovascular efficiency
4. Improves coronary blood flow
5. Reduces atherogenic risk factors for CHD
6. Reduces recurrent CHD events
7. Improves psychological well-being and quality of life

duced pulmonary function; and increased risk of thromboembolism.[9,10] Early mobilization, progressive ambulation, and exercise training counteract these pathophysiologic effects.

Improvement in Functional Capacity

Improvement in functional capacity is also discussed in Chapter 6.

Reduced maximal cardiac output and stroke volume due to loss of myocardium and myocardial dysfunction further contribute to the decline in physical work capacity and $\dot{V}O_2$max levels in patients following acute myocardial infarction. Residual myocardial ischemia induced by physical exertion or emotional reactions can further compromise functional capacity, even when not associated with angina pectoris (silent or asymptomatic ischemia). Ischemia generally is induced at a relatively fixed and reproducible threshold during exercise testing, indicated by the product of heart rate and systolic blood pressure, the so-called rate–pressure product (RPP) or "double-product," a major determinant of myocardial oxygen requirements.

Patients recovered from myocardial infarction, coronary artery bypass graft surgery (CABG), or PTCA typically demonstrate a considerable improvement in $\dot{V}O_2$max levels during coronary rehabilitation exercise programs, ranging from 10 to over 60% after 3 to 6 months of training.[12,13] The lower the pretraining $\dot{V}O_2$max level, the greater is the expected improvement. However, not all improvement in $\dot{V}O_2$max can be attributed to exercise training in patients several months following acute myocardial infarction. A major contribution results from the natural process of healing and the resumption of routine daily activities.[1,14] The incremental contribution of exercise training to improvement of functional capacity for most CHD patients appears to be predominantly due to peripheral adaptations, resulting in an increase in oxygen extraction and utilization by active skeletal muscles and an associated increase in arteriovenous oxygen difference.[1,6,12–15] However, prolonged vigorous exercise training for 1 year or more at 85% of the maximal heart rate reserve, in carefully selected patients after myocardial infarction, has been demonstrated by Ehsani et al.[16] to improve left ventricular contractile function and to substantially increase maximal stroke volume and cardiac output. The RPP also may increase with vigorous training, perhaps as a result of an increase in maximal coronary blood flow. Such vigorous training is appropriate only for a select few CHD patients with good left ventricular function and coronary flow reserve who are at low risk for recurrent CHD events.

Improvement in Cardiovascular Efficiency

Improvement in cardiovascular efficiency is also discussed in Chapter 6.

Although much attention has been paid to improving the maximal aerobic capacity, the usual patient with CHD generally has little direct requirement for increased capacity for peak performance, as at work (see also Ch. 30). Instead, the principal advantage of an augmented $\dot{V}O_2$max level is improved tolerance for daily life activities that require repeated submaximal levels of physical exertion. An increase in $\dot{V}O_2$max enables the patient with CHD to accomplish ordinary tasks at a lower percentage of $\dot{V}O_2$max, resulting in greater vigor and less exertional fatigue and dyspnea. This can considerably enhance the quality of life. Furthermore, submaximal efforts after training are usually accomplished at a lower heart rate, systolic blood pressure, and RPP, thereby reducing myocardial oxygen requirements and raising the threshold for exertional ischemia.[12,15] Thus, after exercise training, patients with angina pectoris may be able to accomplish considerably more physical activity before becoming symptomatic. The reported improvement in the symptom-limited $\dot{V}o_2max$ level in patients with angina pectoris ranges from 32 to 56% following exercise training.[12] The potential for serious cardiac arrhythmias also is reduced by the rise in ischemic threshold, as discussed below.

Improvement in Coronary Blood Flow

A slowing of the heart rate as a result of endurance exercise training prolongs the diastolic phase of the cardiac cycle, during which period coronary blood flow is at its peak. Also, the reduction in heart rate at rest and during physical exertion reduces the associated myocardial oxygen demands and coronary blood flow requirements.

In a number of animal species,[17–21] exercise training augments myocardial capillary density and enlarges the luminal areas of the main and collateral coronary arteries. For example, monkeys that were on atherogenic diets and jogged three times a week on motorized treadmills had substantially larger coronary luminal areas, reduced severity of coronary atherosclerosis, and fewer CHD events compared with matched sedentary control animals on a similar diet.[22] Experiments in intact dogs and pigs have demonstrated that exercise training potentiates the development of coronary collateral arteries induced by gradual or chronic occlusion of a major coronary artery.[19–21,23]

It has been difficult to confirm that exercise enhances myocardial vascularity in patients with CHD.[24–26] Indirect supporting evidence of the ability of exercise to enhance myocardial blood flow in humans is the demonstration of a higher RPP after training prior to development of angina[12,27,28] or regression of ischemic electrocardiographic (ECG) changes (ST segment displacement) at the same or higher RPP[16,29] in some, but not all, patients. Thus, available human data suggest but cannot confirm that exercise training may improve myocardial perfusion in some patients with CHD.[30–32]

Reduction of Atherogenic Risk Factors for CHD

Reduction of risk factors for CHD is also discussed in Chapters 4 and 5.

Favorable effects of exercise training on coronary risk factors, documented predominantly in studies involving healthy volunteers,[33] include loss of excess weight and body fat, increase in high-density lipoprotein cholesterol levels, reduction in blood pressure levels, and improvement in glucose–insulin dynamics. These adaptations may prevent, slow the progression of, or reverse coronary atherosclerotic changes. A recent prospective, randomized, controlled trial involving CHD patients documented that comprehensive lifestyle changes, including exercise training, can reduce the severity of angiographically demonstrated coronary atherosclerosis in CHD patients within 1 year.[34]

Reduction of Recurrent CHD Events

Regular physical activity has been postulated to reduce the risk of initial and recurrent CHD events; proposed mechanisms include reductions in severity of coronary atherosclerosis, in vulnerability to ventricular fibrillation, and in the risk of coronary thrombosis.[33,35] Reduction of CHD risk factors, improved cardiovascular efficiency, and increased coronary flow reserve may contribute to these protective effects.[36,37]

No single randomized secondary prevention trial to test the independent effects of exercise training has demonstrated reduction in morbidity and mortality following myocardial infarction, although most demonstrated a favorable trend for a reduced mortality rate in the exercise compared with the control group.[38–41] In the National Exercise and Heart Disease Project,[38] involving 651 postinfarction men, the cumulative 3-year mortality rate was 4.6% for the exercise group compared with 7.3% for the control group, while the rate for recurrent myocardial infarction was 5.3% for the exercise group compared with 7.0% for the control group. However, some trials included a multifaceted risk factor intervention–health education program.[39,40]

Pooling of existing data from published controlled secondary prevention trials that included an exercise training component, so-called meta-analyses,[42–45] revealed that patients randomly assigned to exercise rehabilitation following myocardial infarction had about 25% lower 1- to 3-year rates of fatal cardiovascular events and total mortality than did control subjects; no differences were observed in the rate of nonfatal recurrent myocardial infarction. However, since most trials included comprehensive coronary rehabilitation, it is impossible to "tease out" the independent contribution of exercise to prevention of future CHD events.

Improvement in Psychological Well-Being

The effect of exercise training on psychological well-being is also discussed in Chapter 28.

There is a common perception that exercise improves psychological well-being by reducing muscular tension, mental depression, and anxiety[46,47]; however, this is difficult to document scientifically in either healthy people or patients with CHD. The National Exercise and Heart Disease Project[48] and other well-controlled trials[49] failed to document long-term psychological benefits with exercise training. A multidimensional 12-week coronary rehabilitation program that included stress management and counseling in addition to exercise training resulted in a significant improvement in psychosocial parameters in a group of predominantly well-educated individuals who had good spouse support.[50] On the basis of available data, scientific evidence is inadequate to attribute to exercise an independent role in improving the psychological well-being of most coronary patients.[6]

CATEGORIES OF CORONARY PATIENTS WHO ARE POTENTIAL CANDIDATES FOR REHABILITATIVE EXERCISE TRAINING

Potential candidates for coronary rehabilitative exercise include CHD patients of all ages recovering from myocardial infarction, CABG, or PTCA and patients with stable angina pectoris or silent myocardial ischemia.[3,6] Other possible candidates include selected patients with left ventricular dysfunction and compensated congestive heart failure or patients following cardiac transplantation.

Patients After Myocardial Infarction

The medical treatment of patients after myocardial infarction has changed dramatically over the past 35 years. Historically, the primary focus of coronary rehabilitation exercise training has been the patient recovering from myocardial infarction. Patients with uncomplicated myocardial infarction typically are enrolled in the inpatient phase of coronary rehabilitation shortly after the acute event (see Ch. 19).[51]

Patients After CABG

Programs for patients after CABG differ from those for patients with myocardial infarction in several ways. Compared with patients with myocardial infarction, patients after CABG who have not sustained myocardial infarction typically begin inpatient exercise rehabilitation sooner, progress at a more accelerated rate, and devote more attention to upper extremity range-of-motion exercises.[51]

Supervised outpatient exercise training results in significant improvements in the functional capacity of CABG patients, similar to that reported for myocardial infarction patients.[52–55] In one randomized, controlled study, CABG patients participating in a supervised exercise program improved their functional capacity 15 to 20% more than did patients in the control group after 1 year of training.[54]

Patients After PTCA

Although patients are generally considered potential candidates for exercise training following PTCA, no major study has evaluated the effects of such a program on this subgroup of patients or compared the effects with the results in CABG patients or patients after myocardial infarction. Approximately 234,000 PTCA procedures were performed in 1988 in the United States; this represents a large group of patients with identified significant CHD who might benefit from coronary rehabilitative services, including exercise training.

Many patients who undergo PTCA had angina pectoris,[56] which may have limited their ability to perform physical activity for some time before PTCA; exercise training would be expected to improve their functional capacity. Exercise training as part of a multidimensional coronary rehabilitation program may reduce CHD risk factors and perhaps slow the progression or reduce the severity of underlying atherosclerosis. Finally, exercise rehabilitation might provide an opportunity for early detection of adverse changes in clinical status suggesting restenosis, usually involving 25 to 35% of patients,[56,57] and early institution of remedial measures.

Patients with Angina Pectoris

Angina pectoris usually occurs in response to increased myocardial oxygen demand, at a reproducible RPP in individual patients,[12] but also may be due to reduced coronary blood flow resulting from coronary artery spasm or abnormal vasodilatation. The severity of angina pectoris may be quantitated by rating scales.[58,59] The use of a rating scale helps to document and quantify functional responses to exercise training. The beneficial effect of exercise training in patients with typical angina pectoris allows them to work or exercise at a higher intensity with a reduced myocardial oxygen cost before reaching the threshold for onset of myocardial ischemia and associated angina pectoris.

Patients with Left Ventricular Dysfunction and Congestive Heart Failure

Exercise training for patients with left ventricular dysfunction and congestive heart failure is discussed in Chapter 21.

Patients with left ventricular dysfunction and compensated congestive heart failure usually become dyspneic or fatigued after even moderate amounts of physical activity, owing to the inability of the heart and peripheral circulation to meet the metabolic needs of the body.[60,61] The major hemodynamic adaptation as a result of exercise training in these patients is an increase in oxygen extraction by exercising muscle with little or no measurable improvement in central coronary function.

Rehabilitative exercise training has improved mean treadmill exercise time[62] and peak oxygen consumption[63] and has significantly reduced the heart rate and RPP at standardized submaximal work loads.[63] Since patients with congestive heart failure have a relatively poor tolerance to physical activity, several modifications must be made in the standard exercise prescription. The usual intensity of exercise must be reduced, and this can be compensated for by increasing the duration of exercise sessions. In addition, the duration of the supervised exercise training program may have to be increased significantly.[5] Appropriately designed exercise programs appear safe and effective in improving exercise tolerance[64,65] in many patients with ventricular dysfunction and compensated heart failure.

Patients After Heart Transplantation

Exercise training after heart transplantation is discussed in Chapter 23.

More than 1,000 cardiac transplantation procedures were performed in 1987,[66] with most common indications being end-stage congestive heart failure (43%) and cardiomyopathy (49%).[5]

Patients with Implanted Pacemakers

Exercise training for patients with implanted pacemakers is discussed in Chapter 24.

PREEXERCISE TRAINING EVALUATION

Preexercise training evaluation is also discussed in Chapters 7 and 8.

The clinical evaluation and exercise testing[67,69] of coronary patients for participation in a rehabilitative exercise program identifies their eligibility, relative risk status, functional capacity in terms of hemodynamic or electrophysiologic (ECG) responses, and perception and tolerance to standardized multilevel exercise tests of known intensities. Measurement of heart rate, blood pressure, $\dot{V}o_2max$,[70] rating of perceived exertion (RPE), ECG, and clinical responses provide the basis upon which an individualized exercise prescription for rehabilitative exercise training is developed. The most common type of exercise prescription for coronary patients utilizes the heart rate to define the lower and upper limits of exercise training intensity (training heart rate zone). Thus, heart rate at rest, during submaximal exercise, and at peak exercise are useful for developing the exercise prescription and for determining appropriate work loads for the exercise prescription. Direct measurement of $\dot{V}o_2$ provides more accurate data than does estimated functional capacity from the duration of the exercise test for the exercise prescription and for counseling the patient regarding appropriate and safe self-care, occupational, and recreational activities; however, $\dot{V}o_2$ measurement is more burdensome to staff and patients and more costly and is not routinely used in clinical practice. RPE using one of two Borg scales[71,72] during exercise testing provides additional information. Assigning an appropriate RPE level provides a means

of fine-tuning the exercise prescription so that the patient exercises at a reasonable and comfortable intensity. RPE also can be useful during exercise training for modifying the exercise prescription because of changes in the clinical status and exercise tolerance of the patient, e.g., the initiation or discontinuation of beta-blocking drug therapy.

If the patient develops significant ischemic ECG changes (≥ 1 mm of ST segment depression) during exercise testing, this information should define training heart rate limits so that the patient exercises below the myocardial ischemic threshold. Likewise, a patient who demonstrates a significant cardiac rhythm disturbance during exercise testing should have the prescribed exercise intensity lowered to a heart rate range at which no cardiac arrhythmias occurred.

Risk Stratification Based on Exercise Test Data

Risk stratification is also discussed in Chapters 7 to 11, 14, and 15.

In patients recovering from myocardial infarction, exercise test findings have prognostic implications related to the risk of future coronary events. Risk stratification has been based on the following characteristics[73–76]: clinical course, myocardial ischemia (at rest or induced), functional capacity, left ventricular ejection fraction, ventricular arrhythmias, and failure of the systolic blood pressure to rise or a fall in systolic blood pressure during exercise. The American Association of Cardiovascular and Pulmonary Rehabilitation (AACVPR) guidelines, based on risk stratification, help determine the type and duration of exercise supervision and the frequency of ECG monitoring needed for patients participating in coronary exercise rehabilitation (Table 20-2).[77]

In general, patients who have at least 1 mm of ischemic ST segment depression, or cannot achieve a peak work load of 4 METs, or cannot increase their systolic blood pressure at least 30 mmHg (or at least to 110 mmHg) during the exercise test are at excess risk for coronary mortality within the first year after myocardial infarction.[73–76] Patients with exercise-induced ischemic ST segment depression within 10 to 21 days

Table 20-2. Guidelines for Risk Stratification for Patients in Coronary Rehabilitative Exercise Programs

Risk Level	Patient Characteristics
Low	Uncomplicated clinical course in hospital
	No evidence of myocardial ischemia
	Functional capacity ≥7 METs
	Normal left ventricular function (EF ≥ 50%)
	Absence of significant ventricular ectopy
Intermediate	ST segment depression ≥2 mm flat or downsloping
	Reversible thallium defects
	Moderate to good left ventricular function (ejection fraction 35–49%)
	Changing patterns of or new development of angina pectoris
High	Prior myocardial infarction or infarct involving ≥35% of the left ventricle
	EF <35% at rest
	Fall in exercise systolic blood pressure or failure of systolic blood pressure to rise ≥10 mmHg on exercise test
	Persistent or recurrent ischemic pain 24 hours or more after hospital admission
	Functional capacity <5 METs with hypotensive blood pressure response or 1-mm ST segment depression
	Congestive heart failure syndrome in hospital
	≥2-mm ST segment depression at peak heart rate ≤135 beats/min
	High-grade ventricular ectopy

(From American Association of Cardiovascular and Pulmonary Rehabilitation,[77] with permission.)

after myocardial infarction have a 3- to 20-fold greater risk of subsequent coronary events than do patients without this finding. Patients unable to achieve a peak work load of 4 METs during exercise testing by 3 weeks after infarction are at significantly higher risk for subsequent recurrent myocardial infarction, coronary death, cardiac arrest, or CABG at a 2-year follow-up than are patients with at least 4 METs functional capacity. Inadequate systolic blood pressure responses at exercise testing after myocardial infarction also identify patients at increased risk for future coronary events, probably reflecting left ventricular dysfunction or myocardial ischemia.[75,76] The abnormal blood pressure response may be a more sensitive predictor of mortality at 1 year than the maximal work load achieved or the presence of angina pectoris, ischemic ST segment changes, or ventricular arrhythmias.[75,76]

Such prognostic data are useful for categorizing patients after myocardial infarction into high-, intermediate-, and low-risk groups. High-risk patients require more intensive medical management, including additional diagnostic and interventional procedures, whereas the low-risk patients often do not require such procedures and can promptly initiate rehabilitative exercise training and resumption of sexual and other physical activities.

Medical Conditions Requiring Stabilization Before Exercise Training

Certain medical conditions are relative or absolute contraindications to exercise training and should be controlled or stabilized before initiation of an outpatient rehabilitative exercise program. Examples include unstable angina pectoris, complex cardiac arrhythmias, uncompensated congestive heart failure, and uncontrolled hypertension or metabolic diseases, such as diabetes mellitus.[3,67,77]

Chronic angina pectoris does not exclude a patient from participating in an exercise training program, but the anginal symptoms should be stable and predictable; it should be possible to identify and maintain a level of exercise and RPP below the threshold which precipitates angina pectoris. If new angina occurs or the pattern of the symptoms changes, exercise training should be discontinued until these symptoms are medically controlled and/or further diagnostic procedures are performed.

Patients with uncompensated congestive heart failure should not participate in a rehabilitative exercise program. Signs and symptoms of uncompensated congestive heart failure include lung rales, a third heart sound, distended neck veins, peripheral edema, dyspnea, an unexplained excessive weight gain (e.g., 3 to 4 lb or more in 1 week), easy fatigability, and/or decreased urinary output. Once congestive heart failure has been medically stabilized, exercise training can be initiated or resumed in selected patients.

Patients with high-grade ventricular arrhythmias at rest or at low levels of exercise should delay or discontinue exercise training until these arrhythmias are adequately controlled. High-grade arrhythmias include frequent ventricular ectopic beats and multiform or serial ventricular ectopic beats.

Poorly controlled hypertension or excessive hypertensive response to exercise are other contraindications to exercise testing and training. Uncontrolled metabolic diseases require stabilization prior to participation in exercise training. Although patients with mild to moderately severe diabetes may benefit from exercise training, metabolic control of severe diabetes (fasting plasma glucose level exceeding 250 to 300 mg/dL and usually associated with ketoacidosis) may be aggravated by exercise. Diabetic patients receiving insulin therapy often must reduce their insulin dosage or increase their food intake when starting exercise training, to avoid hypoglycemia.[78]

Relative and absolute contraindications for exercise are summarized in Table 20-3.

Table 20-3. Contraindications for Exercise for Coronary Patients

Absolute contraindications	**Relative contraindications** (*continued*)
Unstable angina pectoris	Pericarditis associated with CABG
Recent acute myocardial infarction and unstable condition	Resting ST segment depression of >2 mm
	Poorly controlled diabetes mellitus
Uncontrolled hypertension with resting systolic blood pressure of >200 mmHg or diastolic blood pressure of >110 mmHg	Neuromuscular, musculoskeletal, or arthritic disorders that would prevent activity
	Excessive incisional drainage after CABG
Inappropriate asymptomatic postural or exertional blood pressure response	Sinus tachycardia (>120 beats/min) at rest
Serious atrial or ventricular arrhythmias	New ECG changes after CABG or acute myocardial infarction that are diagnostic or suggestive of new infarction
Second- or third-degree heart block	
Recent embolism (systemic or pulmonary)	Ventricular aneurysm
Acute or chronic thrombophlebitis	Symptomatic anemia (hematocrit of <30%)
Dissecting aneurysm	**Conditions requiring special consideration and/or precautions**
Fever of >100°F	
Excessive sternal movement after CABG (contraindication for upper-extremity and trunk ROM exercises)	Conduction disturbances
	Left bundle branch block
	Wolff-Parkinson-White syndrome
Uncompensated heart failure	Lown-Ganong-Levine syndrome
Active pericarditis or myocarditis	Bifascicular block
Severe aortic stenosis (>50 mmHg gradient) and idiopathic hypertrophic subaortic stenosis	Controlled arrhythmias
	Fixed rate pacemaker
Acute systemic illness	Mitral valve prolapse
Relative contraindications	Angina pectoris or other manifestations of coronary insufficiency
Resting diastolic blood pressure of >100 mmHg or resting systolic blood pressure of >180 mmHg	Electrolyte disturbances
	Cyanotic heart disease
Inappropriate increase in blood pressure during exercise	Marked obesity (>50% above standard weight for height)
Hypotension	Renal, hepatic, and other metabolic insufficiency
Moderate aortic stenosis (25–50 mmHg gradient)	Moderate to severe pulmonary disease
Compensated heart failure	Intermittent claudication
Significant emotional stress or psychological disorder	

(Adapted from Pollock and Wilmore,[51] with permission.)

EXERCISE GUIDELINES AND PRESCRIPTION

Overview

An exercise prescription has been defined[67] as the process for recommending a regimen of physical activity in a systematic and individualized manner to help the patient achieve optimal physiologic benefit from exercise training, enhance physical fitness, promote health by reducing risk for future development or recurrence of disease, and ensure safety during exercise participation. The specific aims for participation in exercise training vary with the individual participant's interests (return to work, recreation, etc.), needs, background, and health status and will influence the exercise prescription. The exercise prescription includes the mode, intensity, duration, frequency, and rate of progression of exercise(s) to be used in the training program.

Guidelines for Rehabilitative Exercise Programs

Convalescent/Therapeutic Exercise

Outpatient exercise rehabilitation usually begins shortly after the patient is discharged from the hospital after myocardial infarction, PTCA, or CABG[79]; however, patients who have not been hospitalized but who require exercise supervision also are sometimes referred to exercise training programs. Although the traditional length of this phase of exercise rehabilitation is usually 8 to 12 weeks, some patients may require 6 to 12 months to achieve optimal functional improvement.[6]

These programs are generally conducted in a hospital outpatient facility and less commonly in a community center or university gymnasium in which ECG monitoring, emergency personnel and cardiac care support, and physician supervision are available.

There is a general expectation that coronary patients will increase their $\dot{V}o_2max$ level 10 to 56% with exercise training[6,12,13]; this percentage will vary with the patient's age and clinical status, the specific exercise prescription utilized, and patient compliance with the exercise training program. Supervised exercise programs appear particularly useful for higher-risk patients, for those who perform heavy physical labor in their job and/or vigorous recreational pursuits, and for those who need reinforcement for health behavioral changes and risk factor modification.[1,6,7,80]

ECG monitoring, traditionally used to detect potentially serious rhythm and ischemic ST segment changes and to ensure compliance with heart rate limitations, has recently come under close scrutiny.[3,80,81] In a 1986 survey,[82] no significant differences were observed in rates of cardiac arrest, recurrent myocardial infarction, or fatalities during exercise in programs with continuous ECG monitoring compared with those with either intermittent monitoring alone or initial continuous monitoring for at least three sessions followed by intermittent monitoring. Because continuous ECG monitoring entails substantial cost and personnel requirements, American College of Cardiology guidelines[2,3] and those of the AACVPR[77] indicate a need for ECG monitoring only for moderate- and high-risk coronary patients. Such patients exhibit either significantly depressed left ventricular function, resting or exercise-induced complex ventricular arrhythmias, or decreased systolic blood pressure levels during exercise; are survivors of sudden death or complications following myocardial infarction; or are unable to self-monitor their exercise heart rates. Additional research is required to define the need for and optimal duration of ECG monitoring for intermediate- and high-risk patients. In the interim, it appears prudent to provide variable durations of ECG monitoring based on the patient's clinical status, functional capacity, and prognosis following risk stratification.[6]

A related issue is the feasibility, efficacy, and safety of structured prescriptive unsupervised group or home exercise programs. Home exercise programs, with and without intermittent transtelephonic ECG monitoring, have been shown to be safe and feasible for selected low-risk coronary patients.[83] Although improvement in functional capacity in low-risk patients after myocardial infarction and CABG who undertake home exercise is equivalent to that of patients who exercise in a supervised coronary rehabilitation program,[83–86] issues other than physiologic improvement must be considered when comparing supervised group programs with home exercise.[87] Supervised group programs offer advantages over home exercise for teaching coronary patients about risk reduction, promoting compliance with the overall medical program, and permitting verification of the patient's ability to implement the exercise program safely and effectively. Also, group programs provide psychosocial support, promote an opportunity for better understanding of the coronary disease and its management, and provide an atmosphere that reduces anxiety and depression.[6,67] In addition, group programs provide social reinforcement through camaraderie and companionship that may enhance adherence to the rehabilitation program. Even with home exercise, contact with a nurse or allied health professional can improve patient compliance.[88]

A symptom-limited exercise test usually is performed between weeks 3 and 6 of a therapeutic program. The results of this evaluation are used to adjust the patient's exercise prescription, to evaluate the need for continued ECG monitoring during exercise, and to assess the adequacy of the patient's physical capacity to return to work. An exercise capacity of 5 METs or more, without abnormal cardiac symptoms or signs, is generally considered sufficient to allow most coronary patients to return to light to moderate physical activities.[67] It is further recommended that patients who are asymptomatic and without exercise test abnormalities at a 9-MET level do not require supervised exercise rehabilitation with ECG monitoring.[6,80,89] Significant abnormalities in the exercise test indicate the need for further medical evaluation and treatment and continued medical supervision and ECG monitoring during exercise training.

Table 20-4 suggests criteria for successful completion of a supervised exercise program and graduation to a maintenance phase.

Maintenance Exercise

Maintenance exercise programs typically are based in a community recreational facility such as a YMCA or a university gymnasium. Guide-

Table 20-4. Suggested Criteria for Successful Completion of a Convalescent Therapeutic Outpatient Coronary Rehabilitation Program

Parameter	Level Desired
Functional capacity	≥5 METs
Medical status	Normal hemodynamic response to exercise (appropriate increase in blood pressure; normal or unchanged ECG at peak exercise; absent or stable arrhythmias: medically acceptable or stable ischemic response)
	Absent or stable angina pectoris
	Stable and/or controlled resting heart rate and blood pressure (<90 beats/min and <140/90 mmHg, respectively)
Physical fitness	Adequate level of comprehensive physical fitness to meet the demands for daily activities and occupational tasks
Education	Satisfactory understanding of: Basic pathophysiology of specific cardiovascular disease
	Rationale for the intervention plan
	Lifestyle characteristics associated with low risk of CHD
	Reasons for any prescribed cardiovascular medications and possible side effects
	Range of safe activities permitted including sexual activity and vocational and recreational pursuits
	Individualized exercise prescription guidelines and demonstrated ability to exercise within the limits prescribed
	Signs and symptoms of exertional intolerance

(Adapted from American College of Sports Medicine: Guidelines for Exercise Testing and Prescription,[67] with permission.)

lines for maintenance rehabilitation exercise programs have been published by the American College of Sports Medicine (ACSM)[67] and the AACVPR,[77] among others. These community-based exercise programs ideally accept low-risk coronary patients who have left the hospital following a coronary event 6 to 12 weeks earlier and who have clinically stable or decreasing angina pectoris, absent or medically controlled arrhythmias during exercise, a knowledge of coronary symptoms, and the ability to self-regulate their exercise intensity. At times, low-risk coronary patients with good functional capacity are directly referred to a maintenance program without prior exercise supervision.[6] It is common to require a minimal functional capacity of 5 METs for participation in a maintenance program. Patients typically participate in such programs for 4 to 6 months, during which time efforts are made to gradually reduce supervision and promote self-regulation of a lifelong physical activity program. Exercise testing and medical evaluation are repeated at 3- to 6-month intervals and eventually on an annual basis or as medically necessary.

Lifelong (Unsupervised) Exercise

Lifelong unsupervised exercise has the primary goal of maintenance of existing fitness levels. Patients participating in these programs should have at least a 5-MET capacity.[67] This phase of exercise rehabilitation is commonly conducted at home or at a community facility that offers a variety of exercise modalities.

Basic Components of the Exercise Prescription

The exercise prescription is the cornerstone of rehabilitative exercise training. It provides form and guidelines for exercise recommendations. The exercise prescription used for outpatient coronary rehabilitation should be individualized on the basis of the results of an exercise test. Individualization allows for adjustments for interpatient variation in physiologic responses such as resting and peak heart rates, chronotropic effects of the exercise stimulus, resting and exercise blood pressure levels, and symptoms. The exercise prescription also may have to be modified according to the individual's responses to scheduled reevaluation exercise tests, adaptations to exercise training, and changes in clinical condition during exercise training.

The components of the exercise prescription for coronary patients have been described in detail elsewhere[51,67,79,90]; this section summarizes the major principles involved. In applying these principles of exercise prescription to the coronary patient, the wide variety of patients with CHD who can benefit from exercise training must be considered. These patients vary greatly in their severity of CHD, degree of ventricular dysfunction, and symptoms at rest or during exercise. In addition, patients recovering from CABG, myocardial infarction, PTCA, permanent pacemaker insertion, or other coronary surgical procedures each require special considerations during exercise training, as described above.

Warm-Up and Cool-Down Phases

Each exercise training session should have three phases: a warm-up phase, an aerobic phase, and a cool-down phase. The warm-up session typically lasts 10 to 15 minutes. Activities appropriate for the warm-up phase include low-level calisthenics and stretching to limber up the musculoskeletal system, and low-level dynamic, cardiorespiratory activity. The most logical cardiorespiratory warm-up involves performing the prescribed mode of exercise at a lower intensity. Achieving a heart rate during the warm-up phase within 20 beats/min of the target heart rate prescribed in the exercise prescription is recommended.[90] Warm-up prior to the training session reduces the risk of exercise-related cardiovascular complications and musculoskeletal injuries during exercise training. Sudden abrupt strenuous exertion without a warm-up may produce ischemic ST segment changes and arrhythmias,[91,92] as well as a decrease in left ventricular ejection fraction,[93] even in healthy people. Warm-up exercise reduces such cardiovascular abnormalities in response to strenuous exercise.

The cool-down phase should last 5 to 10 minutes and usually includes slow walking and other low-intensity dynamic exercise. During the cool-down phase, the continued low-level dynamic activity permits the appropriate return of pooled venous blood to the heart and a gradual decrease in the heart rate, cardiac output, systolic blood pressure, and myocardial oxygen requirements.

Aerobic (Endurance) Phase

The aerobic phase follows the warm-up phase. Prescription for this phase includes recommendations for the intensity of exercise, its duration, frequency, and mode of exercise. Guidelines for each of these components are discussed below.

Methods for Prescribing Intensity of Exercise. To achieve improvement in aerobic power during formal exercise training, the intensity of endurance exercise should be maintained between 40 and 85% of functional capacity (see Chs. 7 and 8), for 15 to 60 minutes. However, humidity, ambient temperature, anxiety, and fatigue may disturb the relationship between heart rate and body oxygen uptake; on the other hand, since exercise heart rate correlates well with myocardial oxygen uptake (see Chs. 7 and 8), the intensity of exercise should be decreased when such conditions are present.

Heart Rate.   There are three acceptable methods used to calculate an appropriate heart rate for exercise training. The first, frequently used in coronary rehabilitation programs, is the *heart rate reserve* or *Karvonen method*.[94] This involves calculating the difference between the maximal and resting heart rates (defined as the heart rate reserve), multiplying the difference by a percentage between 60 and 80% (equivalent to 60 to 80% of functional capacity), depending on the desired intensity level, and then adding this to the resting heart rate. A prerequisite for using this method is accurate measurement of resting and maximal heart rate during an exercise test. The Karvonen method results in higher training heart rates than subsequent methods described below.

A second method used to determine the training heart rate (THR) for exercise training is simply to multiply a fixed percentage (70 to 85%) by the maximal heart rate achieved during an exercise test. This fixed percentage range is equivalent to 60 to 85% of functional capacity.

A third exercise prescription method involving heart rate requires plotting the relationship between exertional heart rate and $\dot{V}O_2$, expressed either in METs or in milliliters of oxygen uptake adjusted for body weight.[95] Using this method, the THR is equal to the heart rate which occurred at a given level of $\dot{V}O_2$ during exercise testing. The specific THR is selected from heart rates corresponding to 40 and 85% of $\dot{V}O_2$, depending on the desired initial exercise intensity. This method requires an accurate measurement of ex-

ercise heart rate and direct measurement of $\dot{V}O_2$ during exercise and is therefore used infrequently in clinical practice.

The principles of prescribing exercise intensity for coronary patients are applied below to two case studies. Methods of calculating heart rates are shown in Figure 20-1.

CASE 1 was a 54-year-old woman who underwent CABG and was given a symptom-limited exercise test 15 days after surgery. Her resting heart rate and blood pressure were 97 beats/min and 136/82 mmHg, respectively. The symptom-limited exercise test duration was 8.0 minutes using a modified Bruce protocol, beginning at 1.7 mph and 0% grade. Peak exercise values were as follows: heart rate, 137 beats/min; blood pressure, 190/94 mmHg; estimated METs, 6; RPE, 17; and RPP product, 20,030. The patient stopped exercising because of dyspnea and fatigue. Asymptomatic ST segment depression of 1 to 2 mm was noted on the exercise ECG at a heart rate of about 130 beats/min.

CASE 2 was a 59-year-old man who was given a symptom-limited exercise test 16 days following acute myocardial infarction in preparation for entering an outpatient exercise program. The resting heart rate was 70 beats/min, and the blood pressure was 126/74 mmHg. The exercise test duration was 11.0 minutes using a modified Bruce protocol. The patient achieved the following peak values: heart rate, 138 beats/min; blood pressure, 142/70 mmHg; estimated METs, 9; RPE, 17; and RPP, 27,832. The endpoint for the test was patient fatigue; no significant ST-T changes or rhythm abnormalities were noted on the ECG.

Note that the peak heart rate multiplied by a fixed percentage always results in a lower THR range than does the Karvonen method. Therefore, the former method is a more conservative approach, but may result in a diminished training effect than that for the Karvonen or the heart rate-$\dot{V}O_2$ plot methods.

Anaerobic Threshold.   The concept of anaerobic threshold (AT) also is relevant to the prescription of exercise intensity. AT is defined as the level of $\dot{V}O_2$ during exercise above which aerobic energy production is supplemented by anaerobic mechanisms, and it is reflected by an increase in

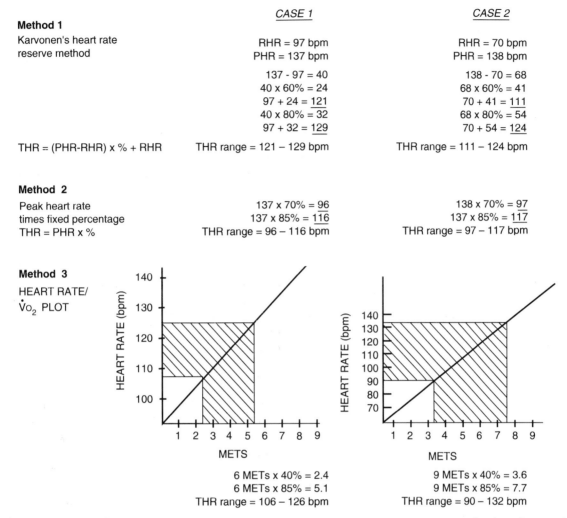

Method 1

Karvonen's heart rate
reserve method

CASE 1

RHR = 97 bpm
PHR = 137 bpm

137 - 97 = 40
40 x 60% = 24
97 + 24 = 121
40 x 80% = 32
97 + 32 = 129

CASE 2

RHR = 70 bpm
PHR = 138 bpm

138 - 70 = 68
68 x 60% = 41
70 + 41 = 111
68 x 80% = 54
70 + 54 = 124

THR = (PHR-RHR) x % + RHR

THR range = 121 – 129 bpm

THR range = 111 – 124 bpm

Method 2

Peak heart rate
times fixed percentage
THR = PHR x %

137 x 70% = 96
137 x 85% = 116
THR range = 96 – 116 bpm

138 x 70% = 97
137 x 85% = 117
THR range = 97 – 117 bpm

Method 3

HEART RATE/
$\dot{V}O_2$ PLOT

6 METs x 40% = 2.4
6 METs x 85% = 5.1
THR range = 106 – 126 bpm

9 METs x 40% = 3.6
9 METs x 85% = 7.7
THR range = 90 – 132 bpm

Fig. 20.1. Calculating the appropriate heart rates for exercise training in cases 1 and 2 (cited in text) using three methods. Abbreviations: THR, training heart rate; PHR, peak heart rate; RHR, resting heart rate.

lactate levels in muscle and arterial blood.[96] In the past, anaerobic threshold was determined by direct measurement of arterial or arterialized capillary blood lactate values during and immediately following exercise. There has been a recent trend toward estimating AT noninvasively by respiratory gas measurements during exercise. This procedure determines the anaerobic threshold by identifying the $\dot{V}O_2$ level just below the point of a nonlinear increase in ventilation, carbon dioxide production, and respiratory quotient during exercise.[96] By plotting the $\dot{V}O_2$ level at which the anaerobic threshold occurred against the heart rate response to exercise, the heart rate at the AT can be determined. The optimal training intensity should be slightly below the heart rate corresponding to the AT, which ensures that the exercise is aerobic. The AT in coronary patients typically occurs at about 60% of maximal oxygen uptake, or 60 to 70% of maximal heart rate (Fig. 20-2).

Rating of Perceived Exertion. RPE during exercise can also be used to judge exercise intensity. The concept of systematically describing perceived effort during exercise was introduced by Borg[71,72]

Table 20-5.   Comparison of the Borg RPE Scales[85,86]

15-Point Scale		10-Point Scale	
6			
7	Very, very light	0.5	Very, very weak
8			
9	Very light	1	Very weak
10			
11	Fairly light	2	Weak
12		3	Moderate
13	Somewhat hard	4	Somewhat strong
14		5	Strong
15	Hard	6	
16		7	Very strong
17	Very hard	8	
18		9	
19	Very, very hard	10	Very, very strong
20	Maximal[a]		Maximal[a]

[a] Maximal effort or exhaustion.

with his introduction of RPE scales. These scales consist of either 15 successive numeric values beginning with 6 and ending with 20 (the original scale) or a more recent scale ranging from 0 to 10 (Table 20-5). Descriptive phrases help the individual choose the number that best describes the effort during physical exertion.

The current ACSM guidelines[67] recommend that coronary patients exercise within an RPE range of 12 to 16 ("somewhat hard" to "hard") on the original Borg scale (which corresponds to 3 to 7 on the modified Borg scale). This should approximate 60 to 85% of the maximal heart rate and is consistent with intensity levels prescribed by heart rate. Interestingly, an aerobic training effect typically occurs at an average RPE of 13.5 in coronary patients, which falls in the middle of the recommended 12 to 16 range.

Metabolic Requirements. Another approach to determining exercise intensity for prescriptive purposes is based on the metabolic requirements over resting levels during exercise (METs). The metabolic cost of most types of exercise has been defined in terms of the $\dot{V}O_2$ required to sustain the activity. These metabolic costs are commonly

expressed as multiples of resting metabolic requirements or METs, with 1 MET equaling about 3.5 ml of O_2/kg/min. The appropriate range for the exercise prescription, expressed in METs, is usually between 40 and 85% of an individual's maximal functional capacity.

Using the exercise test data for cases 1 and 2 cited above, the following training intensities would result using the metabolic requirements method. The peak METs achieved in case 1 were 6. Multiplying 6 by 40% and 85% results in a training intensity range of 2.4 to 5.1 METs. The patient in case 2 achieved a peak MET value of 9, and the 40 to 85% training intensity range would therefore be 3.6 to 7.7 METs.

The primary limitation of this method of prescribing exercise intensity is the variability in the energy cost of given physical activities because of ambient environmental conditions such as temperature, wind, humidity, and geographic difference. Again, the RPE or heart rate response can be used as an indicator of exertional intensity for maintaining a prescribed exercise intensity under changing environmental circumstances.

Duration of Exercise.   The generally recommended duration of the dynamic exercise phase of training sessions for coronary patients in an outpatient setting is 20 to 60 minutes.[52,67] A minimum of 20 minutes at the usually prescribed exercise intensity of 50 to 85% of $\dot{V}O_2$max is necessary to either improve or maintain functional capacity. Since there is an inverse relationship between exercise intensity and duration, the lower the intensity of the exercise session, the longer the required exercise duration and vice versa.

The exercise training session may include either continuous or intermittent aerobic physical activity, the choice of which also affects the required overall duration of the session. Continuous activity implies that the patient exercises continuously during the endurance phase of the exercise session at the THR or within the THR range. The advantage of a continuous exercise format is a more rapid improvement in cardiorespiratory endurance than with intermittent exercise. Intermittent exercise consists of alternat-

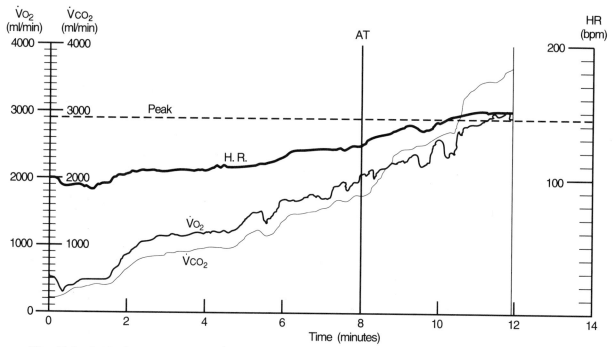

Fig. 20-2. A 106 kg patient with a $\dot{V}O_2$max of 28 ml/kg/min and a maximal heart rate of 151 beats/min was found to have an anaerobic threshold (AT) at 18 ml/kg/min. His heart rate at the anaerobic threshold was 100 beats/min. An optimal training intensity for staying below the anaerobic threshold would be about 16 ml/kg/min, corresponding to a maximal training heart rate of 85 beats/min. Abbreviations: AT, anaerobic threshold; HR, heart rate; bpm, beats per minute; $\dot{V}O_2$, oxygen uptake; $\dot{V}CO_2$, carbon dioxide production.

ing periods of exercise and rest, systematically spaced throughout the exercise session. The total exercise time in an intermittent session should at least equal the exercise time prescribed for a continuous format. A work-to-rest ratio of approximately 1:1 with exercise and rest periods each longer than 2 minutes for each cycle are recommended for aerobic training with coronary patients.[67]

There are several advantages of intermittent training for coronary patients.[97] First, the intermittent format allows a patient to achieve a higher exercise intensity and a greater total work load during exercise sessions with less fatigue, since the rest periods minimize the accumulation of lactic acid as compared with continuous exercise, in which only a single mode of exercise per session is used. In addition, intermittent exercise provides a greater number of training stimuli to the heart during each session than does contin-

uous exercise because of repeated increases in stroke volume, venous return, and intracardiac pressures.

Frequency of Exercise. The usual frequency of exercise for coronary patients is three to five sessions per week[51,67] varying with the intensity and duration of the exercise. If the duration of exercise is low (less than 20 minutes per session) or the intensity of exercise is low (less than 60% of maximal heart rate or heart rate reserve), the frequency of exercise sessions should be at the higher end of the guideline range.

Among 254 coronary patients who participated in three 60-minute exercise training sessions per week, those who averaged 2.2 to 3.0 sessions or more per week showed significantly greater mean improvement in aerobic power than did patients who averaged two sessions or less per week. In addition, patients who averaged 3.5 to

5.0 sessions per week demonstrated no greater improvement in aerobic capacity than those who averaged 2.2 to 3.0 sessions per week.[97] These data suggest that three sessions per week is an ideal frequency for usual outpatient coronary rehabilitation exercise programs.

Types of Exercise.   Two major types of exercise can be used in an exercise training program: dynamic (isotonic) exercise and static, resistive, or isometric exercise. More details on the latter type of training are given later in this chapter.

Isotonic or dynamic exercise involves alternate contraction and relaxation of large muscle groups of the lower or upper extremities and torso, which causes body movement. This type of training results in an increase or maintenance of the cardiorespiratory endurance or aerobic component of functional capacity, $\dot{V}o_2max$. Examples of dynamic exercise include walking, jogging, swimming, cycling, minitrampoline rebounding, rope skipping, cross-country skiing, and aerobic dancing.

The training effects of several types of aerobic exercise, i.e., running, walking, and cycling, were compared in healthy, middle-aged, sedentary men[98]; all three modes of exercise training were equally effective in increasing $\dot{V}o_2max$ levels. Special concerns about usual modes of dynamic exercise in coronary rehabilitation programs are discussed below.

Walking.   Barring significant orthopedic problems or physical handicaps involving the lower extremities, walking and jogging are the most natural, accessible, and easiest forms of exercise to regulate for improving cardiorespiratory fitness. Advantages of a walking program over more vigorous forms of endurance exercise include the following: (1) it involves tolerable exercise intensities even for deconditioned patients; (2) there is a lower risk of significant musculoskeletal and orthopedic problems; (3) it can be done both outdoors in pleasant weather and indoors during cold or inclement weather; and (4) it requires no special equipment other than a good pair of walking shoes. Walking on level ground accommodates a wide range of functional capacities (3 to 8 METs at 3.0 to 5.5 mph) and therefore is appropriate for most coronary patients exercising in outpatient programs at a variety of prescribed intensities.[99] Walking uphill or climbing stairs can significantly increase the exercise intensity and metabolic requirements.

Jogging.   Jogging is not recommended in the initial stages of outpatient rehabilitation for coronary patients since the metabolic requirements are too high, typically ranging between 8 and 16 METs.[51,67] The main advantage of jogging over walking is that the intensity of exercise is higher, thereby reducing the duration of exercise required to increase $\dot{V}o_2max$ levels. Jogging, like walking, can be performed either outdoors or indoors and is a relatively inexpensive form of exercise except for the necessity of a well-made pair of running shoes. However, it is associated with a higher risk of orthopedic injuries and cardiac problems than walking, particularly in older individuals.

Swimming.   Swimming is an excellent dynamic exercise. The advantage over walking and jogging is that swimming incorporates both upper- and lower-extremity muscular activity. Other advantages of swimming include the following: (1) the patient is in a low-gravity situation, which facilitates venous return; (2) the risk of musculoskeletal injuries is low; and (3) swimming can be used to train coronary patients who have concomitant arthritis, orthopedic limitations, or intermittent claudication. The major problem with prescribing swimming for coronary patients is the wide variation in skill levels and the resultant variability in energy costs between patients, which results in a wide range of exercise heart rates for standardized swimming activities. Even swimming relatively slowly can result in near-maximal $\dot{V}o_2$ and heart rate levels in some myocardial infarction patients.[100,101] The MET requirements for swimming range from 4 to greater than 8 METs. Water activities other than swimming, such as walking or jogging in the water and aqua-aerobics, are good alternative modes of exercise for coronary patients and provide the advantages of water activity with an opportunity to regulate training intensity more easily.

Cycling.   Cycling can be performed either on a bicycle outdoors or on a stationary cycle ergometer indoors. The energy requirements for outdoor bicycling at a typical recreational pace and conditions range from 3 to 8 METs. The use of calibrated cycle ergometers is recommended for coronary patients rather than the less expensive, uncalibrated ergometers, because of the greater accuracy, which allows regulation of exercise intensity and greater reproducibility of exercise intensity from session to session. To enhance patient comfort and performance on either a bicycle or a cycle ergometer, the seat height should be adjusted to a point that results in a slight bend in the knee when the pedal is at its lowest position.

Minitrampoline Rebounding.   Rebounding involves the use of minitrampolines with patients running in place, bouncing, or performing selected calisthenics. Usual mean heart rates and $\dot{V}O_2$ during rebound running in sedentary young to middle-aged subjects were reported as 116 beats/min and 17 ml/kg/min, respectively.[102] These values are equivalent to walking at approximately 4 mph. Our group[103] found that a mean of 76 to 80% of the $\dot{V}O_2max$ level obtained on a treadmill exercise test could be obtained during minitrampoline rebounding. Rebounding is a good activity for coronary patients with low fitness levels and patients with selected musculoskeletal conditions, since it minimizes the shock transmitted to lower-extremity joints compared with walking or jogging on hard surfaces. However, a much smaller increment in $\dot{V}O_2max$ is reported with minitrampoline training in deconditioned individuals than with other modes of exercise training, i.e., generally less than a 10% increase in $\dot{V}O_2max$.[104] Another relevant problem in prescribing this exercise is shared with rope skipping and is discussed below.

Rope Skipping.   Rope skipping is a relatively inexpensive aerobic activity, easily accessible to most individuals, but one that requires physical skill and coordination. Another disadvantage of rope skipping for coronary patients is its high energy cost, which ranges from 9 to 12 METs.[67]

An additional potential problem[105] related to prescribing rope-skipping exercise for coronary patients is that it is difficult to significantly increase the metabolic costs and heart rate response during rope skipping by increasing the skipping rate; i.e., $\dot{V}O_2$, heart rate, and energy expenditure levels were essentially the same at skipping rates of 125, 135, and 145/min. Similar observations[103] were made during bouncing on the minitrampoline; in fact, there was an inverse relationship between the bouncing rate and RPE. These findings reduce the usefulness of rope skipping and minitrampoline bouncing in exercise rehabilitation programs. Additionally, if rope skipping is the desired mode of activity for the highly fit coronary patient, an interval exercise training format is recommended, with each exercise phase of less than 5 minutes duration, because of the high intensity of rope skipping.

Cross-Country Skiing.   Cross-country skiing is an excellent low-impact aerobic activity that incorporates both lower- and upper-extremity activity. It is a popular mode of exercise training in coronary rehabilitation programs in Scandinavian countries, where cross-country skiing is commonly used for exercise and as a mode of transportation. Disadvantages include the necessity for snow, accessibility to skiing areas, and the required development of skiing skills and techniques. Another potential disadvantage for coronary patients is the high energy requirement of 6 to 12 METs,[67] which means that skiing is unsuitable for low-fitness coronary patients. Also, energy requirements vary greatly depending on skiing efficiency, ambient temperatures, the terrain, snow conditions, and altitude. An acceptable alternative is the use of stationary ski ergometers such as the Nordic Track (Nordic Track, Chaska, MN), which simulates cross-country skiing. A mean 12% improvement in $\dot{V}O_2max$ levels with 19 weeks of Nordic Track training occurred in deconditioned healthy young women.[106]

Aerobic Dance.   Aerobic dance, as a dynamic exercise, has the advantage of incorporating muscle activity of the upper and lower extremities and torso simultaneously or in selected combinations. Aerobic dance is best performed in a group setting and, for the coronary patient, should be of the low-impact type. Since the typical MET range for aerobic dance routines is 6 to 9,[67] this activity is appropriate only for coronary patients with moderate or high baseline fitness levels.

Rate of Progression of Exercise Training. The rate at which a coronary patient progresses through an exercise training program is important. On the one hand, patients should exercise vigorously enough to improve their $\dot{V}O_2$max level. On the other hand, exercising too vigorously too soon may place the patient at risk for cardiovascular complications or musculoskeletal injuries or can make exercise an unpleasant experience because of the discomfort during exercise and muscle soreness after exercise. Such negative experiences minimize the chances of long-term adherence to an exercise program. Thus, it is important for the exercise leader to appropriately adjust the exercise intensity, duration, and frequency in a manner that will optimize the chances of patient enjoyment.

ACSM guidelines[67] outline three stages in the progression of an exercise training program: initial, improvement, and maintenance stages. The initial stage starts with light calisthenics and low-level aerobic activities. During this initial stage, it is best to be conservative in terms of the intensity and duration of exercise, while the frequency of sessions is increased. To remove the risk of ventricular arrhythmias and ischemic injury, the exercise intensity for coronary patients should be maintained below the threshold for cardiovascular symptoms or ECG abnormalities as demonstrated during exercise testing. This initial stage includes all in-hospital and early posthospital convalescent-phase exercise training. In general, patients recovering from PTCA and CABG can initially progress faster than those recovering from myocardial infarction, for at least up to 4 to 8 weeks,[51,79] since they usually have no associated myocardial damage.

The second training stage, the improvement phase, is usually initiated after 4 months or more of exercise training. During this stage, the patient may progress more rapidly. The exercise leader should appropriately increase the exercise intensity and session duration to remain safe and enjoyable for the patient. The training improvement stage typically takes place during the middle and later stages of in-hospital exercise and continues throughout therapeutic exercise training.

The final stage of an exercise program is the maintenance phase. This generally begins after 6 months of training, at which time there no longer is a need to systematically increase the training stimulus. Patients should be informed that they will attain minimal further improvement in functional capacity and that the goal is to maintain their current fitness levels. Introducing different exercise activities helps keep exercise enjoyable and minimizes patient dropout.

Low-risk patients after uncomplicated myocardial infarction can safely enter outpatient exercise training programs within 2 weeks of the acute event. Such programs typically continue for 8 to 12 weeks.

Patients after CABG who have not sustained recent heart muscle damage can often progress through an exercise training program more rapidly than patients after acute myocardial infarction. CABG patients also can begin outpatient exercise within 2 weeks of surgery, but often complete the program within 6 to 8 weeks. Programs for these patients usually emphasize exercise to enhance and maintain upper-body flexibility after surgery.

Although patients who have undergone PTCA are generally considered potential candidates for exercise training, little information is available about the effects of such a program for this subgroup of patients. Theoretically, they could begin outpatient exercise training within 1 week of PTCA if no myocardial damage had occurred immediately prior to PTCA. This type of patient generally can progress rapidly through a 4- to 6-week exercise program.

Patients with angina pectoris can begin exercise training as soon as their cardiac symptoms are stable. These patients should exercise at an intensity below their anginal threshold and, as a result, may have to progress slowly through a 12-week program. If the intensity of exercise is very low (less than 50% according to the Karvonen heart rate reserve method), the duration of the aerobic phase of the exercise sessions may have to be increased beyond the usual 20 to 30 minutes or the frequency of exercise increased beyond the typical three to five times per week.

Special Considerations for Arm Exercise

Arm exercise is also discussed in Chapters 6 and 8.

Traditionally, coronary exercise rehabilitation

programs have emphasized training the lower extremities. The resulting physiologic changes are predominantly specific to the muscle groups used (i.e., leg training results in a substantial decrease in the heart rate response to leg exercise, but not to arm exercise).[107] Despite the well known concept of muscle specificity of training[108] and although most coronary patients, and the general population as well, perform most of their daily occupational and recreational activities with their arms, upper-extremity exercise training often has been restricted in coronary rehabilitation programs. The early rationale for discouraging arm exercise was based on the false belief that upper-extremity exercise was more likely to increase myocardial oxygen demand and induce ischemia than lower-extremity exercise.

An appropriate arm exercise prescription for coronary patients should consider three variables: (1) the appropriate exercise heart rate; (2) the work load that will elicit a sufficient metabolic stress for training; and (3) the proper training equipment or modalities.[109] Ideally, target heart rates for arm exercise training should be calculated from the results of an arm ergometry test. However, this is not practical in many clinical settings, and arm exercise training heart rates are often based on data from a treadmill or bicycle exercise test. When prescribing arm exercise intensity from leg ergometry test data, the THR obtained from the test should be reduced by about 10 beats/min. It also is important to realize that heart rate, blood pressure, $\dot{V}O_2$, ventilation, and RPE are similar for arm and leg exercise when expressed as a percentage of peak work load for each, but differ significantly when expressed in terms of the true $\dot{V}O_2max$ level[109,110] (see also Chs. 7 and 8). A work load approximately 50% of that used for leg training[111] is generally recommended as an appropriate work load for arm training in coronary patients.

There are also gender and age differences among healthy subjects in response to arm ergometry exercise.[112] Men generally achieved significantly higher power outputs and $\dot{V}O_2$ levels than did women during arm exercise. However, the heart rate response to total body oxygen demand during arm ergometry was generally significantly higher in women than in men. Among subjects aged 22 to 59 years, the younger ones usually achieved a significantly higher peak power output during arm work than did older subjects, although $\dot{V}O_2$ data were similar for the younger and older groups. These aspects should be considered when prescribing arm exercise for coronary patients without specific arm ergometry testing.

Either specially designed or modified exercise equipment can be used to provide upper extremity exercise. Equipment specific for upper extremity training includes the Monark Rehab Trainer (Monark, Varberg, Sweden) and Cybex UBE (Lumex, Inc., Ronkonkoma, NY). As an alternative, most leg cycle ergometers can be securely mounted to a table or countertop and used for arm ergometry exercise.

A variety of cycle ergometer exercise equipment is available that combines upper- and lower-extremity exercise. Examples of this type of cycle ergometer are Schwinn Air-Dyne (Excelsior Fitness Equipment Company, Northbrook, IL), Tunturi Dual Action Aircycle (Tunturi, Pilispanristi, Finland), and the Ross Futura (Ross, Farmingdale, NY). Although rowing ergometers exercise primarily the upper extremities, they also involve the lower extremities. Examples of rowing ergometers include the Concept II (Concept II, Morrisville, VT), Tunturi AirRower (Tunturi), and the liferower (Bally Fitness Products Corp., Irvine, CA). Other types of exercise equipment that incorporate upper- and lower-extremity exercise include cross-country skiing simulators, such as the Nordic-Track, and vertical climbing devices, such as the Versa-Climber (Heart Rate, Inc., Costa Mesa, CA).

Weight Training and Resistive and Isometric Exercise

Weight training, combining isometric and dynamic work, can be an important component of coronary rehabilitative and general fitness programs by improving skeletal muscle strength and muscular endurance. These adaptations can help prepare coronary patients to return to selected vocational and recreational activities. However, there has traditionally been concern about the safety of weight training for coronary patients.

Variable-resistance exercise in coronary patients is described[113] to elicit peak heart rates that were only 56 to 64% of maximal heart rates obtained during an exercise test. Contrary to popular belief, this was not associated with any arrhythmias, abnormal blood pressure responses, ST segment depression on the ECG, or cardiovascular symptoms. Other studies have demonstrated that the long-term effects of strength training are similar for coronary patients and normal subjects.[114,115]

Circuit training is another approach to combining upper- and lower-extremity exercise training to improve muscular strength and cardiorespiratory fitness. The duration of a single circuit usually varies between 7 and 12 minutes for a 10-station routine, depending on the rest interval between exercises (15 to 60 seconds) and the number of repetitions performed per exercise (6 to 15 repetitions). Circuit weight training may include conventional free weights and barbells; stacks of weight plates that permit variable resistance exercise; or cam-and-pulley devices and exercise machines that incorporate hydraulic cylinders to provide both variable speed and resistance.[116]

In a recent study[117] of circuit training in coronary patients, the training program included 12 to 20 repetitions at 30 to 40% of one maximal repetition. There was no change in the mean values for systolic or diastolic blood pressure when measured immediately before, halfway through, or upon completion of the repetition session. Training resulted in a significant 22% increase in muscular strength. On the basis of these and other similar data, circuit weight-training exercise appears safe for selected coronary patients. Exclusion criteria for weight training in coronary patients include abnormal hemodynamic responses or ischemic changes on the ECG during an exercise test, hypersensitive carotid sinus reflex, poor left ventricular function, peak exercise capacity less than 6 METs, uncontrolled hypertension, or baseline arrhythmias.

Guidelines[67,118] for incorporating resistive exercise or weight training into coronary rehabilitation exercise programs identify that low-level resistance training may be initiated as early as 7 to 8 weeks following an acute coronary event, provided that a symptom-limited exercise test has ensured that the exclusion criteria cited were absent. Although a THR range may be useful during weight training, the RPP is recommended as a better indicator of myocardial oxygen demand; therefore, monitoring of the RPP is suggested for coronary patients during weight training.

Several methods are available for determining the initial weight to use for initiating weight training.[67] According to Franklin et al.,[118] lifts should involve smooth controlled movements with no breath holding. A light weight should be used initially and progressively incremented as few times as possible to determine the greatest load that the patient can lift at least twice, but not three times. This is estimated to be 90% of a maximal effort, and 40% of this weight is used as the starting weight. Another approach involves monitoring the heart rate and RPP response during or immediately after 10 repetitions with the lowest weight on the weight-training machine. If the patient tolerates this level of exercise, the weight is increased to the next level and so on until an appropriate weight, based on RPP response, is determined for the particular exercise.

The exercise prescription for weight training includes three sets of exercise, with each set consisting of 12 to 15 repetitions. The weight training should be conducted in an interval manner with 30 seconds of work followed by 30 seconds of rest between each type of exercise. Prior to initiating weight training, coronary patients must be thoroughly oriented to the weight-training equipment. Patients should be instructed on proper body position, speed and range of movement, and correct breathing patterns in order to avoid a Valsalva maneuver. Commercially available machines that can be used for circuit weight training include Nautilus (Nautilus Medical and Sports Supply, Dallas, TX), Cybex Eagle (Lumey, Inc., Ronkonkoma, NY), and Universal (Universal Gym Equipment, Cedar Rapids, IA).

Traditionally, static or isometric exercise has been contraindicated for coronary patients on the basis of evidence that isometric exercise decreases venous return because of the absence of an active skeletal muscle pump[119] and that isometric exercise results in significantly elevated systolic, diastolic, and mean blood pressure levels with a relatively small concomitant increase in heart rate.[120] Such cardiovascular responses to isometric exercise are often referred to as "pressor responses." This pressor response is accompanied by only a modest increase in $\dot{V}O_2$, heart rate, and cardiac output levels as compared with dynamic exercise. However, the magnitude of such physiologic changes depend on both the percentage of the maximal voluntary contraction used and the muscle mass involved in the isometric exercise.[67]

In practice, there is little difference in blood pressure response between isometric and dynamic exercise when similar types of activities are compared. In a study comparing handgrip and double-legged knee extension, higher systolic, diastolic, and mean arterial blood pressure levels occurred during knee extension than with handgrip exercise.[121] Two additional studies that evaluated the response of CHD patients to isometric exercise showed no significant difference in the frequency or intensity of angina pectoris, ischemic ST segment depression on the ECG, or ventricular arrhythmias elicited by isometric exercise and with dynamic exercise.[122,123]

These observations suggest that it appears safe and reasonable to incorporate weight training as well as static exercise in medically supervised exercise training programs for low-risk coronary patients. These types of exercises must be prescribed in appropriate intensities as outlined above. Inclusion of weight training and isometric exercise can help the coronary patient become more efficient in safely performing many leisure and occupational activities that require strength and static work as part of the daily routine.

Occupational Considerations.

Occupational considerations in exercise training are also discussed in Chapter 30.

An occupational assessment as part of an exercise training program provides valuable data as to the feasibility for a return to previous employment within a reasonable period. It also can identify potential occupational problem areas that can be addressed within the scope of the exercise prescription. This assessment process includes a job analysis, exercise testing, and exercise training as outlined by Sheldahl et al.[124]

Job analysis is used to determine the physiologic and psychological demands of the patient's job. This includes identification of the type of work performed as dynamic or static-dynamic combinations and upper- or lower-extremity work. The estimated energy requirements of the work tasks, based on standardized tables,[125] can be compared with the patient's estimated or measured functional capacity during exercise testing. The work tasks must also be considered in terms of ambient temperature, humidity, and psychological stresses that affect myocardial oxygen requirements.

Exercise testing is the second major component of a comprehensive occupational assessment. This can include several possible types of tests. A symptom-limited exercise test is useful because it directly measures the patient's functional capacity. The obtained value in METs or energy expenditure in kilocalories per minute (kcal/min) can be compared with the estimated average and peak job energy requirements. The average energy demands over an 8-hour working day should not be greater than 40% of a patient's maximal functional capacity. In addition, it is usually recommended that the highest work intensity for 30 to 60 minutes should not exceed 70 to 80% of the patient's functional capacity.

Two simulated work tests described by Sheldahl et al.[126,127] are useful adjuncts to a standard exercise test. The first is a weight-carrying test; during this test, patients walk on a treadmill at approximately 2 mph at no elevation with the work load varying from carrying no weight up to carrying 50 lb. During the test, the load is increased in 10-lb increments for each test stage. The length of each test stage is 3 minutes, with 2 to 3 minutes of rest between stages. Heart rate, ECG, and blood pressure are monitored during testing. A second simulated work test is a repetitive weight-lifting test. During this test, patients lift between 30 and 50 lb repetitively for 6 minutes followed by 2-minute rest intervals between each of four lifting stages. The weights are lifted from the floor to a height of 33 in. Again, heart rate, ECG, and blood pressure are monitored during the test.

The third component of occupational assessment is the response to exercise training. The information gathered from the previous job assessment tests should be incorporated into the patient's exercise training prescription. This will not only help prepare the patient physiologically for returning to work, but will also help psychologically, by improving self-confidence and decreasing anxiety in anticipation of return to work.

ALTERATION OF EXERCISE PERFORMANCE AND PRESCRIPTION BY CARDIOVASCULAR DRUGS

The effect of cardiovascular drugs on exercise testing and training is also discussed in Chapter 16.

Overview

Most patients in coronary exercise rehabilitation programs receive cardiac medications, many of which can alter exercise performance or its safety. These include drugs to control angina pectoris or other ischemic manifestations, arrhythmias, hypertension, or congestive heart failure. Information about medications and their potential effects on exercise performance is needed to correctly interpret the results of exercise tests and to properly prescribe or modify exercise programs.[67,128] In general, when exercise testing a coronary patient for determining an exercise prescription prior to initiating an exercise program, it is best to have the patient continue taking all prescribed medications to determine their effect on exercise performance. This is in contrast to exercise testing for diagnostic purposes, as for detection of ischemia, when some anti-ischemic and other types of drugs may have to be temporarily withdrawn.

Modification of the exercise prescription should be considered when a drug known to affect exercise performance is added or deleted during an exercise training program. Ideally, the exercise test should be repeated, because changes in drug therapy often reflect changes in clinical status, but this is not always feasible. An alternative is to monitor the patient's next few exercise sessions to determine a new appropriate THR based on the patient's heart rate response, RPE, or symptoms.[67] Specific considerations for major cardiovascular drugs are discussed below.

Beta-blocking Drugs

Beta-adrenergic receptor-blocking agents are frequently prescribed for coronary patients[129,130] because long-term beta blockade substantially reduces the risk of subsequent cardiovascular mortality in patients following myocardial infarction for whom its administration is deemed appropriate.[42] Beta-blocking drugs are commonly prescribed to control angina pectoris, hypertension, and certain arrhythmias. Different classes of beta-blocking drugs have similar general pharmacologic cardiovascular effects, but show subtle differences in modifying heart rate, myocardial contractility, peripheral circulation, ventilatory capacity, and metabolic functions.

At rest, beta-blocking agents exert a dose-dependent reduction in cardiac output by attenuating the heart rate and myocardial contractility. Both systolic and diastolic blood pressure levels also are reduced, particularly in patients with preexisting hypertension. Several mechanisms appear to contribute to blood pressure reduction, including a reduction in cardiac output and inhibition in release of norepinephrine following sympathetic nerve stimulation with an associated decrease in renin secretion.

Both nonselective and selective beta-blocking agents generally attenuate the heart rate response by 15 to 60 beats/min at a given work load, depending on the dose, time of administration prior to exercise, and individual variability in responsiveness during submaximal levels of dynamic exercise up to 90% $\dot{V}O_2max$.[130] Above 90% $\dot{V}O_2max$, beta-1 cardioselective agents suppress the heart rate more than nonselective drugs do, although all preparations lose cardioselectivity at higher dosage ranges. Beta-blocking drugs with intrinsic sympathomimetic activity (ISA) attenuate heart rate to a lesser extent than do those without ISA, both at rest and during submaximal exercise, but this differential becomes smaller as

$\dot{V}O_2max$ is approached. Beta-blocking drugs also attenuate the heart rate and pressor response to submaximal and peak static and arm exercises.[130]

Blood pressure levels are reduced to a similar extent during dynamic and static exercise with both selective and nonselective beta-blocking drugs, with and without ISA. An increase in peripheral vascular resistance by unopposed alpha-adrenergic stimulation may help prevent a precipitous decline in blood pressure levels during prolonged dynamic exercise. Although this adaptation reduces blood flow to most tissues, this reduction is compensated for during chronic drug administration by increased peripheral oxygen extraction by muscle and other tissues, increasing the arteriovenous oxygen difference.[131] In addition, cardiac output is restored to the pretreatment level or to a level only slightly below usual levels during submaximal exercise by an increase in stroke volume almost in direct proportion to the negative chronotropic heart rate response.[130] The capacity for prolonged (1 to 8 hours) submaximal dynamic exercise appears to be reduced with both selective and nonselective beta-blocking drugs,[130] related to metabolic changes that reduce the availability of substrates (blood glucose and free fatty acids) for fuel to the active skeletal muscles.

Administration of beta-blocking drugs to patients whose exercise performance is limited by angina pectoris significantly increases the peak exercise capacity prior to development of symptoms.[131] This results from a reduction in myocardial oxygen demands and coronary blood flow requirements through attenuation of the heart rate, systolic blood pressure, and the RPP response to exercise. In contrast, the effects of beta-blockade on $\dot{V}O_2max$ levels are variable, with some studies showing a reduction and others showing no effect on $\dot{V}O_2max$ levels. An important variable in determining the effect of beta-blockade on $\dot{V}O_2max$ appears to be the pretreatment $\dot{V}O_2max$ level.[130] Studies in hypertensive subjects showed that those with high baseline $\dot{V}O_2max$ levels were more likely to experience significant reductions in $\dot{V}O_2max$ with beta-blockade; in contrast, subjects with average or below-average initial $\dot{V}O_2max$ levels often had no attenuation of $\dot{V}O_2max$ with beta-blockade, whereas

those with moderately high levels had a variable response, i.e., either no change or a decline. Reported decrements in $\dot{V}O_2max$ levels ranged from 4 to 18% with both nonselective and selective beta-blocking agents in hypertensive and CHD patients.[130,132,133] However, even with such reductions in $\dot{V}O_2max$, the usual relationship persists during exercise between heart rate and the percentage of $\dot{V}O_2max$[51] (See also Chs. 7 and 8). Thus, a similar exercise training prescription, based on resting and symptom-limited maximal heart rate (i.e., heart rate reserve) can be used for patients taking beta-blocking drugs as is used for patients not receiving such agents. Similarly, the relationships between the RPE and percentage of $\dot{V}O_2max$ or maximal heart rate are not significantly altered by beta-blockade, despite the depression of heart rate at each work load.[51,134] Hence, RPE also can serve as the basis of an exercise prescription as in the non-beta-blocked patient.

Beta-blocking drug therapy prolongs exercise duration before the development of symptoms in patients with exercise-induced ischemia, thereby enabling patients to achieve a greater level of exercise. A substantial number of patients with CHD receiving either a selective or nonselective beta-blocking drug, who do not have exercise-induced ischemia or contraindications for exercise, respond with improvement in $\dot{V}O_2max$ level during exercise training when prescribed exercise in a similar manner as CHD patients not receiving beta-blocking agents.[130,132,135,136] Improvements in $\dot{V}O_2max$ levels with exercise training in such CHD patients receiving beta-blocking agents range from 12 to 36% (as compared with reported improvements of 7 to 21% in healthy young sedentary men trained while on beta-blocking agents).[130] The oxygen pulse also is substantially improved as a result of an exercise training program in patients with CHD receiving beta-blocking drugs.[132] An increase in the arteriovenous oxygen difference is probably the major factor contributing to increased $\dot{V}O_2max$ and improved exercise tolerance with endurance exercise training in patients with CHD who are taking beta-blocking agents, similar to patients with CHD who are not receiving beta-blocking drugs.

Exercise training has been suggested to attenuate the adverse blood lipid changes described in patients receiving propranolol.[137]

Nitrate Drugs

Sublingual nitrate preparations are useful for the prevention or acute relief of anginal episodes. Sublingual nitroglycerin, administered immediately before exercise, may reduce the likelihood of anticipated exertional angina, thereby enhancing exercise tolerance. Many patients with angina also receive long-acting nitrate preparations either in oral form or transdermally as an ointment or patches to prevent anginal episodes.

The anti-ischemic effects of nitrate preparations result primarily from their ability to increase coronary blood flow and to reduce myocardial oxygen demand, both via a decrease in preload through venodilatation and afterload through peripheral arteriolar vasodilatation. Increased coronary collateral flow may also help attenuate ischemic episodes.

Acute administration of sublingual nitroglycerin before exercise necessitates careful surveillance of patients for exertional hypotension, which may result in reflex tachycardia. On the other hand, long-term administration of nitrate drugs usually is accompanied by a reduction in levels of heart rate, systolic blood pressure, and RPP at a given submaximal workload.[67,128,138] This results in an improvement in exercise tolerance by increasing the amount of exercise that can be performed before the onset of myocardial ischemia, as manifested by ST-T wave abnormalities on the ECG and by angina pectoris. Since the relationship of maximal exercise heart rate, RPP, and Borg score for RPE before the onset of myocardial ischemia and angina is not significantly altered during long-term administration of nitrate drugs, the exercise prescription usually does not require alteration with initiation of nitrate drug therapy.[67,138]

Possible adverse responses to nitrate drugs may impair exercise performance. Postural hypotension with dizziness, weakness, and/or loss of consciousness is an occasional side effect that may require reduced dosage; this occurs more commonly when hypovolemia is present, as with excessive diuretic therapy or dehydration for other reasons.

Calcium Channel-blocking Agents

This class of drugs, which includes verapamil, diltiazem, nifedipine, and nicardipine, has beneficial effects on angina pectoris, hypertension, and supraventricular arrhythmias.[67,128] Calcium channel-blocking drugs reduce transsarcolemmal calcium ion influx through slow calcium channels into cardiac, skeletal, and smooth muscle cells.[139] Cardiovascular effects include vasodilatation of the peripheral and coronary arteries, a negative inotropic effect, a variable heart rate response, and reduced atrioventricular conduction.[67,140] These agents differ in their vasodilatation and negative inotropic effects, as well as effects on atrioventricular conduction and heart rate. Side effects include light-headedness, reflex tachycardia due to hypotension during exertion, and peripheral edema.[67]

These drugs improve dynamic exercise tolerance in patients with CHD by increasing the ischemic threshold; in healthy individuals they do not adversely affect $\dot{V}O_2$max levels, skeletal muscle strength or endurance, or either anaerobic or aerobic power.[139] Because of possible alterations in heart rate, prescriptions for exercise training should be based on exercise test data performed with patients on their usual drug dosage.[67] The limited data available suggest that calcium channel-blocking drugs do not alter the expected training response to endurance exercise training.

Diuretic Drugs

Diuretic drugs are commonly given as antihypertensive agents and in the management of congestive heart failure. They include thiazide and thiazidelike diuretic drugs (e.g., hydrochlorothiazide and chlorothalidone), "loop" diuretic drugs (furosemide and ethacrynic acid), and potassium-sparing diuretic drugs (spironolactone and triamterene). Their principal pharmacologic effect is to increase renal excretion of sodium and extracellular fluid. Thiazide diuretic drugs also reduce peripheral vascular resistance, decreasing the blood pressure level with no effect on heart rate at rest or during exercise.[67]

Although no alteration in the exercise prescription is required for patients taking diuretic drugs and there is no effect on the exercise training response, there are a number of concerns related to exercise. Excessive fluid loss may result in hypotension. Thiazide and "loop" diuretic drugs produce a loss of potassium from the body and may result in hypokalemia with subsequent muscular fatigue, weakness, ST-T wave abnormalities on the ECG, false-positive exercise test ECG changes, and predisposition to arrhythmias.[67] Other adverse metabolic effects with thiazide diuretic drugs include elevation of serum cholesterol levels, glucose levels, and elevation of serum uric acid levels that may precipitate acute gouty arthritis. Risk of dehydration and heat injury during exercise also is increased in individuals receiving diuretic drugs.

Digitalis

Digitalis preparations are used in the management of congestive heart failure and atrial fibrillation, as well as other arrhythmias. They increase myocardial contractility by limiting sodium–potassium exchange across the myocardial cell, resulting in a parallel increase in sodium-coupled calcium transport within the cell. They also decrease atrioventricular (A-V) conduction. Digitalis-induced ST-T wave abnormalities on the ECG make exercise ECG testing less reliable in detecting ischemia.

Digitalis slows the heart rate by increasing vagal tone, which may alter the exercise prescription. Exercise tolerance is improved by digitalis therapy in patients with congestive heart failure and when arrhythmias are controlled.

Digitalis toxicity is of particular concern in patients receiving diuretic drugs because of possible associated hypokalemia. Exercising coronary patients receiving digitalis require surveillance of potassium blood levels, particularly when receiving concomitant diuretic drug therapy.

Vasodilator Drugs

This is a broad class of drugs with various mechanisms for producing peripheral vasodilatation; these drugs are used in the management of hypertension and heart failure.[128] The principal concern for the exercising patient is the potential for postexercise hypotension, which is diminished by an adequate cool-down period during exercise recovery. Patients are also susceptible to problems arising from hypovolemia.

Angiotensin-converting Enzyme Inhibitors

Angiotensin-converting enzyme (ACE) inhibitors are frequently used in the treatment of hypertension and congestive heart failure. Their mechanism of action is through peripheral vasodilatation,[67] accomplished by inhibition of the enzyme responsible for conversion of angiotensin I to the potent vasoconstrictor angiotensin II and destruction of the potent vasodilator bradykinin. These drugs improve exercise capacity and reduce the mortality rate in patients with congestive heart failure.[67] They otherwise have no effect on exercise prescription and exercise training effects. Since blood pressure levels may be reduced during dynamic exercise with ACE inhibitors, precautions similar to those with other vasodilator agents should be taken to avoid postexercise hypotension.[128]

SAFETY OF EXERCISE IN CORONARY PATIENTS

Prevalence of Cardiac Complications

Cardiac complications, although uncommon, during coronary exercise rehabilitation include cardiac arrest, cardiac arrhythmias requiring cardioversion, myocardial infarction, pulmonary embolism, pulmonary edema, cardiogenic shock, and unstable angina.[13,82] Cardiac arrest, although rare, is the most serious complication and is seven times more frequent than recurrent nonfatal myocardial infarction. A comprehensive study of cardiovascular complications during exercise rehabilitation recently reported[82] was based on data obtained from 167 randomly selected supervised outpatient exercise programs throughout the United States involving 51,303 patients, who exercised for a total of more than 2 million hours during 1980 to 1984. A total of 21 cardiac arrests (18 successfully resuscitated and 3 fatal) and 8 nonfatal myocardial infarctions were reported, for a complication rate of one cardiac arrest per 111,996 hours, one nonfatal myocardial infarction per 293,900 hours, and one fatality per 783,976 hours of prescribed supervised exercise. This relatively high level of safety was attributed to high standards of medical screening and assessment of patients, proper education and treatment of patients, careful exercise prescription, appropriate ECG monitoring and exercise supervision, well-trained personnel, and rapid and effective handling of emergencies.

Medical Screening and Assessment

CHD patients at high risk for recurrent events or complications should be identified early after a coronary event. High-risk coronary patients include those with severely depressed left ventricular function, prior cardiac arrest, complex ventricular arrhythmias, markedly reduced exercise capacity, ischemic ST segment depression at low levels of exercise, exercise-induced hypotension, and nonoperated or inoperable left main or triple-vessel coronary artery disease.[3,14,67,77] Such high-risk patients, referred for exercise rehabilitation after diagnostic evaluation and medical and/or surgical therapy that was unable to reverse their high risk status, require careful monitoring and supervision during exercise training sessions.

Patient Education about Exercise

Patients participating in rehabilitative exercise programs must be educated regarding the importance of compliance with their exercise prescription. This includes adherence to proper warm-up and cool-down phases, exercising within the prescribed THR range, compliance with prescribed medical therapy, and the prompt reporting of cardiovascular symptoms to the supervising physician or exercise program staff.

Adherence

Patient compliance is a key factor that affects the success of most long-term secondary intervention programs. Since adherence to training plays an important role in determining the magnitude of the response, the factors that affect adherence must be considered in any prescription. Exercise testing and training are often overemphasized at the expense of the counseling, leadership, education, and motivation phases of the program. As a result, negative aspects often outweigh the positive factors that contribute to sustained participant interest (Fig. 20-3), adherence declines, and the effectiveness of the program diminishes. Many individuals enter exercise programs with high expectations, achieve a small training effect, and ultimately leave the program or become irregular in their attendance. Whereas most people who leave exercise programs intend to continue to exercise, many apparently lose enthusiasm and return to preprogram activity patterns and physiologic status.[141] Adherence and attendance rates for long-term preventive and rehabilitative exercise programs are not encouraging (Table 20-6).

Psychosocial factors that relate to exercise noncompliance include (1) perception of the program, (2) personal convenience factors, and (3) family lifestyle components.[142,143] Exercise noncompliers generally lack enthusiasm for the program and frequently report high levels of postexercise fatigue. Similarly, dropouts find it more difficult to arrive on time for exercise sessions, perceive their job to interfere more with their attendance, and vice versa. Those who find it difficult to relax after work and those whose incomes had not reached their expectations have higher dropout rates. Adherence rates among participants whose spouses are neutral or negative toward the exercise program are lower than among those whose spouses are supportive.[144]

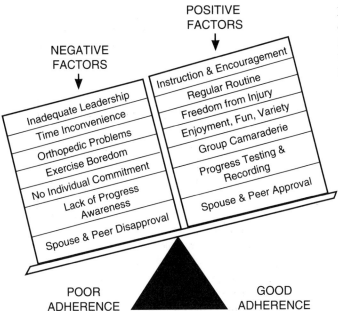

Fig. 20-3. Factors affecting adherence to a physical conditioning program. Negative factors often outweigh positive factors, resulting in poor adherence.

Table 20-6. Adherence and Attendance Rates of Coronary Risk and Postmyocardial Infarction Patients Participating in Exercise Training Programs

Program	Adherence[a] (%)	Attendance[b] (%)	Length of Program (Months)
Taylor et al.[155]	62–75	45	18
Pyorala et al.[156]	86	72	18
Oldridge[157]	50	70	18
	40	74	48
	30	79	84
Mann et al.[158]	59	83	6
Bruce et al.[159]	42	N/G[c]	6–9
Knapp et al.[160]	39	63	12
Sanne and Rydin[161]	39	63	9
	29	N/G	24
Oldridge et al.[145]	53	71	12
	48	80	24
	27	75	36
Gottheiner[162]	60	N/G	36

[a] Adherence = number of persons still in program at a given time compared with total intake.
[b] Attendance = number of sessions attended per unit of time compared with total possible number of sessions during that time.
[c] N/G, not given.

Recent research has focused on identifying potential exercise dropouts (early and late) in an attempt to initiate compliance-improving strategies to improve the likelihood that treatment goals will be achieved.[145,146] Principal factors related to early noncompliance included type A personality, cigarette smoking, inactive leisure time, and a history of at least two previous myocardial infarctions.[145] These characteristics suggest that individuals leaving exercise programs early may have been those at the greatest risk of a future coronary event. Principal factors related to long-term noncompliance were cigarette smoking, blue-collar employment, inactive leisure time, and inactive occupation.[147] The noncompliance rate increased progressively, from 59% with smoking alone, the single most discriminating variable, to 95% with all four variables present.

Adherence (Table 20-6) to long-term exercise programs varies widely.[148,149] More successful programs have recognized and made provision for the following important factors to increase long-term exercise motivation and compliance[147]: comprehensive program design; exclusion of subjects with specific contraindications; regularity of sessions; supervision; minimizing musculoskeletal injuries by a moderate frequency and duration of exercise[150]; avoiding overemphasis on regimented calisthenics; including a variety of activities and modified recreational games that maximize participant success; providing participants with positive feedback and follow-up evaluation (retesting); using progress charts to record goals and achievements; using a reward system with recognition and symbols of accomplishments of participants; stimulating camaraderie by promoting group as opposed to individual exercise commitments[151,152]; and fostering positive attitudes of spouses toward the program.[144] Compliance-improving behavioral strategies, such as contracting, goal setting, self-monitoring, and education, may also offer potential for improving exercise adherence.[153] The physician and other health professionals must be "aware of the likelihood of noncompliance in the individual patient and make strong efforts to detect problems and persuade patients of the importance of adherence to a program designed to reach and maintain stated,

and often negotiated, therapeutic goals. It is the physician's responsibility to teach, motivate, and strengthen the patient to maximize compliance. . . ."[154]

Patient Supervision

The extent of patient supervision during exercise training sessions depends on the risk status of the patient. Guidelines for ECG monitoring of high- and moderate-risk coronary patients in rehabilitative exercise programs were discussed earlier in this chapter. Adequate supervision also implies ensuring compliance with the exercise prescription guidelines, adjustment of the exercise prescription as warranted by changes in the clinical status and drug therapy of the patient, and supervision of patients during postexercise recovery, as cardiovascular complications often occur in the immediate postexercise period.[82,163]

The high success rate of resuscitation of coronary patients who experience cardiac arrest during or immediately after exercise training in supervised sessions is well documented.[82,163,164] It is imperative to have adequately trained staff and functioning medical emergency equipment and supplies immediately available during exercise training sessions for coronary patients.

Supervised Versus Unsupervised Exercise Training

The issues of patient safety just discussed raise the additional question of supervised and unsupervised outpatient exercise training for patients recovering from acute myocardial infarction or CABG.[84,86,87] When outpatient exercise training programs were beginning to become commonplace in the mid-1970s, exercise sessions were generally supervised. This was logical, since little was known at that time about the safety of exercising coronary patients or about risk stratification following myocardial infarction. As experience in this area has grown during the past 15 to 20 years, the practice of routinely supervised outpatient exercise sessions, including

ECG monitoring, for all patients has been questioned.

The type and duration of patient supervision and ECG monitoring during exercise can be determined by the patient's risk status. The AACVPR recently published guidelines for exercise supervision based on risk stratification[77] (Table 20-2). High-risk patients who require supervised exercise training sessions and often continuous ECG monitoring can be identified by applying these guidelines based on risk stratification.

In addition to the AACVPR guidelines,[77] the American College of Cardiology has published criteria for use of ECG monitoring during exercise-training sessions for coronary patients.[3] Criteria for ECG monitoring include:

1. Severely depressed left ventricular function (ejection fraction of less than 30%)
2. Resting complex ventricular arrhythmias (Lown type 4 or 5)
3. Appearance or increasing frequency of ventricular arrhythmias during exercise
4. Decrease in systolic blood pressure with exercise
5. Survivors of sudden cardiac death
6. Hospital course of acute myocardial infarction complicated by congestive heart failure, cardiogenic shock, and/or serious ventricular arrhythmias
7. Severe coronary heart disease and marked exercise-induced ischemia
8. Inability to self-monitor exercise heart rate (or use rating of perceived exertion)

Although there is general agreement on the need to supervise exercise sessions for high-risk patients, the picture is less clear for low- and moderate-risk patients. Several studies have compared unsupervised or home exercise training with supervised programs.[83,85] The results regarding adherence to the exercise regimen are variable, but improvement in functional capacity is documented to be comparable[85] with unsupervised and supervised exercise. These studies also found that patient safety was not compromised by unsupervised exercise.

There are several advantages to unsupervised exercise. The availability of exercise training is greater for all patients, regardless of how far they live from a major medical center. Unsupervised exercise is also convenient for patients, since they do not have to follow a program schedule or spend time commuting to and from the program site. Also, costs are generally significantly lower, and this in turn may help to increase the availability of exercise training to more patients.

Furthermore, unsupervised exercise training has a potential advantage for selected hospitals and other facilities that might provide outpatient exercise training services without the associated requirements and costs of space, equipment, and staff if the services were provided on-site. Consequently, some institutions that might otherwise not be able to provide rehabilitative exercise services would be able to do so by using an unsupervised format for low-risk coronary patients.

There also are disadvantages to unsupervised exercise training. There may be limited or no opportunity to teach patients the skills to adequately self-monitor their exercise program or the signs and symptoms of exercise intolerance. There are also limited opportunities to teach patients about strategies for reducing their overall risk for future coronary events. Unsupervised exercise may also eliminate the peer support inherent in supervised programs; this may have a negative effect on exercise adherence. The reduced possibility of successful management of exercise-related medical emergencies in the unsupervised setting is a potential disadvantage. Although such occurrences are rare, a patient would not have the benefit of immediate professional assistance in the event of a medical emergency.

Unsupervised exercise should be augmented by some type of contact with health care professionals. Scheduled telephone calls by health care professionals to the patient at home can be used to discuss the progress of the exercise prescription or issues related to coronary risk factor reduction. Periodic contact with health care professionals provides a systematic way for patients to have their positive behaviors reinforced and their questions answered. Newly available videocassettes are a means to have professional information available in the patient's home in a more lively and entertaining format than printed materials. There are home exercise and educational videocassettes specifically designed for patients recuperating from myocardial infarction and CABG.

The current trend in outpatient exercise training seems to be moving away from routine standardized supervised exercise sessions with ECG monitoring for all patients. Instead, supervision and ECG monitoring are used more selectively, on an individualized basis, for the higher-risk coronary patients. Further study is necessary to determine the best model for delivering this individualized outpatient programming to the coronary patient.

SUMMARY

Medically prescribed and supervised exercise as part of a comprehensive rehabilitation program is an accepted standard of care for coronary patients, particularly following acute myocardial infarction or coronary revascularization procedures, or for patients with angina pectoris without an acute event. The exercise training program, which now commonly provides a blend of dynamic and resistive exercises and includes upper-extremity exercise, usually results in beneficial physiologic adaptations that help the patients resume active productive lives. Comprehensive lifestyle changes fostered by good coronary rehabilitation programs may help decrease the risk of recurrent CHD events and premature mortality.

The safety of coronary rehabilitative exercise is well documented and is attributed to high standards of medical screening and patient assessment, proper patient education and medical management, careful exercise prescription, appropriate supervision by well-trained personnel, and prompt and proper handling of medical emergencies as they arise.

REFERENCES

1. National Center for Health Services Research and Health Care Technology Assessment: Health Technology Assessment Reports. Cardiac Rehabilitation Services. DHHS Publication no. (PHS)88:3427, U.S. Department of Health and Human Services, Rockville, MD, 1957

2. Hellerstein HK, Ford, AB: Rehabilitation of the cardiac patient. JAMA 164:225, 1957

3. American College of Cardiology Task Force: Recommendations of the American College of Cardiology on cardiovascular rehabilitation. J Am Coll Cardiol 7:451, 1986

4. Wenger NK, Balady GJ, Cohn LH, and the Ad Hoc Task Force on Cardiac Rehabilitation: Cardiac rehabilitation services following PTCA and valvular surgery: Guidelines for use. Cardiology 19:4, 1990

5. Wenger NK, Haskell WL, Kanter K, and the Ad Hoc Task Force on Cardiac Rehabilitation: Cardiac rehabilitation services after cardiac transplantation: Guidelines for use. Cardiology 20:4, 1991

6. Leon AS: Position Paper of the American Association of Cardiovascular and Pulmonary Rehabilitation. Scientific evidence of the value of cardiac rehabilitation services with emphasis on patients following myocardial infarction. I. Exercise conditioning component. J Cardiopulmonary Rehabil 10:79, 1990

7. Health and Public Policy Committee, American College of Physicians: Cardiac rehabilitation services. Ann Intern Med 109:671, 1988

8. Miller NH, Taylor CB, Davidson DM et al: Position Paper of the American Association of Cardiovascular and Pulmonary Rehabilitation. The efficacy of risk factor intervention and psychosocial aspects of cardiac rehabilitation. J Cardiopulmonary Rehabil 10:198, 1990

9. Wenger NK: Rehabilitation of the patient with acute myocardial infarction during hospitalization: Early ambulation and patient education. p. 405. In Pollock ML, Schmidt DM (eds): Heart Disease and Rehabilitation. 2nd Ed. John Wiley & Sons, New York, 1986

10. Bloch A, Maeder J-P, Haissly J-C et al: Early mobilization after myocardial infarction. A controlled study. Am J Cardiol 34:152, 1974

11. Jorgensen CR, Gobel FL, Taylor HL, Wang Y: Myocardial blood flow and oxygen consumption during exercise. Ann NY Acad Sci 301:213, 1977

12. Clausen JP: Circulatory adjustments to dynamic exercise and effect of physical training in normal subjects and in patients with coronary artery disease. p. 39. In Sonnenblick EH, Lesch M (eds): Exercise and Heart Disease. Grune & Stratton, New York, 1977

13. Thompson PD: The benefits and risks of exercise training in patients with chronic coronary artery disease. JAMA 259:1537, 1988

14. DeBusk RF, Blomqvist CG, Kouchoukos NT et al: Identification and treatment of low-risk patients after acute myocardial infarction and coronary-artery bypass graft surgery. N Engl J Med 314:161, 1986

15. Detry J-M, Rousseau M, Vandenbroucke G et al: Increased arteriovenous oxygen difference after physical training in coronary heart disease. Circulation 44:109, 1971

16. Ehsani AA, Biello DR, Schultz J, et al: Improvement of left ventricular contractile function by exercise training in patients with coronary artery disease. Circulation 74:350, 1986

17. Leon AS, Bloor CM: Effects of exercise and its cessation on the heart and its blood supply. J Appl Physiol 24:485, 1968

18. Leon AS, Bloor CM: The effect of complete and partial deconditioning on exercise-induced cardiovascular changes in the rat. Adv Cardiol 18:81, 1976

19. Leon AS: Comparative cardiovascular adaptations to exercise in animals and man and their relevance to coronary heart disease. p. 143. In Bloor CM (ed): Comparative Pathophysiology of Circulation Disorders. Plenum, New York, 1972

20. Scheuer J: Effects of physical training on myocardial vascularity and perfusion. Circulation 66:491, 1982

21. Froelicher VF: Exercise, fitness and coronary heart disease. p. 429. In Bouchard C, Shephard RJ, Stephens T et al (eds): Exercise, Fitness, and Health. A Consensus of Current Knowledge. Human Kinetics, Champaign, IL, 1990

22. Kramsch DM, Aspen AJ, Abramowitz BM et al: Reduction of coronary atherosclerosis by moderate conditioning exercise in monkeys on atherogenic diet. N Engl J Med 305:1483, 1981

23. Bloor CM, White FC, Sanders TM: Effects of exercise on collateral development in myocardial ischemia in pigs. J Appl Physiol Respir Environ Exercise Physiol 56:656, 1984

24. Rose G, Prineas R, Mitchell JR: Myocardial infarction and the intrinsic calibre of the coronary arteries. Br Med J 29:548, 1967

25. Ferguson RJ, Petticlerc R, Choquette G, et al: Effect of physical training on treadmill exercise capacity, collateral circulation and progression of coronary disease. Am J Cardiol 34:764, 1974

26. Conner JF, LaCamera F, Jr, Swanick EJ et al: Effects of exercise on coronary collateralization– angiographic studies of six patients in a supervised exercise program. Med Sci Sports Exercise 8:145, 1976

27. Sim DN, Neill WA: Investigation of the physiological basis for increased exercise threshold for angina pectoris after physical conditioning. J Clin Invest 51:763, 1974

28. Redwood DR, Rosing DR, Epstein SE: Circulatory and symptomatic effects of physical training in patients with coronary artery disease and angina pectoris. N Engl J Med 286:959, 1972

29. Ehsani AA, Heath GW, Hagberg JM et al: Effects of 12 months of intense exercise training on ischemic ST-segment depression in patients with coronary artery disease. Circulation 64:1116, 1981

30. Froelicher V, Jensen D, Genter F et al: A randomized trial of exercise training in patients with coronary heart disease. JAMA 252:1291, 1984

31. Sebrechts CP, Klein JL, Ahnve S et al: Myocardial perfusion changes following 1 year of exercise training assessed by thallium-201 circumferential count profiles. Am Heart J 112:1217, 1986

32. Myers J, Ahnve S, Froelicher V et al: A randomized trial of the effects of 1 year of exercise training on computer-measured ST segment displacement in patients with coronary artery disease. J Am Coll Cardiol 4:1094, 1984

33. Leon AS: Effects of exercise conditioning on physiologic precursors of coronary heart disease. J Cardiopulmonary Rehabil 11:46, 1991

34. Ornish D, Brown SE, Scherwitz LW et al: Can lifestyle changes reverse coronary heart disease? The Lifestyle Heart Trial. Lancet 336:129, 1990

35. Leon AS: Physical activity levels and coronary heart disease. Analysis of epidemiologic and supporting studies. Med Clin N Am 69:3, 1985

36. Berlin A, Colditz GA: A meta-analysis of physical activity in the prevention of coronary heart disease. Am J Epidemiol 132:612, 1990

37. Leon AS: Leisure-time physical activity levels and risk of coronary heart disease and death. The Multiple Risk Factor Intervention Trial. JAMA 258:2388, 1988

38. Shaw LW: Effects of a prescribed supervised exercise program on mortality and cardiovascular morbidity in patients after a myocardial infarction. The National Exercise and Heart Disease Project. Am J Cardiol 48:39, 1981

39. Vermeulen A, Lie KI, Durrer D: Effects of cardiac rehabilitation after myocardial infarction: Changes in coronary risk factors and long-term prognosis. Am Heart J 105:798, 1983

40. Kallio V, Hamalainen H, Hakkila J, Luurila OJ: Reduction in sudden deaths by a multifactorial intervention programme after acute myocardial infarction. Lancet ii:1091, 1979

41. Rechnitzer PA, Cunningham DA, Andrew GM et al: Relation of exercise to the recurrence rate of myocardial infarction in men. Ontario Exercise-Heart Collaborative Study. Am J Cardiol 51:65, 1983

42. May GS, Eberlein KA, Furberg CD et al: Secondary prevention after myocardial infarction: A review of long-term trials. Prog Cardiovasc Dis 24:331, 1982

43. Pollock ML: Benefits of exercise: Effect on mortality and physiological function. p. 189. In Kappagoda CT, Greenwood PV (eds): Long-Term Management of Patients After Myocardial Infarction. Martinus Nijhoff, Boston, 1988

44. Oldridge NB, Guyatt GH, Fischer ME, Rimm AA: Coronary rehabilitation after myocardial infarction. Combined experience of randomized clinical trials. JAMA 260:945, 1988

45. O'Connor GT, Buring JE, Yusuf S et al: An overview of randomized trials of rehabilitation with exercise after myocardial infarction. Circulation 80:234, 1989

46. Dishman RK: Medical psychology in exercise and sport. Med Clin N Am 69:123, 1985

47. Hughes JR: Psychological effects of habitual aerobic exercise. A critical review. Prev Med 13:66, 1984

48. Stern MJ, Cleary P: The National Exercise and Heart Disease Project. Long-term psychological outcome. Arch Intern Med 142:1093, 1982

49. Blumenthal JA, Emery CF, Rejeski WJ: The effects of exercise training on psychosocial functioning after myocardial infarction. J Cardiopulmonary Rehabil 8:183, 1988

50. Dracup K, Moser DK, Marsden C et al: The effect of a multidimensional cardiopulmonary rehabilitation program on psychosocial functioning. Am J Cardiol, in press

51. Pollock ML, Wilmore JH: Exercise in Health and Disease. Evaluation and Prescription for Prevention of Rehabilitation. 2nd Ed. p. 485. WB Saunders, Philadelphia, 1990

52. Hartung GH, Rangel R: Exercise training in post-myocardial infarction patients: Comparison of results with high risk coronary and post-bypass patients. Arch Phys Med Rehabil 62:147, 1981

53. Waites TF, Watt EW, Fletcher GF: Comparative functional and physiologic status of active and dropout coronary bypass patients of a rehabilitation program. Am J Cardiol 51:1087, 1983

54. Froelicher V, Jensen D, Sullivan M: A randomized trial of the effects of exercise training after coronary artery bypass surgery. Arch Intern Med 145:689, 1985

55. Robinson G, Froelicher VF, Utley JR: Rehabilitation of the coronary artery bypass graft surgery patient. J Cardiopulmonary Rehabil 4:74, 1984

56. American College of Cardiology/American Heart Association: A report of the American College of Cardiology/American Heart Association Task Force on Assessment of Diagnostic and Therapeutic Cardiovascular Procedures (Subcommittee on Percutaneous Transluminal Coronary Angioplasty): Guidelines for percutaneous transluminal coronary angioplasty. Circulation 78:486, 1988

57. King SB: Current status of percutaneous transluminal coronary angioplasty. Cardiovasc Rev Rep 9:27, 1988

58. Campeau L: Grading of angina pectoris. Circulation 54:522, 1976

59. Borg G, Holmgren A, Lindblad I: Quantitative evaluation of chest pain. Acta Med Scand Suppl 644:43, 1981

60. Sullivan MJ, Knight JD, Higginbotham MB, Cobb FR: Relation between central and peripheral hemodynamics during exercise in patients with chronic heart failure. Muscle blood flow is reduced with maintenance of arterial perfusion pressure. Circulation 80:769, 1989

61. Wasserman K: The peripheral circulation and lactic acid metabolism in heart, or cardiovascular, failure. Circulation 80:1084, 1989

62. Conn E, Williams RS, Wallace AG: Exercise responses before and after physical conditioning in patients with severely depressed left ventricular function. Am J Cardiol 49:296, 1982

63. Coats AJ, Adamopoulos S, Meyer TE et al: Effects of physical training in chronic heart failure. Lancet 335:63, 1990

64. Dubach P, Froelicher VF: Cardiac rehabilitation for heart failure patients. Cardiology 76:368, 1989

65. Miller HS, Morley D: Low functional capacity. p. 281. In Skinner JS: Exercise Testing and Exercise Prescription for Special Cases. Theoretical Basis and Clinical Application. Lea & Febiger, Philadelphia, 1987

66. Schroeder JS, Hunt S: Cardiac transplantation. Update 1987. JAMA 258:3142, 1987

67. American College of Sports Medicine: Guidelines for Exercise Testing and Prescription. 4th Ed. Lea & Febiger, Philadelphia, 1991

68. Hamm LF, Crow RS, Stull GA, Hannan P: Safety

and characteristics of exercise testing early after acute myocardial infarction. Am J Cardiol 63:1193, 1989

69. Hamm LF, Stull GA, Serfass RC, Ainsworth B: Prognostic endpoint yield of high-level versus low-level graded exercise testing. Arch Phys Med Rehabil 69:86, 1988

70. Sullivan M, McKirnan MD: Errors in predicting functional capacity for post-myocardial infarction patients using a modified Bruce protocol. Am Heart J 107:486, 1984

71. Borg G: Physical Performance and Perceived Exertion. Gleerup, Lund, Sweden, 1962

72. Borg G: Perceived exertion as an indicator of somatic stress. Scand J Rehabil Med 2:92, 1970

73. Theroux P, Waters DD, Halphen C et al: Prognostic value of exercise testing soon after myocardial infarction. N Engl J Med 301:341, 1979

74. Weld FM, Chu K-L, Bigger JT, Rolnitzky LM: Risk stratification with low-level exercise testing 2 weeks after acute myocardial infarction. Circulation 64:306, 1981

75. Fioretti P, Brower RW, Simoons ML et al: Prediction of mortality in hospital survivors of myocardial infarction. Comparison of predischarge exercise testing and radionuclide ventriculography at rest. Br Heart J 52:292, 1984

76. Krone RJ, Gillespie JA, Weld FM et al: Low-level exercise testing after myocardial infarction: Usefulness in enhancing clinical risk stratification. Circulation 71:80, 1985

77. American Association of Cardiovascular and Pulmonary Rehabilitation: Guidelines for Cardiac Rehabilitation Programs. Human Kinetics, Champaign, IL, 1991

78. Leon AS: Patients with diabetes mellitus. p. 118. In Franklin BA, Gordon S, Timmis GC (eds): Exercise in Modern Medicine. Williams & Wilkins, Baltimore, 1989

79. Metier CP, Pollock ML, Graves JE: Exercise prescription for the coronary artery bypass graft surgery patient. J Cardiopulmonary Rehabil 6:85, 1986

80. Greenland P, Chu JS: Efficacy of cardiac rehabilitation services with emphasis on patients after myocardial infarction. Ann Intern Med 109:650, 1988

81. Wenger NK: Exercise rehabilitation for coronary patients. Is ECG monitoring necessary? Cardiovascular Perspect 2:4, 1988

82. Van Camp SP, Peterson RA: Cardiovascular complications of outpatient cardiac rehabilitation programs. JAMA 256:1160, 1986

83. DeBusk RF, Haskell WL, Miller NH et al: Medically directed at-home rehabilitation soon after clinically uncomplicated acute myocardial infarction: A new model for patient care. Am J Cardiol 55:251, 1985

84. Stevens R, Hanson P: Comparison of supervised and unsupervised exercise training after coronary artery bypass surgery. Am J Cardiol 53:1524, 1984

85. Miller NH, Haskell WL, Berra K, DeBusk RF: Home versus group exercise training for increasing functional capacity after myocardial infarction. Circulation 70:645, 1984

86. Hands ME, Briffa AT, Henderson K et al: Functional capacity and left ventricular function: The effect of supervised and unsupervised exercise rehabilitation soon after coronary artery bypass graft surgery. J Cardiopulmonary Rehabil 7:578, 1987

87. Wenger NK: Home versus supervised exercise training after myocardial infarction and myocardial revascularization procedures. Pract Cardiol 15:47, 1989

88. King AC, Taylor CB, Haskell WL, DeBusk RF: Strategies for increasing early adherence to and long-term maintenance of home-based exercise training in healthy middle-aged men and women. Am J Cardiol 61:628, 1988

89. Haskell WL, Brachfeld N, Bruce RA et al: Task Force II: Determination of occupational working capacity in patients with ischemic heart disease. J Am Coll Cardiol 14:1025, 1989

90. Franklin BA, Hellerstein HK, Gordon S, Timmis GC: Exercise prescription for the myocardial infarction patient. J Cardiopulmonary Rehabil 6:62, 1986

91. Barnard RJ, Gardner GW, Diaco NV et al: Cardiovascular responses to sudden strenuous exercise—heart rate, blood pressure, and ECG. J Appl Physiol 34:833, 1973

92. Barnard RJ, MacAlpin R, Kattus AA, Buckberg GD: Ischemic response to sudden strenuous exercise in healthy men. Circulation 48:936, 1973

93. Foster C, Anholm JD, Hellman CK et al: Left ventricular function during sudden strenuous exercise. Circulation 63:592, 1981

94. Karvonen MJ, Kentala E, Mustala O: The effects of training on heart rate. Ann Med Exp Biol Fenn 35:307, 1957

95. Wilmore JH, Haskell W: Use of the heart rate-energy expenditure relationship in the individualized prescription of exercise. Am J Clin Nutr 24:1186, 1971

96. Wasserman K, Hansen JE, Sue DY, Whipp BJ

(eds): Principles of Exercise Testing and Interpretation. Lea & Febiger, Philadelphia, 1987

97. Hellerstein HK, Franklin BA: Exercise testing and prescription. p. 197. In Wenger NK, Hellerstein HK (eds): Rehabilitation of the Coronary Patient, 2nd Ed. John Wiley, New York, 1984

98. Pollock ML, Dimmick J, Miller HS et al: Effects of mode of training on cardiovascular function and body composition of adult men. Med Sci Sports Exercise 7:139, 1975

99. Pollock ML, Pels AE, Foster C, Ward A: Exercise prescription for rehabilitation of the cardiac patient. p. 477. In Pollock ML, Schmidt DH (eds): Heart Disease and Rehabilitation. 2nd ed. John Wiley & Sons, New York, 1986

100. Fletcher GF, Cantwell JD, Watt EW: Oxygen consumption and hemodynamic response of exercises used in training of patients with recent myocardial infarction. Circulation 60:140, 1979

101. Magder S, Linnarsson D, Gullstrand L: The effect of swimming on patients with ischemic heart disease. Circulation 63:979, 1981

102. Katch VL, Villanacci JF, Sady SP: Energy cost of rebound-running. Res Q Exercise Sport 52:269, 1981

103. Gerberich SG, Leon AS, McNally C et al: Analysis of the acute physiologic effects of minitrampoline rebounding exercise. J Cardiopulmonary Rehabil 10:395, 1990

104. Edin JB, Gerberich SG, Leon AS et al: Analysis of the training effects of minitrampoline rebounding on physical fitness, body composition, and blood lipids. J Cardiopulmonary Rehabil 10:401, 1990

105. Town GP, Sol N, Sinning WE: The effect of rope skipping rate on energy expenditure of males and females. Med Sci Sports Exercise 12:295, 1980

106. Jacobsen DJ, Leon AS, Wang D et al: The effects of simulated cross-country skiing on physical fitness and blood lipid levels. Med Sci Sports Exercise 18(suppl. 2):S10, 1986

107. Clausen JP, Trap-Jensen J, Lassen NA: The effects of training on the heart rate during arm and leg exercise. Scand J Clin Lab Invest 26:295, 1970

108. Sharkey BJ: Specificity of exercise. p. 55. In American College of Sports Medicine (ed): Resource Manual for Guidelines for Exercise Testing and Prescription. Lea & Febiger, Philadelphia, 1988

109. Franklin BA, Hellerstein HK, Gordon S, Timmis GC: Cardiac patients. p. 44. In Franklin BA, Gordon S, Timmis GC (eds): Exercise in Modern Medicine. Williams & Wilkins, Baltimore, 1989

110. Levandoski SG, Sheldahl LM, Wilke NA et al: Cardiorespiratory responses of coronary artery disease patients to arm and leg cycle ergometry. J Cardiopulmonary Rehabil 10:39, 1990

111. Franklin BA, Scherf J, Pamatmat A, Rubenfire M: Arm exercise testing and training. Pract Cardiol 8:43, 1982

112. Balady GJ, Weiner DA, Rose L, Ryan TJ: Physiological responses to arm ergometry exercise relative to age and gender. J Am Coll Cardiol 16:130, 1990

113. Vander LB, Franklin BA, Wrisley D, Rubenfire M: Acute cardiovascular responses to Nautilus exercise in cardiac patients: Implications for exercise training. Ann Sports Med 2:165, 1986

114. Kelemen MH, Stewart KJ, Gillilan RE et al: Circuit weight training in cardiac patients. J Am Coll Cardiol 7:38, 1986

115. Butler RM, Beierwaltes WH, Rodgers FJ: The cardiovascular response to circuit weight training in patients with coronary diseases. J Cardiopulmonary Rehabil 7:402, 1987

116. Katch FI, Freedson PS, Jones CA: Evaluation of acute cardiorespiratory responses to hydraulic resistance exercise. Med Sci Sports Exercise 17:168, 1985

117. Sparling PB, Cantwell JD, Dolan CM, Niederman RK: Strength training in a cardiac rehabilitation program: A six-month follow-up. Arch Phys Med Rehabil 71:148, 1990

118. Franklin BA, Bonzheim M, Gordon S, Timmis GC: Resistance training in cardiac rehabilitation. J Cardiopulmonary Rehabil 11:99, 1991

119. Asmussen E: Similarities and dissimilarities between static and dynamic exercise. Circ Res 48:I-3, 1981

120. Lind AR, McNicol GW: Muscular factors which determine the cardiovascular responses to sustained and rhythmic exercise. Can Med Assoc J 96:706, 1967

121. Lewis SF, Snell PG, Taylor WF et al: Role of muscle mass and mode of contraction in circulatory responses to exercise. J Appl Physiol 58:146, 1985

122. DeBusk RF, Valdez R, Houston N, Haskell W: Cardiovascular responses to dynamic and static effort soon after myocardial infarction. Application to occupational work assessment. Circulation 58:368, 1978

123. Ferguson RJ, Cote P, Bourassa MG, Corbara F: Coronary blood flow during isometric and dynamic exercise in angina pectoris patients. J Cardiac Rehabil 1:21, 1981

124. Sheldahl LM, Wilke NA, Tristani FE: Exercise prescription for return to work. J Cardiopulmonary Rehabil 5:567, 1985

125. Fox SM, Naughton JP, Gorman PA: Physical activity and cardiovascular health. III. The exercise prescription: Frequency and type of activity. Mod Concepts Cardiovasc Dis 41:21, 1972

126. Sheldahl LM, Wilke NA, Tristani FE, Kalbfleisch JH: Response of patients after myocardial infarction to carrying a graded series of weight loads. Am J Cardiol 52:698, 1983

127. Sheldahl LM, Wilke NA, Tristani FE, Kalbfleisch JH: Response to repetitive static-dynamic exercise in patients with coronary artery disease. J Cardiopulmonary Rehabil 5:139, 1985

128. Lowenthal DT, Stein D, Hare TW et al: The clinical pharmacology of cardiovascular drugs during exercise. J Cardiopulmonary Rehabil 3:829, 1983

129. Wilmore JH: Exercise testing, training and beta-adrenergic blockade. Physician Sportsmed 16:45, 1988

130. Mehta J, Feldman RL, Marx JD, Kelly GA: Systemic, pulmonary, and coronary hemodynamic effects of labetalol in hypertensive subjects. Am J Med 75:32, 1983

131. Opie LH, Sonnenblick EH, Kaplan NM, Thadani U: Beta blocking agents. p. 1. In Opie LH (ed): Drugs for the Heart. Grune & Stratton, Orlando, FL, 1984

132. Stuart RJ, Koyal SN, Lundstrom R et al: Does exercise training alter maximal oxygen uptake in coronary artery disease during long-term beta-adrenergic blockade? J Cardiopulmonary Rehabil 5:410, 1985

133. Agre JC, Leon AS, Hunninghake DB et al: The effects of methyldopa and propranolol on the response to dynamic and static exercise during treatment of mild hypertension in men. J Cardiopulmonary Rehabil 6:214, 1986

134. Hartzell AA, Freund BJ, Jilka SM et al: The effects of beta-adrenergic blockade on ratings of perceived exertion during submaximal exercise before and following endurance training. J Cardiopulmonary Rehabil 6:444, 1986

135. Wilmore JH, Wambsgans KC, Kunkel RC et al: Effects of beta-adrenergic blockade on achievement of the trained state in post-MI patients: Nonselective vs beta$_1$-selective blockers. J Cardiopulmonary Rehabil 10:50, 1990

136. Blood SM, Ades PA: Effects of beta-adrenergic blockade on exercise conditioning in coronary patients: A review. J Cardiopulmonary Rehabil 8:141, 1988

137. Dressendorfer RH, Smith JL, Hollingsworth V et al: Propranolol treatment and the effectiveness of exercise training after myocardial infarction in patients not limited by exertional symptoms: Improved maximal oxygen uptake and high-density lipoprotein cholesterol. J Cardiopulmonary Rehabil 10:409, 1990

138. Wayne VS, Fagan ET, McConachy DL: The effects of isosorbide dinitrate on the exercise test. J Cardiopulmonary Rehabil 7:239, 1987

139. Lehnhard RA, Lehnhard HJ, Kirby TE, Muir WW: Calcium antagonists and skeletal-muscle function in man. J Cardiopulmonary Rehabil 8:45, 1988

140. Cummings DM, Amadio P, Jr, Nelson L, Fitzgerald JM: The role of calcium channel blockers in the treatment of essential hypertension. Arch Intern Med 151:250, 1991

141. MacKeen PC, Franklin BA, Buskirk ER: Eighteen-month follow-up of participants in a physical conditioning program for middle-aged women. Med Sci Sports 10:52, 1978

142. Andrew GM, Oldridge NB, Parker JO et al: Reasons for dropout from exercise programs in post-coronary patients. Med Sci Sports 13:164, 1981

143. Andrew GM, Parker JO: Factors related to dropout of post myocardial infarction patients from exercise programs. Med Sci Sports 11:376, 1979

144. Heinzelmann F, Bagley R: Response to physical activity programs and their effects on health behavior. Public Health Rep 85:905, 1970

145. Oldridge NB, Wicks JR, Hanley C et al: Noncompliance in an exercise rehabilitation program for men who have suffered a myocardial infarction. Can Med Assoc J 118:361, 1978

146. Oldridge NB: Compliance of post myocardial infarction patients to exercise programs. Med Sci Sports 11:373, 1979

147. Franklin BA: Motivating and educating adults to exercise. J Phys Ed Recreation 49:13, 1978

148. Hellerstein HK: Exercise therapy in coronary disease. Bull NY Acad Med 44:1028, 1968

149. Wilhelmsen L, Sanne H, Elmfeldt D et al: A controlled trial of physical training after myocardial infarction: Effects on risk factors, nonfatal reinfarction, and death. Prev Med 4:491, 1975

150. Pollock ML, Gettman LR, Milesis CA: Effects of frequency and duration of training on attrition and incidence of injury. Med Sci Sports 9:31, 1977

151. Kavanagh T, Shephard RJ: Exercise for post coronary patients: An assessment of infrequent supervision. Arch Phys Med Rehabil 61:114, 1980

152. Oldridge NB, Spencer J: Exercise habits and health perceptions after graduating or dropping out of cardiac rehabilitation. Med Sci Sports 15:120, 1983

153. Oldridge NB, Jones NL: Contracting as a strategy to reduce dropout in exercise rehabilitation. Med Sci Sports 13:125, 1981

154. Anderson RJ, Kirk LM: Methods of improving patient compliance in chronic disease states. Arch Intern Med 142:1673, 1982

155. Taylor HL, Buskirk ER, Remington RD: Exercise in controlled trials of the prevention of coronary heart disease. Fed Proc 32:1623, 1973

156. Pyorala K, Karava R, Punsar S et al: A controlled study of the effects of 18 months physical training in sedentary middle-aged men with high indexes of risk relative to coronary heart disease. p. 261. In Larsen OA, Malmborg RO (eds): Coronary Heart Disease and Physical Fitness. University Park Press, Baltimore, 1971

157. Oldridge NB: A program of physical activity for the coronary-prone individual—a seven-year follow-up. Presented at the Human Kinetic Symposium, University of Guelph, Ontario, Canada, 1974

158. Mann GV, Garrett HL, Farki A et al: Exercise to prevent coronary heart disease: An experimental study of the effects of training on risk factors for coronary disease in man. Am J Med 46:12, 1969

159. Bruce EH, Frederick R, Bruce RA et al: Comparison of active participants and dropouts in CAPRI cardiopulmonary rehabilitation programs. Am J Cardiol 37:53, 1976

160. Knapp D, Gutmann M, Squires R et al: Exercise adherence among coronary artery bypass surgery (CABS) patients. Med Sci Sports Exercise 15:120, 1983

161. Sanne H, Rydin C: Feasibility of a physical training program. Acta Med Scand 551(suppl.):59, 1973

162. Gottheiner V: Long-range strenuous sports training for cardiac reconditioning and rehabilitation. Am J Cardiol 22:426, 1968

163. Hossack KF, Hartwick R: Cardiac arrest associated with supervised cardiac rehabilitation. J Cardiac Rehabil 2:402, 1982

164. Haskell WL: Cardiovascular complications during exercise training of cardiac patients. Circulation 57:920, 1978

POPULATIONS WITH SPECIAL NEEDS FOR EXERCISE REHABILITATION

21

Patients with Left Ventricular Dysfunction and Congestive Heart Failure

Nanette K. Wenger, M.D.

Congestive heart failure is not a diagnosis with a specific etiology, but rather is the end stage manifestation of a variety of progressive cardiovascular diseases whose primary effects may be on the coronary arteries, the cardiac valves, or the myocardium. Many patients with compensated congestive heart failure are asymptomatic at rest, but characteristically develop exertional dyspnea and/or fatigue with progressive levels of activity. This premature onset of exertional symptoms limits their tolerance for physical activity.[1] Activity intolerance occurs gradually and progressively; thus, the patient's perception of exercise impairment, as described by the New York Heart Association functional classification based on the symptomatic response to "usual" levels of activity, may be misleading. As habitual levels of physical activity progressively decline, the patient's perception of the intensity of "usual" physical activity decreases concomitantly; the Specific Activity Scale may provide a more reproducible assessment of functional status.[2] The patient's functional capacity is determined by the extent of cardiac dysfunction and the resulting beneficial and unfavorable compensatory adjustments.[1]

During the past decade, newer medical therapies have not only alleviated disabling symptoms of patients with congestive heart failure but also favorably altered the prior generally poor prognosis.[3–5] These include treatment with nitrate drugs and hydralazine[4] and with angiotensin-converting enzyme inhibitors[5]; these vasodilator drugs, often added to therapy with digitalis and diuretics, have improved both symptomatic and functional status, slowed cardiac deterioration, and modestly prolonged survival.[6] Vasodilator therapy was based on an improved understanding of the compensatory mechanisms in congestive heart failure; these drugs are designed to modify the deleterious neurohumoral responses to the low cardiac output state engendered by depressed cardiac function that result in peripheral vasoconstriction and sodium retention.

Although dramatic short-term symptomatic improvement has been described in patients with severe heart failure treated with nondigitalis positive inotropic agents, particularly the phosphodiesterase inhibitors that effect both a positive inotropic and a vasodilator response, this class of drugs has not improved the prognosis and indeed may shorten survival. Accumulating evidence suggests that the failing heart responds better to vasodilator therapy, which decreases energy expenditure, than to positive inotropic agents, which may worsen the prognosis either by increasing myocardial energy demands or by exacerbating cardiac arrhythmias.[7]

Labetalol, a combined alpha- and beta-block-

403

ing drug, improved symptoms, exercise capacity, and exercise hemodynamics (increased cardiac output and decreased systemic vascular resistance) in a short-term study of patients with idiopathic dilated cardiomyopathy.[8]

Thus, appropriate contemporary goals in the management of patients with congestive heart failure include both the alleviation of disabling symptoms and the prolongation of survival. The quality of that survival and the patient's functional status can be enhanced by rehabilitative care.

PATHOPHYSIOLOGIC MECHANISMS IN CONGESTIVE HEART FAILURE

The decreased cardiac output of the patient with severe left ventricular dysfunction (ejection fraction < 30%) and chronic congestive heart failure stimulates both the renin-angiotensin-aldosterone system and the sympathetic nervous system. The compensatory vasoconstriction and increase in systemic vascular resistance may both limit cardiac performance and diminish the delivery of blood and oxygen to exercising muscle. Peripheral vasoconstriction and sodium retention increase the work load on the already impaired ventricle, promoting the progressive downward spiral of heart failure. Often tachycardia and elevation of the pulmonary capillary wedge pressure occur even at rest. Atrial natriuretic peptide and other natriuretic substances can promote vasodilatation and sodium excretion in the early stages of heart failure, but appear inadequate to counteract the peripheral vasoconstriction and sodium retention with advanced congestive heart failure.

In addition to the cardiac hemodynamic abnormalities, a number of peripheral mechanisms, including impaired vasodilator ability and altered skeletal muscle metabolism, determine the symptoms of congestive heart failure. When cardiac output is reduced, regional changes in blood flow selectively direct the limited cardiac output to the heart and brain. Patients with heart failure have impairment of blood flow and oxygen de-

livery to exercising skeletal muscle; abnormal regional regulation of blood flow may further limit skeletal muscle circulation. Many manifestations of heart failure probably relate to the diversion of blood flow from skeletal muscle, but factors regulating regional blood flow remain poorly understood.

Symptoms of activity intolerance and limitation of exercise capacity are the hallmarks of heart failure; most of these appear related to altered skeletal muscle metabolism, resulting in a low anaerobic threshold,[9,10] rather than to the severity of the ventricular dysfunction or indexes of resting and exertional hemodynamic abnormalities. Some patients maintain a normal exercise capacity despite severely impaired ventricular systolic function. Hypoperfusion of skeletal muscle may be due to abnormalities of regional blood flow, intrinsic skeletal muscle abnormalities,[11] or excess sympathetic stimulation or stimulation of the renin-angiotensin-aldosterone mechanism.

RESPONSE TO EXERCISE OF PATIENTS WITH CONGESTIVE HEART FAILURE

The response to exercise of patients with congestive heart failure is also discussed in Chapter 6.

In prior years, exercise testing and training were not recommended for patients with chronic congestive heart failure and severe left ventricular systolic dysfunction because of concern of adverse responses including arrhythmias, angina pectoris in coronary patients, and exacerbation of the severity of the ventricular dysfunction. Data acquired during the past decade suggest that most patients with congestive heart failure appear to tolerate exercise testing with few complications[12]; also, complications have not been prominent during the exercise training of selected patients with heart failure, even when severe ventricular dysfunction was present. However, the response to exercise varies substantially.

The symptomatic endpoints of dyspnea and of fatigue lead to the premature termination of exercise. However, hemodynamic data (including peak pulmonary capillary wedge pressure) cannot differentiate patients with heart failure who terminate their exercise because of dyspnea from those whose exercise endpoint is fatigue. The exercise capacity of patients with severe left ventricular systolic dysfunction correlates poorly with measures of ventricular preload or afterload.

Dyspnea, previously attributed to increased left atrial pressure, does not correlate directly with elevation of the pulmonary capillary wedge pressure. At any level of exercise, the patient with heart failure has an increased level of ventilation.[13] Breathing is shallow and rapid with increased ventilation of the dead space, and an increase in minute ventilation maintains adequate alveolar ventilation. Associated with this is the increased work of breathing as a result of abnormal pulmonary compliance. Ventilation and effort tolerance both appear more related to the pulmonary capillary wedge pressure at rest than at peak exercise. Patients with heart failure have maximal oxygen extraction by exercising skeletal muscle in the early stages of exercise, with early transition to anaerobic metabolism; metabolic receptors have been implicated as causing dyspnea.

Because the failing heart cannot increase its cardiac output in response to increasing levels of exercise, fatigue was, in earlier reports, attributed to inadequate tissue perfusion, i.e., lack of nutritive blood flow to exercising skeletal muscle, but fatigue does not relate directly to the decrease in cardiac output and oxygen supply. Inability of the peripheral vasculature to adequately dilate may limit skeletal muscle blood flow, with a resultant change to anaerobic glycolysis and lactate accumulation; metabolic alterations unrelated to hypoxia may also raise lactic acid levels.[14] The resultant increase in lactate levels may contribute to or produce fatigue, as the impairment of blood flow alone is inadequate to explain all the abnormalities.[15] However, reduction in vasodilator capacity was not demonstrated during forearm exercise in patients with severe heart failure.[16] Intracellular acidosis may also contribute to the limited exercise capacity. Thus, fatigue may represent various combinations of alterations in muscular oxidative metabolism, changes in substrate utilization, inadequate vasodilator response, and

abnormalities of autonomic regulation of the circulation, among others.

There is also a change in skeletal muscle type in chronic heart failure, with an increase in fast-twitch, glycolytic, easily fatiguable type IIb fibers and a reduced percentage of slow-twitch type I fibers; the oxidative enzyme capacity also decreases.[9] It is uncertain how much deconditioning due to lack of exercise contributes to these intrinsic alterations in skeletal muscle,[9] although deconditioning is characterized by reduced skeletal muscle mass and strength.

In individuals with normal ventricular function, pulmonary vascular resistance falls in response to exercise; this does not occur in patients with heart failure.[17] Both pulmonary vascular resistance and resting right ventricular ejection fraction correlate with exercise capacity in patients with left ventricular dysfunction and heart failure.[18] Since right ventricular function is substantially afterload-dependent, drugs that dilate the pulmonary vascular bed can improve the exercise tolerance of patients with congestive heart failure.

Maintenance of exercise tolerance in patients with ventricular dysfunction and compensated congestive heart failure relates to several variables: (1) ability to increase heart rate, thereby maintaining cardiac output when stroke volume cannot be further increased, i.e., maintenance of chronotropic competence; (2) ability to tolerate elevation of the pulmonary capillary wedge pressure without experiencing undue dyspnea; (3) capacity to dilate the ventricle to enable an increase in stroke volume; (4) maintenance of right ventricular function[18]; and (5) ability to decrease peripheral vascular resistance in response to upright exercise.

The exercise capacity and exercise endpoints of patients with heart failure also depend substantially on the pace at which physical activity is performed.[19] Although symptoms of dyspnea and fatigue seem characterized by the same hemodynamic abnormalities, some reports show that slow incremental exercise is typically terminated owing to fatigue, whereas dyspnea appears to be the exercise endpoint after rapid increases in exercise workload.[20] Patients with heart failure display substantial differences in oxygen uptake at comparable workloads; these depend significantly on the efficiency of exercising, which can be improved with training.

Even after cardiac transplantation and restoration of a normal or near-normal cardiac output, the exercise tolerance of the patient with prior severe heart failure fails to improve for weeks or months; the mechanism or mechanisms responsible for this delayed response are not yet delineated but may relate to factors that limit blood flow to skeletal muscle.

EVALUATION BY EXERCISE TESTING

Evaluation by exercise testing is also discussed in Chapters 7–10.

Cardiopulmonary exercise testing is increasingly used in the evaluation of patients with congestive heart failure when appropriate monitoring conditions and qualified personnel are available. In addition to assessing the severity of the cardiocirculatory impairment, exercise testing provides an objective, replicable, and safe measure of activity tolerance; enables evaluation of the responses to pharmacotherapy; and determines the change in functional capacity resulting from exercise rehabilitation and other therapeutic interventions.[21] Exercise testing before and after pharmacotherapy is of value in evaluating the functional impact of these agents on patients with congestive heart failure. Testing also permits differentiation of cardiac and pulmonary limitations to exercise.

Despite earlier concerns about the safety of exercise testing in patients with ventricular dysfunction and chronic heart failure, complications of repeated exercise testing were minimal in patients with stable congestive heart failure in the Veterans Administration Cooperative Study–Vasodilator Heart Failure Trial.[12] There were no major adverse effects during almost 3,000 tests in 607 patients; exercise-induced hypotension was rare, even after the application of vasodilator therapy. Ventricular arrhythmias were also uncommon, with exercise testing terminated in

fewer than 2% of patients because of this complication.

The optimal method for the exercise testing of patients with heart failure is not known; indeed, different methods of exercise testing may be preferable for different purposes. Modification of the usual exercise test protocol may provide more information about the severely impaired patient, particularly initiating the graded exercise test at very low intensity and providing small increments of increase in work demand, often 1 MET of exercise per work load. Rest periods between exercise stages, i.e., an intermittent exercise test protocol, may permit the test to be terminated as a result of cardiorespiratory endpoints rather than local muscle fatigue. Additionally, an adequate exercise duration may be attained to enable differentiation between levels of exercise limitation and improvement by therapeutic interventions.[22] As an example, exercise testing to evaluate the ability of a patient with compensated congestive heart failure to return to work (or, conversely, to determine whether the impairment is too great for this to be accomplished, as in disability determinations) may be best done by an intermittent test protocol that more nearly mimics activities at work. However, intermittent testing may not be feasible for arm test protocols, as the resistance in some arm-testing systems to be overcome in initiating higher levels of arm exercise may discourage patients from attempting the next step or stage.

Data derived from exercise testing, however, may not predictably reflect the extent to which performance of usual daily activities is limited by exercise-related symptoms. The termination of exercise testing usually is based on the occurrence of severe symptoms, whereas more modest symptoms typically induce cessation of usual daily activities. Further, many exercise test protocols involve continuous work of progressive intensity, whereas the performance of usual daily activities, particularly in patients with ventricular dysfunction, is intermittent and is characterized by marked variations in pace and in intensity.

Whereas a continuous exercise test protocol, even with small incremental increases in exercise intensity, may adequately measure the maximal exercise performance, it is uncertain whether small benefits from a therapeutic intervention can be readily detected. Also, for patients with heart failure who have a reasonable exercise tolerance, the need to perform a large number of exercise steps or stages with small increments of intensity may engender muscle fatigue, generating an endpoint that does not represent a cardiovascular limitation.

The addition of respiratory gas analyses may complement the exercise testing; measurement of lactate levels can also be helpful. Although there is reasonable correlation of exercise duration with oxygen consumption, exercise duration can be increased at repeated exercise testing, owing to an increased efficiency of exercising, without a corresponding increase in work load.

There is great variability in the relationship between the exercise capacity as objectively determined at exercise testing and the degree of impairment of resting left ventricular systolic function (ejection fraction)[23–24]; factors contributing to this variability in exercise performance are not well delineated. However, the maximal oxygen uptake (as determined at exercise testing) and the left ventricular ejection fraction appear as independent prognostic variables in patients with congestive heart failure.[4] Neither is there direct correlation among other hemodynamic measurements at rest, i.e., cardiac output, diastolic volume, or pulmonary capillary wedge pressure and exercise tolerance; nor do these correlate with the clinical classification of functional status by symptoms. Inadequate oxygen delivery to working muscle, rather than central hemodynamic abnormalities, contributes significantly to fatigue and diminished exercise capacity[25]; however, as previously noted, the factors regulating blood flow to skeletal muscle require investigation.

When functional capacity is based on exercise testing, patients with congestive heart failure in exercise class I (no functional impairment) have a maximal oxygen uptake in excess of 20 ml/kg/min; those in exercise class II (mild functional impairment) have an uptake of 15 to 19.9 ml/kg/min; those in exercise class III (moderate functional impairment) have an uptake of 10 to 14.9 ml/kg/min; and those in exercise class IV (severe functional impairment) have an uptake below 10 ml/kg/min.[26]

Further, many cardiac medications that improve symptoms of heart failure (e.g., digitalis glycosides, dopamine, and dobutamine) do not improve exercise capacity. Despite improvement in the hemodynamic response to exercise with the *acute* administration of these drugs and with a variety of vasodilator agents (e.g., hydralazine, prazosin, nitrate drugs, etc.), these also fail to improve exercise tolerance acutely. Exercise capacity appears to improve with the *chronic* administration of nitrate and other vasodilator drugs; one suggested mechanism is that the decrease in symptoms encourages a spontaneous increase in physical activity that results in a training effect.[27]

There has been continued interest in the anaerobic threshold at exercise testing, the point of increase in the lactate and ventilatory responses to increasing exercise. Anaerobic threshold has been defined either as the oxygen uptake beyond which the lactate concentration increases consistently above resting values or as the point beyond which the ventilatory equivalent for oxygen ($\dot{V}E/\dot{V}O_2$) increases without an increase in the ventilatory equivalent for carbon dioxide ($\dot{V}E/\dot{V}CO_2$).[14]

Lactate production may increase in response to exercise without a change in blood lactate levels, as a result of changes in metabolism and clearance. The lactate threshold can also be influenced by habitual activity level, independent of changes in circulatory function; inactivity decreases the lactate threshold, whereas exercise training can increase lactate clearance without a change in lactate production. Additionally, oxygen consumption can change without an associated change in the anaerobic threshold; this may reflect a change in patient motivation to exercise rather than an absolute change in functional capacity. Lactate production can also occur under fully aerobic conditions, dependent on recruitment of fast-twitch muscle fibers and differences in substrate utilization. Although the anaerobic threshold is a good measure of submaximal exercise tolerance in healthy individuals, this concept has been challenged for patients with heart failure in whom the anaerobic threshold occurs earlier. Nevertheless, beyond this threshold, which may have multiple determinants in patients with heart failure, further physical activity results in rapid exhaustion.

RESPONSE TO EXERCISE TRAINING: SEVERE SYSTOLIC LEFT VENTRICULAR DYSFUNCTION

The mechanisms underlying the improvement in exercise cardiac output in patients with congestive heart failure may vary depending on the etiology of the heart failure. Improved exercise tolerance results from increased maximal blood flow to exercising muscle, improved muscle vasodilatation, and avoidance of deconditioning.[8] When the underlying disease is cardiomyopathy, the increase in cardiac output appears due predominantly to an increase in stroke volume, with little or no change in ventricular end-diastolic volume. In the patient with coronary heart disease, there is little change in ejection fraction, with the improved cardiac output enabled by an increase in left ventricular end-diastolic and systolic diameters.[28] The decrease in myocardial oxygen demand in response to exercise training evident at any submaximal work level is due to the lower double product, i.e., decrease in the heart rate and systolic blood pressure responses to exercise. As previously stated, the mechanism of functional improvement in response to training relates predominantly to peripheral adaptations that enable an increase in peak blood flow to exercising muscle and an improvement in the oxidative capacity of trained skeletal muscle with increased peripheral oxygen extraction. This is predominantly a muscle-specific effect, although maximal oxygen uptake also increases with training. The decrease in myocardial oxygen demand can lessen exercise-induced myocardial ischemia in patients whose etiology of heart failure is coronary heart disease and ischemic ventricular dysfunction.

Small study populations, heterogeneity of causes and severities of heart failure, frequent lack of control groups, and different exercise interventions limit generalizations about results of exercise training.[29–30]

Exercise training of patients with a very low ejection fraction can produce a peak increase in exercise oxygen consumption of about 20%, with increases in work load and in peak heart rate also described. Lean body mass may increase. The muscle myoglobin level increases. Alterations in skeletal muscle mitochondria and increased aerobic enzyme content enable more efficient use of energy substrates. This capacity to increase peripheral oxygen extraction is attenuated with aging, so that elderly patients with congestive heart failure can be expected to have greater exercise intolerance because of limitation of this compensatory response.

Therefore, most exercise-related adaptations are considered to be primarily or exclusively due to peripheral mechanisms, because little or no improvement in ventricular function is generally described. There is no significant change in central hemodynamic parameters at rest as a result of exercise training of patients with heart failure: no change in stroke volume, left ventricular ejection fraction, cardiac index, cardiac volumes, mean arterial pressure, pulmonary capillary wedge pressure, or intracardiac pressures. The increase in arteriovenous oxygen difference reflects a redistribution of blood flow; the relative contributions of the vasodilator capacity of exercising muscle versus the vasoconstriction in nonexercising muscle or other vascular beds are uncertain and may vary with different classes of cardiovascular drugs used to treat heart failure.

There is no significant change in exercising-leg blood flow with training, except at peak exercise; however, there is a substantial training-induced decrease in lactate production, reflecting an increased capacity for aerobic metabolism at any given muscle blood flow; the ventilatory anaerobic threshold is increased. This increase in anaerobic threshold is associated with improved exercise performance, because most daily activities involve submaximal exercise levels. Additionally, there is an improved exercise duration at a fixed submaximal level, with decreased resting and submaximal exercise heart rate responses and a decreased respiratory exchange ratio (RER).[29] RER may be a good way to quantify functional capacity in patients with chronic heart failure. The catecholamine response to exercise also appears to decrease with training; exercise training produces an overall reduction in sympathetic stimulation, which may then decrease renin and resultant vascular tone and vasoconstriction, increasing the capacity for vascular redistribution with exercise. The decrease in resting heart rate also may be due to decreased sympathetic tone, with up-regulation of beta receptors.

An increase in peak $\dot{V}O_2$ is frequently associated with an improved exercise capacity; however, some pharmacologic interventions can improve exercise duration without improving peak $\dot{V}O_2$. One explanation is that improved peripheral (muscular) vascular vasodilation with training permits an increase in muscle blood flow at peak exercise, may delay lactate accumulation in skeletal muscle, and allows a longer exercise duration. Thus, exercise training appears to improve peripheral vasodilatation in patients with heart failure, as it does in normal subjects.

Exercise training occurs gradually, over a period of months; there seem to be few arrhythmic complications. A significant training effect can be safely achieved in patients with substantial systolic dysfunction without an apparent adverse effect on left ventricular geometry and volumes.[29,31–33] Although there is no gross adverse effect on left ventricular function, deterioration of ventricular function has been reported in patients with recent large anterior myocardial infarction who undergo early exercise training.[34,35] Some reports[17,30] suggest that, in addition to peripheral adaptations to exercise training, central hemodynamic adaptations may occur with longer-term, higher-intensity exercise training of patients with well-compensated ventricular dysfunction, resulting in increases in peak cardiac output. The capacity for central adaptation appears dependent on the severity of myocardial failure in that exercise training has been found to increase ventricular volume and cause myocardial hypertrophy in some patients with mild or moderate ventricular dysfunction. The long-term effects of exercise training on morbidity and mortality in patients with heart failure remain unknown. Also unknown is whether patients with severe ischemic or unstable heart failure syndromes should participate in exercise training.

VASODILATOR DRUG THERAPY AND EXERCISE CAPACITY

Vasodilator drug therapy and exercise capacity are also discussed in Chapter 16.

Vasodilator drug therapy is undertaken to reverse the excessive compensatory vasoconstriction that limits cardiac performance and decreases the delivery of blood to exercising muscle in patients with chronic congestive heart failure. Vasodilator drugs decrease ventricular filling pressures as well. Although most vasodilator drugs improve the symptomatic status and produce hemodynamic benefit at rest in patients with congestive heart failure, the activity-related symptoms and the improvement in exercise capacity may be significantly influenced by the type of vasodilator drug used.[3,23,26,27,36–38] A confounding feature is that any therapy that improves the symptoms of heart failure both at rest and with exercise is likely to encourage an increased spontaneous activity level among patients so treated; the training effect that results from this spontaneous activity, characteristically begun by previously sedentary patients, may also improve the vasodilator capacity of exercising muscle and increase skeletal muscle oxidative enzymes.

Different mechanisms of vasodilatation result from different classes of vasodilator drugs. Vasodilator preparations that act directly on arteriolar smooth muscle, independent of the mechanism producing vasoconstriction, such as hydralazine and the calcium entry-blocking drugs, decrease the work load on the left ventricle by generalized vasodilatation to counteract the excessive compensatory vasoconstrictive response to congestive heart failure. However, the normal response to exercise involves vasoconstriction in the renal and splanchnic vascular beds, effecting an exercise-induced redistribution of cardiac output to provide optimal blood flow to exercising muscle. This important adaptation is limited by nonspecific vasodilator drugs that do not permit these regional changes in blood flow to occur and thereby engender suboptimal delivery of blood to exercising muscle. Vascular alpha-adrenergic vasoconstriction appears to be the most important mechanism enabling the redistribution of blood flow with exercise; therefore, alpha-adrenergic-blocking vasodilator drugs, such as prazosin, result in generalized vasodilatation and an increased need for cardiac output; energy is wasted in perfusing the viscera during exercise, with a resultant lack or limitation of improvement in the exercise capacity of patients with congestive heart failure treated with this type of vasodilator preparation.

Administration of angiotensin-converting enzyme inhibitor drugs counteracts the excessive compensatory vasoconstriction of heart failure by decreasing the levels of angiotensin II, vasopressin, and norepinephrine, thereby producing vasodilatation. This mechanism does not impede the normal regulation of sympathetic control of vascular tone during exercise and permits an increase in blood flow to exercising skeletal muscle and limitation of blood flow to the viscera during exercise. This difference may, at least in part, explain the dramatic improvement in exercise capacity of patients with congestive heart failure treated with angiotensin-converting enzyme inhibitors.[39] Favorable improvements in left ventricular pressure–volume relationships during diastole are described as well.

Although positive inotropic agents may improve myocardial contractility in patients with heart failure, the inotropic effect may be desirable only during activity; in patients so treated who are asymptomatic at rest, an unnecessary increase in cardiac work is effected at rest.

GUIDELINES FOR EXERCISE TRAINING

Protracted bed rest is no longer the recommended approach to treating patients with congestive heart failure, as deconditioning unfavorably alters vascular reactivity and skeletal muscle oxidative capacity, among others. Usual well-tolerated activities are not restricted once heart failure has been stabilized, and there is increasing application of prescriptive exercise training for appropriately selected patients, designed to enhance their activity tolerance. Both the safety and benefits[40] of exercise training for

patients with ventricular dysfunction and congestive heart failure have substantially exceeded the initial expectations.[41]

Reports of exercise rehabilitation, undertaken by small groups of selected patients with moderate to severe congestive heart failure of various etiologies, document that functional aerobic capacity is frequently improved. However, no pre-training variables have yet been identified that can predict which patients with heart failure will benefit from exercise training. Although considerable exercise supervision was usual in the initial phase of exercise training, exercise-related complications were limited, even with subsequent unsupervised exercise, and the training effected a substantial improvement both in exercise duration and in peak oxygen consumption,[29] as well as in oxygen extraction from the blood during exercise. Although neither the resting nor the exercise left ventricular ejection fraction improved with exercise, deterioration of ventricular function was generally not encountered,[29,42–43] even among patients with ventricular aneurysm.[42]

In stable patients with a low functional capacity, exercise training should involve a longer duration of low-intensity exercise, with consideration of greater frequency of exercise as well.[44] Several features that appear to determine the safety of exercise training for patients with ventricular dysfunction and compensated congestive heart failure include the stability of the cardiovascular status; the severity and the etiology of the underlying cardiovascular disease; the occurrence and complexity of ventricular arrhythmias; the proximity of undertaking training to an acute event, particularly in patients with coronary heart disease; and the intensity of the exercise training. The safety of home-based training was cited in a small, controlled, randomized trial involving patients with ischemic ventricular dysfunction without arrhythmias at exercise testing.[33]

Initially, a 5- or 10-minute session each day may be optimal, with the duration of exercise increased before the exercise intensity is augmented. Warm-up and cool-down periods should be prolonged. Interval training is often advisable. Improvement in physical work capacity has been effected by this long-term, low-intensity exercise training, a regimen that is within the ability and the safety guidelines for most patients with chronic congestive heart failure. Patients with heart failure should limit their food intake before exercise. Weight loss to near ideal body weight is an added factor in improving exercise capacity. Blood pressure control should be serially evaluated. Alcohol intake should be avoided as it can further depress myocardial contractility.

EFFECTS OF EXERCISE REHABILITATION

Exercise capacity, symptoms, functional class, and $\dot{V}o_2$ max can be improved safely by exercise training, even in patients with significant ventricular systolic dysfunction.[33] Clinical benefit appears sustained, but often requires a more protracted training period than for patients without congestive heart failure. A variety of adaptations in cardiac function, skeletal muscle, the circulatory system, and the nervous system may result from exercise training to effect this improved exercise capacity. Severely impaired patients benefit from exercise training by being better able to tolerate daily-life activities; despite the relatively small absolute increases in exercise performance, the relative improvements that occur in severely functionally impaired patients are sizable.[33] Psychosocial benefits are also described. The improvement in quality of life described with exercise training appears associated both with an actual improvement in exercise tolerance and with an improved perception of personal health status.

Other components of the training effect include a lower heart rate for a comparable work intensity, without deterioration of ejection fraction or end-diastolic volume. Therefore, exercise training in patients with severe left ventricular dysfunction can improve cardiovascular fitness without associated adverse responses. Although the safety of this intervention is increasingly established, the mechanisms by which training improves exercise capacity are only incompletely understood. Mechanisms of benefit also require

delineation in terms of whether they differ with age, gender, or etiology of the ventricular dysfunction, among others.

It remains uncertain whether patients with different etiologies of ventricular dysfunction have comparable responses to exercise training. Neither is it known whether the etiology of the heart failure influences the risk of exercise-related malignant ventricular arrhythmias. The optimal modes, intensity, duration, and surveillance of exercise training have yet to be determined, as have the guidelines for surveillance and electrocardiographic (ECG) monitoring of this training. The relationship of exercise training to the varied drug therapies for congestive heart failure has had only limited examination to identify potential exercise–drug interactions. Importantly, the long-term functional and prognostic outcomes of exercise training must be ascertained; in addition to the effects of exercise training on morbidity and mortality, the effect on ventricular geometry and other aspects of ventricular function must be examined.

The goals of management of patients with chronic congestive heart failure include improvement in symptomatic status and enhancement of functional capabilities. Exercise training, predominantly because of peripheral adaptations, can decrease activity-related symptoms and improve physical work capacity.

REFERENCES

1. Jennings GL, Esler MD: Circulatory regulation at rest and exercise and the functional assessment of patients with congestive heart failure. Circulation 81(suppl. II):II-5,1990
2. Goldman L, Cook EF, Mitchell N et al: Pitfalls in the serial assessment of cardiac functional status. How a reduction in "ordinary" activity may reduce the apparent degree of cardiac compromise and give a misleading impression of improvements. J Chron Dis 35:763, 1982
3. The Captopril-Digoxin Multicenter Research Group: Comparative effects of therapy with captopril and digoxin in patients with mild to moderate heart failure. JAMA 259:539, 1988
4. Cohn JN, Archibald DG, Ziesche S et al: Effect of

vasodilator therapy on mortality in chronic congestive heart failure. Results of a Veterans Administration Cooperative Study. N Engl J Med 314:1547, 1986

5. The CONCENSUS Trial Study Group: Effects of enalapril on mortality in severe congestive heart failure. Results of the Cooperative North Scandinavian Enalapril Survival Study (CONCENSUS). N Engl J Med 316:1429, 1987

6. Pfeffer MA, Lamas GA, Vaughan DE et al: Effect of captopril on progressive ventricular dilatation after anterior myocardial infarction. N Engl J Med 319:80, 1988

7. Uretsky BF, Jessup M, Konstam MA et al, for the Enoximone Multicenter Trial Group: Multicenter trial of oral enoximone in patients with moderate to moderately severe congestive heart failure. Lack of benefit compared with placebo. Circulation 82:774, 1990

8. Leung WH, Lau CP, Wong CK et al: Improvement in exercise performance and hemodynamics by labetalol in patients with idiopathic dilated cardiomyopathy. Am Heart J 119:884, 1990

9. Sullivan MJ, Green HJ, Cobb FR: Skeletal muscle biochemistry and histology in ambulatory patients with long-term chronic heart failure. Circulation 81:518, 1990

10. Cohen-Solal A for the VO$_2$ French Study Group: Improving exercise tolerance in patients with chronic heart failure: Should we treat the heart or the periphery? Eur Heart J 10:866, 1989

11. Mancini DM, Coyle E, Coggan A et al: Contribution of intrinsic skeletal muscle changes to ^{31}P NMR skeletal muscle metabolic abnormalities in patients with chronic heart failure. Circulation 80:1338, 1989

12. Tristani FE, Hughes CV, Archibald DG et al, for the VA Cooperative Study: Safety of graded symptom-limited exercise testing in patients with congestive heart failure. Circulation 76(suppl. VI):VI-54, 1987

13. Sullivan MJ, Higginbotham MB, Cobb FR: Increased exercise ventilation in patients with chronic heart failure: Intact ventilatory control despite hemodynamic and pulmonary abnormalities. Circulation 77:552, 1988

14. Tavazzi L, Gattone M, Corra U, De Vito F: The anaerobic index: Uses and limitations in the assessment of heart failure. Cardiology 76:357, 1989

15. Massie BM, Conway M, Rajagopalan B et al: Skeletal muscle metabolism during exercise under ischemic conditions in congestive heart failure. Evidence for abnormalities unrelated to blood flow. Circulation 78:320, 1988

16. Arnold JMO, Ribeiro JP, Colucci WS: Muscle blood flow during forearm exercise in patients with severe heart failure. Circulation 82:465, 1990

17. Sullivan MJ, Knight JD, Higginbotham MB, Cobb FR: Relation between central and peripheral hemodynamics during exercise in patients with chronic heart failure: Muscle blood flow is reduced with maintenance of arterial perfusion pressure. Circulation 80:769, 1989

18. Baker BJ, Wilen MM, Boyd CM et al: Relation of right ventricular ejection fraction to exercise capacity in chronic left ventricular failure. Am J Cardiol 54:596, 1984

19. Feinstein AR, Joseph BR, Wells CK: Scientific and clinical problems in indexes of functional disability. Ann Intern Med 81:641, 1986

20. Lipkin DP, Canepa-Anson R, Stephens MR, Poole-Wilson PA: Factors determining symptoms in chronic heart failure: comparison of fast and slow exercise tests. Br Heart J 55:439, 1986

21. Wilson JR: Exercise and the failing heart. Cardiol Clin 5:171, 1987

22. Wenger NK, Frishman WR, Tanaka T et al: Exercise testing of patients with low functional capacity: continuous vs intermittent test protocol. In preparation

23. Franciosa JA: Epidemiologic patterns, clinical evaluation, and long-term prognosis in chronic congestive heart failure. Am J Med 80(suppl. 2B):14, 1986

24. Guyatt GH: Methodologic problems in clinical trials in heart failure. J Chron Dis 38:353, 1985

25. Roubin GS, Anderson SD, Shen WF et al: Hemodynamic and metabolic basis of impaired exercise tolerance in patients with severe left ventricular dysfunction. J Am Coll Cardiol 15:986, 1990

26. Franciosa JA: Exercise testing in chronic congestive heart failure. Am J Cardiol 53:1447, 1984

27. Leier CV, Huss P, Magorien RD, Unverferth DV: Improved exercise capacity and differing arterial and venous tolerance during chronic isosorbide dinitrate therapy for congestive heart failure. Circulation 67:817, 1983

28. Shen WF, Roubin GS, Hirasawa K et al: Left ventricular volume and ejection fraction response to exercise in chronic heart failure: differences between dilated cardiomyopathy and previous myocardial infarction. Am J Cardiol 55:1027, 1985

29. Sullivan MJ, Higginbotham MB, Cobb FR: Exercise training in patients with severe left ventricular dysfunction. Hemodynamic and metabolic effects. Circulation 78:506, 1988

30. Ehsani AA: Adaptations to training in patients with exercise-induced left ventricular dysfunction. Adv Cardiol 34:148, 1986

31. Kellermann JJ, Ben-Ari E, Fisman E et al: Physical training in patients with ventricular impairment. Benefits/limitations—open questions. Adv Cardiol 34:131, 1986

32. Hoffman A, Duba J, Lengyel M, Majer K: The effect of training on the physical working capacity of MI patients with left ventricular dysfunction. Eur Heart J 8(suppl. G):43, 1987

33. Coats AJS, Adamopoulos S, Meyer TE et al: Effects of physical training in chronic heart failure. Lancet 335:63, 1990

34. Judgutt BI, Michorowski BL, Kappagoda CT: Exercise training after anterior Q wave myocardial infarction: Importance of regional left ventricular function and topography. J Am Coll Cardiol 12:362, 1988

35. Iskandrian AS: Exercise training after anterior Q wave myocardial infarction: harmful or beneficial? J Am Coll Cardiol 12:373, 1988

36. Captopril Multicenter Research Group: A placebo-controlled trial of captopril in refractory chronic congestive heart failure. J Am Coll Cardiol 2:755, 1983

37. Lipkin DP: The role of exercise testing in chronic heart failure. Br Heart J 58:559, 1987

38. Engel PJ: Effort intolerance in chronic heart failure: What are we treating? J Am Cardiol 15:995, 1990

39. Tan LB: Clinical and research implications of new concepts in the assessment of cardiac pumping performance in heart failure. Cardiovasc Res 21:615, 1987

40. Shabetai R: Beneficial effects of exercise training in compensated heart failure. Circulation 78:775, 1988

41. Dubach P, Froelicher VF: Cardiac rehabilitation for heart failure patients. Cardiology 76:368, 1989

42. Giordano A, Giannuzzi P, Tavazzi L: Feasibility of physical training in post-infarct patients with left ventricular aneurysm: a haemodynamic study. Eur Heart J 9(suppl. F):11, 1988

43. Cobb FR, Williams RS, McEwan P et al: Effects of exercise training on ventricular function in patients with recent myocardial infarction. Circulation 66:100, 1982

44. Mathes P: Physical training in patients with ventricular dysfunction: choice and dosage of physical exercise in patients with pump dysfunction. Eur Heart J 9(suppl. F):67, 1988

POPULATIONS WITH SPECIAL NEEDS FOR EXERCISE REHABILITATION

22

Elderly Coronary Patients

Nanette K. Wenger, M.D.

HABITUAL PHYSICAL ACTIVITY OF ELDERLY INDIVIDUALS

Many elderly persons, often unintentionally, decrease their habitual levels of physical activity as a result of combinations of musculoskeletal instability; concomitant illnesses; decreased muscular mass and contractile strength; peripheral vascular disease; cardiovascular symptoms; anxiety, depression, and/or loss of motivation; and inappropriate admonitions from family, friends, and medical personnel. This decreased level of physical activity threatens their continued independent living[1] and potentiates anxiety and depression, which may result in a further decrease in activity levels. In addition to the inactivity-related deconditioning and cardiac limitations to exercise capacity, the physical activity of elderly coronary patients can be further adversely affected by arthritis and other orthopedic problems; decreased pulmonary function; neurologic problems; nutritional deficiencies; psychological problems; and a distorted perception of exertion,[2] among others. Despite the decrease in pulmonary function with aging, ventilatory factors do not limit physical work capacity in the absence of coexisting lung disease. This decrease in habitual physical activity is greater among elderly women than elderly men; with the comparable occurrence of myocardial infarction among men and women in the seventh and eighth decades, elderly women with coronary disease must be en-couraged to participate in exercise rehabilitation to maintain and enhance their exercise capacity. Teaching energy-conserving techniques for household work constitutes an added feature of rehabilitation for both elderly men and women with symptomatic coronary heart disease who have residual functional impairment following a coronary event.

CHANGES IN CARDIOVASCULAR STRUCTURE AND FUNCTION AND IN THE CARDIOVASCULAR RESPONSE TO EXERCISE IN THE ELDERLY

Among the cardiovascular changes of aging that contribute to the decreased habitual physical activity level of elderly individuals is the age-related decrease in aerobic capacity. The performance of any submaximal task is perceived as requiring increased work because it entails a greater percentage of the lowered functional capacity, i.e., an increased relative energy cost. However, this decrease in maximal oxygen uptake in elderly populations is not as pronounced as previously described, when maximal oxygen uptake values are corrected for the decreased lean body mass characteristic of aging.[3] The extent of the decrease in muscle mass related to

415

aging per se and that due to inactivity and a relatively sedentary lifestyle remains uncertain; nevertheless, reversal of the sedentary lifestyle, even among the very elderly, can increase muscle mass, maximal oxygen uptake, and resultant functional status, retarding the age-related decline in aerobic capacity.[1,4] Even among frail nonagenarians in a nursing home, high-intensity resistance exercises produced a substantial increase in muscle mass and strength and in functional mobility[5]; however, these improvements rapidly regressed on cessation of the strength training. The decreased compliance of the aged ventricle, which limits early diastolic filling, may further contribute to exercise-induced dyspnea, even at low intensities of exercise,[6] causing elderly individuals to further overestimate the intensity of their activity. Finally, the increased work of breathing characteristic of the aging lung additionally enhances the perception of a greater work intensity demand of any submaximal task. Thus, much of the decrease in cardiovascular reserve in elderly populations results from a sedentary lifestyle, rather than from aging per se or disease; almost half of all persons older than age 60 in the United States describe themselves as sedentary.

The cardiovascular response to exercise (see also Ch. 6) also differs between elderly and younger persons. There is an increased dependence on diastolic filling, particularly late diastolic filling, to maintain exercise cardiac output in the elderly. There is also a decreased responsiveness to beta-adrenergic stimulation with aging such that, with advanced age, the increase in exercise cardiac output is not catecholamine-mediated via an increase in heart rate and a decrease in end-systolic volume (as in the young), but places greater reliance on the Frank-Starling mechanism. With aging, there is an accentuated rise in cardiac filling pressures with exercise, as an adjustment to the decreased myocardial distensibility and increased left ventricular mass; both of these latter features place the aging heart at a mechanical disadvantage, rendering it less functionally efficient. The increased filling pressure with exercise contributes to the increase in stroke volume, compensating for the decrease in cardiac compliance. The larger end-diastolic volume enables this increase in stroke volume and

is the major contributor to the enhanced cardiac output needed for exercise.[7]

As in younger coronary patients, the exercise training-induced hemodynamic adaptations are predominantly or exclusively peripheral in origin; substrate needs for exercising muscle are met by improved extraction of oxygen from the perfusing blood by trained muscle (rather than by an increase in blood flow and pressure), with a resultant reduction in cardiac work. The decrease in systemic vascular resistance, coupled with adaptations of skeletal muscle and the autonomic nervous system, decreases the rate–pressure product and thus the myocardial aerobic requirement for any submaximal exercise intensity, characteristic of the activities of daily living. Even following myocardial infarction, the reduction in myocardial oxygen requirement that results from exercise training increases the anginal threshold, lessening the likelihood of the activity-induced angina that often limited everyday activities prior to exercise training. Trained patients function farther from their ischemic threshold in the conduct of daily tasks, with the increase in exercise tolerance enabling increased independence. Because trained elderly coronary patients require a lesser percentage of the increased physical work capacity for the performance of their usual daily activities, improved stamina and endurance are described, because routine activities are accomplished with less fatigue.

Physiologic adaptations to exercise training are comparable in elderly patients recovering from myocardial infarction and those recovering from myocardial revascularization procedures, despite the greater clinical stability and lesser ischemia of the latter group. Even most of the medically complex elderly coronary patients can attain a substantial improvement in physical work capacity as a result of exercise training. Lower intensity, increased frequency, and longer duration exercise training regimens are often needed, with electrocardiographic (ECG) monitoring indicated for selected high-risk patients. This intervention may, nevertheless, prove cost-saving, in that it can increase the ability to perform daily living activities and thereby maintain independent community living, as well as improve the elderly coronary patient's quality of life.

EARLY AMBULATION AFTER MYOCARDIAL INFARCTION AND CORONARY ARTERY BYPASS SURGERY

Early ambulation after myocardial infarction and coronary artery bypass surgery is also discussed in Chapters 12 and 19.

Elderly individuals are particularly susceptible to the adverse effects of continuous bed rest, even for as little as several days. Early mobilization of an elderly patient following a coronary event helps limit or avert the hypovolemia that results from protracted bed rest; this problem typically presents as orthostatic intolerance and reflex tachycardia and underlies the impairment of function when activity is resumed. The gravitational stress of sitting in bed or in a bedside chair for 15 to 20 minutes several times daily, an activity level well tolerated by most elderly patients, provides an adequate orthostatic stimulus to induce neurohumoral adaptive responses and prevent these problems. Walking after a meal was able to reverse the hypotensive effects of digestion in elderly nursing-home residents; this intervention may limit postprandial hypotension and resultant falls.[8] Favorable psychological responses to early ambulation also occur; the demonstration that self-care and limited physical activity do not produce cardiac symptoms provides reassurance and offers promise of maintenance of relative independence.

Stretching and range-of-motion warm-up exercises can be initiated on subsequent days, followed by gradually progressive increases in the pace and distance of walking. The subsequent maintenance of an appropriate level of physical activity requires reenforcement and encouragement, both from the physician and other health professionals and from family and friends.

GUIDELINES FOR EXERCISE TRAINING OF ELDERLY CORONARY PATIENTS

Although in the early years of coronary exercise rehabilitation the age of 65 years or older was arbitrarily considered an exclusion criterion, an ever-increasing proportion of elderly coronary patients are currently enrolled in supervised exercise rehabilitation programs or independent exercise is more frequently recommended by physicians to aid in the recovery of their elderly patients following a coronary event.[9] Regular physical activity is recognized to help maintain physical work capacity into old age. The improvement in aerobic capacity resulting from exercise training of elderly patients is comparable to that characteristic of younger age patients,[10,11] with only modest adaptations and modifications of the exercise prescription, exercise training techniques, and standard program components typically applied to younger coronary patients[12,13] (see also Ch. 20). However, recommendations for activity levels and energy expenditure must include consideration of the cardiovascular changes associated with aging, those related to physical inactivity, and those reflecting the cardiac dysfunction caused by coronary heart disease.

In encouraging the participation of older coronary patients in physical activity regimens, several distinctive features of their responses to activity must be appreciated. A greater emphasis on and more time for warm-up and cool-down activities are appropriate for elderly patients[14]; warm-up activities, which include flexibility and range-of-motion exercises, enable musculoskeletal and cardiorespiratory readiness for exercise. Cool-down activities allow gradual dissipation of the heat load of exercise and subsidence of the exercise-induced peripheral vasodilatation; exercising elderly patients are at greater risk from venous pooling owing to the slower baroreceptor responsiveness with aging. The exercise heart rate returns more gradually to resting values in elderly patients, so that longer rest periods are required between components of exercise or for low-intensity activity when alternated with episodes of higher exercise intensity.

Aerobic training is initially begun at low level, 2 to 3 METs, with gradual increases in intensity and duration to limit discomfort and injury. Exercise training sessions should not engender more problems than mild fatigue. Musculoskeletal complications can be substantially lessened by avoidance of running, jumping, and other high-impact activities. Elderly patients who remain asymptomatic at lower intensities of exercise and who have no contraindications to more strenuous exercise (based on the results of pretraining exercise testing) may progress gradually to higher, albeit still moderate, intensities of activity. The absence of angina cannot be assumed to indicate that exercise-induced myocardial ischemia is not present, in that many elderly patients have asymptomatic ischemia[15]; dyspnea is often an anginal equivalent. Painless ischemia at exercise testing indicates a level of exercise that may prove hazardous during exercise training. An intensity range for exercise training of 60 to 75% of the heart rate safely achieved at recent exercise testing is associated with greater comfort and enjoyment and with fewer musculoskeletal complications than encountered at the 70 to 85% heart rate range. It is also characterized by greater safety during unsupervised exercise and an improved adherence to long-term maintenance exercise training, yet entails an effective stimulus for aerobic metabolism and improved endurance.

Although an ideal exercise regimen for an elderly population has not yet been determined, the exercise undertaken should be dynamic, enjoyable, easily accessible, and without adverse sequelae[16]; brisk regular walking is an excellent prototype of a readily accessible form of exercise for achieving aerobic fitness, with gradual increases recommended in the pace of walking and the distance walked. No special equipment, facilities, exercise skills, or training are required; and walking allows for socialization during exercise as well. Whereas brisk walking requires an insufficient percentage of the maximal oxygen uptake of most younger individuals (except for extremely sedentary persons) to stimulate a training effect, it requires a substantial percentage of the lower maximal oxygen uptake of the aged patient and is therefore an effective and safe physical conditioning stimulus.[17] Arm exercises should be added to the regimen because training of arm muscles is needed to effect improvement in the exercise response to arm work. Strength training, designed to improve muscle function and increase muscle mass, thereby also improving aerobic capacity, is an additional component of value in the exercise rehabilitation of the elderly coronary patient.[14]

The skin blood flow decreases with aging, with resultant lessened efficiency of sweating and temperature regulation during exercise; this warrants reduction of the intensity of exercise for elderly patients in hot or humid environments.[13] Enclosed shopping malls provide ideal sites for walking for elderly coronary patients who do not require supervision of their exercise, as such areas offer a level surface in a temperature- and humidity-controlled environment. Patients can control the intensity of their exercise by pulse counting or by use of the rating of perceived exertion[18]; my preference is for the "talk test," wherein patients are instructed to exercise only to an intensity that will permit them to continue to talk with an exercising companion.

The energy costs of recreational activities determine which of these enjoyable pastimes are appropriately included in recommendations for exercise rehabilitation.[19] For example, an energy cost of only 1 to 2 METs is required for walking at a speed of 1 mile/hr, sewing, knitting, or painting while seated. Activities such as riding a lawn mower, driving a car, light woodworking, and playing the piano and many other musical instruments entail an energy expenditure of 2 to 3 METs. Included in the 3- to 4-MET range are horseshoe pitching, golfing using a golf cart, bowling, and pushing a light lawn mower. Cycling at about 8 miles/hr on level ground, swimming, slow dancing, gardening, and raking leaves are in the 4- to 5-MET range; walking at 4 miles/hr and ice or roller skating are activities in the 5- to 6-MET range that are recommended by the U.S. National Council on Fitness and Aging for elderly coronary patients with a well-preserved exercise capacity. Swimming provides excellent exercise for elderly patients, as the buoyancy of the water may lessen musculoskeletal discomfort.

BENEFITS OF EXERCISE TRAINING FOR ELDERLY CORONARY PATIENTS

The major benefit of exercise training is an improvement in physical work capacity and endurance, which can prolong the duration of an active lifestyle[16] and may retard or obviate disability and dependency and the need for costly custodial care. The enhancement of flexibility, joint mobility, balance, stability, muscle strength and tone, and neuromuscular coordination may lessen the propensity for falls, as well as enabling increased participation in daily activities. Physical fitness appears to be a major determinant of bone mass and density[20]; moderate exercise can retard bone demineralization and resultant osteoporotic fractures,[20] a particularly important consideration for elderly women. Further, participation in an exercise regimen often encourages coronary risk modification (see also Ch. 5) and the increased energy expenditure of exercise can aid in weight control, as well as serving as an adjunct to dietary therapy, especially when giving up smoking. Exercise training is associated with an improvement in self-confidence, sense of well-being, mental relaxation, and self-image and a lessening of anxiety, depression, and loss of motivation[21] (see also Ch. 28); some studies describe an exercise-related improvement in cognitive function and psychomotor speed.[22] Elderly coronary patients who participate in exercise training programs report an increase in leisure activities, an increase in sexual interest and function, better sleep status, and improved optimism; these multifaceted benefits can enhance the quality of life of elderly coronary patients.

Paul Dudley White was a proponent of the benefits of exercise for elderly coronary patients: "... exercise of almost any kind, suitable in degree and duration ... can and does play a useful role in the maintenance of both physical and mental health of the aging individual ..."[23]

EDUCATION AND COUNSELING OF ELDERLY CORONARY PATIENTS

Education and counseling of elderly coronary patients are also discussed in Chapters 25 and 26.

GOALS OF EXERCISE REHABILITATION FOR ELDERLY CORONARY PATIENTS

The rehabilitative goals for elderly coronary patients address limitation of the physical and psychosocial invalidism often associated with coronary heart disease. They include the preservation of physical function (mobility and self-sufficiency) needed for an active way of life; maintenance of mental function (self-respect, self-image, and alertness); limitation of anxiety, depression, and sick role behavior; attainment and maintenance of functional independence; and facilitation of readjustment to and participation in prior community and societal roles.[24] Elderly patients value functional independence; therapies directed to achieve this goal can be both beneficial and cost-effective.

REFERENCES

1. Council on Scientific Affairs: Exercise programs for the elderly. JAMA 252:544, 1984
2. Shephard RJ: Habitual physical activity levels and perception of exertion in the elderly. J Cardiopulmonary Rehabil 9:17, 1989
3. Fleg JL, Lakatta EG: Role of muscle loss in the age-associated reduction in VO_2 max. J Appl Physiol 65:1147, 1988
4. Blumenthal JA, Emery CF, Madden DJ et al: Cardiovascular and behavioral effects of aerobic exercise training in healthy older men and women. J Gerontol 44:M147, 1989
5. Fiatarone MA, Marks EC, Ryan ND et al: High-intensity strength training in nonagenarians. Effects on skeletal muscle. JAMA 263:3029, 1990
6. Lakatta EG: Cardiovascular system aging. p. 199. In Kent B, Butler RN (eds): Human Aging Research: Concepts and Techniques. Raven Press, New York, 1988
7. Weisfeldt M: Left ventricular function. p. 297. In Weisfeldt M (ed): The Aging Heart. Raven Press, New York, 1981
8. Jonsson PV, Lipsitz LA, Kelley M, Koestner J: Hypotensive responses to common daily activities in

institutionalized elderly. A potential risk for recurrent falls. Arch Intern Med 150:1518, 1990

9. Wenger NK: Rehabilitation of the coronary patient: a preview of tomorrow. J Cardiopulmonary Rehabil 11:93, 1991

10. Williams MA, Maresh CM, Aronow WS et al: The value of early out-patient cardiac exercise programmes for the elderly in comparison with other selected age groups. Eur Heart J 5(suppl. E):113, 1984

11. Ades PA, Grunvald MH: Cardiopulmonary exercise testing before and after conditioning in older coronary patients. Am Heart J 120:585, 1990

12. Shephard R: The scientific bases of exercise prescribing for the very old. J Am Geriatr Soc 38:62, 1990

13. William MA, Esterbrooks DJ, Sketch MH: Guidelines for exercise therapy of the elderly after myocardial infarction. Eur Heart J 5(suppl. E):121, 1984

14. Pollock M, Wilmore J (eds): Exercise in Health and Disease: Evaluation and Prescription for Prevention and Rehabilitation. 2nd Ed. WB Saunders, Philadelphia, 1990

15. Gottlieb SO, Gottlieb SH, Achuff SC et al: Silent ischemia on Holter monitoring predicts mortality in high-risk postinfarction patients. JAMA 259:1030, 1988

16. Larson EB, Bruce RA: Exercise and aging. Ann Intern Med 105:783, 1986

17. Bruce RA, Larson EB, Stratton J: Physical fitness, functional aerobic capacity, aging, and responses to physical training or bypass surgery in coronary patients. J Cardiopulmonary Rehabil 9:24, 1989

18. Borg G: Psychophysical bases of perceived exertion. Med Sci Sports Exercise 14:377, 1982

19. Wolfel EE, Hossack KF: Guidelines for the exercise training of elderly healthy individuals and elderly patients with cardiac disease. J Cardiopulmonary Rehabil 9:40, 1989

20. Pocock NA, Eisman JA, Yeates MG et al: Physical fitness is a major determinant of femoral neck and lumbar spine bone mineral density. J Clin Invest 78:618, 1986

21. Taylor CB, Sallis JF, Needle R: The relation of physical activity and exercise to mental health. Public Health Rep 100:195, 1985

22. Dustman RE, Ruhling RO, Russell EM et al: Aerobic exercise training and improved neuropsychological function of older individuals. Neurobiol Aging 5:35, 1984

23. White PD: The role of exercise in the aging. JAMA 165:70, 1957

24. Wenger NK, Marcus FI, O'Rourke RA (eds): 18th Bethesda Conference Report: Cardiovascular disease in the elderly. J Am Coll Cardiol 10(suppl. A):2A, 1987

POPULATIONS WITH SPECIAL NEEDS FOR EXERCISE REHABILITATION

23

Cardiac Transplantation Patients

William L. Haskell, Ph.D.

Cardiac transplantation has become a generally accepted form of therapy for patients with end-stage heart disease. Following the development of more effective medical regimens to detect, prevent, and treat episodes of organ rejection in the early 1980s and the agreement of medical insurors to cover most of the costs of the surgery and postoperative care, cardiac transplantation has been instituted by a number of major medical centers throughout the world. In 1989, 2,437 heart transplants were performed worldwide, 1,600 of which were performed in the United States. Given a median patient survival of approximately 6 years, it is estimated that there are about 9,500 cardiac transplant patients living in the United States, most of them eligible for rehabilitation services. It is expected that this number will continue to slowly increase throughout the 1990s. Thus, professionals working in cardiac rehabilitation must become aware of the special considerations required for the safe and effective rehabilitation of these patients.

The main objective of this chapter is to familiarize physicians and other health care personnel with the physical rehabilitation of patients following cardiac transplantation, especially medical personnel who have had limited or no contact with these patients. The major hemodynamic and metabolic responses of cardiac transplant patients to dynamic and static exercise and the ways in which these responses differ from those of nontransplant patients are reviewed. Next, available data on the responses of cardiac transplant patients to exercise training are presented, with

special emphasis on measures of cardiopulmonary function and physical performance. On the basis of the differences in their acute and chronic responses to exercise as a result of cardiac transplant surgery and its sequelae, special considerations regarding the design of an exercise prescription and the monitoring of exercise for these patients are discussed. Finally, specific guidelines for exercise prescription and monitoring are provided.

CARDIAC TRANSPLANTATION IN THE 1990s

Two basic cardiac transplantation surgical procedures have been used in humans. *Orthotopic transplantation* involves removal of the recipient's heart and the anastomosis of the donor heart to the recipient's great vessels and posterior wall of the atria. *Heterotopic transplantation* involves placing the donor heart "piggyback" style in the recipient's chest without removing the recipient's heart. Orthotopic transplantation is by far the dominant procedure, with fewer than 1% of patients having a heterotopic procedure. The preferred donor heart is from a relatively young person free of cardiopulmonary disease and matched for blood type and general body size with the recipient. The major features related to the surgery that must be considered in cardiac rehabilitation are that the donor heart is denervated and remains that way, there is no pericardium, the heart is prone to acute and chronic rejection, and owing to immunosuppressive medication, the patient is highly susceptible to infections, hypertension, neoplasm, and accelerated coronary atherosclerosis.

Following cardiac transplantation, most patients have a hospital stay of 4 to 8 weeks and then remain in the vicinity of the hospital where the surgery was performed for another several months. During this time their medical status is monitored, with special attention to recovery from the thoracic surgery and detection of cardiac rejection episodes or infections. After patients become medically stable and their immunosuppressant medication regimen is established, they usually return to their private internist or cardiologist for ongoing medical care. In most instances, patients return to the medical center where the transplant surgery was performed for comprehensive cardiac evaluations annually or more frequently if clinically indicated evaluations or therapy are required.

SPECIAL CONSIDERATIONS FOR EXERCISE REHABILITATION

The Surgical Procedure

The challenge to therapy and rehabilitation posed by the surgical procedure of cardiac transplantation is placing the donor heart, a relatively large mass of foreign tissue, into the body of the recipient and leaving it there without innervation. Cardiac denervation itself only slightly alters cardiorespiratory performance and produces minor limitations in functional capacity. The functional capacity of the transplanted heart may be reduced if there was ischemic exposure during transfer from the donor to the recipient, if the donor had a substantially smaller body size than the recipient, or if the recipient's pulmonary vascular resistance was elevated. If it were not for medical complications of tissue rejection and its treatment with immunosuppressant medications, the cardiac transplant patient would present few therapeutic and rehabilitative challenges other than some psychological issues.

Medical Treatment and Complications

During the first 4 to 8 weeks after cardiac transplantation, patients generally incur medical complications related to tissue rejection and require substantial medical care, including percutaneous transvenous endomyocardial biopsies to assess acute rejection. Most medical centers currently use a three-drug protocol for chronic immunosuppression: cyclosporine, prednisone, and azathioprine.[1] The overall goal of any regimen is to maintain effective immunosuppression at the lowest possible doses of agents without incurring overlapping toxicity. Many programs also incorporate a prophylactic course of polyclonal antithymocyte globin or monoclonal anti-T-cell OKT3 antibody therapy during the first several weeks after surgery. Since most long-term complications are related to the dosage of steroids, attention is directed to minimizing the dose of steroids or to eliminating their use altogether.

Graft Rejection

With cyclosporine-based immunosuppression, rejection of a cardiac allograft generally is not accompanied by any clinical indications. Prior to the introduction of cyclosporine, rejection episodes usually could be detected by changes in the resting electrocardiogram (ECG) that included QRS voltage reduction, new S3 gallop sounds, signs of congestive heart failure, or atrial arrhythmias. None of these clinical signs usually appears early in the rejection process of patients receiving cyclosporine.[1] Right ventricular biopsies are needed for early detection. Currently, these biopsies are performed weekly and then monthly for the first 6 months after transplantation and then every 3 months on an indefinite basis. Since the major treatment for rejection is to increase the steroid dosage, the major therapeutic goal is to keep rejection episodes to a minimum. During periods of acute rejection, exercise training is contraindicated.

Drug Toxicity

Each drug used for immunosuppression has its specific toxicity. Side effects of long-term use of corticocosteroid hormones include muscle atrophy, osteoporosis, glucose intolerance, and cataract formation. Azathioprine suppresses the bone marrow in a dose-dependent fashion. The major adverse effect of cyclosporine is nephrotoxicity, resulting in interstitial fibrosis and progressive glomerular sclerosis with a steady rise in systemic arterial pressure that frequently is severe and difficult to control. Many patients require high doses of several antihypertensive drugs. Cyclosporine and prednisone also contribute to increased plasma total cholesterol and low-density lipoprotein (LDL) cholesterol concentrations. Increased lipid levels are not easily managed by diet or drugs; bile acid-binding resins are contraindicated because of their possible interference with absorption of cyclosporine, and higher levels of lovastatin are associated with increased rhabdomyolysis.[2]

Infections

Cardiac transplant patients are highly susceptible to infections with a variety of opportunistic pathogens. Although the overall incidence of infection, as well as death from infection, has been lower since the advent of cyclosporine-based immunosuppression, rejection remains the most common cause of death after cardiac transplantation. Patients are at highest risk early after surgery and for a time after treatment for acute bouts of rejection. The most common site of infection is the lung; thus, screening chest x-rays are frequently used and close attention should be paid to symptoms suggesting pulmonary infection.

Graft Atherosclerosis

Probably the most vexing problem in the medical management of patients following cardiac transplantation is that of graft atherosclerosis.[3] This process is characterized by its speed of development in the coronary arteries of the donor heart, its diffuseness, and the lack of coronary collateral vessel formation. Diffuse concentric atherosclerosis affects all major epicardial coronary arteries and their branches. The development of this atherosclerosis is associated with established risk factors for coronary heart disease (family history, hypertension, smoking, diabetes, lipoprotein profile). The process is believed to be immunologic in origin, involving immune injury to the coronary endothelium that exposes a thrombogenic surface and leads to platelet aggregation, lipid infiltration, and fibrous scarring, resulting in occlusive arterial disease.[4] The actual mechanisms to explain why this process occurs rapidly in some patients and not in others have not been identified. Because cardiac denervation is permanent, these patients do not experience angina pectoris even with severe occlusive disease. Myocardial infarction is frequently "silent," detected only by changes in serial ECGs, myocardial enzyme levels, the onset of congestive heart failure, or sudden cardiac death. Standard noninvasive testing is not very sensitive in detecting coronary atherosclerosis; hence, annual coronary angiography is used in many centers. Given the diffuseness of the disease and the absence of coronary collateral vessels, the atherosclerosis generally is not amenable to coronary bypass surgery (CABG) or percutaneous transluminal coronary angioplasty (PTCA). The major treatment for advanced disease is retransplantation.[1]

Psychological Responses to Transplantation

The total process of cardiac transplantation usually has a profound psychological impact on the patient and family. The fact that transplantation is medically indicated identifies to patients, sometimes for the first time, the immediate threat to their survival. Although the idea of transplant surgery is frightening to most patients, very few refuse the procedure. The period between acceptance for transplantation and the actual surgery, which typically lasts months, can be highly emotional, with extremes of elation, anxiety, and depression. This emotional roller coaster frequently continues during the first few months following surgery, with elation at the prospects of improved function and a longer life intertwined with the anxiety and depression in response to initial rejection episodes, the extensive medication regimen required, and the general setbacks frequently associated with major surgery. Considerable effort is required by the transplant team, personal physician, and family to provide psychological support to patients before and after surgery, with an emphasis on helping them to regain independence and to become productive members of society.[5–7]

HEMODYNAMIC AND METABOLIC RESPONSES OF TRANSPLANT PATIENTS TO EXERCISE

The altered hemodynamic and metabolic responses to exercise of patients following cardiac transplantation appear due primarily to the chronic denervation of the donor heart. Also, the lack of an intact pericardium, the ischemic state of the donor heart during transport and surgery, and myocyte necrosis as a result of repeated rejection episodes all contribute to some depression of cardiac function in most patients at rest and during exercise.[8,9] Later, rapid development of coronary atherosclerosis may interfere with cardiac function.[3] A summary of the major hemodynamic and metabolic changes observed after transplantation is presented in Table 23-1.

Hemodynamic Characteristics at Rest

At rest, the most notable hemodynamic feature of the transplant patient is a high resting heart rate, which usually is close to the inherent rate of the sinoatrial node.[10] This high heart rate is accompanied by a reduced stroke volume and a cardiac output that is normal or slightly low.[11,12] During supine rest, the cardiac transplant patient has a reduced end-diastolic volume and increased filling pressure, suggesting abnormal cardiac compliance.[12] Pulmonary artery, pulmonary capillary wedge, and right atrial pressures are also elevated.[13]

Dynamic Exercise

As a result of denervation, the normal increase in heart rate at the onset of dynamic exercise is substantially delayed in the transplanted heart.

Table 23-1. Cardiorespiratory and Metabolic Responses to Dynamic Exercise in Patients Following Cardiac Transplantation

Heart Rate
  Delayed increase at onset of exercise
  Slow increase during exercise
  Low peak heart rate
  Delayed return to rest after cessation of exercise
Stroke Volume
  Initial increase due to increase in LVEDP
  Maintained during submaximal exercise but reduced LVEF (higher LVEDV and LVESV)
  Decreased at peak exercise
Vascular Pressures
  Increased LVEDP
  Increased pulmonary artery, wedge, and right atrial pressures
  Frequent increase in systemic arterial pressures at rest and during exercise as a result of immunosuppressant therapy
Cardiac Output
  Increases from rest, but is low at any submaximal work rate or $\dot{V}O_2$
  Low peak cardiac output
Oxygen Uptake
  Slow oxygen uptake kinetics
  Low at any submaximal work rate
  Low peak oxygen uptake
Pulmonary Function
  Increased ventilatory equivalents for oxygen and carbon dioxide
  Reduced anaerobic threshold
  Increased blood lactate concentrations at rest and peak exercise.

Abbreviations: LVEDP, left ventricular end-diastolic pressure; LVEF, left ventricular ejection fraction; LVEDV, left ventricular end-diastolic volume; LVESV, left ventricular end-systolic volume; $\dot{V}O_2$, oxygen uptake.

During exercise, the heart rate increases much more slowly than in the innervated heart, with the initial rise apparently due to intrinsic regulation via pacemaker stretch; later on, the heart rate increase is dependent on the increase in circulating catecholamines. The peak heart rate achieved is usually lower than for age-matched control subjects, but with a wide variation among patients. Thus, most transplant patients have a substantially decreased chronotropic reserve. Following exercise, the heart rate does not demonstrate the characteristic rapid decrease seen in the innervated heart, but remains elevated for several minutes and slowly returns to preexercise rates in conjunction with a decrease in plasma catecholamine concentrations.[8]

At the onset of exercise, the stroke volume is increased as a result of an increase in venous return and end-diastolic volume, allowing cardiac output to increase without a significant rise in heart rate (Frank-Starling mechanism).[11] As exercise continues, the stroke volume is maintained and a further increase in cardiac output is achieved by the delayed increase in heart rate. This increase in cardiac output is lower at any given workload or oxygen uptake than is seen in healthy persons, and peak cardiac output is also below normal. During dynamic exercise, the left ventricular ejection fraction is usually below normal with no decrease or a very limited decrease in end-systolic volume.[14,15] During supine exercise, there is an increase in left ventricular end-diastolic pressure, pulmonary artery and capillary wedge pressures, and right atrial pressure.[12,13] These increases in pressure are abnormal, since they do not occur in patients with innervated hearts.

The ventilatory and metabolic responses to exercise are significantly altered following cardiac transplantation. The lower cardiac output during submaximal exercise is compensated for by an increase in arteriovenous oxygen difference, owing to a lower mixed venous oxygen concentration and an increase in anaerobic metabolism.[8,12] At any given level of oxygen uptake there is a higher pulmonary ventilation resulting in an abnormally high O_2 ($\dot{V}E/\dot{V}O_2$) and CO_2 ($\dot{V}E/\dot{V}CO_2$) ventilatory equivalent and respiratory exchange ratio (RER).[16] The early increase in anaerobic metabolism is indicated by the increase in plasma lactate concentration during submaximal exercise and the higher-than-average peak lactate values achieved during maximal treadmill exercise.[16] During submaximal exercise, oxygen uptake at a given work output on the treadmill or cycle ergometer is lower than expected; the peak $\dot{V}O_2$ is decreased an average of 20 to 30% compared with age-matched sedentary but healthy persons; and the oxygen debt is greater.

Isometric Exercise

The predominant response to static (isometric) exercise in patients with *innervated* hearts is a rapid rise in systemic arterial pressure (diastolic, mean, and systolic), with the increase being proportional to the intensity of the contraction expressed as a percentage of capacity. This increase in pressure is produced by an increase in cardiac output as a result of an increase in heart rate (but not stroke volume) and arterial vasoconstriction in nonexercising muscle as a result of vagal withdrawal and increased sympathetic activity. In contrast, during static exercise the cardiac transplant patient has a normal rise in systemic arterial pressure, despite no increase in heart rate or cardiac output.[17] The pressure increase is the result of an increase in peripheral vascular resistance. The ability of the cardiac transplant patient with an otherwise normal heart to perform brief static exercise appears to be unimpaired.[18]

RESPONSES TO EXERCISE TRAINING

Exercise conditioning has become a standard component of the postsurgery treatment program for cardiac transplant patients. Many of these patients are extremely deconditioned by extended periods of inactivity or bed rest. They usually have substantial anxiety regarding their "new" heart and how well it functions, and they lack confidence regarding exercise. Other aspects of the transplantation procedure that increase the need for exercise training include the restriction of normal movement after thoracic surgery and the skeletal muscle atrophy caused by the prednisone used as a component of immunosuppressant therapy.

Carefully controlled randomized trials of physical rehabilitation are difficult to conduct with cardiac transplant patients because relatively few patients are available at any one center and recurrent bouts of organ rejection and changes in immunosuppressant therapy interfere with the training regimen and objective evaluation of its

Table 23-2. Effects of Exercise Conditioning in Patients Following Cardiac Transplantation

Heart Rate
  Possible decrease in donor resting heart rate if training is of sufficient intensity and duration
  Decrease in heart rate at submaximal exercise
  Frequent increase in peak heart rate

Oxygen Uptake and Ventilation
  Increase in peak oxygen uptake
  Increase in anaerobic threshold
  Increase in peak ventilation volume
  Decrease in $\dot{V}E/\dot{V}O_2$ and $\dot{V}E/\dot{V}CO_2$ at submaximal exercise
  Delay in lactate increase at start of exercise

Hemodynamics
  Decrease in rest (possible) and submaximal exercise systolic blood pressure
  Increase in peak blood pressure
  Increase in blood volume

Other
  Increase in peak work rate
  Decrease in RPE at submaximal exercise
  Possible increase in lean body mass
  Possible improvement in psychological function

Abbreviations: $\dot{V}E/\dot{V}O_2$, ventilatory equivalent for oxygen; $\dot{V}E/\dot{V}CO_2$, ventilatory equivalent for carbon dioxide; RPE, rating of perceived exertion.

effects. However, a small series of studies that evaluated the effects of endurance training on peak work rate, hemodynamic and metabolic responses at rest, and submaximal and peak exercise, generally show benefit similar to that reported for patients following acute myocardial infarction or CABG surgery[19] (Table 23-2).

The initial reports of exercise training of cardiac transplant patients were made in 1983. Squires and colleagues demonstrated the feasibility of exercise training for cardiac transplant patients, reporting their experience with two patients who participated in a 7- to 8-week outpatient supervised exercise program that began 6 weeks after transplantation.[20] Moderate-intensity exercise (Borg scale 12 to 13) (see also Chs. 6 and 20) was performed by using a treadmill and cycle ergometer. The major results were a lower rating of perceived exertion (RPE) and systolic blood pressure during exercise testing after exercise.

The second report, from Savin and colleagues at Stanford,[21,22] involved a 16-week training program for five cardiac transplant recipients and

seven normal controls. Training consisted of at least 30 minutes of stationary cycling at 75% peak heart rate 5 or more days per week. Adherence to the training regimen was excellent in both groups. The transplant patients were men with a mean age ($\pm$SD) of 39.3 $\pm$ 9.7 years and were free of acute rejection. A series of measurements was made at rest and during exercise, before and after training. Exercise training produced several classic adaptations to exercise, without significant differences between the two groups. Transplant patients had a significant increase in peak work rate of 240 kpm/min and a 14 beat/min decrease in heart rate at a submaximal work load. Peak oxygen uptake increased 3.6 ml/kg/min, but did not reach significance. These results were similar in magnitude to those achieved by patients with innervated hearts. Of interest, the resting heart rate decreased significantly in controls (-12 bpm; $P < 0.05$) but not transplant patients. Other significant changes in transplant patients included a significant increase in blood volume, a decrease in $\dot{V}E/\dot{V}O_2$ during exercise and recovery, a decrease in RER at submaximal exercise, and a delayed onset of lactate production during exercise. All these changes somewhat normalize the cardiac transplant patients' response to dynamic exercise. No significant changes occurred in cardiac dimensions at rest as determined by two-dimensional (2-D) echocardiography; and no changes occurred in stroke volume, left ventricular ejection fraction, or cardiac output at submaximal exercise by the myocardial marker technique.[22]

The effects of long-term exercise training in patients following orthotopic cardiac transplantation have been presented by Kavanagh et al.[23] They evaluated 36 men before and after a 16-month program of walking and slow jogging, with a target of continuous exercise for 48 minutes five times per week. All patients progressed to walking and jogging an average distance of 24 km/week, at an average pace of 8.5 min/km. No nonexercising control patients were included in the study. Compared with pretraining values, transplant patients had significant increases in peak oxygen uptake (4.0 ± 6.0 ml/kg/min; $P < 0.001$), work rate (49 ± 34 W; $P < 0.001$), and heart rate (13 ± 17 bpm; $P < 0.001$). At submaximal exercise, there were significant decreases in ventilatory equivalent (VE) and rating of perceived exertion (RPE). At rest, heart rate and both systolic and diastolic blood pressures decreased significantly. Greater changes were observed in highly compliant patients.

Other exercise training data for patients following *orthotopic* cardiac transplantation include a brief report by Degre et al.[24] on three patients who trained three times per week (60 to 80% peak exercise intensity) for 150 days. The peak work rate increased by 50% and the peak $\dot{V}O_2$ increased by 40%, with heart rate (11%) and pulmonary ventilation (32%) decreasing during submaximal exercise. No improvement was noted in two transplant patients who did not exercise. Niset et al.[5] reported early postsurgery exercise rehabilitation of 62 transplant patients. Patients began walking, cycle ergometry, and calisthenics on day 4 after surgery. At 1 year, patients completing exercise training increased their maximal exercise intensity by 34%, peak $\dot{V}O_2$ by 33%, peak systolic blood pressure (SBP) by 18%, and peak heart rate by 11%. The $\dot{V}E/\dot{V}O_2$ during submaximal exercise decreased by 25%. No control group data were presented. Similar results have been reported by Sieurat et al.,[25] who trained eight transplant patients starting soon after surgery and observed an increase in maximal working capacity and peak heart rate. Keteyian et al.[26] also provided preliminary data on the exercise rehabilitation of cardiac transplant patients for 6 to 12 weeks during the first year after surgery. Improvements were similar to those reported by other investigators, with modest increases in peak work rate and oxygen uptake achieved.

Following *heterotopic* cardiac transplantation in ten patients at Harefield Hospital in Middlesex, England, Kavanagh et al.[27] conducted an 18-month walking and jogging exercise training program. Results were compared with those from 14 similarly trained, age-matched, male *orthotopic* transplantation recipients. Compliance with the training regimen was poorer in the heterotopic group owing to a higher incidence of medical complications. Training effects were evident in both groups of patients and were generally commensurate with the distance walked and jogged and the training intensity achieved. The recipient but not the donor heart rate at rest decreased significantly in the heterotopic patients. During cycle ergometry, both groups showed a significant increase in peak work rate (heterotopic, 33%; orthotopic, 52%), peak oxygen uptake (heterotopic, 23%; orthotopic, 30%) and ventilatory anaerobic threshold (heterotopic, 16%; orthotopic, 30%). As with other postsurgery exercise training studies that do not include nonexercising controls, it is difficult to know whether the changes observed are due exclusively to the training or in part to the normal recovery from a period of inactivity and the effects of the surgery.

Prednisone is still prescribed for most cardiac transplant patients, especially during bouts of acute rejection. There is preliminary evidence from studies of renal transplant patients that prednisone-induced myopathy can be alleviated somewhat by physical training. Horber et al.[28] used computed tomography (CT) and isokinetic testing before and after 50 days of heavy resistance exercise training in 12 patients treated with prednisone (12.6 ± 33 mg/day). Patients trained one leg but not the other and experienced a significant increase in thigh muscle area and total work output of the trained leg after exercise. Since the increase in peak torque was inversely related to the prednisone dosage, it is not known whether these results apply to patients on higher doses of corticosteroid hormones. In the two training studies reported by Kavanaugh et al.,[23,27] a significant increase in body weight but not in body fat was estimated from skin fold measurements. The authors suggest that this indicates an increase in lean body mass, but data are inadequate as to the increase in muscle mass. Whether and to what extent different exercise training regimens can influence skeletal muscle mass and function in patients following cardiac transplantation remains to be defined.

GUIDELINES FOR EXERCISE REHABILITATION

General guidelines for the exercise rehabilitation of patients following cardiac transplantation are similar to those recommended for patients following acute myocardial infarction or CABG surgery. They include careful evaluation of the clinical and functional status of each patient, development of an individualized exercise plan that includes both the prescription and proscription of specific activities, a specific plan of medical supervision or monitoring of the program, and a plan for periodic reevaluations. As with exercise programs for other cardiac patients, to be most effective, the exercise component must be well integrated into the patient's overall medical management.[29,30]

Exercise Considerations Pretransplantation

Once patients are accepted for transplant surgery, they may be on a waiting list for up to a year. Typically these patients are in New York Heart Association class IV and, if ambulatory, have a very limited functional capacity. During this time, it is potentially valuable to institute a preoperative physical conditioning program of ambulation or in-bed exercises similar to that used for in-hospital exercise conditioning following myocardial infarction or cardiac surgery. Most of these patients have congestive heart failure and are symptomatic at rest. The primary exercise objectives are to prevent cardiorespiratory and musculoskeletal deconditioning and depression. Passive and active exercise in bed may be required; walking, even for a minute or two sporadically throughout the day, is highly desirable. These activities are not designed to train the heart, but to maintain more normal function of other systems that will play an important role in the successful recovery of the patient following transplant surgery. Recent studies have shown improvement in aerobic capacity from exercise training of patients with congestive heart failure.

Early Postsurgery Exercise

Once medically stabilized after surgery, all patients should be provided with an individualized exercise plan that takes into account the altered hemodynamic characteristics of the denervated heart, the impact of thoracic surgery, and the very low functional capacity of many patients as a result of extended periods of inactivity. Also, the potential for acute rejection episodes and infection requires appropriate monitoring. Patients usually remain in a supervised exercise rehabilitation program at a tertiary medical center for 1 to 2 months as a routine part of their intensive postoperative medical monitoring and treatment. During this time, patients are considered at intermediate risk during exercise; there should be supervision to guide the intensity and duration of the exercise, although continuous ECG monitoring may not be necessary.[31]

Owing to the delayed increase in cardiac output with exercise and its slow response to changes in exercise intensity, warm-up activities are important. The use of RPE may be more appropriate than the heart rate to help guide exercise intensity.[32] Patients should be instructed on how to use heart rate, RPE, and general sense of effort to help guide their exercise intensity both during and unrelated to the exercise program. The heart rate reserve method (Karvonen method) is preferred (see also Ch. 20). The primary endurance exercise should be walking, with stationary cycling as an alternative. Also included should be stretching activities, especially those to aid in recovery of function following thoracic surgery, and muscle-strengthening exercises to help overcome deconditioning due to prolonged inactivity and the muscle-wasting effect of corticosteroid therapy. Supervision and counseling about exercise and citation of specific limitations are critical to prevent overexertion. Of prime importance is the reminder that, with cardiac denervation, myocardial ischemia is not heralded by angina pectoris; other symptoms of ischemia such as shortness of breath, increased fatigue, or signs such as exercise-induced ECG ST-T depression must be monitored more closely.

Long-Term Exercise

Many transplant patients have the potential to attain an exercise capacity of 10 METs or higher after 2 or 3 months of exercise rehabilitation. This is an adequate exercise capacity for activities of daily living and most occupations and for enjoyment of many recreational activities. For these patients, a maintenance exercise program is recommended, which can either occur in a supervised setting or be performed at home, following specific guidelines. Patients should be recommended to exercise three to five times each week, with an exercise session lasting 30 to 60 minutes at an intensity of 50 to 75% of exercise capacity or heart rate reserve and an RPE of 12 to 15. Walking is preferred to running, and moderate-intensity resistance exercise should be included. By using light weights, this component of the program can be completed in 5 to 10 minutes, three times per week. Contraindications to exercise conditioning include acute bouts of rejection, infection, or any symptoms that suggest a decrease in cardiac performance or functional capacity.

For patients who have repeated episodes of rejection or infection, involvement in a progressive program of rehabilitation is difficult because of the numerous periods of bed rest or inactivity. Ideally, these patients will continue to be enrolled in a supervised rehabilitation program that includes patient and family psychological counseling and coronary risk factor education and modification, as well as exercise training. Exercise must be carefully monitored, with many patients having to regain their exercise tolerance very gradually.

Frequent evaluations are exceedingly important even for patients who initially recover quickly from surgery, because of their risk for developing hypertension and cardiac graft atherosclerosis. Particularly for patients who have physically active jobs or recreational pursuits, ECG-monitored exercise testing should be performed at least annually, if not every 6 months. Such testing may help detect the early onset of hypertension and clinically significant coronary atherosclerosis.

By 3 to 6 months following transplantation,[5,33] the psychological status of patients is usually rated as good. This favorable status is due in part to the careful selection of transplant candidates who demonstrate psychological stability and a good social support system. Also, close follow-up after surgery with instruction regarding skills in dealing with the medical regimen, stress man-

agement, and general coping skills is an important component of rehabilitation.[34,35] The effectiveness of these sessions is greatly enhanced when family members are actively involved.[36]

REFERENCES

1. Valantine HA, Schroeder JS: Cardiac transplantation. Intensive Care 15:283, 1989
2. East C, Alivizatos PA, Grunder SM et al: Rhabdomyolysis in patients receiving lovastatin after cardiac transplantation. N Engl J Med 318:47, 1988
3. Gao SZ, Schroeder JS, Alderman EL et al: Clinical and laboratory correlates of accelerated coronary artery disease in the cardiac transplant patient. Circulation 76(suppl. V):V-56, 1987
4. McDonald L, Rector TS, Braunlin EA et al: Association of coronary artery disease in cardiac transplant recipients with cytomegalovirus infection. Am J Cardiol 64:359, 1989
5. Niset G, Coustry-Degre C, Degre S: Psychosocial and physical rehabilitation after heart transplantation: 1 year follow-up. Cardiology 75:311, 1988
6. Bergeret A, Dureau G, Chuzel M, Normand JC: Qualité de vie et reinsertion social après transplantation cardiaque. Presse Med 16:2207, 1987
7. Baumgartner WA, Augustine S, Borkon AM et al: Present expectations in cardiac transplantation. Ann Thorac Surg 43:585, 1987
8. Savin WM, Schroeder JS, Haskell WL: Response of cardiac transplant recipients to static and dynamic exercise: a review. Heart Transplant 1:72, 1983
9. Labovitz AJ, Drimmer AM, McBride LR et al: Exercise capacity during the first year after cardiac transplantation. Am J Cardiol 64:642, 1989
10. Jose AD, Collison D: The normal range and determinants of the intrinsic heart rate in man. Cardiovasc Res 4:160, 1970
11. Pope SE, Stinson EB, Daughters GT et al: Exercise response of the denervated heart in long-term cardiac transplant recipients. Am J Cardiol 46:213, 1980
12. Stinson EB, Griepp RB, Schroeder JS et al: Hemodynamic observations one and two years after cardiac transplantation. Circulation 45:1183, 1972
13. Pflugelder PW, Purves PD, McKenzie FN et al: Cardiac dynamics during supine exercise in cyclosporine-treated orthotopic heart transplant re-

cipients: Assessment by radionuclide angiography. J Am Coll Cardiol 10:336, 1987

14. Verani MS, George SE, Leon CA et al: Systolic and diastolic ventricular response at rest and during exercise in heart transplant recipients. J Heart Transplant 7:145, 1988

15. Borow KM, Neumann A, Arensman FW, Yacoub MH: Left ventricular contractility and contractile reserve in humans after cardiac transplantation. Circulation 71:866, 1985

16. Savin WM, Haskell WL, Schroeder JS, Stinson EB: Cardiorespiratory responses of cardiac transplant patients to graded, symptom-limited exercise. Circulation 62:55, 1980

17. Savin WM, Alderman EL, Haskell WL et al: Left ventricular response to isometric exercise in patients with denervated and innervated hearts. Circulation 61:897, 1980

18. Haskell WL, Savin WM, Schroeder JS et al: Cardiovascular responses to handgrip isometric exercise in patients following cardiac transplantation. Circ Res 48:156, 1981

19. Squires RW: Cardiac rehabilitation issues for heart transplantation patients. J Cardiopulmonary Rehabil 10:159, 1990

20. Squires RW, Arthur PR, Gau GT et al: Exercise after cardiac transplantation: A report of two cases. J Cardiopulmonary Rehab 3:S70, 1983

21. Savin WM, Gordon E, Green S et al: Comparison of exercise training effects in cardiac denervated and innervated humans. J Am Coll Cardiol 1:722, 1983

22. Savin WM: Role of the adrenergic nervous system in the production of cardiovascular training effects in men. Doctoral dissertation, Stanford University, Stanford, CA, 1983

23. Kavanagh T, Yacoub MH, Mertens DJ et al: Cardiorespiratory responses to exercise training after orthotopic cardiac transplantation. Circulation 77:162, 1987

24. Degre S, Niset G, Desmet JM et al: Effects de l'entrainment physique sur le coeur humain dénervé après transplantation cardiaque orthotopique. Ann Cardiol Angeiol 35147, 1986

25. Sieurat P, Roquebrune JP, Grinneiser D et al: Surveillance et réadaption des transplantes cardiaques heterotropiques à la periode de convalescence. Arch Mal Coeur 79:210, 1988

26. Keteyian S, Ehrman J, Fedel F, Rhoads K: Rehabilitation following heart transplantation. Med Sci Sports Exercise 21:555, 1989

27. Kavanagh T, Yacoub MH, Mertens DJ et al: Exercise rehabilitation after heterotopic cardiac transplantation. J Cardiopulmonary Rehabil 9:303, 1989

28. Horber FF, Scheldegger JR, Grunig BE, Frey FJ: Evidence that prednisone-induced myopathy is reversed by physical training. J Clin Endocrinol Metab 61:83, 1985

29. American Heart Association: Exercise standards: A statement for Health Professionals from the American Heart Association. Circulation 82:2286, 1990

30. American Association of Cardiovascular and Pulmonary Rehabilitation: Scientific evidence of the value of cardiac rehabilitation services with emphasis on patients following myocardial infarction. Section I. Exercise conditioning component. J Cardiopulmonary Rehabil 10:79, 1990

31. Wenger NK, Haskell WL, Kanter K et al: Cardiac rehabilitation services after cardiac transplantation: Guidelines for use. Task Force Report for the American College of Cardiology. Cardiology 20:4, 1991

32. Keteyian S, Ehrman J, Fedel F, Rhoads K: Heart rate-perceived exertion relationship during exercise in orthotopic heart transplant patients. J Cardiopulmonary Rehabil 10:287, 1990

33. Mai FM, McKenie FN, Kostuk WJ: Psychiatric aspects of heart transplantation: preoperative evaluation and postoperative sequelae. Br Med J 292:311, 1986

34. Jones BM, Chang VP, Esmore D et al: Psychological adjustment after cardiac transplantation. Med J Aust 149:118, 1988

35. Gier MD, Levick MD, Blazina PJ: Stress reduction with heart transplant patients and their families: a multidisciplinary approach. J Heart Transplant 7:342, 1988

36. Rogers KR: Nature of spousal supportive behaviors that influence heart transplant patient compliance. J Heart Transplant 6:90, 1987

24

Patients with Implanted Pacemakers or Implanted Cardioverter Defibrillators

Fredric J. Pashkow, M.D.

The elements of cardiac rehabilitation are exercise, secondary prevention, education, and psychosocial support. The coronary patient population is changing, as are expectations for outcome and need for risk stratification and electrocardiographic (ECG) monitoring in cardiac rehabilitation programs.[1] A growing population of patients has had devices implanted for the control of cardiac arrhythmias, both bradycardia and tachycardia.[2] The follow-up and management of these patients can be greatly enhanced with a cardiac rehabilitation program.[3]

BRADYCARDIA PACING

Understanding the Technology

A bradycardia pacemaker works fundamentally like a thermostat. When the recipient's heart rate slows below a predetermined level, the pacer turns on and electrically stimulates the heart muscle to contract. Although pacemakers have become progressively smaller, they have also become increasingly sophisticated, with more technical features and potential benefits.

Important parameters of pacer function, such as the amount of electrical energy used to stimulate the myocardium, are programmable from outside the body by use of a special transmitted radiofrequency code ("telemetry"). Many pacers are now "interactive," i.e., are capable of making internal measurements and transmitting this information for monitoring purposes.

Recent technology can provide more physiologic pacing. Pacemakers, rather than being limited to acting as a rate "thermostat," are increasingly capable of emulating the "normal" electrical events that enable a more natural efficient pumping action of the heart.[4]

The goal of modern pacemaker therapy is the emulation of normal heart responses under varying physiologic conditions, such as during sleep or while physically active.[5–7] To accomplish this, the devices must integrate well with the human recipient and take advantage of the rapidly expanding technology.

Physiology

The physiologic aspects of exercise training for patients with implanted pacemakers are identical to those for patients who are not paced. What is unique is the way in which the native physiology of the patients integrates with the implanted technology. "Chronotropy" refers to the ability to alter heart rate relative to metabolic need.[8] "Atrioventricular synchrony" refers to the sequential activation and contraction of the atria and ventricles that provides optimal priming of the pump for adequate cardiac output.[9,10]

Although the relative contribution of chronotropy to cardiac output is generally appreciated, the preeminent relationship of rate versus atrioventricular synchrony during progressive levels of exercise has to be emphasized.[11] An appropriate heart rate response during exercise accounts for the majority of the required increase in cardiac output. Stroke volume, the determinants of which are preload and afterload, accounts for the other increased third of cardiac output. As heart rate increases, the relative contribution from atrioventricular synchrony decreases.[12]

Maintaining Atrioventricular Synchrony

Cardiac atrioventricular synchrony is attained by the placement of two pacing leads, usually one in the right atrium and one in the right ventricle. This type of pacing is often referred to as "dual-chamber" pacing. For some pacemaker patients, the placement of the two leads is sufficient to virtually duplicate the normal cardiac timing relationships. Others, however, do not do well without the addition of variable heart rate pacing.[12]

Chronotropic Competence and Incompetence

Chronotropic competence is the ability to attain a heart rate appropriate for a given level of metabolic activity, such as for exercise or for performing heavy physical work.[8] For practical purposes, the lack of chronotropic competence appears to be of two types: absolute and relative.[4] Patients with absolute chronotropic incompetence have a low, rigidly fixed rate; when paced, the pacemaker rate is the actual rate, exceeding the rate of the sinus node. This is often the primary indication for pacemaker implantation. However, some patients can increase their heart rate somewhat, but the developed rate is inappropriate for a given level of metabolic demand. These individuals have relative chronotropic incompetence, and its presence is often a secondary consideration in pacemaker selection.

Technologic Considerations

A rate-adaptive or rate-responsive pacer uses parameters or physiologic variables other than the physiologic ones that drive one's native pacemaker to control the pacing rate. Several technologic substitutes for the native pacemaker are currently available or under investigation. These technologies are referred to as "sensors." The sensor can be located in the lead wire or within the pacemaker. Sensors fall into four basic categories:

1. *Detecting body motion or activity.* This kind of sensor, the first to be approved for general use in the United States, is relatively simple to implement and works well in physically active patients.
2. *Measuring alterations in flow of electrical current through the heart or other tissues.* These electrical changes are independent of changes related to alteration in rate per se. Examples include sensors that measure changes in minute ventilation, stroke volume, or the repolarization portion (ST-T complex) of the ECG signal. These sensors work well both for increases in metabolic demand that are load related and for certain nonexercise situations such as emotional excitement.
3. *Utilizing changes in body chemistry that correlate well with increased metabolic needs.* Examples are altered states in the blood hemoglobin associated with the burning of oxygen and fuel consumption to provide energy for exercise.
4. *Sensing temperature or pressure changes of the blood pool.* Burning fuel to produce energy generates of heat that is detectable by tiny, sensitive thermometers built into the pacing lead.

These sensors each have relative advantages and disadvantages.[13] One sensor may work better for one person than another because of activity preferences or lifestyles (Table 24-1). Some sensors require more programming to properly fit the individual patient, and some consume more battery energy than others.

What of the future? Sensor technology continues to evolve rapidly. Both the combination of two or more sensors and the incorporation of sen-

Table 24-1. Sensors for Rate-Responsive Pacemakers

Sensor Type	Parameter Measured	Mode of Action	Sensor Characteristics
Activity	Vibration	Piezo crystal	First sensor available in United States; not physiologic
Minute ventilation	Thoracic impedance	Ohm's law	Highly physiologic; simple programming
Temperature	Core body temperature	Thermistor	Requires special lead; complex programming
Stroke volume	Blood impedance	Ohm's law	Physiologic, requires special lead, other uses
Evoked potential	Area under T of ECG	Reflcts catechols	Self-adjusting (closed loop); must pace to work

sors into dual-chamber devices are currently under way.

Applying the Technology

Modes of cardiac pacing are variably appropriate for different cardiac problems (Fig. 24-1). Despite the availability of DDD and DDDR dual-chamber devices, patients most commonly receive VVIR or single-chamber rate-adaptive pacing devices. VVIR pacing works well in patients who have reasonably intact left ventricular function. For those with high-degree atrioventricular block and poorly functioning ventricles, especially with problems of compliance or ob-

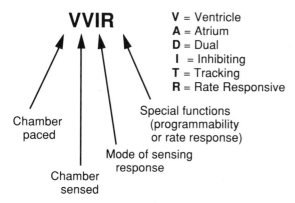

Fig. 24-1. Code for indication of pacing modes. (Data from Report of the Mode Committee of the North American Society of Pacing and Electrophysiology.[13a]).

struction to outflow, DDD pacemakers are more appropriate. DDD pacers are almost "physiologic" in patients with normal sinus node function, in whom the ventricle can track on normal sinus node activity.

If the indication for the pacemaker is "pure" solitary sinus node dysfunction, as in the sick sinus syndrome (SSS), and no atrioventricular block is present or suspected, AAIR pacing is appropriate. However, SSS may also involve abnormalities of the atrioventricular junction and the atrioventricular junctional escape pacemaker may be inadequate clinically. DDDR pacing is becoming more readily available. Although the most fitting indication for DDDR pacing is binodal disease, more commonly these devices will be used in individuals who can benefit from dynamic control of their atrioventricular interval and postventricular atrial refractory period (PVARP), enabling them to track on normal P waves to higher sinus rates without developing iatrogenically induced heart block. The common pacing modes are summarized in Table 24-2.

Special considerations for patients with coronary heart disease include programming of the upper heart rate limit in DDD, DDDR,[14] and VVIR devices below the patient's ischemic threshold; avoiding the induction of second-degree atrioventricular block in patients who are AAIR paced by setting the upper rate below the level of potentially induced atrioventricular block; and optimizing the PR interval by using noninvasive diagnostic means. Patients with significant left ventricular dysfunction need careful assessment of the upper heart rate limit to be sure

Table 24-2.   Common Pacing Modes and Their Indication

Mode	Primary Indication	Secondary Indication	Comment
AAI	Paroxysmal sinus arrest[a]	None	Not to be used in pts with evidence of AV block
VVI	High-degree AV block	Atrial fibrillation	May not be tolerated in pts with intact retrograde AV conduction
DDD	High-degree AV block	Sinus node dysfunction with clinically unacceptable slow ventricular response rate	Physiologic in pts with chronotropically competent SA node

[a] Sinus node dysfunction including SSS (sick sinus syndrome), tachycardia-bradycardia syndrome, and bradycardia syndrome.
Abbreviations: AV, atrioventricular; SA, sinoatrial.

that systolic pressure is maintained and no arrhythmias are induced with the increased catecholamines associated with exercise.

Evaluation Before and After Pacemaker Implantation

Evaluation before[15] and after implantation of a rate-adaptive pacer is important for its successful application. Exercise testing[16] and 24-hour ambulatory ECG monitoring are the main techniques, but telemetry monitoring (as during exercise training) and other technologies such as Doppler ultrasonography may be helpful.[17]

The pacemaker may initially be programmed on the basis of age, predicted maximal heart rate, and estimated activity. However, because of chronotropic incompetence and myocardial ischemia at low heart rates in patients with coronary heart disease, exercise testing of some type, even "informal," is required for accurate adjustment of the device and proves the efficacy of the sensor at its current settings. The various sensor types and the most appropriate means of exercise evaluation and therapy are listed in Table 24-3. "Parameters" refers to the minimal number of components that must be adjusted to program the sensor.

Selection of the appropriate exercise test protocol and the mode of exercise are important (Table 24-3). In the population of patients with pacemakers, the Bruce protocol often has the disadvantage of beginning at a MET energy level

Table 24-3.   Evaluation and Follow-up of Rate-Responsive Pacemakers

Sensor Type	Initial Evaluation	Follow-up Evaluation	Parameters	Appropriate Exercises
Activity	Treadmill	Ambulatory ECG, rate histograms[a]	Slope, sens, on/off	Walk, jog, aerobics; not climb
Minute ventilation	Treadmill, bicycle	Treadmill, bicycle, ambulatory ECG	Slope	Endurance, e.g., bicycle, climb
Temperature	Treadmill, bicycle	Ambulatory ECG, treadmill	Slope, sens, on/off[b]	Endurance: not swim or ski
Stroke volume	Treadmill, bicycle	Ambulatory ECG, treadmill	Slope, sens, on/off	Any: e.g., weights, climb
Evoked potential	Not required	Ambulatory ECG, treadmill	Self-adjusting	Any: e.g., walk, swim

[a] Not available in all makes and models of activity-sensing devices.
[b] These devices frequently have a stand-by rate, an intermediate rate that rapidly occurs with any change in sensor function.
Abbreviations: sens, sensor sensitivity; on/off, sensor onset/offset.

higher than the patient's exercise capability.[18] This results in premature fatigue and an inaccurate estimate of the sensor's physiologic capacity. Certain sensors have significant disadvantages when evaluated by a particular mode of exercise. For example, activity sensing devices respond sluggishly to kinesiologically "smoother activities" such as bicycle riding, or slowly climbing a steeper incline at a steady speed. They also do not reflect the increasing metabolic workloads associated with carrying added weight, such as a suitcase; during walking, the patients must move their arms for the sensor to function reliably. The temperature sensor may be confused by loss of body heat during activities such as swimming or prolonged cold exposure.

Exercise Therapy

Patients who are properly selected, and whose pacing devices are properly programmed almost always notice significant symptomatic improvement.[18] More than 150,000 patients have received these devices, attesting to the prominence and acceptance of these newer technologies in contemporary pacing therapy.

Since the sensor design may limit the effectiveness of the type of exercise prescribed, exercise prescriptions for patients with rate-modulating pacers should be carefully designed with respect to the type of exercise prescribed and its frequency, duration and intensity. Exercise intensity can be measured by using the three classical approaches: Karvonen's method, which bases training heart rate on the achievement of a percentage of heart rate reserve; a rating of perceived exertion (RPE); and the estimation of activity level by using MET level equivalents (see also Ch. 20).

Allied health professionals and exercise specialists are increasingly involved in the selection of patients with devices for exercise training and in patient education and the follow-up process.[2] Although paced patients require little reassurance concerning the safety of their technologies, an understanding of these devices by the cardiac rehabilitation professional allows optimal use of the technology's potential.

Follow-up

Once optimal programming has been achieved with a rate-responsive device, the sensing characteristics have long-term stability. An annual exercise test can document the stability of the sensor and the patient's tolerance of currently programmed values of upper rate and sensor response. If 24-hour ambulatory ECG monitoring is used, the importance of the patient-kept diary in recording activities and symptoms must be stressed. Transtelephonic ECG monitoring during exercise has also been used for this purpose.[19]

Many devices now have the ability to store summaries of the number of beats that occur at a given rate. These summaries, called rate histograms, are useful for documenting the appropriate activity of the sensor.[14] "Slow walk/fast walk" protocols were derived from the regimens used during clinical investigation of the various devices. The patient is asked to walk a prescribed distance at a comfortable pace. The rate histogram is then telemetered and analyzed. The distribution curve for achieved heart rate should be reasonably consistent for the low level of work performed (slow walk), the patient's age, and any other physical limitations. If not, the sensor response should be reprogrammed. For example, if the curve is skewed to the left, the sensitivity of the sensor must be increased. The patient is then asked to walk the prescribed distance at a fast pace, and the sequence of analysis and programming is repeated. With this method, most devices are adjustable without the use of formal exercise testing, but the device must have histogram capability.

IMPLANTABLE CARDIOVERTER DEFIBRILLATORS

Clinical Considerations

Drugs for the suppression of lethal or potentially lethal arrhythmias have proven an incomplete solution to the problem, whereas implantable devices that use direct-current shocks have proven remarkably effective.[20] Such devices,

Table 24-4. Clinical Characteristics of Patients Receiving ICDs

Characteristic	Finding
Male gender	77%
Mean age	60 ± 10 years
Previous myocardial infarction	83%
Cardiomyopathy	8%
Valvular heart disease	3%
No heart disease	6%
Mean left ventricular ejection fraction	36 ± 14%
NYHA functional class I	49%
NYHA functional class II	42%
NYHA functional class III	9%
Sustained VT/VF with cardiac arrest	63%
Sustained symptomatic VT	37%

Abbreviations: NYHA, New York Heart Association; VT, ventricular tachycardia; VF, ventricular fibrillation. (From Fogoros et al,[23] with permission.)

called implantable cardioverter defibrillators (ICDs), although initially limited to patients with histories of sudden cardiac death, are now increasingly implanted in individuals identified as having a susceptible substrate, for example, a prior extensive myocardial infarction[20] and/or left ventricular dysfunction,[21] in whom sustained ventricular tachycardia or fibrillation can be induced in the electrophysiologic (EP) laboratory.[22]

As a result of the limitations of drug therapy and with the availability of EP data predictive of ventricular tachycardia and ventricular fibrillation, the population with these devices is rapidly increasing. Table 24-4 summarizes the clinical characteristics of patients receiving ICDs.[23]

How the Technology Works

An ICD is basically a battery-operated cardioverter defibrillator that monitors the patient's heart rate and rhythm and is capable of electrically shocking the heart through instructions, or algorithms, that are internally programmed into the device.

Recently, an ICD with back-up bradycardia

and antitachycardia pacing entered clinical trials, and several others are about to start in clinical trials. Combination devices of this sort are likely to be common in the future. Another likely innovation will be the capability of controlling electrical discharges with sensors similar in concept to those developed for the control of rate-modulated pacers. In this case they would monitor changes in stroke volume or cardiac output and include this information in the logic process with the rate/rhythm algorithms.

Evaluation After Implantation

Since most algorithms currently involve rate dependency, the patients must be exercise tested to ascertain that their intrinsic rate will not exceed the threshold rate of the device and inadvertently cause it to fire during physical activity. Many patients are concomitantly treated with drugs, so that while this is unlikely, such testing must be done. Table 24-5 summarizes the experience (unpublished) of Thomas Guarnieri and associates at the Johns Hopkins Hospital with respect to the heart rate criterion observed in over 100 patients with ICDs. Since the average patient receiving an ICD is 60 years of age, an exercise training heart rate of 120 bpm should exceed the rate criterion in fewer than 2% of patients implanted with these devices.

Patients are often concerned that they may be

Table 24-5. Rate Criterion in Reprogramming of ICDs

Rate Criterion (bpm)	% Patients Programmed
110–115	0.5
120–125	2.5
130–135	3.8
140–145	8.7
150–155	25.1
160–165	13.5
170–175	25.1
180–185	11.1
190–195	5.4
200+	3.4

shocked by the device during an exercise test. However, they should be reassured that this will not occur since the ICD has been programmed to prevent inappropriate defibrillation. Medications such as beta-adrenergic blocking drugs or calcium channel-blocking drugs can be prescribed to ensure that the exercise-induced heart rate will remain below the ICD rate set for discharge. In the absence of rate-controlling medication, the device can be programmed "off" for the duration of the exercise test and the patient reassured that an inappropriate defibrillation will not occur.

Once evaluated by exercise testing, the exercise prescription can be written to accommodate the heart rate limits of the device. No other major adaptations to the presence of an internal defibrillator are necessary.

Role of Cardiac Rehabilitation

Pacemaker/ICD patients are excellent candidates for cardiac rehabilitation programs that have supervision by medical professionals and telemetry monitoring capability, at least until the likelihood of inadvertent defibrillation has been ruled out by sufficient experience.[24] Patients also benefit from the group support and the socialization.[25] Most patients who were employed before ICD implantation are able to return to work after the procedure.[26]

The implantation of such a potent device into an individual can have significant psychological ramifications.[27] The opportunity to share experiences and to be regarded by others as "normal" is, for many, a significant benefit. Formal group psychotherapy can be offered to patients identified as having significant adjustment problems.

The cardiac rehabilitation program staff and other patients should be aware that the ICD will not harm someone in physical contact with a patient while it is discharging. An understanding of how the device can temporarily be turned off (usually by a magnet) is also necessary. Because of the potentially increased difficulty of external cardioversion in rare instances of ICD failure, owing to the location of the ICD patches on the heart, anterior and posterior paddle positions are

recommended. Again, this detailed knowledge, as well as an understanding of the underlying disease process and thorough preparation for the management of emergencies, leads to the projection of an air of confidence by the program staff that is reassuring to these often anxious patients.

REFERENCES

1. Wenger NK: Rehabilitation of the coronary patient: A preview of tomorrow. J Cardiopulmonary Rehabil 11:83, 1991
2. Pashkow FJ: Complicating conditions. p. 228. In Pashkow FJ, Pashkow PS, Schafer MN (eds): Successful Cardiac Rehabilitation: The Complete Guide for Building Cardiac Rehab Programs. HeartWatchers Press, Loveland, CO, 1988
3. Tamarisk NK: Enhancing activity levels of patients with permanent cardiac pacemakers. Heart Lung 17:698, 1988
4. Pashkow F: Rate responsive pacing: practical application. Cardiology 6:89, 1989
5. Humen DP, Kostuk WJ, Klein GJ: Activity sensing, rate-responsive pacing: improvement in myocardial performance with exercise. PACE 8:52, 1985
6. Rickards AF, Donaldson RM: Rate responsive pacing. Clin Prog Pacing Electrophysiol 1:12, 1983
7. Rickards A: Rate-responsive pacing. p. 799. In Barold S (ed): Modern Cardiac Pacing. Futura Publishing, Mount Kisco, NY, 1985
8. Wilkoff BL, Corey J, Blackburn G: A mathematical model of the cardiac chronotropic response to exercise. J Electrophysiol 3:176, 1989
9. Haskell RJ, French WJ: Physiological importance of different atrioventricular intervals to improved exercise performance in patients with dual chamber pacemakers. Br Heart J 61:46, 1989
10. Mehta D, Gilmour S, Ward DE, Camm AJ: Optimal atrioventricular delay at rest and during exercise in patients with dual chamber pacemakers: a non-invasive assessment by continuous wave Doppler. Br Heart J 61:161, 1989
11. Benditt DG, Mianulli M, Fetter J et al: Single-chamber cardiac pacing with activity-initiated chronotropic response: evaluation by cardiopulmonary exercise testing. Circulation 75:184, 1987
12. Kristensson BE, Arnman K, Ryden L: The haemodynamic importance of atrioventricular syn-

chrony and rate increase at rest and during exercise. Eur Heart J 6:668, 1985

13. Lau CP, Butrous GS, Ward DE, Camm AJ: Comparison of exercise performance of six rate-adaptive right ventricular cardiac pacemakers. Am J Cardiol 63:833, 1989

13a.Report of the Mode Committee of the North American Society Pacing and Electrophysiology. PACE 7:395, 1984.

14. Hayes DL, Higano ST, Eisinger G: Utility of rate histograms in programming and follow-up of a DDDR pacemaker. Mayo Clin Proc 64:495, 1989

15. Benditt DG, Mianulli M, Fetter J et al: An office-based exercise protocol for predicting chronotropic response of activity-triggered, rate-variable pacemakers. Am J Cardiol 64:27, 1989

16. Faerestrand S, Breivik K, Ohm OJ: Assessment of the work capacity and relationship between rate response and exercise tolerance associated with activity-sensing rate-responsive ventricular pacing. PACE 10:1277, 1987

17. Lau CP, Camm AJ: Role of left ventricular function and Doppler-derived variables in predicting hemodynamic benefits of rate-responsive pacing. Am J Cardiol 62:906, 1988

18. Kay GN, Bubien RS, Epstein AE, Plumb VJ: Effect of catheter ablation of the atrioventricular junction on quality of life and exercise tolerance in paroxysmal atrial fibrillation. Am J Cardiol 62:741, 1988

19. Hayes DL, Christiansen JR, Vlietstra RE, Osborn MJ: Follow-up of an activity-sensing, rate-modulated pacing device, including transtelephonic exercise assessment. Mayo Clin Proc 64:503, 1989

20. Mirowski M: The automatic implantable cardioverter-defibrillator: An overview. J Am Coll Cardiol 6:461, 1985

21. Tchou PJ, Kadri N, Anderson J et al: Automatic implantable cardioverter defibrillators and survival of patients with left ventricular dysfunction and malignant ventricular arrhythmias. Ann Intern Med 109:529, 1988

22. Mirowski M, Mower MM, Reid PR et al: The automatic implantable defibrillator: new modality for treatment of life-threatening ventricular arrhythmias. PACE 5:384, 1982

23. Fogoros RN, Elson JJ, Bonnet CA: Actuarial incidence and pattern of occurrence of shocks following implantation of the automatic implantable cardioverter defibrillator. PACE 12:1465, 1989

24. Cooper DK, Valladares BK, Futterman LG: Care of the patient with the automatic implantable cardioverter defibrillator: a guide for nurses. Heart Lung 16:640, 1987

25. Badger JM, Morris PL: Observations of a support group for automatic implantable cardioverter-defibrillator recipients and their spouses. Heart Lung 18:238, 1989

26. Kalbfleisch KR, Lehmann MH, Steinman RT et al: Reemployment following implantation of the automatic cardioverter defibrillator. Am J Cardiol 64:199, 1989

27. Pycha C, Gulledge AD, Hutzler J et al. Psychological responses to the implantable defibrillator. Psychosomatics 27:841, 1986

EDUCATION AND COUNSELING OF THE PATIENT AND FAMILY

25

Education of the Coronary Patient and Family: Principles and Practice

Patricia McCall Comoss R.N., B.S.

In a broad sense, education of the coronary patient can be thought of as the collection of activities that an organized program of health care provides to assist participants in that program in achieving health-related goals. Activities range from simple sheets of instructions to sophisticated series of classes. Teaching and learning are the functions inherent in all educational activities. In coronary rehabilitation, where the ultimate goal is achievement and maintenance of each patient's optimal level of health,[1] education is increasingly recognized as an essential service in contributing to attainment of specific goals.

Historically, the educational component of coronary rehabilitation was loosely structured and largely based on practitioner philosophy and experience. Educational efforts were often secondary to exercise programs. Currently, educational endeavors are acknowledged as being at least equal in importance to exercise.[2] Educational programs are built on established principles of adult education.

Recent research supports the value of education of the patient in coronary rehabilitation. Education of coronary patients during the hospital stay has been shown to increase knowledge and decrease anxiety,[3,4] improve compliance with instructions given at discharge,[5] and reduce self-imposed limitations after discharge.[6] Additionally, education of the coronary patient after leaving the hospital has been documented to be effective in improving self-care[7] and decreasing the degree of coronary disability.[8]

Professional organizations endorse the need for education in coronary rehabilitation. In their *Guidelines for Cardiac Rehabilitation*, the American Association of Cardiovascular and Pulmonary Rehabilitation recommends that "an increased emphasis be placed on educational and counseling components in addition to exercise rehabilitation."[9]

The purpose of this chapter is to apply the principles of adult education to the coronary rehabilitation population and to recommend practical approaches for teaching of the patient and appropriate family members in both inpatient and outpatient coronary rehabilitation settings. It is expected that after reading this chapter, the cardiac rehabilitation professional will be able to do the following:

1. Discuss the importance of education as a standard component of any coronary rehabilitation program.
2. Describe three important principles of adult education and give examples of how each can be applied to teaching of the coronary patient.
3. Outline how to assess a patient's readiness to learn.
4. Prepare a set of lesson plans to be used for teaching coronary patients.

439

5. Evaluate the appropriateness of proposed handout materials for the patient.
6. Develop and use a method for identifying the learning priorities of patients.
7. Set appropriate goals for teaching within the constraints of current inpatient settings.
8. Recommend a plan for sharing responsibility for teaching coronary inpatients.
9. Draft a teaching flowsheet.
10. Set appropriate goals for teaching within the constraints of current outpatient settings.
11. Recommend a plan for providing both elementary and supplementary teaching to coronary outpatients.
12. Draft a quality assurance instrument to evaluate the appropriateness of education.
13. List expected learning outcomes for both inpatient and outpatient coronary rehabilitation programs.

PRINCIPLES OF TEACHING AND LEARNING IN CORONARY REHABILITATION

How Coronary Patients Learn

Successful education of the patient and family in coronary rehabilitation begins with an understanding of what learning is and how it can be facilitated in patients recovering from a coronary illness.

Defining the Learning Experience

Learning is best defined by what it produces—a change in behavior.[10] The behavior may be a decision made and/or an action taken because of newly acquired knowledge, recently practiced skills, reshaped attitudes, or any combination of such events. Exactly how this change occurs is the subject of a number of learning theories from the classic work of Pavlov[11] to the contemporary concept of Bandura[12] (discussed in detail in Ch. 26). However, although the internal process is still controversial, the external result is clear: to learn is to change.

Learning is not passive. It is not just the absorption of information or the robotic repetition of a task. It is not mandatory attendance at a class or completion of a required course of study. Learning is an active process that produces change.

Change is inherent in the purpose of coronary rehabilitation. Patients who are involved in rehabilitation programs have to learn in order to accomplish individual changes in their health status. Further, when patients accept the opportunity to participate in coronary rehabilitation, they have the right to know why change is recommended. By virtue of these needs and rights, patients in programs of coronary rehabilitation are cast in the role of learners.

The threatening, confusing nature of a sudden coronary or other cardiac event quickly turns the patient's family members into learners as well. Spouses, in particular, become learners from two perspectives. First, they must learn for themselves. The learning needs of spouses have been documented to be unique to their situation.[13–15] Second, spouses must learn how to help their mate, now a coronary patient. Cardiac rehabilitation professionals who provide educational efforts to family members as well as patients are likely to realize a dual benefit. Not only will the family learn and change, but also the patient will be supported and encouraged by the family's effort and involvement. Support of the spouse has been shown to be the single most important psychosocial factor in the recovery and rehabilitation of coronary patients.[16]

Projecting Learning Outcomes

Learning is best focused by asking and answering the question of what specific change is sought from the proposed education. Once the desired result, or expected outcome, is clarified, teaching and learning activities that best contribute to achievement of that outcome can be selected. In other words, patient and family education in coronary rehabilitation is outcome driven.

Expected learning outcomes are statements describing what the learner will be able to do as a result of learning.[17] Their purpose is to express the sought-after behavior change in such a way that it will be recognized by educational observers when it occurs. Commonly, such outcomes take the form of "the learner will . . . ," where the

Table 25-1. Relationship Between Behavior Domains and Teaching and Learning Actions

Domain	Teaching Method	Learning Outcome
	The teacher will	The learner will
Cognitive Information, knowledge	inform instruct lecture provide materials	explain describe discuss define
Affective Attitudes, emotions	counsel model reinforce provide peer exchange	express affirm choose share
Psychomotor Skills, performance	demonstrate coach guide provide practice	perform do produce use

verb that follows is selected to express an observable action as well as to reflect the general type of behavior change involved with the learning experience.

Three major aspects of behavior have been identified as being involved with learning. In an educational context, these aspects are referred to as domains of learning.[18] Identification of the domain involved with a particular educational effort helps with the formation of expected learning outcomes as well as with the selection of appropriate teaching methods. Table 25-1 displays the relationship between domains and teaching and learning actions.

Complete outcome statements contain both an action verb and a content phrase specifying what the learner will do. Examples of expected learning outcomes are shown in the sample lesson plan (Fig. 25-1), as well as in the introduction to this chapter. Although the lesson sample addresses patients and the chapter sample addresses professionals, the format is the same since, in both cases, outcomes seek behavioral change.

Applying Principles of Adult Education

Learning is best facilitated through use of established principles of adult education. It would be a mistake for cardiac rehabilitation profession-

als to attempt to teach their patients in the same way they teach their children or for them to replicate the teaching methods they experienced during most of their years of formal education, since both these situations involve pedagogy—the art and science of teaching children.[19] Children learn in different ways and for different reasons than adults. Recognition of these differences has led to a relatively recent development in the field of education called andragogy—the art and science of teaching adults.[19] Recognition and use of the principles of adult education are essential to effective teaching in coronary rehabilitation.

The andragogic model in most common use in patient education is the one developed by Malcolm Knowles.[20] Knowles built his model of adult learning on several ideas about why adults learn differently from children.[19] The major principles of his adult learning theory are summarized in Table 25-2, along with some basic examples of how each can be applied to coronary teaching. As can be seen from the examples in Table 25-2, active participation of the patient is the key ingredient in education of adult coronary patients and family members. Rehabilitation professionals must actively involve patients in their own learning process.

Recognizing Readiness to Learn

Learning is best accomplished when the individual patient is ready to learn. Readiness to learn is included in the principles summarized in Table 25-2. However, readiness is so important to effective learning that an expanded discussion is in order.

Readiness to learn is defined as being both willing and able to learn.[21] Ability to learn can be correlated with physical condition, whereas willingness to learn considers the patient's psychologic state. According to the published articles on education of coronary patients, failure to recognize readiness is a common reason for ineffective teaching.[22] Mistakes are made in both directions—teaching when the patient is not ready, and not teaching when the patient is ready. Both situations can be prevented if rehabilitation professionals assess patient readiness before proceeding with any educational exchange. A readiness check is not time-consuming. Once familiar

HOW TO HANDLE A SUDDEN HEART PROBLEM
(EMERGENCY PLANNING)

Purpose of Lesson
To prepare patient to have a
plan of action in the event of
a coronary emergency at home.
(Length of lesson=20 mins.)

Timing of Lesson
1. As requested by patient
   or family member
2. For inpatients, required
   with discharge planning

Expected Learning Outcomes
As a result of this lesson, the coronary patient/family will
1. recall and compare his/her own presentaion of heart attack to common signs and symptoms
2. describe proper sequence of steps to be taken should similar/suspicious symptoms occur (including use of
   nitroglycerine if ordered)
3. state the importance of not wasting time waiting and wondering
4. choose some form of emergency identification

Lesson Content Outline
I.   Lesson Purpose

II. Symptom Recognition
     1. ask patient to describe own symptoms with acute event
     2. review common signs/symptoms of heart attack, relating to patient's own experience
     3. focus on chest pain/discomfort features since recurrence of pain is a common concern (if, when, etc.)
     4. reassure patient that another event is unlikely, but that "what if" planning is wise for everyone

III. Plan of Action
     1. instruct the patient that should he/she experience signs/symptoms of another heart attack, he should
        a. stop whatever he is doing
        b. quickly sit or lie down
        c. if the symptom does not begin to lessen in 1–2 minutes, then
           IF NITROGLYCERIN PRESCRIBED
           • place one tablet under the tongue
           • expect relief in 3–5 minutes
           • if discomfort persists or worsens, place a second tablet under the tongue
           • wait another 5 minutes; repeat nitroglycerin a third time if necessary
           • if no relief after 3 tablets every 5 mins.,
        OR IF NITROGLYCERIN NOT PRESCRIBED
           • summon help immediately; shout for anyone nearby and have them call 911
           • request emergency transport to the nearest hospital emergency room
           • time is of the essence to minimize heart damage!
           • **do not waste time** trying to get through to the physician's office
           • **do not attempt to drive yourself to the hospital**
           • **do not worry that this may be a false alarm and you will unnecessarily bother the hospital staff**

IV. Means of Identification
     1. show patient emergency ID items (e.g., Medic Alert bracelet, Nitro pendant, mini ECG)
     2. suggest that patient consider choosing and purchasing one of these (provide information once choice is
        made)

Fig. 25-1. Sample Lesson Plan. *(Figure continues.)*

**HOW TO HANDLE A SUDDEN HEART PROBLEM
(EMERGENCY PLANNING)** *(Continued)*

V. Questions and Answers
Teaching Method
Domain=cognitive;
one-to-one discussion with
patient and/or family

Teaching Aids
a. AHA brochure–Heart Attack & Stroke: Signals and Action
b. hospital instruction sheet on nitroglycerin (if applicable &
   not already given)

Learning Evaluation
WHEN: decided by teacher
_____ upon completion of the lesson
_____ the next day (inpatient)
_____ upon next visit (outpatient)

WHAT: expected outcomes
a. ask patient to verbally respond to #1–3 under
   Expected Learning Outcomes
b. ask patient to make choice of #4 (emergency identification)

Fig. 25-1 *(Continued).*

Table 25-2.   Adult Learning Theory in Coronary Teaching

Principle	*Application*
1. Adults should be self-directing, participate in decisions about their health and treatment, and be actively involved in the learning process	Plan teaching activities to include as much patient participation and decision-making as possible. Offer choices of *when* to teach: "Mr. Smith, I can be available at either 11 a.m. or 2:15 p.m. today to discuss the blood pressure information you requested earlier"; suggest alternative learning experiences: "Would you prefer to go to this afternoon's class on heart-healthy eating or have a private appointment with the dietitian when your wife can be here?"
2. Adults have cumulative experience that acts as a resource by either helping or hindering learning	Assess what, if any, exposure the patient has had to the subject matter; what is his or her current understanding; is she or he receptive or resistant: "Mr. Smith, last evening you mentioned that your brother died of a heart attack while having sex; that story has probably raised many questions in your mind; I suggest that we set aside some time today to talk about guidelines for sexual activity and clear up any doubts that you may have."
3. Adults have a problem-solving orientation and learn best from material that can be used in the immediate time frame	Plan to teach coronary topics in order of patient priority and concern; as a coronary teacher, remind yourself often that what you want to teach is not necessarily what the patient wants to learn right now.
4. Adults learn *only* if and when they are ready to learn	Assess the patient's readiness to learn before each teaching encounter; if the patient is not ready, do not proceed with the planned teaching, but instead document assessment findings and the reason why teaching was deferred.

(From Comoss PM: Optimizing patient recovery: Inpatient cardiac rehabilitation in the 1990s. Ch. 73. In Clochesy JM, Breu CS, Cardin S et al (eds): Critical Care Nursing. WB Saunders, Philadelphia, 1991, with permission.)

to the professional, such a check can be done mentally in just a few minutes. Built on the above definition of readiness, Table 25-3 lists suggested readiness checkpoints.

Determining when patients are ready to learn justifies both proceeding with teaching when it is appropriate to do so and deferring teaching when it is inappropriate to proceed. In the latter circumstance, the reason for lack of readiness should be documented to explain the aborted educational attempt as well as to facilitate any necessary follow-up of the problem identified.

How Rehabilitation Professionals Teach

Successful education of patients in coronary rehabilitation recognizes that teaching and learning are distinct functions but that teaching, when properly planned and executed, can influence learning and facilitate desired change.

Defining the Teaching Function

Teaching is best defined as a form of communication specially structured and sequenced to produce learning.[10] Teaching is not a one-sided delivery of information, nor authoritative issuing of commands. Like coronary rehabilitation itself, it is a structured process designed to achieve its goal of change toward health. And like the larger process in which it occurs, it requires interaction between the patient and the professional.

Most coronary rehabilitation programs do not have access to or necessarily need a full-time health educator. Therefore, rehabilitation professionals with various backgrounds—nurses, physiologists, nutritionists, and others—assume the role of teacher. Although all these potential teachers are experts in the content of their respective specialty, they may have little or no training in how to teach coronary patients, their potential learners.

Teaching of coronary patients is an important and serious role. To take on the teaching role is to make a commitment to knowing and applying the principles of learning discussed above and the process of teaching described below.

Preparing the Teacher

Teaching is best performed by rehabilitation professionals who have developed their expertise and organized their teaching tools to optimize the outcome of the teaching–learning interaction.

Professional Background.   Teaching expertise is a functional blend of knowledge and skills. As applied to coronary rehabilitation patients, the knowledge base includes both an understanding of the principles of teaching and learning and a working knowledge of a variety of coronary-related topics from the definition of a heart attack to the latest interventional techniques available for treating coronary disease. (*Note:* although a number of teaching topics are referred to or discussed herein, a complete content description for each topic is beyond the scope of this chapter.)

Skills needed for coronary teaching include interpersonal communication capability and consistent utilization of the teaching process. Clear, concise, accurate articulation of the subject matter is required, as is the ability to quickly gain the patient's trust and cooperation. The stronger the rapport between professional and patient, the more effective the teaching.[23]

The teaching process, based on a scientific method, has four functional steps: assessment, planning, implementation, and evaluation.[24] Ap-

Table 25-3.   Checklist for Assessing Patient Readiness to Learn

Is the Patient Ready to Learn at This Time?	
Physical Ability Checkpoints	Psychological Willingness Checkpoints
• Stable physical condition (free of pain and complications) • Adequate energy level (not too exhausted or sedated)	• Appropriate emotional state (not too anxious or depressed) • Awareness of actual problem (not in total denial)

plication of the steps of the teaching process must become second nature in each teaching–learning encounter. For many cardiac rehabilitation professionals, the requisite knowledge for teaching is acquired through specific classes or seminars and the necessary skills are honed through general experience over time.

Teaching Tools. The appropriate background prepares the would-be coronary teacher to be able to teach. That is, before actual teaching can commence, much "homework" must be done to outline topics, or lessons, to be taught and to select related teaching aids.

Lesson plans are brief descriptions of what will be taught to a patient to achieve expected learning outcomes related to the particular topic. Plans contain an outline of content, suggested teaching methods, and a list of preselected teaching aids to be used. Fig. 25-1 presents a sample lesson plan on the topic of "How to Handle a Sudden Heart Problem." To optimize flow and flexibility of coronary teaching, rehabilitation professionals should compose plans that address singular topics as short, stand-alone lessons.

There is a twofold purpose to these prewritten lessons. First, they help ensure consistency of information delivered to different patients or delivered by different cardiac rehabilitation professionals. Second, although lesson preparation requires some start-up time and effort, once lessons are in place they save time by minimizing the amount of educational charting. Instead of writing the detail of all that was taught in an educational exchange, the rehabilitation professional can simply note "taught lesson on How to Handle a Sudden Heart Problem." The homework of development of specific lessons begins with a list of anticipated topics, identified by potential teachers, about which coronary patients may want or need to learn.

Teaching aids are the written and/or audiovisual materials that are selected to supplement the interpersonal educational exchange. Selection of teaching aids is another part of homework to be done by coronary teachers. With the array of teaching materials available on today's market, it is easy to become overwhelmed by the choices. Rehabilitation professionals must frequently re-

mind themselves that the purpose of teaching aids is to supplement and reinforce teaching, not to act as a substitute for teaching–learning interactions.[25] It may be tempting to think that an exciting new video can replace a teacher's worn-out message, but such substitution ignores the importance of the partnership effort and the support and motivation accompanying it. Even the most innovative teaching technology, such as interactive computers, will never replace the human interaction that is the essence of education.[26]

Every potential teaching aid should be scrutinized professionally before being used with a patient. Whether the material is a self-made handout or an interactive computer program, each item must be previewed. Content critique has been common practice among coronary teachers for a number of years. Recent research has also emphasized the critical importance of the reading level in the selection of teaching aids. In their 1983 landmark study, Boyd and Citro identified that 90% of printed cardiac teaching materials in common use were above the reading ability of the patients receiving them.[27] Rehabilitation professionals should not assume that patients can read at the same level as grades completed. Studies have shown that literacy may vary as much as three grades in either direction.[28] Since the average reading level of U.S. adults is about sixth grade, and since patients in most coronary rehabilitation programs are a cross-section of the general population, materials must be selected to meet the average reading level.

A number of formulas are available for evaluating the reading levels of teaching aids being considered.[10] Use of both the FOG and SMOG formulas has been found helpful in reviewing and revising materials for specific cardiac topics.[29,30] When it is known that reading levels above or below the average are likely to be encountered, a few special pieces can be selected and reserved for those exceptional patients. Special materials may also have to be located or developed for coronary patients who are vision impaired, are totally illiterate, do not speak English, or have specific learning disabilities. Fig. 25-2 provides a sample format for critique of potential teaching aids.

Material: Name _____   Reviewed By:
          Source _____   Name _____
          Cost _____   Date _____

CONTENT REVIEW
          Checkpoint   Critique
_____
                                YES   NO   COMMENT
A. Is the information correct?
B. Is the information current?
C. Is the information compatible
   with actual lesson outline?

READABILITY CHECK
          Checkpoint   Critique
_____
                                YES   NO   COMMENT
A. Is visual appearance or
   style acceptable?
B. Is print large and legible?
C. Is reading level in average
   range (grades 5–9)?
_____

RECOMMENDATION
A. ACCEPT as standard teaching aid _____
B. ACCEPT for limited use, describe _____
C. REJECT due to _____
Additional recommendations:

Fig. 25-2. Sample Format for Critique of Coronary Teaching Aids

Identifying Lesson Priority and Sequence

Teaching is best assigned priorities according to what patients want to learn. Like other health care specialists, cardiac rehabilitation professionals often feel that their expertise enables them to know the exact order in which lessons should be presented to rehabilitation patients. However, research on education of the patient during the last decade has clearly demonstrated that there is no best first lesson or natural sequence of lessons.[31] What rehabilitation professionals want to teach is not necessarily what coronary patients should learn.[32–35]

Only a patient knows her or his foremost questions and concerns and the order in which they should be addressed. Rather than trying to impose a teacher-selected artificial order of lesson priorities, the rehabilitation professional should work with the patient to identify priority learning needs and then match the lesson sequence to expressed needs.

Priorities can be assessed verbally by simply asking, "What questions or concerns do you have at this time?" However, some patients may find it difficult to reply spontaneously to such an open-ended question. Therefore, an assessment instrument designed to help patients collect their thoughts about what they want to learn may be helpful (Fig. 25-3). Such a technique can be adapted to either the inpatient or outpatient setting and used with either patients or family members.

Teaching by patient priorities lends itself well to the shortened time frames of both inpatient and outpatient coronary rehabilitation programs. As long as the rehabilitation professional is prepared to teach and has the appropriate teaching re-sources available, involving patients in the decision on the order of lesson priorities enhances the educational experience for learner and teacher alike.

Choosing Methods of Teaching

Teaching is best delivered by a combination of methods. First, an appropriate general format must be selected, and then specific teaching techniques can be selected on the basis of the domain

---

Patient Learning Priorities

Dear Patient:

   Like most people with heart problems, you probably have many questions. During the next few days we want to address those concerns that are uppermost in your mind. So, to help plan the best sequence for our discussions, please place the numbers 1 through 5 (1 = least) in front of the topics for which you would like more information.

_____ CCU machines and treatments

_____ heart structure and function

_____ coronary arteries normal/abnormal

_____ activity progression during hospital stay

_____ what to do for chest pain

_____ emergency planning for home*

_____ heart attack and healing

_____ your risk factors

_____ how to take your pulse

_____ high blood pressure

_____ high blood cholesterol

_____ your medicines

_____ fitness and health

_____ eating for a healthy heart

_____ sexual activity and your heart

_____ emotional changes after heart problems

_____ development of heart disease

_____ stress and your heart

_____ smoking and your heart

_____ alcohol and your heart

_____ guidelines for activities at home*

_____ activity/exercise precautions

_____ heart catheterization procedure

_____ bypass graft surgery

_____ heart balloon procedure (angioplasty)

_____ heart failure

_____ heart rhythms

_____ coronary rehabilitation program

_____ treadmill exercise test

_____ effects of heart problems on families

_____ return to work questions

OTHER QUESTIONS YOU WOULD LIKE TO HAVE ANSWERED:

_____

_____

_____

*These topics will be discussed by the cardiac rehabilitation staff a day or two before you go home.

Fig. 25-3. Sample Assessment Form (From Comoss PM: Optimizing patient recovery: Inpatient cardiac rehabilitation in the 1990s. Ch. 73. In Clochesy JM, Breu CS, Cardin S et al (eds): Critical Care Nursing. WB Saunders, Philadelphia, 1991, with permission).

Table 25-4. Comparison of Teaching Methods in Coronary Rehabilitation

	Individual Exchanges	Group Classes
Advantages	Instant presentation (captures the most teachable moments)	Peer exchange (adds the element of psychological support)
	Personal application (enables content to be individualized to each patient)	Economies of time and effort (means less repetition by rehabilitation professionals doing teaching)
Disadvantages	Lack of sufficient time to teach (by most rehabilitation professionals)	Lack of concurrent readiness to learn (among different rehabilitation patients)

of learning involved (see Table 25-1). Regarding format, both group and individual teaching have been popular with cardiac rehabilitation professionals.[36] Each of these methods has advantages and disadvantages, as summarized in Table 25-4.

Interestingly, recent educational literature confirms patients' preference for one-on-one encounters.[37,38] However, health professionals often view group teaching as more time- and cost-effective. The sections on education of the patient in inpatient and outpatient coronary rehabilitation settings that follow give suggestions of when each teaching method is most appropriate.

THE PRACTICE OF EDUCATION OF THE PATIENT IN CORONARY REHABILITATION

The Inpatient Setting

A walk through the corridors of a progressive care unit (PCU) in almost any hospital affirms the emphasis placed on patient and family education during a coronary patient's recovery. Nurses visiting the patient's room armed with teaching paraphernalia, dietitians setting up conference rooms for family classes, and other similar activities make teaching efforts highly visible. In coronary care areas, patient education is not an exception—it is an expectation.

Setting Educational Goals for Inpatient Coronary Teaching

Inpatient coronary rehabilitation programs have a dual purpose. They are designed both to minimize complications and to optimize recovery from an acute coronary event.[39] Physical deconditioning is reduced and self-care promoted through early ambulation and progressive activity plans. Psychologically, anxiety and depression are lessened through support, encouragement, counseling, and goal-setting. Educational activities are an integral part of accomplishing inpatient program purposes as well.

While a coronary patient is in the coronary care unit (CCU), the educational goal is simply to answer questions and provide explanation and orientation. Most patients are not ready for substantive learning during their brief CCU stay.[40] Upon transfer to the PCU, teaching can usually proceed. From the point of readiness to the time of discharge, the educational goal in the step-down area is to provide teaching that deals with the patient's identified learning priorities.

Meeting the Challenge of Short Hospital Stays

Educational goals for the inpatient coronary rehabilitation program reflect changes in the health care system in recent years. Advances in interventional cardiology, research on the safety of early discharge, and cost containment concerns have all led to shortened hospital stays for coronary patients. Currently, the average length of stay for both uncomplicated myocardial infarction patients and uncomplicated coronary artery bypass graft surgery (CABG) patients is 7 days.[41,42] In some medical centers, patients who are treated with the newest interventions, such as thrombolysis and/or early percutaneous transluminal coronary angioplasty (PTCA), are discharged even earlier.

These short hospital stays are in sharp contrast to lengths of stay in preceding decades, when many inpatient coronary rehabilitation programs were originally established. Then, with 10 to 14 days to teach coronary patients, comprehensive educational agendas could be completed. Now, with less than a week of teaching time available, cardiac rehabilitation professionals are challenged to make their inpatient educational programs as efficient as possible.

In addition to the short hospital stay, teaching opportunities are further limited by the lack of patient readiness to learn during their early days of hospitalization. As discussed in an earlier section of this chapter, readiness is essential to successful learning. Unstable clinical status and overwhelming emotional reactions during the acute phase of coronary illness mean that most patients are not ready to learn while in the CCU, especially while undergoing diagnostic and therapeutic interventions. Once stabilized and transferred to the PCU, patients become increasingly ready, but only a few days remain of their hospital stay. Recognizing the necessity of readiness to learn, cardiac rehabilitation professionals are challenged to make their inpatient educational programs as effective as possible.

Despite the limitations of short stays and delayed readiness of the patient to learn, an effective and efficient educational program can be developed and implemented as a core service of inpatient coronary rehabilitation. To maximize the effectiveness of the program, teaching should proceed only when patients are ready to learn (Table 25-3). To proceed with teaching when patients are not ready is a waste of the professional's time and effort. To maximize the efficiency of the program, teaching must be based on the patient's learning priorities (Fig. 25-3). Addressing the patient's most pressing concerns first makes the best use of limited time.

It is no longer appropriate to conduct coronary teaching programs built on rigid protocols of what to teach on each day or to herd all coronary patients into a mandatory group class. Instead, to do the job well within the constraints of today's hospital environment, coronary teaching must be based on confirmed readiness to learn and expressed priority needs.

Sharing Responsibility for Inpatient Coronary Teaching

Recent staff shortages and cost concerns have prompted inpatient programs to reexamine who should be doing rehabilitation-related teaching.[43] As a result, there is a growing trend toward sharing responsibility for education of coronary rehabilitation inpatients.[44] One common shared structure divides daily responsibility for coronary teaching between bedside nurses and rehabilitation professionals. Bedside nurses, who are with patients 24 hours a day, are in the best position to initiate teaching that answers patients' questions or addresses their concerns in a timely manner. The most common questions patients ask during their first few days in the hospital center around "What happened?", "Why me?", and "Now what?" These questions contain an element of urgency on the part of the patient. The anxious, inquiring patient should not have to wait for a special teacher to arrive later that day to address such basic concerns. The bedside nurse is in a prime position to capture the "teachable moment."[45]

However, some lessons require specific exercise expertise and/or outpatient follow-up and are therefore best taught by coronary rehabilitation specialists working out of the outpatient cardiac rehabilitation department. Examples include guidelines for home activities, instructions for a progressive walking program, and emergency planning (sign and symptom recognition and management) for home. Some of these topics are considered "survival skills,"[45] but their importance may not yet be recognized by coronary patients preparing for discharge. Assigning respon-

Learning Need		Lessons Available	Teaching Done			Outcomes Evaluated	
	P	**BEDSIDE NURSE** (basic coronary information)	R		F		2E
		Orientation to CCU					
		Explanation of Event: _____ heart attack _____ bypass surgery _____ angioplasty _____ angina pectoris OTHER: _____					
		CHD Development					
		Overview of Risk Factors					
		Emotional Changes					
		Family Reactions					
		Procedures/Treatments: specify					
		Complications: specify					
		Cardiac Medications: list _____ _____ _____ _____ OTHER: _____					
		REHABILITATION SPECIALIST (pre-discharge emphasis)					
		Emergency Planning					
		At-Home Guidelines					
		Walking Program					
		Pulse Taking					
		Outpatient Rehabilitation Introduction					
		Sex and the Heart					
		Exercise Test Information					
		OTHER: _____					

Fig. 25-4. Inpatient Coronary Rehabilitation Program: Sample Patient Education Flow Sheet. *(Figure continues.)*

Learning Need		Lessons Available	Teaching Done			Outcomes Evaluated	
	P	REFERRED LESSONS	R		F		2E
		Heart Healthy Eating (dietitian)					
		Stress & Relaxation (psychologist)					
		Smoking Cessation (pulmonary rehabilitation)					
		Job Questions (vocational rehabilitation)					
		Financial concerns (social worker)					
		OTHER: _____					

KEY: P = Priority identified by patient; R = Readiness to learn confirmed; F = Family involved in ed. exchange; 2E = Second evaluation done; (place checkmarks in keyed columns to indicate above information); * = see written comment on reverse side for further explanation; date and initial Need, Teaching, Outcomes columns as performed.

Fig. 25-4 *(Continued).*

sibility for this predischarge teaching to the coronary rehabilitation staff puts them in the position to offer these lessons and influence the patient's learning priorities near discharge.

With the above considerations in mind, responsibilities can be distributed so that bedside nurses do basic coronary teaching to answer initial questions and coronary rehabilitation specialists do predischarge teaching to include survival skills. When they are requested, specialized topics are referred to other appropriate team members. Although this plan designates specific responsibilities to each teacher, it must be remembered that teaching proceeds only if the patient is ready and that topics are presented only when they are an identified priority of the patient. The variability of topics and timing from one patient or family to another make individual teaching the method of choice for today's inpatient setting.[46] Fig. 25-4 is a sample Coronary Teaching Flow Sheet showing the type of lesson distribution discussed here.

Documenting Inpatient Teaching and Learning

Both teaching and learning must be documented in the patient's chart. Forms selected for this purpose must be clear and concise to communicate quickly the requisite information. Flow sheets are commonly used and should be designed to record each step of the educational process (Fig. 25-4). Table 25-5 summarizes the paperwork needed for inpatient coronary teaching and relates its use to the steps of the teaching process.

Evaluation, the final step of the teaching process, is the determination of whether expected learning outcomes have been achieved.[47] It is a measurement and documentation of what the patient has learned.

Methods of evaluation appropriate for coronary inpatients include verbal feedback, return demonstration, and observation of actual behavior. One method of evaluation useful in other educational settings that is inappropriate for coronary patients is written testing.[48] Psychologically,

Table 25-5.   Records and Forms Used in the Process of Coronary Teaching

Process	Records	Samples
Assessment	1. Patient checklist for learning priorities	Fig. 25-3
	2. Educational flow sheet (assessment columns)	Fig. 25-4
		or 25-5
Planning	1. Lesson book with many lesson plans	Fig. 25-1
	2. Teaching aids and handouts (critiqued)	Fig. 25-2
Implementation	1. Educational flow sheet (taught columns, readiness)	(See above)
	2. Notes and comments on reverse of flow sheet	
Evaluation	1. Educational flow sheet (evaluation columns)	(See above)
	2. Educational transfer or discharge summary on reverse of flow sheet	

paper-and-pencil tests are intimidating to many patients. Functionally, the usefulness of pre-post tests has diminished with increased use of priority-based teaching. The content of such tests assumes that certain material will always be covered. Since content now varies with each individual, such general tests are of little use.

In the shared approach to teaching, it is the responsibility of the professional who taught the lesson—bedside nurse, cardiac rehabilitation specialist, other team member—to evaluate the learning. Asking the patient to do what the expected learning outcomes of the particular lesson state is all that is needed. If the patient responds correctly, the outcome has been achieved and the evaluation column of the educational flow sheet should be dated and initialed to record that appropriate feedback was obtained. If the patient responds incorrectly, the desired outcome has not been achieved and a comment to that effect should be written in the educational commentary on the back of the flow sheet. The comment should include the teacher's recommendation for follow-up, e.g., reassess need, reteach lesson, refer to specific specialist, reevaluate outcomes.

The type of documentation described here not only verifies what was taught and what was learned for the patient's record, but also enables continuation of educational efforts after discharge. With this information available, outpatient cardiac rehabilitation professionals can continue where their inpatient colleagues left off.

The Outpatient Setting

A casual visit to an active outpatient coronary rehabilitation center usually leaves the impression that exercise is the prime service offered. Closer observation, though, reveals the equal importance of other care activities that make up outpatient coronary rehabilitation. For example, one patient might be seen sitting in an easy chair in a quiet conference room listening to a relaxation tape, while another patient's wife is looking through labels from food packages with the dietitian. And, in patient dressing rooms and waiting areas, posters announcing an upcoming smoking cessation class might be prominently displayed. In outpatient coronary rehabilitation, patient and family teaching is not an elective service but an essential component of rehabilitative care.

Setting Educational Goals for Outpatient Coronary Teaching

The purpose of outpatient coronary rehabilitation is to provide a program of secondary prevention,[49] that is, to offer coronary patients the means and opportunity to optimize their health and minimize their risk of future coronary events. Physically, the benefits of exercise for coronary rehabilitation patients have been well documented.[50] Psychosocially, research into the long-term effects of behavioral interventions continues.[51] Educational activities are an integral part of accomplishing outpatient program purposes as well.

Specifically, the educational goal of outpatient coronary rehabilitation is to provide and reinforce the knowledge and skills the patient needs for optimal health. Patients and professionals work together to define what is "optimal" in each case and to project when related outcomes can be expected to be achieved.[52] The individualized rehabilitation plan is then implemented over the weeks of program involvement. Unless patients understand why change is necessary, and until they know how to accomplish change, optimal health will remain elusive.

Meeting the Challenge of Conflicting Time Demands

Ten years ago, outpatient coronary rehabilitation programs were 6 to 12 months long. In contrast, today's structured programs last 6 to 12 weeks. A number of factors intervened in the last decade to reduce the outpatient rehabilitation time frame. For example, the American College of Cardiology took the position that 12 weeks was a sufficient program duration for most coronary patients.[53] Additionally, increasing cost concerns forced many insurance companies to limit coverage, including payment to outpatient coronary rehabilitation programs.[54]

At present, in a typical 12-week program, most coronary rehabilitation patients are scheduled to attend outpatient sessions three times per week to meet their exercise needs. Such frequent visits would seem to offer the patient ample contact to work on all rehabilitative goals, including education. However, since most of the patient's appointment time during these visits is spent in exercise training, additional time for formal teaching is not usually available. Although some programs have had success in scheduling an educational hour back-to-back with an exercise hour,[55] other programs find that patients are unwilling to stay for this extra time. Further, attempts to make such outpatient classes mandatory violates the principles of adult education discussed earlier in this chapter. Thus, a major design issue for outpatient coronary rehabilitation programs is to determine how much time should be devoted to education of the patient.

Time conflicts are a common reason why patients drop out of coronary rehabilitation programs.[56] Younger coronary patients return to work earlier than ever and have other life commitments that supersede coronary rehabilitation involvement. Older coronary patients often have transportation problems and surprisingly busy social schedules that interfere with attendance. Under such circumstances, the more time demands that rehabilitation programs make on their patients, the less likely it is that patients will participate in all that is offered. Therefore, understanding the time conflicts that exist in patients' lives and recognizing the competition for time among rehabilitative services, cardiac rehabilitation professionals working in the outpatient setting are challenged to select strategies that will enable them to provide and reinforce patient and family education in a timely and consistent manner.

Selecting Strategies for Outpatient Coronary Teaching

As discussed in the section on inpatients, the shortened hospital stays of recent years have restricted the time available for teaching. At best, patients leave the hospital with only their most urgent needs and highest priorities approached. Seldom are they sufficiently prepared to embark on a modified lifestyle when they return home. Often questions and fears about what to do or not do have gone unanswered. During this confusing period after discharge, patients require access to health professionals who can answer their questions and support their efforts to resume normal living.

Historically, most outpatient coronary rehabilitation programs did not accept patients until 6 to 8 weeks after the coronary event. The rationale for this delayed point of entry was to allow sufficient time for healing from the coronary event or surgery so that patients could exercise safely at training levels. However, recent exercise experience has shown that testing and training levels are appropriate for many patients as early as 3 weeks after the event[57] and that during the first few weeks after discharge, recovering patients can safely exercise at lower (pretraining) levels. As a result, outpatient programs have begun to revise their plans so that patients can start within 2 to 4 weeks of their event. This change in exercise timing and format has facilitated early referrals, which in turn has enabled new strategies for patient teaching.

Elementary Sessions. Ideally, patients are referred to outpatient coronary rehabilitation at the time of hospital discharge. Hour-long outpatient visits during the first 2 or 3 weeks after discharge are scheduled, one-on-one, between the patient and rehabilitation professional. Half of the appointment time is spent on activity progression practice and instructions, and the other half is available for patient and/or family teaching. Of course, the sequence of teaching is determined by the patient's priorities. Clearly, this strategy employs the principles of learning (participation, readiness, and practical need) and teaching (expert teacher, identified priorities, and primary method) in a way that has not often been possible with outpatient formats of the past.[58,59] These elementary sessions provide consistent, individualized, early outpatient education.

Supplementary Sessions. About 1 month after the coronary event, most patients are ready for symptom-limited exercise testing and subsequent advancement to the exercise training program. Since outpatient exercise is conducted in groups of various sizes, there is less opportunity for the elementary (individual, basic) educational sessions described above. Of course, questions are answered and previously taught content is reinforced as patients come and go from exercise sessions, and private teaching sessions can be scheduled when the patient and professional have time. However, the main teaching strategy at this stage of the rehabilitation program is the group educational meeting.

The frequency of educational meetings varies from once per week to once per quarter depending on the needs of the patient group. The main purpose of group presentations is to reinforce what has already been taught through the earlier elementary sessions. Group topics may be selected for general review from available coronary lessons, or specific subjects may be solicited by surveys. Group participants usually include both current coronary rehabilitation patients and recent program graduates, as well as their families and guests. Some rehabilitation programs send special invitations to spouses to encourage their attendance at group meetings. These periodic educational supplements provide all the advantages of group teaching (Table 25-4) as well as timely reinforcement of previous learning. As an added benefit, the peer interaction that occurs at these gatherings provides psychological support to the patient and family alike.

Shared Responsibility. With the two-part strategy of early elementary teaching and ongoing supplementary teaching, each program must decide which rehabilitation professionals best fill related teaching roles. For example, cardiac rehabilitation nurses commonly do one-on-one initial teaching, whereas later in the program, exercise specialists assist patients with planning their ongoing exercise for when they have left the program. However, to maximize the reinforcement benefit of group sessions, the content should be presented by someone other than the rehabilitation professionals who do the basic teaching. Hearing the same message from a different voice affirms previously learned information for the patient. Therefore, other team members—physicians, pharmacists, dietitians, etc.—should be called upon to teach at group sessions. These roles are quite similar to the sharing of teaching responsibility described for inpatients wherein the nurse did basic teaching, the rehabilitation specialist focused on discharge planning, and various members of the team were available by special request.

Documenting Outpatient Teaching and Learning

Since the same teaching process is followed with outpatients as with inpatients, paperwork for documenting outpatient educational efforts is similar to that already described. In fact, when the same rehabilitation professionals are involved with teaching in both settings, forms should be as similar as possible to simplify their use by rehabilitation staff and to increase their familiarity to other professionals who read coronary rehabilitation charts. Figure 25-5 provides a sample pa-

Learning Need		Lessons Available	Teaching Done		Outcomes Evaluated	
	P	CARDIAC REHABILITATION NURSE (basic coronary information)	R		F	2E
		Orientation to Rehabilitation				
		Personal Risk Factors: ____ high blood pressure ____ diabetes ____ elevated lipids ____ overweight ____ stress ____ smoking ____ lack of exercise OTHER: _____				
		CHD Development				
		Homecoming Depression				
		Family Overprotection				
		Emergency Planning				
		Procedures/Treatments: specify				
		Complications: specify Cardiac Medications: list _____ _____ _____ OTHER: _____				
		EXERCISE SPECIALIST				
		Warm-up/Cool-down Cardiovascular Fitness Aerobic Exercise Post D/C Walking Exercise Test Preparation				
		OTHER: _____				

Fig. 25-5. Outpatient Coronary Rehabilitation Program: Sample Patient Education Flow Sheet. (*Figure continues.*)

Learning Need		Lessons Available	Teaching Done			Outcomes Evaluated	
	P	EXERCISE SPECIALIST	R		F		2E
		Exercise Precautions:					
		_____ hot weather					
		_____ cold weather					
		_____ clothes/shoes					
		Home Equipment					
		Sports/Recreation					
		OTHER: _____					
		GROUP SESSIONS (list those attended)					
		_____					
		_____					
		_____					

KEY: P = Priority identified by patient; R = Readiness to learn confirmed; F = Family involved in ed. exchange; 2E = Second evaluation done; (place checkmarks in keyed columns to indicate above information); * = see written comment on reverse side for further explanation; date and initial Need, Teaching, Outcomes columns as performed.

Fig. 25-5 *(Continued).*

tient education flow sheet for outpatient coronary rehabilitation.

In the evaluation of learning in outpatient coronary rehabilitation, the same methods of feedback are used as were recommended for evaluation of inpatient education. Outcomes of learning should be solicited from the patient as each lesson is completed or at the next outpatient visit. However, because of the length of the outpatient program and the use of group reinforcement, one additional evaluation step is suggested. Educational topics that were taught and evaluated early in the program should be evaluated a second time as the patient approaches discharge from the outpatient program. That is, the patient should again be asked to perform the specific outcomes of the lesson to determine how much new information was retained over time. Should major learning lapses be identified, there

is still sufficient time to repeat priority lessons. In addition to completion of the flow sheet, a summary of the educational activities and results must be included in the discharge summary prepared at the conclusion of the outpatient coronary rehabilitation program.

SUMMARY

Education of the patient is an essential part of coronary rehabilitation. It is of equal importance to exercise training and behavior modification. As discussed in this chapter, state-of-the-art educational programs for coronary patients are constructed on well-founded principles of teaching and learning. Given their common foundation, teaching programs for both inpatient and outpatient coronary rehabilitation are more alike than different.

Differences between programs in the two settings are mainly due to differences between patients, or even variations within the same patient, from one point in time to another. For example, patients are more likely to be ready to learn during the latter part of their hospital stay than at the beginning, and patients just discharged from the hospital are most likely to have a long list of ur-

gent learning priorities. Cardiac rehabilitation professionals must recognize and respond to these differences to capitalize on teaching opportunities.

Similarities between inpatient and outpatient educational programs can be seen both in their structure and in the educational process. Structurally, both programs require written policies that address the teaching function, including educational goals and related professional re-

---

Important Aspect of Care: Appropriateness of Patient Education

Rationale: To be "appropriate," patient education in coronary rehabilitation must follow established principles of teaching and learning.

Source of Data: Representative sample of charts of patients discharged from the program during the last quarter; specifically, Educational Flowsheet for Coronary Teaching.

INDICATORS	FINDINGS	
	YES	NO
1. Patient participating in selecting learning priorities evidenced by checkmarks in "Needs" column		
2. Patient's readiness to learn assessed as indicated by checkmark in "Taught" column OR* note on reverse side re: "NOT READY to learn due to ..."		
3. Identified topics taught as outlined in lesson plans (available in each coronary rehabilitation area) and corresponding teaching aids given as indicated by date & initials of cardiac teacher in "Taught" column		
4. Teaching responsibility shared among several professionals (as described in educational policies) as evidenced by different sets of initials in "Taught" column		
5. Learning outcomes achieved as specified per lesson indicated by date and initials of cardiac teacher in "Evaluated" column OR*note on reverse side re: "NOT ACHIEVED due to ..."		

Threshold: 80% (At least 8 out of 10 records are expected to meet all of the above indicators; should the sample score fall below the threshold, cardiac rehabilitation staff will meet to discuss teaching problems and recommend corrective actions.)

Fig. 25-6. Quality Assurance Monitoring Tool for Patient Education in Coronary Rehabilitation

Table 25-6. Expected Outcomes from Patient Teaching in Coronary Rehabilitation Programs

Inpatient Teaching	Outpatient Teaching
Before hospital discharge, the patient will be able to: 1. give a basic explanation of his or her event and treatment 2. perform the specific outcomes of each selected lesson that was taught 3. describe a plan of action to be taken in the event of a coronary emergency at home 4. list some activity do's and don'ts for the first week at home	Before program discharge, the patient will be able to: 1. give a basic explanation of coronary risk factors, name his or her own, and discuss actions underway to reduce risk 2. perform the specific outcomes of each selected lesson taught 3. describe a plan for self-maintenance of an exercise program after discharge

sponsibilities. Each program must also have lesson plans, teaching aids, charting forms, and the like available to support teaching efforts.

The teaching process—assessment, planning, implementation, and evaluation—is the same in both settings. To help ensure consistent application of the process, patient education services should be reviewed as part of a quality assurance program at both rehabilitation sites. The Joint Commission on Accreditation of Healthcare Organizations (JCAHO) recommends that health care providers monitor and evaluate "Important Aspects of Care" on an ongoing basis as part of their quality assurance program.[60] In coronary rehabilitation, patient education qualifies as an important aspect of care because (1) it is a high-volume service, i.e., all patients in the program are assessed for learning needs and offered teaching services; (2) it is a high-risk service, i.e., patients could be at serious risk of consequence or deprived of substantial benefit if the service is not provided; and (3) it is a problem-prone service, i.e., if patient teaching is not delivered appropriately, it is a disservice to patients and a waste of professional resources. A sample quality assurance tool for monitoring appropriateness of patient teaching is provided in Fig. 25-6.

The best test of the value and effectiveness of any patient education program is its outcomes. In general, expected outcomes are also similar between inpatient and outpatient coronary rehabilitation programs (Table 25-6). Of course, specific outcomes are dictated by the individualized lessons that were taught. It is hoped that the principles discussed and strategies suggested in

this chapter will contribute to successful patient education efforts in coronary rehabilitation programs.

REFERENCES

1. Comoss PM, Burke EAS, Swails SH: Cardiac Rehabilitation: A Comprehenesive Nursing Approach. p. 2. JB Lippincott, Philadelphia, 1979
2. Wenger NK: Future directions in cardiovascular rehabilitation. J Cardiopulmonary Rehabil 7:168, 1987
3. Murdaugh C: Using research in practice. Focus, p. 11, June–July 1982
4. Budan LJ: Cardiac patient learning in the hospital setting. Focus Crit Care 10:16, 1983
5. Steele JM, Ruzicki D: An evaluation of the effectiveness of cardiac teaching during hospitalization. Heart Lung 16:306, 1987
6. Raleigh EH, Odtohan BC: The effect of a cardiac teaching program on patient rehabilitation. Heart Lung 16:311, 1987
7. Garding BS, Kerr JC, Bay K: Effectiveness of a program of information and support for myocardial infarction patients recovering at home. Heart Lung 17:355, 1988
8. Hogan CA, Neill WA: Effects of a teaching program on knowledge, physical activity, and socialization in patients disabled by stable angina pectoris. J Cardiac Rehabil 2:379, 1982
9. American Association of Cardiovascular and Pulmonary Rehabilitation: Guidelines for Cardiac Rehabilitation. Human Kinetics Publishers, Champaign, IL, 1990
10. Redman BK: The Process of Patient Education. 6th

Ed. p. 1–20 and 150–175. CV Mosby, St. Louis, 1988

11. Hilgard ER, Bower GH: Theories of Learning. p. 48. Appleton-Century-Crofts, East Norwalk, CT, 1966

12. Bandura A, Walters RH: Social Learning and Personality Development. Rinehart & Winston, New York, 1963

13. Keeling AW: Health promotion in coronary care and step-down units: focus on the family—linking research to practice. Heart Lung 17:28, 1988

14. Newton KM, Killien MG: Patient and spouse learning needs during recovery from coronary artery bypass. Prog Cardiovasc Nursing 3:62, 1988

15. Sikorski JM: Knowledge, concerns, and questions of wives of convalescent coronary artery bypass graft surgery patients. J Cardiac Rehabil 5:74, 1985

16. Bramwell L: Social support and its relevance to cardiac rehabilitation. p. 70. In Jillings CR (ed): Cardiac Rehabilitation Nursing. Aspen Publishers, Rockville, MD, 1988

17. Mager RF: Preparing Instructional Objectives. 2nd Ed. p. 5–7. Lake Publishing, Belmont, CA, 1984

18. Smith CE: Patient Education: Nurses in Partnership with Other Health Professionals. p. 139–151. Grune & Stratton, Orlando, FL, 1987

19. Knowles M: The Adult Learner: A Neglected Species. p. 49–62. Gulf Publishing, Houston, 1984

20. Murdaugh C: The Nurse's Role in Education of the Cardiac Patient. p. 265. In Kern LS (ed): Cardiac Critical Care Nursing. Aspen Publishers, Rockville, MD, 1988

21. Narrow BW: Patient Teaching in Nursing Practice: A Patient and Family-Centered Approach. p. 78–88. John Wiley & Sons, New York, 1979

22. McHatton M: A theory for timely teaching. Am J Nursing p. 798, July 1985

23. Knapp D, Hansen M, Rogowski B, Pollock M: Education of cardiac surgery patients: a comparison of the effectiveness of nurse educators and primary nurses. J Cardiopulmonary Rehab 5:429, 1985

24. Smith CE: Patient Education: Nurses in Partnership with Other Health Professionals. p. 4. Grune & Stratton, Orlando, FL, 1987

25. Falvo DR: Effective Patient Education: A Guide to Increased Compliance. p. 215–234. Aspen Publishers, Rockville, MD, 1985

26. Squyres WD: Anticipating the "bottom line" in patient education in the twenty-first century. p. 30. In Wenger NK (ed): The Education of the Patient with Cardiac Disease in the Twenty-first Century. LeJacq Publishing Inc., New York, 1986

27. Boyd MD, Citro K: Cardiac patient education literature: can patients read what we give them? J Cardiac Rehabil, 3:513, 1983

28. Hussey LC, Gilliland K: Compliance, low literacy, and locus of control. p. 605. In: Nursing Clinics of North America. Vol. 24. WB Saunders, Philadelphia, 1989

29. Miller A: When is the time ripe for teaching? Am J Nursing p. 801, July 1985

30. Evanoski CAM: Health education for patients with ventricular tachycardia: assessment of readability. J Cardiovasc Nursing 4:1, 1990

31. Armstrong ML: Orchestrating the process of patient education. p. 597. In: Nursing Clinics of North America. Vol. 24. WB Saunders, Philadelphia, 1989

32. Gerard PS, Peterson LM: Learning needs of cardiac patients. Cardio-Vasc Nursing 20:7, 1984

33. Karlik BA, Yarcheski A: Learning needs of cardiac patients: a partial replication study. Heart Lung 16:544, 1987

34. Karlik BA, Yarcheski A, Braun J, Wu M: Learning needs of patients with angina: an extension study. J Cardiovasc Nursing 4:70, 1990

35. Grady KL, Buckley DJ, Cisar NS et al: Patient perception of cardiovascular surgical patient education. Heart Lung 17:349, 1988

36. Sivarajan ES, Newton KM: Exercise, education, and counseling for patients with coronary artery disease. Clin Sports Med 3:349, 1984

37. Boyd MD, Feldman RHL: Health information seeking and reading comprehension abilities of cardiac rehabilitation patients. J Cardiac Rehabil 4:343, 1984

38. Alywahby NF: Principles of teaching for individual learning of older adults. Rehabil Nursing 14:330, 1989

39. Wenger NK: Early ambulation after myocardial infarction: rationale, program components, and results. p. 97. In Wenger NK, Hellerstein HK (eds): Rehabilitation of the Coronary Patient. 2nd Ed. John Wiley & Sons, New York, 1984

40. Murdaugh CL: Barriers to patient education in the coronary care unit. Cardio-Vasc Nursing 18:31, 1982

41. Karliner JS: When do you discharge MI patients? Cardiovasc Med, p. 61, June 1985

42. Goulart DT: Educating the cardiac surgery patient and family. J Cardiovasc Nursing 3:1, 1989

43. Linden B: Unit-based phase I cardiac rehabilitation program for patients with myocardial infarction. Focus Crit Care 17:15, 1990

44. Shine KI, Heller WM, Wenger NK: Hospital-based

education of the cardiac patient. p. 376. In Wenger NK (ed): The Education of the Patient with Cardiac Disease in the Twenty-first Century. LeJacq Publishing Inc., New York, 1986

45. Ruzicki DA: Realistically meeting the educational needs of hospitalized acute and short-stay patients. p. 629. In: Nursing Clinics of North America. Vol. 24. WB Saunders, Philadelphia, 1989

46. Scalzi CC, Burke LE: Education of the patient and family: in-hospital phase. p. 704. In Underhill SL, Woods SL, Froelicher ESS, Halpenny CJ (eds): Cardiac Nursing. 2nd Ed. JB Lippincott, Philadelphia, 1989

47. Mager RF: Measuring Instructional Results. 2nd Ed. p. 7–17. Lake Publishing, Belmont, CA, 1985

48. Gessner BA: Adult education: the cornerstone of patient teaching. p. 589. In: Nursing Clinics of North America. Vol. 24. WB Saunders, Philadelphia, 1989

49. Billings JH: How to help cardiac patients reduce risk factors. Physician Sportsmed 17:71, 1989

50. Leon AS, Certo C, Comoss P et al: Scientific evidence of the value of cardiac rehabilitation services with emphasis on patients following myocardial infarction. Section 1. Exercise conditioning component. J Cardiopulmonary Rehabil 10:79, 1990

51. Miller NH, Taylor CB, Davidson DM et al: Scientific evidence of the value of cardiac rehabilitation services with emphasis on patients following myocardial infarction. Section 2. The

psychosocial component. J Cardiopulmonary Rehabil 10:198, 1990

52. DeMuth JS: Patient teaching in the ambulatory setting. p. 645. In: Nursing Clinics of North America. Vol. 24. WB Saunders, Philadelphia, 1989

53. Parmley WW: Position report on cardiac rehabilitation. J Am Coll Cardiol 7:451, 1986

54. Wilson PK: Cardiac rehabilitation: then and now. Physician Sportsmed 16:75, 1988

55. Newton KM, Froelicher ESS: Life-style adjustments. p. 715–738. In Underhill SL, Woods SL, Froelicher ESS, Halpenny CJ: Cardiac Nursing. 2nd Ed. JB Lippincott, Philadelphia, 1989

56. Comoss PM: Nursing strategies to improve compliance with life-style changes in a cardiac rehabilitation population. J Cardiovasc Nursing 2:23, 1988

57. Dennis C, Goins P: Exercise after myocardial infarction: when and how much? Illust Med 4:1, 1989

58. Sivarajan ES, Newton KM, Almes MJ et al: Limited effects of outpatient teaching and counseling after myocardial infarction: a controlled study. Heart Lung 12:65, 1983

59. Morley D, Ribisl PM, Miller HS: A comparison of patient education methodologies in outpatient cardiac rehabilitation. J Cardiac Rehabil 4:434, 1984

60. Joint Commission on Accreditation of Healthcare Organizations: Quality assurance. p. 211–217. In: Accreditation Manual for Hospitals. Joint Commission on Accreditation of Healthcare Organizations, Chicago, 1990

26

The Behavioral Approach

C. Barr Taylor, M.D.
Nancy Houston Miller, R.N., B.S.

Helping people adopt and maintain health behavior changes, particularly long-term changes that may involve major alterations in lifestyle, is a challenge for even the most experienced counselor and motivated patient. Yet, over the last 20 years, much has been learned about how to institute and develop behavioral programs than can help patients with coronary heart disease (CHD) adopt a healthy lifestyle and adhere to medical regimens. For most coronary patients a healthy lifestyle includes (1) a change in dietary habits, (2) some weight loss and maintenance of "normal body weight," (3) smoking cessation, (4) routine exercise, (5) stress management, (6) adherence to medication, (7) moderate or no use of alcohol, (8) and appropriate response to symptoms. In this chapter we discuss the behavioral approaches to these areas, review data on the effectiveness of the behavioral approaches in coronary rehabilitation, and provide examples of programs.

The earliest theoretical models that guided behavior therapy evolved from operant and classical conditioning.[1] These models focused on behavior and paid little attention to social systems and cognition. More recently, models of health behavior change have been developed that include social and cognitive factors. The most widely cited and applied model is social learning theory, a comprehensive analysis of human functioning in which human behavior is assumed to be developed and maintained on the basis of three interacting systems: behavioral, cognitive, and environmental.[2] Social learning theory emphasizes the human capacity for self-directed behavior change. Willingness to change is related to self-efficacy—a person's confidence that he or she can undertake a particular task or behavior. Self-efficacy is influenced by four main factors: persuasion from an authority, observation of others, successful performance of the behavior, and physiologic feedback.[3] As applied to the coronary patient, persuasion from an authority refers to the information and instructions that health care professionals impart to their patients or the way they educate patients. Chapter 25 discussed the principles involved in teaching coronary patients. From a social learning theory perspective, this teaching is a critical step in behavior therapy. In the early phases of rehabilitation, what patients are told to expect and how the various tests they undergo are interpreted to them is as important as their actual experience. Many of us learn by watching others and "modeling" our behavior after them. In coronary rehabilitation programs, patients learn facts and adopt attitudes and behaviors based on their observation of other patients. Of course, for most patients their past and current experience continues to guide their actions. After myocardial infarction or a coronary surgical procedure, as patients begin to move about, they rapidly gain a sense of efficacy that influences their willingness to resume customary activities.

The treadmill exercise test has a powerful ef-

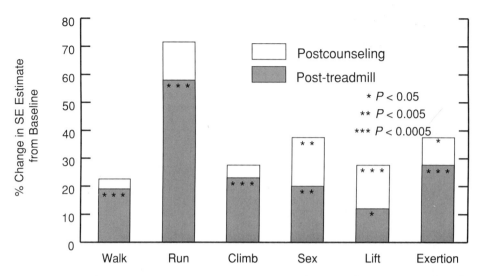

Fig. 26-1. Increases in Self-efficacy (SE) After Treadmill and Counseling Compared with Baseline Values Obtained Before Treadmill Exercise and Before Counseling, Respectively. (From Ewart et al,[4] with permission.)

fect on patients' self-efficacy, particularly if patients are provided with information about their heart rate, blood pressure, and electrocardiographic (ECG) responses during the treadmill test. The post-test counseling and feedback about functional capacity, abnormalities, prognosis, and exercise prescription guidelines amplify the impact on efficacy in helping patients return to routine activities.[4] As seen in Fig. 26-1, increases in self-efficacy were significant following the treadmill exercise test for confidence in walking, running, and general exertion. However, further changes occurred following counseling, particularly in areas where the effects and results of the treadmill test may not have been apparent for patients, such as returning to previous sexual functioning, lifting, and exertion.

Other theories relevant to changes in health behavior have focused more on belief systems,[5] attitudes,[6] the process of change,[7] or relapse.[8] These theories, in conjunction with social learning theory, are useful in helping us understand why people change their behavior. On the other hand, the methods and strategies for effecting and maintaining behavior change have largely been derived from the practice of behavior therapy.[1,9] Many excellent and detailed discussions of behavior change programs are available.[10,11]

ELEMENTS OF A SUCCESSFUL BEHAVIORAL PROGRAM

The basic elements of a successful behavioral program are listed below.

1. *Build a positive, realistic, and accurate expectancy about results.* A patient may know how to do something (high self-efficacy and skills) but be unlikely to do so because of low expectancy of favorable results. The outcome a patient expects from adopting or changing a behavior influences how likely he or she is to make and sustain that change (e.g., a reduction in blood cholesterol level). For instance, a patient is more likely to adopt a low-fat diet if he or she thinks that doing so will have long-term benefits. Yet, if the expectation is that the diet will reduce the blood cholesterol level by 20%, but only a 5% reduction is achieved, the patient is likely to become discouraged and may not continue to comply.

Physicians and most health care professionals make decisions about benefit on the basis of knowledge of coronary risk factors and the probable benefit from making changes. However, the notion of a coronary risk factor is too abstract for many patients unless the information is given in terms that can be easily understood. For instance, patients are more likely to understand that smoking after myocardial infarction doubles their chance of another infarction rather than that their absolute risk increases from 5 to 10%. Also, patients are motivated more by immediate benefits (in weeks) rather than long-term ones (in months). For instance, adoption of a low-fat, low-calorie diet has immediate benefits on losing weight. This is often more appealing to patients than reducing their risk of a heart attack by a few percentage points. As with self-efficacy, expectancy is influenced by information and instruction from an authority, models, and previous experience. Health care professionals can determine whether they have created favorable expectancy by asking a question such as: "What do you think will happen (expect) if you do . . . (e.g., eat less meat)?" Such questions can reveal unanticipated areas of misinformation and allow one to provide realistic information.

2. *Precisely define the behavior to be changed.* Global recommendations (e.g., adopt a low-fat diet, lose weight, exercise more), are rarely useful unless they are accompanied by specific instructions on how to change the behavior. To save time, information about what and how the patient should change can be presented in video format or in pamphlets. In many behavior programs, self-observation instruments are used to help define the behaviors that should be changed.

3. *Set realistic goals.* Patients should be encouraged to establish realistic goals. The goals should be realistic in terms of both the time required to achieve them and the magnitude of change. For instance, patients should be encouraged to lose only 1 to 2 lb (0.5 to 1 kg) of weight per week, which means that for a patient who must lose 30 lb, a course of weight loss may last 10 to 20 weeks or longer. It is often appropriate to have patients set intermediate goals, e.g., a 10-lb weight loss over 2 months, rather than a 30-lb loss over 6 months to a year. Because achieving a goal is very reinforcing and failure to do so lacks reward, the health care professional and patient should set very achievable goals. One way to assess the likelihood of reaching a goal is to ask the patient: "On a scale of 0 to 100 (0 = no confidence; 100 = absolute confidence), how likely are you to be able to . . . (e.g., lose 10 lb in 3

months)?" If the patient is not 70% or more confident of achieving the goal, he or she is unlikely to do so and the goal and/or the method of achieving it must then be changed to enhance success.

4. *Enhance commitment through contracting.* Written contracts with a family member, friend, or health care professional are also extremely useful in maintaining change and helping a patient continue with a program. The contract should be realistic and likely to be achieved. Contracts should be written cooperatively with the patient. An example of a contract for a smoker attempting to quit can be seen in Fig. 26-2. Other incentives, such as having patients reward themselves for goals achieved, can also be useful in enhancing commitment.

5. *Prepare for lapses and relapses.* In the early stages of cessation, as ex-smokers struggle to resist urges to smoke, they may occasionally slip. It is important to prepare patients for these lapses or relapses, a process called "relapse prevention training." The principles of relapse prevention are (1) to identify situations, feelings, or events when lapse (from a new, good habit) or relapse (back to an old habit) may occur; (2) to develop skills to cope with these situations; (3) to practice these skills; and (4) to continue to monitor threats to lapse or relapse and to further develop and/or implement strategies to deal with these situations. Relapse prevention is most useful for changes in addictive behaviors.

6. *Model the desired behavior.* At times, patients need a better understanding of what and how to make a change or may be motivated in other ways by watching others. A variety of videotapes are available to model various behaviors such as how to prepare low-fat foods, request special menus in restaurants, ask a family member or friend not to smoke in one's home, etc.

7. *Prompt the practice of the desired behavior.* If the health behavior requires practice, prompting it can be helpful. Prompts can be as simple as a dot or a sticker on a watch or a telephone reminding a patient to practice the behavior, a chart on the refrigerator, or a note in a datebook. Telephone-prompting programs have been developed to remind patients of appointments, to take medications, or to continue with exercise.

8. *Provide feedback regarding progress.* Feed-

The Contract

Before you carry on with the rest of the program, sign this contract in front of a witness. The witness can be a spouse, relative, close friend or health professional — somebody who will stand by you if you need help.

I, _____ , promise that I will try to remain a nonsmoker for the next year.

If by any chance I should slip up, I will immediately contact the witness whose name is below. With his or her help, I will return to my life as a nonsmoker.

Signed _____   Date _____

Witness _____   Date _____

Fig. 26-2. Sample of a Contract Used to Help Smokers Commit to Quitting.

back strongly influences behavior change. From a behavioral standpoint, feedback should focus on the behaviors undergoing change as well as on the final outcome one is hoping to achieve. The behavioral variables include exercise adherence, confidence to cope with smoking urges, percentage of fat in the diet, and medications. These behaviors, rather than the results they are meant to produce, should be the primary source of feedback, although longer-term measures such as periodic exercise tests and serum cholesterol and weight measurement, which reflect these behaviors, are also important.

9. *Use problem-solving solutions.* Most behavior therapists use a problem-solving approach to help patients overcome difficulties with their health behavior change. The problem-solving approach involves these basic steps:

Specify the problem to be solved in concrete, specific terms

Identify possible solutions

Develop a plan for implementing these solutions

Try out the solutions

Evaluate the results

Repeat the process if the initial solutions have not been successful

10. *Reward achievement.* Positive reinforcement—rewarding achievement—has a very strong influence on behavior. For this reason, many behavioral programs include monetary, interpersonal, or accomplishment rewards. However, we find that patients are rarely successful in developing and implementing a reward system on their own. Therefore, if a reward system is to be used, it will probably require help and monitoring from a health care professional or someone else in the patient's social network.

11. *Enlist social support as needed and as appropriate.* Social isolation has been associated with increased mortality from CHD.[12] Furthermore, the provision of social support has been

shown to increase patient compliance. Involvement of the patient's spouse, for example, in an exercise program may reduce conflict between patient and spouse as a result of greater concordance regarding expectations. Moreover, using a buddy system (e.g., using nonsmokers to help smokers with cessation) may improve compliance with health-related behaviors. It has also been noted that the spouse's approval of participation in an exercise program and his or her commitment to be supportive may positively influence a patient's compliance with coronary rehabilitation.[13] Therefore, encouraging active participation by spouses, friends, and family members is an important element of a successful behavior change program.

Table 26-1 illustrates how the various principles have been incorporated into the management of diet in a large multifactorial risk reduction trial for myocardial infarction patients.

Table 26-1. Hyperlipidemic Diet Intervention for Patients after Myocardial Infarction at Stanford University

Elements	Examples
Build a Positive and Accurate Expectancy About Results	Nurses meet in hospital with post-infarction patients to discuss importance of dietary change.
	A workbook reviews reasons and benefits for lowering serum cholesterol.
	The AHA Active Partnership diet videotape is used to supplement dietary instruction.
Precisely Define the Behavior to be Changed	Patients assess baseline fat and cholesterol intake by using a semiquantitative FFQ.
Set Realistic Goals	At 3 weeks postinfarction, the patient and his or her spouse meet with program nurse to set goals by using feedback from an individualized progress summary sheet generated by computer from their FFQ.
Enhance Commitment	No specific interventions, but the patient's motivation is assessed during each encounter
Prepare for Lapses and Relapses	Counseling session at 3 weeks focuses on identifying possible situations in which patient may lapse from diet.
	At 6 months patient is given a self-monitoring form related to his or her dietary goals. The form includes tips for handling high-risk situations for lapse.
Model the Desired Behavior	Multifit does not include interventions to model desired behavior. An interactive video disc program that models many behaviors related to behavior change is being developed, and patients have the AHA Active Partnership diet tape.
Prompt the Practice of the Desired Behavior	Telephone calls occur at monthly intervals during the first 3 months to determine the patient's success in meeting goals, apply problem-solving to lapses, and to answer questions about diet.
Provide Feedback Regarding Progress	Patients complete two additional FFQs and are given a computer-generated progress report providing feedback about dietary changes and success in reaching goals. The progress summary report is discussed in follow-up telephone calls.
	Serum cholesterol level is measured at 60, 90, 180 and 360 days.
Problem-solve Solutions	Occurs with each face-to-face and telephone contact. Telephone algorithms include problem-solving guidelines.
Reward Achievement	Changes in diet are reinforced by the nurses, appear on the computerized reports, and are evident through reductions in serum lipid levels.
Enlist Social Support as Appropriate	Nurses and dieticians encourage the patient's spouse to attend sessions and join in phone calls.

Abbreviations: AHA, American Heart Association; FFQ, food frequency questionnaire.

DEVELOPING A BEHAVIORAL PROGRAM

Stages of Change

The principles and procedures described above should be organized into a program. The process of health behavior change can be conceptualized as occurring in three basic stages: antecedents, adoption, and maintenance.[9] Antecedents refer to all the factors that can help initiate, hinder, or support change. A patient's motivation or intention to change is one critical antecedent. Motivation should be considered dynamic and not fixed: a patient may be motivated to do something at one time and not another. Motivation or intention is influenced by many of the factors discussed under social learning theory. Greater self-efficacy is associated with greater motivation to change, and efficacy is influenced by information, instructions, perceived benefit, etc. Once a patient intends to make a behavior change and has high confidence that the change will be successful, the adoption of the health change is often precipitated by "cues to action." Certain environmental and physical prerequisites are often necessary for the adoption of health behavior change, such as having the appropriate shoes and clothing prior to embarking on an exercise program, and they should be discussed with the participant. Once a behavior is adopted, different factors determine whether it is maintained. Behaviors generally are maintained if they are satisfying (reinforcing) or if not doing them causes more discomfort (perceived or actual) than doing them. Many of the principles listed in the first section, such as contracting, preventing relapses, setting goals, and using rewards, are useful for enhancing maintenance.

Delivering the Program

A program consists of two basic parts: the adoption and maintenance components and how they are sequenced and integrated, and the interaction with the health care behavior (if any) involved with facilitating the program. Several considerations about delivery should be addressed.

Personal Contact

What is the optimal amount of face-to-face or group contact needed to deliver a program? Despite extensive studies, the extent of face-to-face or group contact that is optimal or even necessary to deliver a behavior program remains uncertain. Many patients do very well with printed materials and need little professional contact to undertake extensive changes. For instance, a recent study of smokers found that most smokers stopped on their own.[14] However, more heavily addicted smokers seem to benefit from smoking cessation programs and from advice by physicians. At the other extreme, patients with multiple medical and psychiatric problems who require extensive help may actually show little change with intensive effort. Often, health professional will devote too much time to such individuals, thus reducing the professionals' feelings of efficacy. Many successful programs provide some face-to-face contact with referral to more specialized providers for recalcitrant or hard-to-manage individuals.

Site of Delivery

Rehabilitation programs have traditionally used a group format to provide exercise training, smoking cessation, stress management, and even psychological counseling. Groups have the advantages of being more cost-effective than individual counseling from the standpoint of instructor time, allowing for the sharing of information and experience and modeling of presumably desired behaviors, providing social support, and structuring a patient's exercise or other experience. On the other hand, in many settings the patient flow is inadequate to create groups, groups are not available, and/or patients do not choose to participate in them for a variety of logistical or personal reasons. There has been recent interest in home-based programs, particularly for exercise, as an alternative to group-based programs. Controlled studies have found that home-based and group exercise programs achieve comparable adherence and functional-capacity outcomes in uncomplicated myocardial infarction patients at 6 months after the event.[15] Home programs with telephone monitoring and feedback provide a cost-effective model for behavior change.

Intervention Modalities

The Telephone.   The telephone is perhaps the most underutilized behavior change tool. Many studies have shown that health care professionals can use the telephone for instituting and maintaining behavior change.[15,16] In a recent study, a smoking cessation treatment program, delivered by nurses making telephone calls to myocardial infarction patients who had smoked before the infarction, achieved a 71% abstinence rate at 1 year compared with a 45% abstinence rate in a usual care group. Several studies in which the telephone was used to help post-infarction patients adhere to exercise regimens have also reported adherence rates of 70 to 80% in the first 6 months after the infarction. Some studies use algorithms to help guide the telephone interventions.[17] In the future, the telephone, linked to data bases and home electronic systems, may become a critical behavior change tool.

Bibliotherapy.   Printed materials are an excellent method of conveying information to patients if they are designed to be readable by patients and if the patient is told how and when to use the material. Even the simplest presentations of educational materials are often not sufficiently tailored to a patient's needs and abilities. For instance, 90% of the materials used in a sample of coronary rehabilitation programs were written at levels above the projected mean reading level of the targeted population.[18] The reader must be involved and considered in all steps of program development so that language, illustrations, skills, examples, etc., are appropriate. When this occurs, the written materials are more likely to be useful and used by the potential consumers.

Technology.   Audiotapes, videotapes, and computers can reduce the work and increase the effectiveness of education for patients with CHD.[19] Many of the steps in Table 26-1 are readily adaptable to computer technology. For instance, computers can help patients assess their knowledge, attitudes, behavior, and skills related to a particular risk factor; then provide information, corrective feedback, and further assessment as needed; and, finally, establish specific goals for change. Many computer programs with these character-

istics have been developed.[20] For instance, a new computer system for dietary feedback has been developed whereby patients complete a food frequency assessment of their eating habits, mail it to a facility for computer entry, and receive an individualized progress summary report of their eating habits. The report summarizes food items of high saturated fat and cholesterol in the diet and has built-in goals to help the patient begin dietary changes. New interactive video/computer formats offer even greater potential for more interesting, yet personal, instruction.[21] Another new interactive laser video disc system for diet allows patients to sit at a computer terminal and assess their knowledge of food content of cholesterol and saturated fats, determine personal behavior through a food frequency assessment, set goals for dietary change, and prepare for relapse through assessment of high-risk eating habits. Patients are then provided with a printout of their eating plan. However, despite their potential, computers have achieved little use in most clinical practice settings. A recent survey found that fewer than 4% of physicians use computers for educating their patients.[22] There are many reasons for this low rate of use: physicians and other health care professionals are not knowledgeable about computers, the computers and computer programs are expensive, the programs are often unimaginative, interactive programs are expensive to produce, and health care professionals worry that their patients react negatively to the use of computers for education and behavior change. However, all these factors are rapidly changing. Computers are becoming more "user friendly" and ubiquitous. More and better software programs are being developed. The cost of developing computer programs is dropping. Studies have shown that patients react favorably to computer education.[23]

Evaluation
Evaluation of the behavior therapy program is critical. Each behavior targeted for intervention should be monitored, not only to provide feedback to the patient but also to determine how well a program is succeeding overall in terms of smoking cessation, exercise adherence, weight and diet changes, and adherence to medication or other targeted behaviors. In addition, partici-

pants should be encouraged to provide feedback about how the program could be changed or improved.

EFFECTIVENESS OF BEHAVIORAL PROGRAMS IN CORONARY REHABILITATION

The efficacy of behavior modification programs in altering behaviors related to coronary risk in patients at risk for but without overt coronary illness has been well established in a number of studies.[24] Less is known about the effectiveness of such interventions in patients with coronary disease, but, as discussed below, the evidence suggests that risk factors can be successfully reduced in these patients. Four recent reviews and reports address the effectiveness of behavior modification programs in populations with coronary disease.[25–28] Our conclusions are based on these reviews and our assessment of the literature. Some studies have focused on individual risk factors; others have focused on multiple interventions. We begin with an overview of the former.

Diet

A number of dietary trials in healthy individuals have shown that plasma cholesterol levels can be reduced by 5 to 10% through dietary change and to a greater extent by lipid-lowering medications.[29–31] Trials of diet modification have also been conducted in patients with coronary disease and have shown similar results.[32] Most of the successful diet interventions have involved relatively frequent and long-term contact with health professionals.

The principles involved in diet change are similar in patients with and without coronary disease. Four conclusions about dietary change in coronary patients seem in order: (1) coronary patients are often highly motivated to make major changes in their diet, and such changes, particularly in patients consuming a relatively high-fat, high-cholesterol diet, can significantly reduce

plasma cholesterol levels; (2) diet change is a complicated process involving alterations in patterns that have been firmly established by culture, family, and personal factors; (3) although diet change appears to require some face-to-face contact and long-term follow-up, the optimal "dose" and "timing" of initial and follow-up contacts are not known; (4) and the majority of coronary patients with substantial hyperlipidemia will require medication to achieve the serum cholesterol goals set forth by the National Cholesterol Education Project. Therefore, behavioral programs should focus on adherence.

Exercise

Helping patients adopt and maintain an exercise program is one of the most challenging aspects of the rehabilitation of the patient with CHD. Dropout rates greater than 50% by 1 year are typical for exercise rehabilitation programs. However, some programs have reported exercise participation rates of 80% or greater in myocardial infarction patients at 6 months after hospitalization.[15,33] The characteristics of successful exercise programs involve use of the principles listed in the first section of this chapter.

Obesity/Weight Reduction

Alterations in weight are strongly related to changes in diet and exercise. Losing weight and maintaining weight loss are difficult for most people. However, a recent review of 21 behavioral studies in healthy individuals reported a mean weight loss between 7 and 9 kg immediately after treatment.[34] The weight loss was more closely related to the length of the program than to the technique used. Eight recent studies also reported a 75% maintenance of post-treatment weight losses at 1 year follow-up. The successful programs are longer, have multiple components, and emphasize regular exercise for weight loss.

Weight changes have been used as outcome measures in a number of intervention trials of patients with coronary disease.[35,36] One of these trials found a significantly greater weight loss in the treatment group than the control group.[35] Once again, effective weight loss programs appear to require some initial face-to-face contact and multiple follow-up sessions.

Smoking Cessation

Among coronary populations, cessation rates of 50% or more have been reported by a number of groups in which the physician and medical team are committed to smoking cessation. According to Mulcahy,[37] smoking cessation rates of 46% in the period 1961 to 1963 increased to 58% in the period 1973 to 1975 and to as high as 70% in the 1980s. In a review of several studies, 0 to 35% difference between treatment and control patients was found at 6 months or later after acute myocardial infarction.[16,38] The American Association of Cardiovascular and Pulmonary Rehabilitation report[27] noted that (1) most smokers quit on their own; (2) interventions combining multiple components are more successful than those relying on a single component; (3) use of nicotine gum combined with behavioral counseling may increase cessation rates; (4) for individuals successful at quitting, the greatest problem is relapse, preparation for which must be included in the overall cessation plan; and (5) health care professionals can be powerful facilitators of smoking behavior change.

Hypertension

Treatment of hypertension in coronary patients has focused on weight reduction, alterations in diet, and adherence to medication. In a meta-analysis, Mullen et al.[24] found that behavioral programs were effective in helping to control blood pressure levels in hypertensive patients.

Adherence to Medical Regimens

Behavioral interventions to enhance adherence to drug therapy in post-infarction patients have been less well studied than those focusing on single or multifactorial risk factor change. In an analysis of 23 studies involving multiple illnesses, Mullen et al.[24] found significant improvement in adherence with behavioral interventions. The Lipid Research Clinic Coronary Primary Prevention Trial[30] demonstrated that multiple, face-to-face interactions with clinic staff can help achieve long-term, high rates of adherence to diet and medication regimens. Further work is needed to determine the effectiveness of behavioral procedures designed to improve adherence to hyperlipidemic medications in coronary patients.

Combined Interventions

Many interventions to reduce coronary risk factors have involved alterations in several risk factors simultaneously, by using both behavioral and pharmacologic interventions. For instance, in the Oslo Diet Heart Study[29] involving 1,232 healthy men, dietary manipulation was associated with a 13% decrease in plasma cholesterol in the treatment group compared with the control group. The study found that 25% of smokers in the treatment group stopped smoking, compared with 17% in the control group. In the Coronary Drug Project,[39] combinations of diet and drugs resulted in significant reductions in plasma lipid levels. More intensive interventions have produced even greater changes in risk factors.

Because the more successful programs have been labor-intensive, it is easy to conclude that more effort results in more effect. In fact, the "dose" of face-to-face intervention required to effect behavior change is not known: although intensive interventions involving multiple face-to-face contacts are sufficient for extensive and long-term behavior change, they may not be necessary. For instance, behavior change initiated through face-to-face contact can be maintained through telephone and mail contact.[15,16,40] Also, it is not possible to conclude from the previous studies which components of a behavioral intervention are necessary or sufficient for behavior change.

SUMMARY

Behavioral interventions are successful in reducing coronary risk factors and in improving adherence to medication regimens. Although the optimal amount of face-to-face contact to achieve behavior change is not known, at least some initial face-to-face contact is necessary. Because of cost, the widespread implementation of behavior change interventions in patients with CHD will require innovation in delivery. Media and computer technology can significantly reduce cost without compromising effectiveness. Implementation of interventions in nonclinical settings may vastly expand the access and acceptability of behavior change programs.

REFERENCES

1. Agras WS, Kazdin AE, Wilson GT: Behavior Therapy: Toward an Applied Clinical Science. WH Freeman, San Francisco, 1979
2. Bandura A: Social Learning Theory. Prentice-Hall, Englewood Cliffs, NJ, 1977
3. Bandura A: Social Foundations of Thought and Action: A Social Cognitive Theory. Prentice-Hall, Englewood Cliffs, NJ, 1986
4. Ewart CK, Taylor CB, Reese LB, DeBusk RF: Effects of early postmyocardial infarction exercise testing on self-perception and subsequent physical activity. Am J Cardiol 51:1076, 1983
5. Becker MH: The health belief model and personal health behavior. Health Educ Monogr 2:236, 1974
6. Ajzen I, Fishbein M: Understanding Attitudes and Predicting Social Behavior. Prentice-Hall, Englewood Cliffs, NJ, 1980
7. Prochaska JO, DiClemente CC: Stage process of self-change of smoking: toward an integrative model of change. J Consult Clin Psychol 51:390, 1983
8. Marlatt GA, Gordon JR (eds): Relapse Prevention: Maintenance Strategies in the Treatment of Addiction. Guilford Press, New York, 1985
9. Taylor CB, Miller NH, Flora J: Principles of health behavior change. p. 323. In SN Blair, Painter P, Pate RR et al (eds): Exercise Testing and Prescription Guidelines: A Resource Manual. American College of Sports Medicine. Lea & Febiger, Philadelphia, 1988
10. Watson DL, Tharp RG: Self-directed Behavior Change. Brooks/Cole, Monterey, CA, 1981
11. Goldfried M, Davison CC: Clinical Behavior Therapy. Holt, Rinehart and Winston, New York, 1976
12. Ruberman W, Weinblatt E, Goldberg JD, Chaudhary BS: Psychosocial influences on mortality after myocardial infarction. N Engl J Med 311:552, 1984
13. Janis IL: The patient as the decision-maker. In Gentry WD (ed): Handbook of Behavioral Medicine. The Free Press, New York, 1977
14. Fiore MC, Novotny TE, Pierce JP et al: Methods used to quit smoking in the United States. JAMA 263:2760, 1990
15. DeBusk RF, Haskell WL, Miller NH et al: Medically directed at-home rehabilitation soon after clinically uncomplicated myocardial infarction: a new model for patient care. Am J Cardiol 55:251, 1985
16. Taylor CB, Miller NH, Killen J, DeBusk RF: Smoking cessation after acute myocardial infarction: effects of a nurse-managed intervention. Ann Intern Med, 113:118, 1990
17. Gillis CL, Doordan AM: Data gathering by telephone: an application in a study of clinical nursing. Prog Cardiovasc Nursing 4:107, 1989
18. Duncan BM, Citro K: Cardiac patient education literature: can patients read what we give them? J Cardiac Rehabil 3:513, 1983
19. Wenger NK, Cleeman JI, Herd JA, McIntosh HD: Education of the patient with cardiac disease in the twenty-first century: an overview. Am J Cardiol 57:1187, 1986
20. Taylor CB, Ironson G, Burnett K: Adult medical disorders. p. 371. In Bellack AS, Hersen M, Kazdin AE (eds): International Handbook of Behavior Modification and Therapy. 2nd Ed. Plenum, New York, 1990
21. Brand S: The Media Lab. Viking Press, New York, 1987
22. Ellis LBM: Computer-based patient education. Primary Care 12:547, 1985
23. Agras WS, Taylor CB, Feldman DE et al: Developing computer-assisted therapy for the treatment of obesity. Behav Ther 21:99, 1990
24. Mullen PD, Velez R, Mains DA et al: Meta-analysis of patient education for cardiovascular disease patients, submitted
25. Siegel D, Grady D, Browner WS, Hulley SB: Risk factor modification after myocardial infarction. Ann Intern Med 109:213, 1988
26. Blumenthal JA, Levenson RM: Behavioral approaches to secondary prevention of coronary heart disease. Circulation 76(suppl. I):I-130, 1987

27. Miller NH, Taylor CB, Davidson DM et al: The efficacy of risk factor intervention and psychological aspects of rehabilitation. J Cardiopulmonary Rehabil, 10:198, 1990

28. Godin G: The effectiveness of interventions in modifying behavioral risk factors of individuals with coronary heart disease. J Cardiopulmonary Rehabil 9:223, 1989

29. Hjerman L, Holme I, Velve Byre K, Leren P: Effects of diet and smoking intervention on the incidence of coronary heart disease: Report from Oslo study group of a randomized trial in healthy men. Lancet ii:1303, 1981

30. The Lipid Research Clinic Coronary Primary Prevention Trial Results. I. Reduction in incidence of coronary heart disease. JAMA 251:351, 1984

31. Blankenhorn DH, Johnson RL, Mack WJ et al: The influence of diet on the appearance of new lesions in human coronary arteries. JAMA 263:1646, 1990

32. Arntzenius AC, Kromhout D, Barth JD et al: Diet, lipoproteins, and the progression of coronary atherosclerosis. The Leiden Intervention Trial. N Engl J Med 312:805, 1985

33. Oldridge NB, Jones NL: Preventive use of exercise rehabilitation after myocardial infarction. Acta Med Scand, Suppl 711:123, 1986

34. Brownell KD, Jeffery RW: Improving long-term weight loss: pushing the limits of treatment. Behav Ther 18:353, 1987

35. Kallio V, Hämäläinen H, Hakkila J, Luurila OJ: Reduction of sudden deaths by a multifactorial intervention program after acute myocardial infarction. Lancet ii:1091, 1979

36. Carson P, Phillips R, Lloyd M et al: Exercise after myocardial infarction: controlled trial. J R Coll Physicians 16:147, 1982

37. Mulcahy R: Influence of cigarette smoking on morbidity and mortality after myocardial infarction. Br Heart J 49:410, 1983

38. Sivarajan ES, Newton KM, Almes MJ et al: The patient after myocardial infarction. Limited effect of outpatient teaching and counseling after myocardial infarction: a controlled study. Heart Lung 12:65, 1983

39. The Coronary Drug Project Research Group: The Coronary Drug Project. Initial findings leading to modifications of its research protocol. JAMA 214:1303, 1970

40. King A, Taylor CB, Haskell WI, DeBusk RF: Strategies for increasing early adherence and long-term maintenance of home-based physical activity in middle-aged men and women. Am J Cardiol 61:628, 1988

EDUCATION AND COUNSELING OF THE PATIENT AND FAMILY

27

Sexual Problems/Interventions

Chris Papadopoulos, M.D.

Successful rehabilitation should include consideration of the sexual activity of the patient. Sex is woven into the everyday life of many patients.

CORONARY EVENTS AND RELATED PROCEDURES

Myocardial Infarction

Percentages of people who do not restart sexual relations after a myocardial infarction vary, but in general, approximately one-quarter of the patients do not resume sexual activity, one-quarter do not change the frequency, and half decrease their sexual activity.[1-3] Reasons for not resuming sexual relations are loss of libido, the patient's or spouse's fears of risk in resuming sexual activity, the patient's or spouse's excuse to stop sexual relations that were not enjoyable before the myocardial infarction, persistence of the patient's cardiac symptoms, the patient's impotence, lack of an available partner, or the patient's depression. The patient's age and that of the partner, the previous level of sexual activity, and discussion of sexual relations between the couple are important factors in resuming sexual activity.[2,3] The frequency of sexual relations may be decreased,[3-5] and there may be a decline in the quality of sexual activity.[3,5,6] Often patients wait 8 to 9 weeks before resumption of sexual relations.[3,7] Fear, depression, and cardiac symptoms may delay resumption. Sexual difficulties reported include

loss of libido, impotence, and premature or retarded ejaculation.[1,8] The patients may report cardiac symptoms with sexual activity, but the frequency has varied in various reports.[9]

Concerns and fears develop after a myocardial infarction and affect the patient and his or her partner. Understanding by health professionals of the physiologic factors, the psychosocial adjustment, and the effects of drugs after myocardial infarction is vital for their patients.

Most experts agree that there are few, if any, physiologic reasons for the coronary patient not to achieve sexual satisfaction.[10] The physiologic load of sexual relations is not significant.[5,11] Sex play is relaxing and healthful, whereas anxious preoccupation, frustration, and avoidance may actually be greater risk factors than the mild physical effort involved in coitus or coital alternatives.[12]

It is generally safe to allow a patient to resume sexual activity if he or she can perform exercise at levels of 6 to 8 kcal/min without symptoms, abnormal pulse rate, or blood pressure or electrocardiographic (ECG) changes.[5] Studies have shown that the equivalent oxygen cost of the maximal activity during sexual intercourse approximated 6 kcal/min (5 METs) for less than 30 seconds and about 4.5 kcal/min during the preorgasmic and postorgasmic periods.[5,13] The study by Larson et al.[14] supported the clinical use of a two-flight stair-climbing test (10 minutes of rapid walking, followed by climbing two flights of steps in 10 seconds) as a physiologic test of readiness to resume sexual activity after an acute myocardial infarction. More accurate evaluation of the physical capacity of the patient can be estimated by a treadmill or bicycle exercise test. Exercise training can lessen the peak coital heart rate,[15] and this may lead to a decrease in symptoms and improvement of sexual function and enjoyment.

Masturbation is not an uncommon sexual practice for the coronary patient and other adults. Noncoital activities have lower energy expenditures than coitus.[16]

The potential for cardiac arrhythmias during sexual activity exists, but is small.[5,17–19]

Unquestionably, an important factor that may affect the sexual function of patients after myocardial infarction, percutaneous transluminal coronary angioplasty (PTCA), or coronary artery bypass grafting (CABG) is their psychological status. In a psychiatric evaluation of patients in a coronary care unit, the three most frequent reasons for psychiatric referral were anxiety, depression, and behavior management.[20] The patient may develop anxiety and fears after discharge from the hospital; these fears have been described by coronary patients in various studies.[3,4] Fear of resumption of sexual activity was expressed by 31% of male patients and 51% of female patients.[1,3] Such fears were not uncommon among spouses, varying from 44 to 68%.[1–3] The major fears expressed about resuming sexual activity were chest pain, another heart attack, coital death, poor quality of sexual activity, sexual unattractiveness of the patient to the partner after the infarction or discovery of a previously existing extramarital sexual relationship of the patient. Although fear may prevent resumption of sexual relations by some couples, at times it is counteracted by the young age of the couple, the level of previous sexual drive, and the level of interpersonal communication of the couple. Fear, however, can decrease the frequency and quality of sexual activity.

Angina Pectoris

Patients who have coronary heart disease (CHD) and angina may experience chest pain or discomfort during sexual activity. Most of them may also have similar symptoms during other daily activities, and occasional patients may exhibit the symptoms only during or after sexual intercourse. Patients who have experienced angina during intercourse may decide to abstain from sexual activity, either because of the discomfort or because of the fear that this may lead to infarction or sudden death.

Coronary Artery Bypass Grafting

Emphasis after CABG is usually concentrated on the relief of angina and on the employment status of the patient. Little attention is often devoted to sexual activity.[21]

Often the results of CABG in regard to sexual activity are not encouraging.[22–24] Postoperative sexual functioning, frequency of sexual activity, and sexual adjustment often deteriorated. The damaged self-image, preoperative impairment, and duration of symptoms may have played a role. However, studies show that over time, more patients make a satisfactory sexual adjustment.

Many CABG patients still view themselves as "heart patients" and, as such, feel fragile, vulnerable, and as if they are living on borrowed time. Some are very reluctant to relinquish the sick role, and, not unexpectedly, these issues militate against a satisfying sex life. Furthermore, some CABG patients may have been cardiac invalids for so long prior to surgery that they are out of practice. After protracted periods of nonindulgence in sex, they may have suppressed any interest, and it may not be able to be resurrected. For some individuals, previous sexual problems may provide a good excuse for abstinence, an excuse unlikely to be forsaken with improvement in symptoms.[25]

In another study,[26] however, after a prolonged period of angina with restricted physical activity, avoidance of excitement, and abstinence from sexual intercourse, the patients showed pronounced improvement in lifestyle and 70% had resumed their previous sexual activity.

In our study of 134 male and female patients who had CABG, 91% of those who were sexually active before surgery resumed sexual activity.[21] The average time of resumption was 7.8 weeks.

Sexual dissatisfaction prior to surgery was a negative factor, whereas return to work, in the group that was previously working, had a positive effect on resuming sexual activity. Of patients who were sexually active before CABG, 17% expressed a fear of resuming sexual activity. They were afraid of a heart attack, chest pain, "hurting" the chest incision, or dying during coitus. The main reasons offered by the few who actually did not resume sexual activity were fear, lack of desire, and impotence. Of those who resumed sexual relations, 51% did not change the frequency, 10% increased the frequency, and 39% decreased the frequency. Among those who continued sexual activity after the surgery, 23% reported symptoms during coitus, mostly shortness of breath, fatigue, chest pain, or palpitations. Overall, it appeared that a higher percentage of the previously sexually active patients resumed sexual activity after CABG than after myocardial infarction and that they had less fear of resumption. More patients increased and fewer patients decreased the frequency of sexual activity after CABG than after infarction.[1,3]

Percutaneous Transluminal Coronary Angioplasty

A review of life adaptation after PTCA[27] revealed that after 6 months, the patients who had undergone PTCA functioned better at work and during sexual performance and related better with their families than did those who had CABG. The improvements in work functioning continued at 15 months, but the differences in family and sexual domains became insignificant by that time.

Cardiac Transplantation

During the past several years, transplantation of the heart has emerged as a reliable therapeutic alternative for end-stage congestive heart failure in coronary patients. Little is known, however, about the sexual adaptation of these patients. One report[28] found that impotence and diminished libido were of considerable concern for many pa-

tients. Another recent study[29] revealed that only 50% of transplanted-heart recipients were either nearly or completely satisfied with their sexual life. Sexual activity had increased for 20% and decreased for another 29% of patients.

Implanted Pacemakers

Patients who are still sexually active prior to receiving a permanent pacemaker often develop sexual concerns. In one study, however, pacemaker treatment did not influence the quality of sexual activity in the majority (68%) of patients. A small percentage perceived improvement, whereas a corresponding number reported deterioration in sexual activity following the pacemaker implantation.[30]

Automatic Implantable Cardioverter Defibrillator

Patients who receive an automatic implantable cardioverter defibrillator (ICD) have physical, social, and psychological alterations, often developed during previous resuscitations and hospitalizations. Fears and limitations are common, and sexual abstinence was reported in 41% of patients.[31]

CORONARY COITAL DEATH

Cases of coital death have been reported.[32,33] Accurate data are often difficult to obtain since the partner in an extramarital relationship disappears and then calls the police and the partner in marital situations may be hesitant to report the real circumstances. Although the true incidence of new infarction or sudden death during intercourse is difficult to establish, a study conducted in Japan[32] indicated that coitus accounted for only 34 of 5,559 cases (0.6%) of sudden death and that death was due to heart disease in about half of these cases. In 70% it occurred during or after intercourse with a partner other than the wife and in a place other than their home. In a study of 100 sudden deaths from CHD,[34] no patient was recorded as having died soon after or during coitus.

Experiences of medical examiners are that when cases of coital death come to their attention, they usually occur in an illicit sexual connection, in unfamiliar surroundings, and after a large meal and high alcohol intake.[33] Superimposed on the demands of the sexual act simultaneously with the digestive process are the psychological effects of sexual excitement, guilt, fear of discovery, and the concern about possible impotence.

CARDIOVASCULAR DRUGS

Drugs may have a negative impact on the patient's quality of life as a result of possible adverse effects, not only on sexuality, but on the physical state, emotional well-being, and social and cognitive function. Sexual dysfunction may adversely affect the overall health of the individual since sexuality is woven into the everyday life of most people and good sexual function is vital for emotional satisfaction.[35]

Pharmacologic agents may affect the libido and the erectile and orgasmic phases of sexuality. Most drugs have side effects of some sort or degree, depending on the dosage, the unique reaction of each individual (personality, age, gender, diet, underlying disease process, and genetic factors), and duration of drug consumption.[36] Frequently, inadequate attention is paid to the sexual side effects of drugs.

Although such psychological causes as deterioration of the interpersonal relationship, poor communication, and interpsychic factors play a role in sexual dysfunction, disease processes, specific lesions, and pharmacologic agents can profoundly affect sexual function.[35] The emotional state of the patient, as well as the function of the vascular, neurologic, and endocrine systems is involved in the integrity of normal sexual function. Cardiovascular drugs affect the neurogenic, hormonal, and vascular mechanisms.

Cardiovascular drugs taken by coronary patients may affect their sexuality.[37] Diuretic, antihypertensive, antiarrhythmic, antianginal, and hypolipidemic drugs may have sexual side effects in some patients. They may result in diminished libido, impotence, ejaculatory and orgasmic difficulties, inhibited vaginal lubrication, menstrual irregularities, and gynecomastia (in men) or painful breast enlargement in women. Other medications such as sedatives, antidepressants, tranquilizers, antispasmodics, and histamine H_2-receptor antagonists may also have negative sexual impact in certain patients.

On the other hand, these medications may often have a beneficial effect on the sexuality of some patients. In patients with angina during sexual activity, the use of beta-blocking drugs and sublingual nitrate drugs has proven beneficial. Antiarrhythmic drugs, in patients who develop arrhythmias during sexual activity, may reduce the concern of the patients who have palpitations during intercourse. Antihypertensive medications, when properly selected, may allow better quality of sexual life by controlling blood pressure in the hypertensive patient. Psychotropic drugs may alleviate anxiety or depression and allow the patient a more acceptable approach to sexual life.

THE CORONARY PATIENT'S SPOUSE

The spouse of the coronary patient is often subjected to a tremendous amount of stress. Role reversal occurs in both the family and the marital unit and often persists after hospitalization. During the home-bound phase of recovery it is a threat to the patient's sexuality.[38] The impact of the illness usually appears to depend on the quality of the marital relations before its onset.[39]

A report, based on interview with 100 wives of post-infarction patients, revealed that the spouse's sexual concerns were the risk of intercourse, the patient's sexual difficulties and change in sexual patterns, the patient's symptoms during intercourse, the emotional relationship of the couple, and poor sexual instructions by the health professionals.[2] While their husbands were still hospitalized, one-third of the wives had concerns about future sexual activity. Most of them wondered whether intercourse would be too strenuous. After discharge of the patients, all of the wives developed concerns and nearly all who were fearful of resuming sexual activity expressed fear of their husband having chest pain or another infarction. Several wives, in a group who did not resume sexual activity, expressed sexual anxieties and frustrations. Others, however, saw the termination of sexual relations as an opportunity to end previously unwelcome sexual activity. There was a significant association between the emotional relationship of the husband and wife and the resumption of sexual activity. Failure to communicate sexually often leads to communication failure in other areas of marriage. Many wives felt that they had not received adequate instructions and information about sexual activity. Many couples eliminated variety in their sexual activity, eliminating several previously used positions.

The concerns and questions of wives of convalescent CABG patients were investigated in a study of 30 women during the second or third week after their husbands were discharged from the hospital.[40] Although the wives had knowledge of generally recommended physical activities, they lacked information about sexual activity. They were concerned about the safety, the time of resumption, and the welfare of their husbands during sexual relations. Increased expression of feelings, a greater appreciation of each other, and a positive change in their husband's attitude were, however, reported. The shared experience of the uncertainty of the surgery might have fostered more openness and appreciation of each other. Many of the wives enjoyed the husband's improved physical capabilities and reduction or absence of angina.

SEXUAL COUNSELING AND REHABILITATION

Sexual rehabilitation is part of the overall, comprehensive coronary rehabilitation. Attention to the sexual concerns and needs of the coronary patient and partner is vital for complete rehabilitation. Sexual activity may be gradually integrated into the program of physical and psychological rehabilitation. Too often the psychosexual effects of myocardial infarction or CABG on the patient are neglected because of the overriding concern for the medical aspects of the illness or because of lack of time. The number of patients who are fearful and who request sexual counseling remains large.[1,3,41] Since sexuality has an important place in the lives of these patients and their partners, specific information on the return to sexual functioning should be included in the rehabilitation process.[42] It is important that physicians provide a sensitive atmosphere so that patients with sexual concerns will be sufficiently comfortable to express them. The physicians must also recognize that some patients will not be able to introduce the topic of sex, regardless of the quality of the patient–physician communication, and should be prepared to approach the subject as a matter of routine. Physicians and other health care professionals should be aware that not all coronary patients will have sexual problems and that some who report no such problems may be denying their existence.

A sexual history, obtained as a routine part of the data base from all coronary patients, is important in providing counseling, as is provision of thorough sexual instructions to the patient and partner with specific attention to their sexual concerns and needs. Sexual instructions should be based on the pre-illness sexual history. Sexual preferences, desires, and concerns should be explored. In considering the patient's sexual response to the disease, the state of the individual before the illness, the pathophysiologic effect of the coronary disease, the psychological state of the patient, the effect of treatment upon the patient, and the response of the patient's partner to the illness should be considered.[43] Furthermore, the age of the patient, the duration of the marriage, and the previous sexual drive and satisfaction are significant factors in the interest and decision of the patient to resume sexual activity. The presence of such associated conditions as hypertension and diabetes mellitus may also affect the patient, as may older age.

Sexual instructions are often not specific and comprehensive and may not alleviate the fears of the patient.[1–3] Physicians should, in discussing the subject of sex, avoid generalities and answer questions concerning the resumption, position, and frequency of coitus and the side effects of drug therapy.

Advice about sexual activity should be provided through printed material or auditory or visual tapes, in addition to personal communication, with consideration of the patient's ability to read and comprehend. Specific instructions given to the patient in written or printed form also should be explained clearly to provide the best method of comprehensible and effective communication.

Sexual counseling should be supportive and reassuring to the couple and should strive to facilitate communication between the patient and the partner. Failure to communicate sexually often leads to communication failure in other areas of the marriage. The quality of family life and marriage is markedly associated with sexual satisfaction and appears to be an important determinant of the psychological and social outcome of the patient.[44] Each patient should receive sexual instructions individually and together with his or her partner and have the opportunity to deal with any fears. Ignoring the spouse can only be counterproductive to successful coronary rehabilitation. When a wife or husband indicates concern about continuing sexual relations, the interviewer must take a careful history to help determine whether the concern is genuine or merely an excuse to stop an unwanted activity.

In addition to the initial sexual counseling before discharge from the hospital, there should be further follow-up during the first visit of the patient to the physician's office and periodically thereafter as necessary. Nurses in rehabilitation programs and at home visits may also provide counseling. When reservations, ambiguities, or anxieties persist beyond 4 to 6 weeks after the start of counseling and continue to block progress, complex interpersonal psychopathology should be considered and may require more analytical or specialized behavior techniques. At this point, referral to a psychiatrist or psychologist experienced in the management of sexual dysfunction may be indicated.[45]

For a couple who wish to restart sexual activity after myocardial infarction or CABG, the following categories of general advice can be given[9]:

1. *Time of resumption.* When a patient's condition has become stable and asymptomatic, sexual activity may be resumed within 3 to 6 weeks. The time, however, may vary depending on the libido of the couple. It should be pointed out that the extent of recovery from sexual inertia or from other causes of unsuccessful coitus depends upon the duration of the period of abstinence.[45] An exercise program may encourage an earlier return to sexual activity. Women, however, are less likely to participate in structured coronary rehabilitation programs and also seem to resume sexual activity later than men.[46] Menopause is another factor that may influence the return of a female patient to sexual activity because of psychological and physiologic changes that may occur. In recent years, studies have shown a wide spectrum of reactions to menopause, ranging from a nonspecific sense of liberation to a feeling of loss of femininity and sexual desire.[47]

2. *Initial contacts.* In the convalescent coronary patient's first contact with the partner, non-demand, non-genital touching, and in some cases masturbation to partial arousal may suffice. This may build the patient's self-confidence, provided that there are no complaints of chest pain, shortness of breath, or palpitations. Nonorgasmic, exciting forms of stimulation should be progressively repeated and extended over the next week. As the libido and confidence of the patient improve and if he or she remains physically comfortable, it is permissible to proceed with coitus. Foreplay is desirable and as important as the "warm-up" period before any exercise. Rest preceding sexual activity and intercourse is advisable, and, often, marital relations may be preferable after a restful sleep.

3. *Partner.* The patient may be reassured that the return to sexual activity with a long-term partner will not involve any excessive physical or emotional demand on the heart.

4. *Environment.* Sexual activity in the usual surroundings of one's home and comfortable room is advisable. Extremes of air temperatures, humidity, restrictive clothing, and cold bed sheets should be avoided.

5. *Other precautions.* Avoid vigorous sexual activity and intercourse soon after physical or

emotional stress, after eating a heavy meal, and after drinking excessive amounts of alcohol.

6. *Positions.* It is not invariably necessary to recommend transition to unfamiliar sexual positions, especially if the patient may feel that this affects his masculine or her feminine role. Most patients do not make changes in patterns of foreplay or position adopted during coitus.[2,17] However, if it is acceptable to the couple, the patient may assume the bottom position, which may be more restful, or the patient may consider the side-by-side, face-to-face, or face-to-back positions. In certain situations, especially if the patient develops shortness of breath when lying down, he or she may be more relaxed sitting in a chair with the partner sitting on the patient's lap.

7. *Warning signals.* The patient should recognize and report to the physician rapid heart rate and rapid breathing that persist for 10 to 15 minutes after coitus; a feeling of extreme fatigue that may persist until the next day; irregular heart beating, dizziness, lightheadedness or "blacking out"; chest pain during or after coitus; and sexual dysfunction.

Counseling of the patient who undergoes CABG should start preoperatively and should address the physical, occupational, and psychosocial benefits and problems that may occur after surgery. The patient should know about the thoracotomy and sternotomy, the healing of the bone and wound, and be reassured about the potential discomfort that may linger for a while. Counselors should encourage return to work and address concerns about recreational and sexual activity after surgery. Postoperatively, the treating staff should be alerted to symptoms of anxiety, depression, and paranoid tendency and should inquire about social and sexual patterns of withdrawal and passive dependency.[48]

Apparently, CABG does not abolish the misgivings about sexuality that frequently accompany symptoms of CHD, despite their elimination. Having received little or no counseling from staff, patients seem to set their own patterns for sexual behavior, which may represent a considerable deviation from sexual activity engaged in before the illness.[24] Perhaps patients who do not resume pre-illness sexual behavior may benefit from sexual counseling.

If a question arises concerning the patient's physical tolerance and possibility of an arrhythmia, a treadmill or bicycle ergometer exercise test; or ambulatory ECG monitor recording before, during, and after sexual activity can provide objective evaluation for appropriate guidance and medical treatment and the use of antianginal and antiarrhythmic medications when necessary.

The patient will deal better with sexual relations if the anxiety or depression that he or she may experience is recognized by the physician, who can provide encouragement and reassurance. Enrollment in a coronary rehabilitation program or in a support group for post-infarction or CABG patients may be beneficial. When necessary, anxiolytic or antidepressant drugs can be used.[49]

When the patient's condition is stable and the couple is eager to resume sexual activity, but there is persistent sexual dysfunction, referral for sexual therapy is indicated. Certain couples who, because of fear or sexual dysfunction, would not be interested in intercourse should be reassured that the expression of affection by cuddling and caressing may be rewarding.

Attention to the patient's cardiac medications is vital. Once a sexual problem is discovered, an evaluation of its nature and then its cause (organic or psychic) is important. The patient should always be encouraged to contact the physician if any side effects are experienced. The patient's compliance with the medication regimen may easily be affected because of the drug's effect on his or her sexuality and the undesirable impact on marital relations. A reduction in the dosage of the medication or substitution of an equally effective drug with a lesser potential effect on the sexual mechanism may be instituted.

At a time when the lives of the patient and the partner are heavily burdened with fears and anxieties, proper counseling by well-informed physicians, nurses, and other health care professionals will lead to successful rehabilitation and alleviate much of the stress that can interfere with emotional and sexual well being.

REFERENCES

1. Papadopoulos C: A survey of sexual activity after myocardial infarction. Cardiovasc Med 3:821, 1978

2. Papadopoulos C, Larrimore P, Cardin S et al: Sexual concerns and needs of the postcoronary patient's wife. Arch Intern Med 140:38, 1980

3. Papadopoulos C, Beaumont C, Shelley SI et al: Myocardial infarction and sexual activity of the female patient. Arch Intern Med 143:1582, 1983

4. Tuttle WB, Cook WL, Finch E: Sexual behavior in post-myocardial patients. Am J Cardiol (abstract) 13:140, 1964

5. Hellerstein HK, Friedman EH: Sexual activity and the postcoronary patient. Arch Intern Med 125:987, 1970

6. Wishnie HA, Hackett TP, Cassem NA: Psychological hazards of convalescence following myocardial infarction. JAMA 215:1292, 1971

7. Mann S, Yates JE, Raftery EB: The effects of myocardial infarction on sexual activity. J Cardiac Rehabil 1:187, 1981

8. Mehta J, Krop H: The effect of myocardial infarction on sexual functioning. Sex Disabil 2:115, 1979

9. Papadopoulos C: Coronary artery disease and sexuality. p. 1. In: Sexual Aspects of Cardiovasculr Disease. Praeger, New York, 1989

10. Bakker C, Bogdonoff M, Hellerstein H: Heart disease and sex. Response to questions. Med Aspects Hum Sex 5:24, 1971

11. Nemec ED, Mansfield L, Kennedy JW: Heart rate and blood pressure responses during sexual activity in normal males. Am Heart J 92:274, 1976

12. Renshaw DC, Karstaedt A: Is there (sex) life after coronary bypass? Compr Ther 14:61, 1988

13. Douglas JE, Wilkes TD: Reconditioning cardiac patients. Am Fam Physician 11:123, 1975

14. Larson JL, McNaughton MW, Kennedy JW et al: Heart rate and blood pressure responses to sexual activity and a stair-climbing test. Heart Lung 9:1025, 1980

15. Stein RA: The effect of exercise training on heart rate during coitus in the post myocardial infarction patient. Circulation 55:738, 1977

16. Bohlen JG, Held JP, Sanderson MO et al: Heart rate, rate-pressure product, and oxygen uptake during four sexual activities. Arch Intern Med 144:1745, 1984

17. Kavanagh T, Shephard RJ: Sexual activity after myocardial infarction. Can Med Assoc J 116:1250, 1977

18. Johnston BL, Fletcher GF: Dynamic electrocardiographic recording during sexual activity in recent post-myocardial infarction and revascularization patients. Am Heart J 98:736, 1979

19. Barreto DG, Sin-Chesa C, Rivas-Estany E et al: Sexual intercourse in patients who have had myocardial infarction. J Cardiopulmonary Rehabil 6:324, 1986

20. Cassem NH, Hackett TP: Psychiatric consultation in a coronary care unit. Ann Intern Med 75:9, 1971

21. Papadopoulos C, Shelley SI, Piccolo M et al: Sexual activity after coronary bypass surgery. Chest 90:681, 1986

22. Gundle MJ, Reeves BR, Tate S et al: Psychosocial outcome after coronary artery surgery. Am J Psychiatry 137:1591, 1980

23. Kornfeld DS, Heller SS, Frank KA et al: Psychological and behavioral responses after coronary artery bypass surgery. Circulation 66(suppl. III):III-24, 1982

24. Thurer S: Sexual adjustment following coronary bypass surgery. Rehabil Counseling Bull 24:319, 1981

25. Thurer S, Thurer RL: Sex after coronary bypass surgery. Med Aspects Hum Sex 16:68F, 1982

26. Westaby S, Sapsford RN, Bentall HH: Return to work and quality of life after surgery for coronary artery disease. Br Med J 2:1028, 1979

27. Raft D, McKee DC, Popio KA et al: Life adaptation after percutaneous transluminal coronary angioplasty and coronary artery bypass grafting. Am J Cardiol 56:395, 1985

28. Lough ME, Shinn JA: Impact of symptom frequency and symptom distress on self-reported quality of life in heart transplant recipients. Heart Lung 16:193, 1987

29. Harvison A, Jones BM, McBride M et al: Rehabilitation after heart transplantation: the Australian experience. J Heart Transplant 7:337, 1988

30. Mickley H, Petersen J, Nielson BL: Subjective consequences of permanent pacemaker therapy in patients under the age of retirement. PACE 12:401, 1989

31. Cooper DK, Luceri RM, Thurer RJ et al: The impact of the automatic implantable cardioverter defibrillator on quality of life. Clin Prog Electrophysiol Pacing 4:306, 1986

32. Ueno M: The so-called coition death. Jpn J Leg Med 127:333, 1963

33. Massie E, Rose EF, Rupp JC et al: Sudden death

during coitus—fact or fiction? Med Aspects Hum Sex 21:22, 1969

34. Myers A, Dewar HA: Circumstances attending 100 sudden deaths from coronary artery disease with coroner's necropsies. Br Heart J 37:1133, 1975

35. Levine SB: Marital sexual dysfunction: introductory concepts. Ann Intern Med 84:448, 1976

36. Story NL: Sexual dysfunction resulting from drug side effects. J Sex Res 10:132, 1974

37. Papadopoulos C: Cardiovascular drugs and sexuality. p. 69. In: Sexual Aspects of Cardiovascular Disease. Praeger, New York 1989

38. Okoniewski GA: Sexual activity following myocardial infarction. Cardiovasc Nursing 15:1, 1979

39. Skelton M, Dominian J: Psychological stress in wives of patients with myocardial infarction. Br Med J 2:101, 1973

40. Sikorski JM: Knowledge, concerns and questions of wives of convalescent coronary artery bypass graft surgery patients. J Cardiac Rehabil 5:74, 1985

41. Miller NH, Gossard D, Taylor CB: Advice to resume sexual activity after myocardial infarction. Circulation 70(suppl. II):II-134, 1984

42. McLane M, Krop H, Mehta J: Psychosexual adjustment and counseling after myocardial infarction. Ann Intern Med 92:514, 1980

43. Dengrove E: Sexual responses to disease processes. J Sex Res 4:257, 1968

44. Mayou R, Foster A, Williamson B: The psychological and social effects of myocardial infarction on wives. Br Med J 1:699, 1978

45. Cooper AJ: Myocardial infarction and advice on sexual activity. Practitioner 229:575, 1985

46. Boogaard MAK: Rehabilitation of the female patient after myocardial infarction. Nursing Clin North Am 19:433, 1984

47. Dyer R: Menopause—a closer look for nurses. p. 303. In Kjervik DK and Martinson IM (eds): Women in Stress: A Nursing Perspective. Appleton-Century-Crofts, East Norwalk, CT, 1979

48. Heller SS, Frank KA, Kornfeld DS et al: Psychological outcome following open-heart surgery. Arch Intern Med 134:908, 1974

49. Stern TA: The management of depression and anxiety following myocardial infarction. Mt Sinai J Med 52:623, 1985

28

Psychological Problems and Their Management

John L. Shuster, M.D.
Theodore A. Stern, M.D.
George E. Tesar, M.D.

This chapter discusses psychiatric aspects of coronary rehabilitation. The psychological responses that arise and complicate the course of recovery from myocardial infarction will be reviewed. Additionally, the possible contribution of behavior and mood to the genesis and progression of coronary heart disease (CHD), as well as treatment strategies to alter these factors, will be discussed. The interface between coronary disease and concurrent psychiatric disorders will be presented so that proper treatment for these disorders can be initiated when they are present. Brief guidelines will also be given for the use of psychotropic medications in this population. Examination of these issues in detail outlines what psychiatry has to offer in the rehabilitation of patients with coronary heart disease.

PSYCHOLOGICAL CONSEQUENCES OF CORONARY HEART DISEASE AND ITS COMPLICATIONS

Coronary heart disease and myocardial infarction (MI) have emotional as well as cardiovas-cular consequences. Although most coronary patients adjust well to their illness, a significant number of patients develop new or accentuated prior psychiatric symptoms or syndromes such as anxiety, depression, and delirium. These sequelae not only complicate management of patients with CHD, but may also aggravate the coronary illness itself. MI requires rapid adjustment to the presence of chronic disease, acceptance of new physical limitations, and, frequently, major changes in lifestyle. Some patients are unable to make these adjustments easily. Additionally, invasive diagnostic, therapeutic, and life-supporting interventions are often indicated in the care of post-MI patients. These interventions may contribute to the development of psychiatric symptoms.

MI, cardiac arrhythmias, sudden cardiac death, diagnostic procedures (e.g., coronary angiography) and therapeutic procedures (e.g., percutaneous transluminal coronary angioplasty [PTCA], placement of the intra-aortic balloon pump [IABP] or automatic implantable cardioverter-defibrillator [ICD], and coronary bypass [CABG] surgery) may be associated with the development of psychiatric symptomatology.

483

Myocardial Infarction

MI is also discussed in Chapter 11.

The defense mechanism of denial is a major obstacle to the successful management of coronary patients in the acute and rehabilitative phases of illness. In fact, since the majority of MI deaths occur within the first 4 hours after infarction,[1] denial in the form of delayed presentation for emergency care is a possible source of significant mortality. One study[2] found the mean delay time from MI symptom onset to arrival in an emergency room to be 3.9 hours, and one-third of patients studied had not arrived in the emergency room 6 hours after the onset of chest pain. This finding has important implications for the success of newer thrombolytic therapies (e.g., tissue plasminogen activator [t-PA] and streptokinase), which should be initiated within 6 hours of onset of MI to be effective. Patients and their families, who are also subject to the effects of denial, should be educated about the signs and symptoms of the onset of myocardial ischemia leading to MI and given instruction about specific actions to take, even if the patient has previously sustained an infarction and would be expected to know the appropriate response.

In the emergency room and the coronary care unit (CCU), the patient is often overwhelmed by the ambient activity and medical procedures (e.g., catheter insertion, defibrillation, and thrombolysis). Physical discomfort, separation from family members, and fear of death may intensify the patient's anxiety. Invasive interventions such as IABP placement or emergent coronary catheterization and PTCA can also aggravate anxiety. Anxiolytic medication is indicated under such circumstances, but is commonly deferred until transfer to the CCU. Even in the intensive care setting, anxiolytic drugs are frequently underutilized and prescribed on a PRN, rather than a maintenance, schedule.[3]

Anxiety, which is manifest by tension, apprehension, fear, and physical signs (e.g., tachycardia, tachypnea, diaphoresis, insomnia, hypertension, and ventricular ectopy), is the most common reason for psychiatric consultation early in the CCU stay.[4] The realistic threat of death and its premonitory symptoms (chest pain, dyspnea), concern about cardiorespiratory complications (arrhythmias, cardiac or respiratory arrest, hypotension), and the anticipation of a need for lifesaving maneuvers (cardioversion, IABP or pacemaker placement, mechanical ventilation) are common causes of anxiety in the acute setting. Additional anxiety may be provoked by witnessing the cardiac arrest of another patient, experiencing memories of previous admissions to a CCU, identification with a friend or relative who died of coronary disease, or having repeated trips to the catheterization suite for electrophysiologic testing.

In 1971, Cassem and Hackett[4] described a pattern of requests for psychiatric consultation in patients admitted to the CCU. Psychological reactions were correlated with the length of time spent in the CCU. Anxiety, denial, depression, and emergence of chronic character traits were found to occur in a characteristic pattern. Any of these reactions, however, may persist or re-emerge later in the course of recovery. During the past 20 years, psychological reactions of patients with acute MI have become less marked as a result of earlier interventions (thrombolysis, PTCA, CABG, etc.), enhanced survival, shortened hospital stay, subsequent rehabilitation, and secondary preventive measures.[5]

Denial is a common defense against anxiety and often helps to calm the anxious patient. Although it may interfere with the patient's recognition of symptoms and prompt request for medical assistance, denial that does not lead to detrimental behavior may be beneficial. Patients who minimize the impact of their illness, deny fear, and give the appearance of calm have been found to have better survival rates during their CCU stay than those who appear to be worried and preoccupied with their illness.[6,7]

Depression is typically the reason for psychiatric consultation on the third or fourth day in the CCU, as anxiety and denial abate.[4] Depressed patients may show sadness, disinterest, pessimism, hopelessness, weeping, or psychomotor retardation; have thoughts of frustration or anger; and perceive an injury to their self-esteem ("ego infarction").[8] One or more of these symptoms may become evident as patients begin to consider the consequences of coronary illness and its impact on their lives. In some individuals, misconceptions about the implications of an MI (e.g., having to quit work, give up sex, give up sports) can be a source of depression or anxiety. Clarification and supportive discussion with such patients is frequently helpful. Major depression (as described below) or severe anxiety causes suffering that merits specific treatment. Untreated depression and anxiety can deplete physical and emotional reserves and complicate the course of recovery from MI.

In the convalescent phase, patients may be faced with a sense of loss, vulnerability, and depression that can escalate after hospital discharge.[8,9] This has been referred to as "homecoming depression"[2] and is at least partially correlated with the extent to which patients consider themselves disabled. Concerns about disability are common and were formerly complicated by the considerable physical deconditioning that resulted from prescribed periods of extended bed rest. More recently, physical reconditioning has come to be regarded as an important part of physical and psychological recovery from MI.[8,10] Many patients require and benefit from specific instruction about the extent to which they can participate in physical, social, vocational, recreational, and sexual activities and self-care.

Precision in activity recommendations helps dispel myths and inaccurate beliefs held by patients about their achievable levels of activity. Patients in the post-MI state may erroneously believe that even mild exertion is dangerous, that driving is prohibited, that the arms should not be lifted over the head, that sexual intercourse should never again be attempted, and that recurrent MI and sudden death tend to occur at orgasm.[8]

Arrhythmias and Sudden Cardiac Death

Patients who have malignant ventricular arrhythmias often develop psychosocial and neuropsychiatric problems.[11,12] Chronic and acute anxiety, for example, are common sequelae of recurrent, symptomatic ventricular ectopic activity (VEA). Mild to moderate anxiety may progress to extreme apprehension, resistance to tranquilization, and fear of sleep or other sleep disturbances. The evaluation of VEA can also generate anxiety. Furthermore, many antiarrhythmic medications have neuropsychiatric side effects, including anxiety, delirium, and seizures.[13–16]

Patients with recurrent, symptomatic VEA live with constant uncertainty and the continuing threat of sudden cardiac death. Although denial permits some adaptation, anxiety, fearfulness, and extreme vigilance take over if denial fails. Patients with VEA in the hospital commonly become fixated and dependent on their cardiac monitors. Significant separation anxiety can occur when a patient is disconnected from the monitor.[7] An irrational fear of dying during sleep may also develop in patients with VEA, which is then complicated by the effects of sleep deprivation (e.g., irritability and mild paranoia). The presence of such psychological symptoms can be expected to lead to considerable loss of social and occupational functioning.[11]

Survivors of cardiac arrest are also susceptible to adverse psychiatric effects. In addition to concerns raised by having a coronary illness and being rescued from near-death, some of the psychological consequences of cardiac arrest may be due to post-anoxic encephalopathy. When this is severe, features include amnesia, cortical blindness, post-anoxic action myoclonus, as well as confusion and agitation that may follow a lucid interval of several days to weeks after the arrest.[17,18] Even when central nervous system (CNS) injury is not obvious after resuscitation, cardiac arrest increases the risk of brain injury secondary to hypotension and hypoxia. One study[19] found that the majority of arrest survivors suffered from organic brain syndromes, had frightening and violent dreams, and had prominent experiences of "having been dead and reborn." They also demonstrated poor long-term adaptation. Mild hypoxic brain injury may also contribute to persistent behavioral and personality changes that appear to result from poor adjustment or depression.[20]

Impaired CNS function after cardiac arrest is probably not universal.[21,22] Dobson et al.[22] found that only 5 of 20 survivors of cardiac arrest failed to make a satisfactory adjustment and that those who did not seemed to have more difficulty with personality disturbance or unremitting physical disability than with factors related to the arrest.

Diagnostic Procedures

Diagnostic procedures are also discussed in Chapters 7–10, 14, and 15.

The diagnostic evaluation of coronary illness can be an emotionally charged experience for patients. They may feel their cardiac health is at stake and dread even noninvasive tests (e.g., electrocardiograms [ECGs], exercise tests) for fear of bad news. Cardiac catheterization, although generally brief and uneventful, is a stressful and uncomfortable experience for many patients. At times, the fear of pain or possible death intensifies the discomfort associated with the procedure. If admission to the hospital or CCU is required for the evaluation, a spectrum of reactions similar to those seen after MI can occur. Also, if the patient has had a previous MI, return to the hospital may arouse anxiety-laden memories of a previous CCU experience.

Electrophysiologic study, which involves serial drug testing and possibly one or more cardioversions, can be a grueling experience for the patient. The physical discomfort from multiple catheter insertions and chest wall burns from defibrillation, extended duration of study, and anxiety about test outcome combine to make coping difficult. Anticipatory anxiety also tends to be high, but generally abates once the study begins and may lessen with each successive test. Some patients, particularly those with a history of poor adaptation to their coronary illness, demonstrate extreme anxiety and may even refuse completion of testing. Supportive psychotherapy, anxiolytic drugs, and group support have been beneficial to these patients.[23,24] The terms "pass" and "fail" should be avoided as much as possible by the staff, since some patients who "fail" the test can become dejected and perceive themselves as losers in a game with very high stakes.

Therapeutic Procedures

Therapeutic procedures are also discussed in Chapters 11, 16, 17, and 18.

Invasive procedures, such as PTCA and thrombolysis with intravenous streptokinase or t-PA, may cause physical discomfort or difficult-to-control bleeding and aggravate existing anxiety. These procedures are performed on patients who frequently are already in a state of extreme emotional distress and are excessively attentive to unusual physical sensations. Support and reassurance (with or without anxiolytic medications) are effective approaches to reduce anxiety in these patients.

Many patients implanted with an ICD initially have strong psychological reactions to the device. One study[25] found a pattern of preoperative anxiety, ultimately followed by good adaptation in general. Depression, fear, emotional lability, and hyperarousal diminished over time. The patients were quite aware of having a "foreign object" inside them, but generally came to view the device as life-saving and a source of security. Another recent study[26] found high degrees of anxiety and anger in ICD patients. During the course of follow-up, a reduction in anxiety scores was observed, which was temporally related to a reduction in ICD discharges.

Patients often respond to coronary and other cardiac surgery with a mixture of terror and resignation[27,28] and with concerns about life and death. Since extreme preoperative psychological stress and prior psychiatric disorders may adversely affect their outcome, patients should be screened for these problems before surgery. In addition to psychiatric disorders (e.g., depression, anxiety, extreme denial, paranoia, and personality disturbance), substance abuse and cognitive or CNS dysfunction are associated with a poor postoperative outcome (and higher mortality).[29–33] Psychiatric consultation should be obtained for patients at risk. Several studies have demonstrated a beneficial effect of preoperative psychiatric intervention on postoperative outcome.[34–37]

Delirium, one of the most common complications of cardiac surgery, is characterized by alterations in consciousness, orientation, attentiveness, organization of thought, perceptual ability, sleep–wake cycle, memory, and psychomotor activity.[38] Delirium usually has a rapid onset and is considered to be due to a reversible disturbance of brain function. Delirium has been reported in 11 to 70% of cardiac surgery patients.[30,39–41]

Intraoperative factors that have been associated with an increased likelihood of postoperative delirium include the complexity and type (CABG versus valve repair) of operative procedure,[40] total anesthesia time,[30] hypothermia (temperature less than 27°C),[30,42] the type of oxygenator used (more complications with the bubble than the membrane oxygenator),[43] and prolonged intraoperative hypotension.[44–47] The time spent on cardiopulmonary bypass has not been independently correlated with outcome.[40] Postoperative factors that contribute to the development of delirium include complications during recovery,[40] medications administered in the recovery room (particularly anticholinergic agents),[40,48] use of the IABP,[49] and environmental phenomena.[42,50]

The factors associated with postoperative delirium are probably etiologic to the extent that they cause CNS dysfunction. Scanning by positron emission tomography (PET) reveals a critical reduction in cerebral blood flow during cardiac surgery and up to 1 year postoperatively.[51] Reduced cerebral blood flow, which is generally not as pronounced after CABG as after valve replacement, may also cause the subtle but significant cognitive deficits that have been seen after cardiac surgery.[33,52,53] These findings support the general belief that cardiac surgery is associated with diffuse CNS injury and are consistent with the observation that those who come to cardiac surgery with preexisting CNS compromise (e.g., elderly patients) are more likely to experience postoperative delirium.

PSYCHOLOGICAL AND BEHAVIORAL RISK FACTORS FOR CORONARY HEART DISEASE

Type A Behavior Pattern, Hostility, and Depression

The type A behavior pattern (TABP) was first identified by Friedman and Rosenman more than 30 years ago.[54] TABP is characterized by competitiveness, excessive drive, free-floating hostility, status insecurity, polyphasic thinking and performance, and an enhanced sense of time urgency.[55,56] TABP and its relationship to CHD have been studied extensively.

The majority of early research supported the idea that TABP adversely affects the course of CHD. In the Western Collaborative Group Study (WCGS),[57] a prospective 8.5-year follow-up of patients with TABP, the rate of diagnosable CHD was approximately double that identified in those without the TABP. CHD, as measured by coronary angiography, has in some studies correlated positively with TABP.[58–61] A 1978 consensus conference of researchers in the field concluded that there was sufficient evidence to support the TABP as an independent risk factor for CHD.[62]

Although little conclusive evidence exists, several attempts have been made to identify the physiologic mechanisms by which TABP might exert a detrimental effect on CHD. Type A subjects have been reported to exhibit exaggerated responses to mental work by cardiovascular and neuroendocrine measures,[63–65] higher 24-hour testosterone levels,[66] and higher intraoperative blood pressures during CABG.[67] ECG changes and arrhythmias are associated with a variety of CNS processes,[68,69] including cerebrovascular accidents.[70] Arrhythmias, myocardial injury, and coronary vasospasm may result from electrical stimulation of limbic brain nuclei believed to mediate behavior and emotion.[69,71,72] Neuroendocrine substances such as epinephrine and norepinephrine have been shown to cause elevations in blood pressure, cholesterol level, and heart rate[73,74] and to lower the threshold for ventricular arrhythmias.[75] Serum glucocorticoids, associated with stress and depression, have also been linked to an increased risk of CHD.[76]

Not all studies, however, have supported the TABP concept.[77] The Aspirin Myocardial Infarction Study[78] failed to show a correlation between presence of TABP and recurrent coronary events in patients who had sustained an MI. The Multicenter Post-Infarction Group corroborated this finding.[79] The Multiple Risk Factor Intervention Trial (MRFIT)[80] found no correlation between TABP and development of CHD in a population of patients with other risk factors for CHD. In fact, some evidence suggests that TABP may provide a survival advantage by reducing the risk of non-acute death after MI.[81,82]

The contradictory findings among studies of TABP may be due to methodologic errors, particularly those related to the inherent difficulty of measuring TABP. The proposed gold standard of TABP measurement has been evaluation of a videotaped patient interview by using an objective rating scale. Various written and patient-administered measures, such as the Jenkins Activity Survey,[83] have also been used. However, the best method of measuring coronary-prone behavior remains controversial.

Additionally, global assessment of TABP may not be sufficiently specific to measure the variables of personality and behavior that are presumably detrimental to coronary health. Recently, researchers have reanalyzed the components of type A behavior.[56] There is mounting evidence that hostility, cynicism, and suppressed anger are the specific pathogenic features of TABP, while others (e.g., ambitiousness and time urgency) are probably not.[56,84,85]

Hostility, measured by objective scales such as the Cook-Medley subscale of the Minnesota Multiphasic Personality Inventory (MMPI),[86] has been strongly correlated with morbidity and mortality from CHD.[87,88] Patients with suppressed anger and high hostility ratings have demonstrated more severe CHD than patients without these features, and hostility and anger suppression ratings have correlated with CHD as measured by coronary angiography.[61,84,89] Even re-analysis of previous TABP studies has revealed significant associations between hostility or suppressed anger and CHD.[61,89,90] Reexamination of data from both the WCGS and MRFIT studies revealed evidence of a markedly elevated risk of CHD in the hostile patient groups.[91,92] This is especially impressive since the MRFIT data showed no evidence of increased CHD risk associated with global ratings of TABP.

Measurements of hostility as a CHD risk factor may also prove to be insufficiently specific. A recent study found only one subtype of a hostility measure to be positively associated with CHD severity.[93]

The effect of depressive syndromes, particu-

larly major depression, on the course of CHD has long been a subject of study. In an early study, psychiatric inpatients who were depressed had a mortality from coronary disease almost eight times that seen in the general population.[94] More recently, Murphy et al.,[95] in a 16-year prospective follow-up of a large cohort of individuals, found a significant association between overall mortality and affective illness, which was generally true across sexes and age groups. Deaths from circulatory illness in particular were also associated with the presence of affective illness.[95] Avery and Winokur[96] compared mortality in depressed patients who received adequate versus inadequate treatment with antidepressant medications or electroconvulsive therapy (ECT) for their depression. Nonsuicidal death and MI were significantly more common in the inadequately treated group after 3 years of follow-up.

Depression also appears to contribute to the progression of CHD. Depression has been associated with poorer cardiac function after MI, as well as with increased mortality.[10,77,97] Carney et al.[98] found that the presence of major depression in patients with CHD conferred an increased risk of all cardiac events, including CABG and death. Higher scores on scales of depression and anxiety have been found to correlate with the severity of CHD.[60,77]

Depression and emotional stress have also been related to an increased risk of sudden cardiac death from malignant ventricular arrhythmias.[99–102] Prolongation of the QT interval may be an effect of depression in some patients[103] and could predispose them to an increased risk of a ventricular rhythm disturbance.[104] Studies of heart rate variability, as measured by 24-hour ECGs, have suggested that changes in the balance of sympathetic and parasympathetic inputs to the heart (possibly a result of decreased parasympathetic tone) in depressed patients may increase their risk of post-MI cardiac complications (e.g., arrhythmias and death).[105–108]

Treatment

Studies of TABP as a coronary risk factor inevitably led to attempts to reduce TABP and thereby lessen its harmful effects. Many attempts have been made to demonstrate a beneficial effect of various psychotherapeutic treatments on the secondary prevention of CHD and coronary rehabilitation. Most of these studies have design flaws, including small numbers of patients and limited periods of follow-up. In addition to these drawbacks, the studies are also hampered by the above-mentioned difficulties in defining and measuring the targeted symptoms and behaviors (generally TABP in the research to date). Nevertheless, efforts to define and alter the cardiotoxic elements of behavior in patients who have sustained MI have yielded some encouraging results.

TABP in persons without CHD has been shown to respond to relaxation and anxiety management techniques.[109–115] TABP reduction strategies can also promote the reduction of other risk factors for CHD (e.g., hypercholesterolemia and hypertension) in healthy individuals.[109,111,112] Patel et al.[116] studied healthy patients with two or more CHD risk factors. Those randomized to eight sessions of group treatment with meditation, relaxation, stress reduction, and general health education showed greater reductions in blood pressure, cholesterol level, and cigarette use at 8-week and 8-month follow-up than those receiving health education alone. Controls showed more angina, CHD, and MI after 4 years. At this 4-year follow-up, reductions in blood pressure were maintained in the treatment group.

Individual Psychotherapy. Numerous studies have attempted to examine the effect of psychological and psychotherapeutic approaches to coronary rehabilitation in individual patients. Most studies have focused on relaxation programs or a psychological intervention as a component of a complex intervention strategy. However, studies of relatively simple interventions have revealed favorable results.

Guizzetta[117] found that both relaxation and music therapy administered to MI patients in the CCU lowered apical heart rates, peripheral temperatures, and cardiac complications in hospital. Improvements in self-reports of depression, anxiety, coping skills, and sense of well-being have been demonstrated after up to 3 months of social work counseling,[118] brief courses of relaxation training or stress management training,[119,120] and in-hospital counseling and support.[121,122]

Other studies have failed to find a significant beneficial effect of counseling in MI patients. Naismith et al.[123] found that, other than increasing social independence, a course of supportive individual counseling administered by a nurse was effective in improving the psychological functioning in only those MI patients with high scores on a pretreatment test of neuroticism. Mayou et al.[124] found no appreciable benefit of counseling at a 3-month follow-up.

Gruen[125] reported a study of 70 patients, hospitalized for a first MI, who were randomized to either no treatment or daily psychotherapeutic contact during their hospital admission. The treated group had shorter intensive care unit (ICU) and hospital stays, lower nurse ratings of weakness and physician ratings of depression, and fewer episodes of supraventricular arrhythmia and congestive heart failure in hospital. Treated patients also fared better in terms of self-reported physical well-being, anxiety, and residual fears, as well as superior ability to return to normal function at 4-month follow-up.

Dixhoorn et al.[126] studied 156 MI patients randomized to exercise therapy plus relaxation and breathing training or exercise therapy alone. They found improvement in measures of anxiety, sense of well-being, and feelings of invalidism in the patients treated with both therapies and no changes in the group given only exercise treatment.

Oldenberg et al.[127] examined the effect of education and relaxation training in hospitalized patients after a first MI versus the same strategy plus six to ten supportive and behavioral counseling sessions, and compared both with those in a control group of patients receiving routine care. At follow-up (12 months), both treated groups showed improvements in psychological and lifestyle functioning, reported fewer symptoms of CHD, and were less treatment-dependent. Measures of TABP and anxiety were lowered in the treated groups, and treated patients were more physically active. None of these changes was evident in the routine care group.

Frasure-Smith and Prince[128] reported the results of up to 7-year follow-up of a large group of patients randomly assigned to supportive treatment after MI or no treatment. In this simple treatment program, telephone contact between treated patients and a nurse determined which patients needed home visits as a result of high stress. Home visits were individually tailored, continued as long as stress remained high, and were specifically directed at support and reduction of stress. At 1 year after treatment, there was a reduction in cardiac death rates by about 50%, but this effect disappeared with further follow-up. A significant decrease in rates of recurrent MI, however, emerged when long-term follow-up data were examined.

Ornish et al. have evaluated the impact of stress management and other risk factor modification techniques. In one study,[129] 23 patients with CHD received 24 days of training in stress management (stretching and relaxation, meditation, visualization, and environmental manipulation) and a modified vegetarian diet. A control group ($n = 23$) received routine care. The treated group showed increases in exercise duration, total work performed, and left ventricular ejection fraction compared with control subjects. The treated group also showed a decrease in plasma cholesterol level and a reduction in the frequency of angina. Ornish also led an ambitious study of comprehensive lifestyle changes including a low-fat vegetarian diet, smoking cessation, moderate exercise, and stress management training for CHD patients.[130] At the end of the 1-year training period, the experimental group exhibited modest regression in the size of coronary lesions as measured by coronary angiography, while the usual-care control group demonstrated progression of disease. Additionally, the greatest improvement was seen in the most severely stenosed vessels. Although these findings are remarkable and encouraging, the intervention was quite intensive and complicated. It is not possible to sort out the effect of the psychological intervention (stress management training) from the other treatment factors, nor is it clear what contribution, if any, the individual components would have in isolation.

Group Psychotherapy. Several researchers have studied the potential for reduction of coronary-prone behavior in the group psychotherapy setting. One of the earliest attempts was reported by Adsett and Bruhn,[131] who treated a small number of patients with previous MI with 10 weekly group psychotherapy sessions. Compared with a matched control group, treated patients showed improved psychosocial function as rated by the treaters. There were no apparent differences in physiologic measures between the two groups at a 6-month follow-up.

Ibrahim et al.[132] randomized 118 MI patients to either weekly group therapy for 1 year or no treatment. Therapy sessions focused on support and reduction of stress and anxiety. Follow-up measures were taken at 6, 12, and 18 months. Cardiac survival was better among treated patients, although the difference did not achieve statistical significance. This difference was strongest among the most severely ill patients in the study. Although no changes were seen in physical or psychologic measures, treated patients reported a very positive attitude toward treatment and exhibited less social alienation, cynicism, and competitiveness than control subjects.

Rahe et al.[133–135] reported results of a 3- to 4-year follow-up of a group of patients randomly assigned to psychoeducational, supportive group treatment (six biweekly therapy sessions). At 18 months, treated patients showed comparatively fewer cardiac events (coronary insufficiency, CABG, death, and particularly recurrent MI). Three to four years after treatment, these differences in cardiac events persisted, although patients showed little memory of the educational content of the sessions. There was little or no change in CHD risk factors, although a few measured behaviors characteristic of the TABP (overwork, time urgency) were reduced among the treated patients.

Stern et al.[136] studied the response of 106 MI patients to treatment with either 12 weekly sessions of group therapy oriented toward education, stress reduction, and reduction of the TABP, or 12 weeks of supervised exercise. All patients had either exercise capacity rated at no more than 7 METs or evidence of significant depression or anxiety after their MI. Follow-up measurements were taken at 3, 6, and 12 months. Although no effects on mortality were evident at 1 year, exercising patients tended to have fewer cardiovascular sequelae. Exercising patients also showed increased work capacity, stamina, sociability, and independence, as well as improvements in depression and anxiety. Group therapy patients showed less depression and interpersonal friction and improvements in independence, sociability, and sense of friendliness.

Bilodeau and Hackett[137] reported that their patients were very pleased with group treatment. Group members requested continuation of the meetings beyond the scheduled duration. Patients particularly liked the atmosphere of mutual support and relaxation. None of their patients experienced cardiac symptoms during any of the meetings.

Horlick et al.[138] compared 83 MI patients in group treatment with 33 control subjects and found no benefit from therapy. Therapy patients received six weekly sessions in an education/ group discussion format, in addition to the standard coronary education program given to all patients. No differences between groups were seen in health status, social and recreational involvement, family satisfaction, anxiety, depression, and health locus of control. Control group patients tended to show quicker return to work and lower cardiac mortality at follow-up.

The work of Friedman and colleagues[139–142] in the Recurrent Coronary Prevention Project represents the most ambitious and comprehensive attempt to date to assess the feasability of altering coronary-prone behavior (in this case the TABP) and the effect of such a change on recurrent MI and cardiac death in patients who sustained an MI. Their 862 patients were followed for 4.5 years after randomization to either group cardiac counseling or group cardiac counseling in combination with type A behavioral counseling. Another group of patients was followed without intervention after they declined randomization. TABP was significantly reduced in a greater percentage of the patients given type A counseling. Prospective follow-up also revealed a significant reduction in rates of coronary recurrence (both nonfatal MI and cardiac death) in the combined-treatment group (12.9% compared with 21.2% of cardiac-counseling-only patients having coronary recurrences). The final follow-up report found an association between TABP alteration and a reduction in cardiac mortality.

In summary, although most of these studies are hampered by methodologic and other limitations and the data on efficacy (in decreasing mortality and recurrence of coronary events) are mixed, some general observations can be made. Most available studies support a beneficial effect of psychotherapeutic treatments on recovery after MI. In a recent report,[143] meta-analysis of controlled studies of psychotherapeutic treatments for TABP revealed a reduction in 3-year combined mortality and MI incidence of approximately 50% in therapy-treated patients compared with controls. The data also suggested that reduction of angina pectoris may result from these psychological interventions. Evidence also exists that psychological treatments can reduce the risk of recurrent ventricular arrhythmias.[75,144]

Patient satisfaction with the treatments was almost uniformly high.[131,132,137] Subjective (patient-perceived) effects on interpersonal activity and quality-of-life factors have also been generally positive. Even in the absence of a direct beneficial effect on CHD outcome, the positive impact on life satisfaction is an important and laudable product of psychotherapy. Moreover, as evidence mounts regarding the role of such psychological factors as hostility and suppressed anger in the pathogenesis of CHD, improvements in life satisfaction may become even more important.

Some of the curative elements of group psychotherapy, as outlined by Yalom,[145] are particularly evident in groups of post-MI patients. The element of universality ("I am not the only one who feels this way") is particularly beneficial. Instruction about CHD, risk factor management, and strategies for coping are also helpful, and patients are often more receptive to information from another patient with the same experience than from a second-hand source. The groups are usually quite cohesive from the start, and the feeling that all the members are "in the same boat" goes a long way in fostering the group's identity. Members typically become involved and concerned about the health of all members. Seeing the success of others in the group instills hope and may lead to imitation of health-promoting behaviors and attitudes.

In general, psychotherapeutic interventions in

the management of MI have been shown to be beneficial. Patients value these treatments. Some improvement in psychological and/or social function is usually achieved, and a few studies with substantial follow-up periods have demonstrated positive effects on coronary morbidity and mortality. Promptness of intervention is important, but treatments do not necessarily have to be complex to be beneficial. Combinations of treatment techniques (e.g., educational, cognitive, behavioral, or supportive approaches) appear to be most effective.[143] In an analysis of several studies, Mumford et al.[146] concluded that even modest psychological interventions can be beneficial as well as cost-effective.

Pharmacotherapy. Evidence is beginning to accumulate that pharmacologic treatments may be effective in the modification of behavioral risk factors for CHD. Krantz et al.[147] studied the effect of propranolol on patients given structured interviews for TABP and found significant reductions in components of the TABP and in cardiovascular reactivity. Another study[148] found similar results with both propranolol and atenolol in hypertensive patients with the TABP. A third study[149] failed to find a similar effect from propranolol, but detected a reduction in global TABP (as well as ratings of several TABP components) with administration of isoproterenol, a beta-adrenergic agonist.

Alprazolam, a benzodiazepine anxiolytic, reduces levels of circulating catecholamines[150] and, in preliminary studies, reduced blood pressure and cortisol responses to mental stress in type A men.[151]

Low levels of CNS serotonin have been associated with aggressive behavior and hostility.[152] Lithium, which appears to affect CNS serotonin activity, has reduced aggression in male prison inmates.[153] A group from the Massachusetts General Hospital[154] reported results of an open trial of a serotonergic anxiolytic, buspirone, in type A patients. A battery of psychological tests and videotaped structured interviews demonstrated a significant reduction of TABP and hostility after treatment with buspirone.

Smoking

Smoking is also discussed in Chapters 4 and 5.

Reduction or cessation of cigarette smoking after MI is an important goal of treatment. Cigarette smoking has long been known to cause morbidity and mortality from cardiac illnesses.[155] Studies have shown reduced mortality and frequency of MI among patients with CHD who stopped smoking compared with those who did not[156] and greater longevity in patients who chose to give up smoking after MI.[157] The occasion of a patient's MI is an opportunity to begin attempts to achieve this goal. Most studies, as summarized by Blumenthal and Levenson,[158] show that the smoking cessation rate after MI is about 50%. One would hope that active intervention could improve this cessation rate.

Therapeutic approaches, as reviewed elsewhere,[159] have included the use of nicotine chewing gum, lobeline (a nicotine substitute), propranolol, naloxone (an opioid inhibitor), and clonidine. Glassman et al.[160] found clonidine to be effective in reducing the craving for cigarettes during early abstinence. Studies of nicotine gum efficacy have been mixed. The rationale behind this treatment is to prevent withdrawal from nicotine (which has CNS-stimulating properties), thereby permitting the smoker to quit more easily; it avoids the pulmonary effects of smoke inhalation. Some studies have found nicotine gum beneficial in smoking cessation,[161–163] whereas others have not.[164,165]

Multiple psychological and behavioral approaches (including hypnosis, aversive therapy, and self-control techniques) have been used to promote smoking cessation.[159] Powerful suggestion by a faith healer has also been reported to have beneficial effects.[166] Although cessation rates have generally been disappointingly low, one study of a relapse prevention program achieved a 52% remission rate at 1-year follow-up.[167]

Several observations can be made about the success of these interventions. The presence of anxiety and abnormalities detected by MMPI screening[168,169] is predictive of treatment failure in smoking cessation programs. Recent evidence has linked cigarette smoking and depression. Depressed persons are more likely to smoke, and smokers who are depressed are less likely to quit.[170] Additionally, persons with a lifetime history of major depression are more likely to have a history of smoking, and smokers with a history of major depression are less successful in attempts at smoking cessation.[171] The latter study also suggests that depressive symptoms may re-emerge in these patients after smoking cessation, possibly contributing to smoking relapse.

Many smoking cessation strategies have been studied. No therapeutic approach shows a consistent, clear-cut advantage, and all have substantial relapse rates. Despite the somewhat discouraging results of reported smoking cessation trials, some patients benefit from these treatments. Even patients chronically ill with pulmonary and/or cardiac disease have demonstrated good responses to smoking cessation treatment.[172] Some smokers achieve full cessation from a single-treatment approach, whereas others require multiple attempts and different approaches. Some are successful only in reducing the amount of tobacco used. Nonetheless, given the magnitude of the problem of smoking and its adverse health effects, any reduction in smoking behavior is worthwhile. Studies suggest that a physician's strong advice to stop smoking is one of the best and most cost-effective aids to smoking cessation.[173,174]

CARDIAC PRESENTATIONS OF PSYCHIATRIC DISORDERS

Patients frequently attribute somatic symptoms to heart disease in the absence of identifiable cardiac disease. The symptoms are often due to problems in an organ system other than the heart; alternatively, they may be a feature of a psychiatric disturbance. Failure to recognize psychopathology can lead to complicated and frustrating cardiac evaluations that are unnecessary, costly, and potentially harmful to the patient. The presence of a psychiatric disorder can also complicate the management of patients in rehabilitation after MI.

A substantial incidence of psychiatric disorders, including hypochondriasis, somatization, anxiety, and depression, is evident in those who complain of chest pain in the absence of significant CHD.[175-179] For example, high MMPI subscale scores for hypochondriasis have been associated with continued chest pain in the absence of significant CHD.[179] Also, patients with high levels of anxiety and depression were more likely to have a normal exercise test as part of their chest pain evaluation than those without anxiety or depression.[176] However, coronary spasm or abnormal reactivity should be excluded by ergonovine and other provocative tests. Pasternak et al.[180] followed a group of patients with chest pain and normal coronary arteries; a significant number of these patients continued to complain of pain, persisted in their use of antianginal medications, were limited in their activity, and had some impairment in work functioning at 12- to 18-month follow-up.

A variety of psychiatric and neuropsychiatric disorders may present with cardiac symptoms. These include the anxiety, mood, and somatoform disorders, as well as factitious disorders and complex partial seizures.

Anxiety Disorders

Epidemiologic study has demonstrated about a 10% prevalence of significant anxiety in the general population.[181] About 10 to 14% of all patients who present to a cardiologist's office have anxiety-derived complaints.[182] The current classification of anxiety disorders[38] includes panic disorder with and without agoraphobia, agoraphobia alone, social phobia, simple phobia, obsessive-compulsive disorder, post-traumatic stress disorder, and generalized anxiety disorder. Patients with panic disorder and generalized anxiety disorder are particularly likely to present to cardiologists for evaluation, and the course of rehabilitation after MI may be complicated by the presence of an anxiety disorder.

Panic disorder is diagnosed when there are episodes of anxiety marked by intense apprehension or fear of doom, associated with at least four of the following symptoms: dyspnea, dizziness or faintness, palpitations or tachycardia, trembling or shaking, diaphoresis, choking sensations, nausea or abdominal distress, depersonalization or derealization, paresthesias, hot flashes or chills, chest pain or discomfort, and fear of dying or going crazy.[38] Diagnostic criteria also include the spontaneous onset (in the absence of anxiety-provoking stimuli) of at least one of the attacks, rapid symptom development (four of the above symptoms should develop suddenly and increase in intensity within 10 minutes of the onset of the first symptom), and a frequency of at least four attacks within a 4-week period (or one or more attacks followed by at least 1 month of persistent fear of having another). Conditions that meet all other panic disorder criteria but show fewer than four of the somatic features listed above are referred to as limited-symptom panic attacks. Anticipatory anxiety develops rapidly, particularly in women, and may contribute to the development of agoraphobia. Agoraphobia is the fear (and avoidance) of places or circumstances from which escape might be restricted (e.g., tunnels, bridges, elevators, moving automobiles) or in which help might be unavailable in the event of a panic attack.[38]

As is evident from the somatic symptoms listed among the diagnostic criteria, panic attacks can mimic several physical disorders, including symptomatic CHD and cardiac arrhythmias. Up to 30% of those with chest pain and angiographically normal coronary arteries meet diagnostic criteria for panic disorder.[183] Many medical disorders can also cause symptoms identical to those of panic disorder and should be considered and excluded early in the course of treatment.[184] The emergency room or outpatient medical office is the typical setting for evaluation of these episodes, and these patients may undergo a long series of diagnostic tests and see several physicians without a clear diagnosis being established.[185] Panic disorder, however, also occurs in the presence of the disorders it mimics, and a diagnosis of panic disorder does not exclude the possibility of comorbid CHD. In patients with CHD, untreated panic disorder can lead to symptoms difficult to differentiate from episodes of myocardial ischemia or arrhythmia.

Antipanic treatments include a range of pharmacologic alternatives, behavioral therapy, or a combination of the two. Panic disorder typically responds well to high-potency benzodiazepine anxiolytic drugs, which may have to be continued indefinitely. Although tolerance to the sedating effects of benzodiazepines develops quickly at a given dose, similar tolerance to the anxiolytic effects seems not to develop.[186] Antidepressants are equally effective against panic disorder,[187] although they tend to cause more side effects than benzodiazepines. Antidepressants are particularly indicated when anxiety is refractory to benzodiazepines or when abuse of benzodiazepines is a concern.

Generalized anxiety disorder describes a chronically anxious state of at least 6 months' duration during which the patient experiences anxiety more days than not.[38] Evidence of motor tension and sympathetic arousal may be seen in the physical symptoms often present during periods of anxiety (e.g., sweating, tachycardia, dyspnea, hyperventilation, tremulousness, light-headedness). Heightened vigilance, scanning of the environment, and apprehension may lead sufferers to seek medical attention for their physical symptoms. As opposed to those with panic attacks, patients with generalized anxiety disorder are anxious about particular life circumstances, which could include complications of CHD. Treatment often involves behavioral therapy to promote relaxation and to reduce tension and anxiety and the judicious use of anxiolytic medications.

Mood Disorders

Bipolar (manic-depressive) disorder, major depression, cyclothymia, and dysthymia are included in the category of mood disorders. Major depression is of particular interest, given its prevalence (up to 9.3% of all females and up to 3.2% of all males)[38] and its interface with CHD. The diagnostic criteria for major depression[38] include the presence of at least four of the following symptoms for at least 2 weeks: depressed mood, marked loss of interest or pleasure, appetite or weight change, change in sleep pattern, psycho-motor agitation or retardation, loss of energy, feelings of worthlessness or guilt, decreased concentration or increased indecisiveness, and thoughts of death or suicide. Either depressed mood or loss of interest or pleasure must be present to make the diagnosis. Many depressed patients will deny that their mood is depressed; when this occurs, it has been referred to as "masked depression."

Physical complaints and somatic preoccupation are common features of depressive disorders, especially in the elderly. Depressed patients may focus on or amplify physical symptoms or sensations (e.g., fatigue or chest pain). Additionally, major depression is often associated with anxiety and panic attacks, which can, as mentioned above, mimic symptomatic CHD.

The treatment of major depression is primarily somatic. Antidepressant medications and ECT are the standards. Antidepressant medications will not usually show beneficial effects for several days to a few weeks after therapeutic doses are achieved.[188] Inadequate dosage is a common cause of failure to respond to antidepressants.[189] Once remission is achieved, maintenance of antidepressant therapy for about 6 months is recommended to minimize the chances of relapse.[190] Psychotherapy is an important adjunct to pharmacotherapy in the treatment of depressive disorders.

Somatoform Disorders

The somatoform disorders are characterized by physical symptoms that suggest a physical disorder in the absence of evidence for a physical disorder (i.e., organic findings or a known physiologic mechanism) and evidence or presumption of an underlying psychological conflict. The somatoform disorders include body dysmorphic disorder, conversion disorder, hypochondriasis, somatization disorder, somatoform pain disorder, and undifferentiated somatoform disorder.[38] Successful management requires careful evaluation to rule out diagnosable physical problems, recognition of the patient's distress, supportive care, and regular follow-up. The MMPI is a useful test in the evaluation of these disorders and may be especially helpful in the treatment of patients who do not recognize the contribution of psychological factors to their disease. As with anxiety and mood disorders, somatoform disorders can coexist with demonstrable organic disease, such as CHD. It is also important to consider other psychiatric disorders (e.g., anxiety and depression) as alternative diagnoses or comorbid conditions. The somatoform disorders of most concern in coronary rehabilitation include somatization disorder, hypochondriasis, and somatoform pain disorder.

The diagnosis of somatization disorder requires the presence of at least 13 symptoms from a list of 35 in the DSM-III-R.[38] These are generally grouped into symptoms referable to the gastrointestinal and cardiovascular systems (including dyspnea, palpitations, chest pain, and dizziness), pain symptoms, pseudoneurologic symptoms, and sexual and female reproductive symptoms. These symptoms generally begin before age 30 and persist for several years in the absence of an identifiable cause. The complaints are often dramatic and exaggerated and may vary between examinations. Patients with this disorder often see many different physicians and frequently undergo unnecessary and repetitious diagnostic and surgical procedures.

The essential features of hypochondriasis are a preoccupation with disease or being sick, an unrealistic interpretation of physical sensations as abnormal, and a persistent pursuit of medical care and advice despite reassurance and negative evaluations for the same complaint.[38] These features are present for at least 6 months in hypochondriasis. In cardiac patients, this cluster of symptoms is often referred to as cardiac neurosis. Persistent complaints of chest pain have been associated with high scores on the hypochondriasis and hysteria subscales of the MMPI,[178,179] and chest wall tenderness is often present on physical examination of these patients. Hypochondriacal behavior secondary to other psychiatric disorders (e.g., anxiety and depression) is important to consider and exclude, as treatment of the primary problem may lead to remission of hypochondriacal complaints.[191]

Somatoform pain disorder is diagnosed when a patient complains of at least 6 months of pain for which there is no identifiable etiology or that is far in excess of what would be expected from any physical findings present.[38] Temporal association between a stressor or psychological conflict and the onset of the symptoms serves as a clue to the diagnosis, as does evidence of secondary gain or avoidance of circumstances felt by the patient to be undesirable. As with other disorders in this category, somatoform pain disorder can coexist with an organic source of pain.

Thorough evaluation to exclude organic problems that may be mimicked by somatoform disorders is necessary. Although hypochondriasis and somatoform disorders are remarkably stable and treatment-resistant, psychiatric consultation can be helpful. Patients with somatoform disorders often respond best to a supportive approach with regular follow-up visits.[192,193]

Other Disorders

The word *factitious* means not real, genuine, or natural. Patients with factitious disorder with physical symptoms, also known as Munchausen syndrome, or "cardiopathica fantastica" when cardiac symptoms are predominant,[194,195] may present to a cardiologist for evaluation. In contrast to the patients with somatoform disorders, who often have vague histories, these patients typically describe grandiose and fantastic events in great detail. They also tend to lack social supports, have a history of travel to many places, and have had trouble with the law. A thorough and nonthreatening evaluation will usually reveal an underlying personality disorder and features of hostility, masochism, poor impulse control, and self-destructive acting-out. Again, it is important to remember that a diagnosis of a factitious disorder does not preclude a diagnosis of CHD or a past of MI.

Complex partial seizures are characterized by multiple atypical psychiatric symptoms.[196] The presentation of complex partial seizures may also include cardiac signs and symptoms (e.g., chest pain, cardiac rhythm disturbances, cardiac arrest, or syncope due to bradyarrhythmia).[197,198] This diagnosis is made by clinical evaluation, absence of evidence of coronary or myocardial disease,

and evidence of a seizure disorder. Patients with complex partial seizures commonly have normal surface-lead electroencephalograms (EEGs), since the ictal focus may reside in deep limbic structures. The high incidence of sudden death in patients with seizure disorders may be attributable to cardiovascular complications of seizure activity, (e.g., arrhythmias, sinus arrest, and neurogenic pulmonary edema). Although their response to anticonvulsant drugs is variable, patients with complex partial seizures often obtain dramatic relief from these agents.[199]

USE OF PSYCHOTROPIC AGENTS AND ECT IN PATIENTS WITH CHD

Most psychopharmacologic agents exert important effects on the heart and cardiovascular system,[200] as does ECT.[201] The prospect of prescribing these treatments for patients with CHD is understandably disquieting. However, the decision not to treat psychiatric disorders in coronary patients for fear of cardiac side effects surrenders the opportunity to relieve suffering from psychiatric illnesses, which can themselves contribute significantly to cardiac morbidity and mortality.[95,96] Apprehension concerning potential side effects of psychotropic drug treatment probably contributes to the undertreatment of the majority of depressed patients in the general population, according to Keller et al.[189] Fortunately, psychotropic drugs can be safely and effectively administered, given an understanding of their cardiac side effects.

Anxiolytic Drugs

The benzodiazepine anxiolytic drugs have replaced barbiturates as the agents of choice in the treatment of anxiety.[202] This is due to their efficacy and relative safety, as their risk of toxicity in overdose is low.[184] Patients with MI and symptomatic CHD are frequently given these drugs. Clinically important characteristics of benzodiazepines have been reviewed elsewhere.[203]

In addition to their anxiolytic effects, benzodiazepines have beneficial cardiac effects. Intravenously administered diazepam has a nitroglycerinlike effect on the coronary and systemic circulations, reducing myocardial oxygen consumption ($M\dot{V}o_2$) without altering coronary blood flow or coronary vascular resistance.[204] The short-acting parenteral benzodiazepine midazolam produces even greater $M\dot{V}o_2$ reductions.[205] These agents,[206] as well as orally administered alprazolam,[150] decrease sympathetic tone and baroreflex activity. This may be helpful in patients with MI or congestive heart failure, as these conditions are associated with elevations in circulating catecholamines.[207] Excessive stores of catecholamines have also been found in coronary arteries prone to spasm.[208] The antiadrenergic effect of benzodiazepines may become problematic in patients unable to tolerate reductions in sympathetic tone (e.g., those with hypovolemia or those receiving combinations of benzodiazepines and morphine sulfate).[209] Lorazepam may have less effect on sympathetic tone than other benzodiazepines[210] and has been recommended (with haloperidol) for use in agitated patients in an ICU.[211,212] Alprazolam may have an additional benefit for CHD patients, as it inhibits platelet-activating factor-induced aggregation of human platelets.[213]

Antidepressant Drugs

Although treatment of major depression is the most common use for medications marketed as antidepressants, these agents are also useful in the treatment of many other problems, including headache, chronic pain, panic disorder, and obsessive-compulsive disorder. Antidepressants act on central and peripheral adrenergic, cholinergic, serotonergic, and histaminergic systems. Although the precise mechanism of action of antidepressant medications remains to be clarified, activity at some or all of these receptor sites is believed to account for their therapeutic actions and side effects. Cardiovascular side effects of antidepressants include tachycardia, postural hypotension, conduction abnormalities, and pro- and antiarrhythmic effects.[200] The degree to which these effects are seen with various antidepressants varies greatly.[203]

Tricyclic antidepressants (TCAs), in clinical use since the 1950s, are the oldest class of antidepressant drugs. Their cardiovascular effects have been studied more extensively than those of any of the newer antidepressants. Early reports on the adverse effects of overdoses of these drugs (arrhythmias, conduction disturbances, and profound hypotension leading to cardiovascular collapse and death) and later reports of a relatively high death rate among patients treated with amitriptyline[214,215] led to excessive concern about the use of these drugs in cardiac patients. However, TCAs can be prescribed safely in patients with CHD when one is mindful of the relative contraindications to their use.

The principal side effects of TCAs are related to heart rate, blood pressure, electrical conduction, and cardiac rhythm. TCAs typically produce an elevation in heart rate averaging 10 to 15 beats/min. This effect is thought to be mediated by anticholinergic effects and is generally benign. However, it is wise to proceed cautiously (if at all) with TCA treatment of patients in whom a mild elevation of heart rate would be detrimental (e.g., unstable angina, marginally compensated congestive heart failure). Among the TCAs, desipramine has the least anticholinergic potency.[216,217]

Induction or exacerbation of orthostatic hypotension is a serious potential side effect of TCAs.[218] TCA-induced orthostatic hypotension is probably an idiosyncratic phenomenon and does not appear related to age, sex, or TCA dose.[219] It has, however, been reported to occur more frequently in the setting of cardiovascular disorders,[220–223] concomitant use of other medications that lower blood pressure,[218,220,224] and a pretreatment orthostatic drop in systolic blood pressure of more than 15 mmHg.[225] Clinical experience suggests that use of a low initial dose, followed by a gradual increase to the therapeutic dose, reduces the likelihood of these and other side effects.[200] In practice, imipramine seems to be the TCA most likely to cause orthostasis.[200] On the other hand, nortriptyline poses the least risk of orthostatic hypotension in healthy patients, as well as those of advanced age or with cardiac disease,[223,226–229] and is therefore the TCA of choice for depressed patients with cardiovascular disorders. Nortriptyline also has a "therapeutic window" that allows close and reliable monitoring of drug levels.[230]

Conduction changes seen during TCA therapy include lengthening of the QRS complex and the PR and QT intervals and a decrease in T-wave amplitude.[219] The quinidine-like, type 1A antiarrhythmic activity of TCAs causes dose-related slowing of conduction through the His-ventricular segment of the atrioventricular node.[231–233] The dose-dependent slowing of electrical conduction becomes clinically significant in patients with preexisting abnormalities in the His-Purkinje system, particularly bundle branch blocks.[218,220,223] Development of second- and third-degree heart block is a significant risk only in patients with preexisting conduction defects.[218,220] Although doxepin has been advertised as the least likely of the TCAs to produce adverse cardiac conduction effects,[231,233,234] equipotent doses of doxepin slow conduction to the same degree as other TCAs.[235,236]

In toxic doses, TCAs have been associated with various disturbances of cardiac rhythm, including supraventricular tachycardia, atrial fibrillation and flutter, atrial and ventricular premature contractions, junctional and idioventricular rhythms, ventricular tachycardia, and ventricular fibrillation.[237–239] However, at therapeutic serum levels, the quinidinelike (type 1A antiarrhythmic) effects of these agents may confer protection against ventricular arrhythmias.[219,240–242] Type 1 antiarrhythmic agents can also be proarrhythmic.[243] If TCAs share this property with type 1A antiarrhythmics, this could explain the idiosyncratic vulnerability to ventricular arrhythmias that rarely occurs with therapeutic TCA levels.[244]

There is little if any impairment in mechanical heart function or myocardial contractility related to TCAs, whether left ventricular function is normal[220,245] or abnormal.[221,223,236] Ejection fractions in patients with significant impairment of left ventricular function have remained unchanged after treatment with TCAs.[221,223,236] Even toxic concentrations of TCAs have caused no clinically significant effects on left ventricular contractility.[245]

Newer (second-generation) antidepressant agents include trazodone, maprotiline, amoxapine, bupropion, and fluoxetine. Although clinical and research experience with these drugs is not as great as with TCAs, some of them have advantages for the treatment of depressed cardiac patients.[246]

Trazodone may cause improvement in left ventricular function.[247] Little effect is apparent on cardiac conduction until very high doses are achieved.[248] Trazodone is, however, associated with significant orthostatic hypotension[249] and may aggravate preexisting cardiac arrhythmias.[250–252]

The profile of the cardiotoxic effects of maprotiline is similar to that of the TCA desipramine,[200] with important exceptions. At high therapeutic doses, it has been reported to cause torsade de pointes[200] and seizures.[253] In overdose, its cardiac toxicity is difficult to treat,[254] presumably owing to its long elimination half-life.[246]

Amoxapine has dopamine-blocking activities similar to neuroleptic drugs, which may account for the extrapyramidal effects reported with its use (e.g., akathisia, dyskinesias, and parkinsonism).[246] It also has been reported to cause atrial arrhythmias and conduction abnormalities[246] and has been associated with tachyphylaxis.

Bupropion is an activating antidepressant that blocks the reuptake of dopamine. Although apparently devoid of anticholinergic and cardiotoxic effects,[255] it has been reported to cause seizures at normal or slightly toxic doses.[256]

Fluoxetine, a serotonin-specific antidepressant, also has negligible cardiac effects as measured by ECG[257] and appears to be safe in overdose.[258] Some patients become anxious or agitated, especially early in the course of therapy. A small case series[259] has purported an association between fluoxetine treatment and the emergence of violent suicidal ideation. The significance and prevalence of this finding, however, are disputed.[260] In most cases, fluoxetine is well tolerated, but its exceptionally long half-life may excessively prolong the duration of adverse effects.

The monoamine oxidase inhibitors (MAOIs)

have also been in use since the 1950s. The MAOI antidepressants include phenelzine, tranylcypromine, and isocarboxazid. Another MAOI, pargyline, has been used primarily as an antihypertensive agent. Recently, there has been a revival of interest in the MAOIs because of their efficacy in the treatment of panic disorder, agoraphobia, and certain TCA-resistant depressive disorders.[261,262] In fact, MAOIs appear at least as effective against depression as are TCAs.[187] MAOIs commonly lower blood pressure and can cause marked orthostatic hypotension in therapeutic doses,[224,263] an effect that can be dangerous in the elderly and in those with cardiovascular disorders. Strategies used to counteract MAOI-induced orthostasis have included increasing fluid and sodium intake, the wearing of supportive hose, and the use of fludrocortisone acetate or caffeine.[264,265] Although the MAOIs are virtually devoid of cardiotoxic side effects (barring hypotension), many practitioners have been reluctant to use them because of the possible hypertensive crisis that may occur when tyramine-containing foods or stimulant medications are ingested by patients taking MAOIs. Unfortunately, these dietary restrictions have caused many patients to miss the benefits of MAOI treatment.[266] MAOIs are safer than previously thought when patients follow a low-tyramine diet and avoid sympathomimetic drugs.

Psychostimulant Drugs

The psychostimulant drugs, including dextroamphetamine and methylphenidate, have been used successfully to treat depressed and apathetic states in geriatric patients,[267,268] in medically ill patients,[269–271] and in patients recovering from cardiac surgery.[272] Despite a reputation of illicit use, abuse, and addiction, these agents are both safe and useful when prescribed appropriately. Depressed cardiac patients for whom a therapeutic trial of a psychostimulant is indicated include those who have debilitating congestive heart failure, who have been hospitalized for long periods, who require chronic ventilatory support, or in whom other pharmacologic treatments for depression are contraindicated. The advantages

of stimulants over TCAs include rapid onset of action, absence of anticholinergic effects, and no induction of orthostatic hypotension. At the low doses used to treat these patients (5 to 20 mg/day orally of either agent), tachycardia, coronary spasm, arrhythmias, and hypertension rarely occur, even in the presence of cardiac disease.[271,273] Close monitoring of heart rate, blood pressure, and cardiac rhythm is nonetheless advised. Possible contraindications to the use of stimulants include clinically significant hypertension, hypersensitivity, pregnancy, certain seizure disorders, delirium, psychosis, and concomitant use of medications such as alphamethyldopa, MAOIs, and bronchodilator drugs.

Lithium

Lithium carbonate is also used in the treatment of mood disorders, especially mania. Serious cardiotoxicity is rare, but adverse effects occur. Lithium commonly produces flattening or inversion of T waves, which is reversible and probably due to displacement of intracellular potassium.[274] Sinus node dysfunction associated with bradycardia and sinus arrest has also been observed, most commonly in the elderly.[275,276] Reversible first-degree atrioventricular block[277] and ventricular arrhythmias[276,278] have been reported. Lithium toxicity (characterized by nausea, vomiting, diarrhea, ataxia, slurred speech, convulsions, coma, and death) is more likely to occur in patients with hypertension, heart failure, or renal insufficiency. The reduced glomerular filtration, use of thiazide diuretics, and sodium restriction associated with these disorders may cause elevations in serum levels of lithium.[279] Close monitoring of lithium levels, cardiac status, and renal function is indicated. Prescription of a loop diuretic, such as furosemide, however, may not necessitate modification of lithium dose.[280]

Neuroleptic Drugs

Also known as antipsychotics, neuroleptic drugs are indicated for delirium, uncontrolled emesis, benzodiazepine-resistant anxiety, and psychosis. The antidopaminergic activity of these drugs is thought to mediate their antipsychotic effects. Neuroleptics exhibiting a high potency of dopaminergic blockade (e.g., haloperidol, trifluoperazine, fluphenazine, and perphenazine) are generally less cardiotoxic than the low-potency agents (e.g., chlorpromazine and thioridazine). Consequently, the high-potency agents are used almost exclusively in cardiac patients. Neuroleptics also have anticholinergic, quinidinelike, and alpha-adrenergic properties, whose strength tends to be inversely proportional to the dopaminergic potency of the drugs. Therefore, the low-potency agents are associated with tachycardia,[281] orthostatic hypotension,[281,282] conduction defects, repolarization abnormalities, and atrial and ventricular arrhythmias.[281,283,284] Low-potency neuroleptic drugs are relatively contraindicated in patients with preexisting cardiac dysfunction and those receiving drugs with synergistic action (e.g., type 1 antiarrhythmic drugs, diuretics, beta-blocking drugs, and calcium channel-blocking drugs).

High-potency neuroleptic drugs rarely cause clinically significant adverse cardiac effects. Haloperidol, in particular, has a proven record of safety in cardiac patients with both oral and parenteral use,[285,286] even when high doses are used in the treatment of delirious patients.[287–291] The combined use of propranolol and haloperidol, however, was associated with hypotension and cardiac arrest in one reported case.[292]

All neuroleptic agents, especially the high-potency ones, have the potential to produce extrapyramidal symptoms. These are generally of little clinical consequence and are rare with intravenously administered neuroleptics[291,293]; however, laryngeal dystonia can impair respiration.[294,295] Acute dystonias induced by neuroleptic drugs are easily reversed in most cases by administration of parenteral diphenhydramine, 25 to 50 mg, or benztropine mesylate, 1 to 2 mg. Dystonias refractory to this approach may respond to small doses of parenteral lorazepam, but continued laryngeal dystonia may require temporary use of a paralytic agent and intubation.

Electroconvulsive Therapy

ECT, possibly the most efficacious treatment now available for depression, also appears to be one of the safest procedures performed under general anesthesia.[296] ECT is often used in patients who are refractory to pharmacologic approaches, who require emergent treatment of depression, or for whom antidepressant medications are contraindicated. Elderly, hospitalized patients with failure to thrive as a result of severe, debilitating depression are candidates for ECT. This population includes a large number of patients with cardiovascular disorders.

ECT has been reported to cause a variety of cardiovascular effects. These include exaggerated hypertensive responses,[297,298] circulatory collapse,[299] acute MI,[300–302] and a variety of arrhythmias.[298,303] Transient repolarization abnormalities[298,303–305] and ST segment depression have also been reported.[305] Recent MI (within 6 months) is a relative contraindication, as it is with most procedures requiring general anesthesia.[296] However, the use of certain psychotropic drugs may also be contraindicated, such that ECT may be the most appropriate treatment.

Cardiovascular complications were reported by Gerring and Shields[306] in 28% of all ECT-treated patients and 70% of patients with known cardiovascular disease. However, Dec et al.[307] found that ECT was safe, effective, and well-tolerated by a group of elderly, often debilitated patients, one-fourth of whom had cardiovascular disorders (e.g., conduction system disorders, recent MI, and severely impaired left ventricular function), in a prospective study at the Massachusetts General Hospital. Transient ECG abnormalities resolved 4 to 6 hours after treatments, and no evidence of ECT-related myocardial injury was evident as measured by serial determinations of serum creatine kinase and aspartate aminotransferase.

These results and clinical experience show that careful attention to pretreatment evaluation and post-treatment management can make ECT safe, even in patients with known cardiovascular disease. ECT-related morbidity is further reduced by modern-day modifications of seizure stimulus and advanced pharmacologic management of cardiovascular disturbances.[201,308]

REFERENCES

1. Wallace WA, Yu PN: Sudden death and the prehospital phase of acute myocardial infarction. Annu Rev Med 26:1, 1975
2. Hackett TP, Cassem NH: Factors contributing to delay in responding to the signs and symptoms of acute myocardial infarction. Am J Cardiol 24:651, 1969
3. Stern TA, Caplan RA, Cassem NH: Use of benzodiazepines in a coronary care unit. Psychosomatics 28:19, 1987
4. Cassem NH, Hackett TP: Psychiatric consultation in a coronary care unit. Ann Intern Med 75:9, 1971
5. Wenger NK, Hellerstein HK, Blackburn H, Castranova SJ: Physician practice in management of patients with uncomplicated myocardial infarction—changes in the past decade. Circulation 65:421, 1982
6. Froese A, Hackett TP, Cassem NH et al: Trajectories of anxiety and depression in denying and non-denying acute myocardial infarction patients during hospitalization. J Psychosom Med 18:413, 1974
7. Hackett TP, Cassem NH, Wishnie HA: The coronary care unit: an appraisal of its psychological hazards. N Engl J Med 279:1365, 1968
8. Cassem NH, Hackett TP: Psychological rehabilitation of myocardial infarction patients in the acute phase. Heart Lung 2:383, 1973
9. Wishnie HA, Hackett TP, Cassem NH: Psychological hazards of convalescence following myocardial infarction. JAMA 215:1292, 1971
10. Stern MJ, Pascale L, Ackerman A: Life adjustment postmyocardial infarction: determining predictive variables. Arch Intern Med 137:1680, 1977
11. Fricchione GL, Vlay SC: Psychiatric aspects of patients with malignant ventricular arrhythmias. Am J Psychiatry 143:1518, 1986
12. Vlay SC, Fricchione G: Psychosocial aspects of surviving sudden cardiac death. Clin Cardiol 8:237, 1985
13. Saravay SM, Marhe J, Steinberg MD, et al: "Doom anxiety" and delirium in lidocaine toxicity. Am J Psychiatry 144:159, 1987
14. Charness ME, Morady F, Scheinman MM: Frequent neurologic toxicity associated with amiodarone therapy. Neurology 34:669, 1984
15. Deleu D, Schmedding E: Acute psychosis as an idiosyncratic reaction to quinidine: report of two cases. Br Med J 294:1001, 1987
16. Kennedy A, Thomas R, Sheridan DJ: Generalized seizures as the presentation of flecainide toxicity. Eur Heart J 10:950, 1989
17. Bass E: Cardiopulmonary arrest. Ann Intern Med 103:901, 1985
18. Plum F, Posner JB, Hain RF: Delayed neurological deterioration after anoxia. Arch Intern Med 110:56, 1962
19. Druss RG, Kornfeld DS: The survivors of cardiac arrest. JAMA 201:75, 1967
20. Reich P, Regestein QR, Murawski BJ et al: Unrecognized organic mental disorders in survivors of cardiac arrest. Am J Psychiatry 140:1194, 1983
21. Hackett TP: The Lazarus complex revisited. Ann Intern Med 76:135, 1972
22. Dobson M, Tattersfield AE, Adler MW et al: Attitudes and long-term adjustment of patients surviving cardiac arrest. Br Med J 3:207, 1971
23. Menza MA, Stern TA, Cassem NH: The treatment of anxiety associated with electrophysiologic studies. Heart Lung 17:555, 1988
24. Debiaso N, Rodenhausen N: The group experience: Meeting the psychosocial needs of patients with ventricular tachycardia. Heart Lung 13:597, 1984
25. Pycha C, Gulledge AD, Hutzler J et al: Psychological responses to the implantable defibrillator: preliminary observations. Psychosomatics 27:841, 1986
26. Vlay SC, Olson LC, Fricchione GL et al: Anxiety and anger in patients with ventricular tachyarrhythmias: Responses after automatic internal cardioverter defibrillator implantation. PACE 12:366, 1989
27. Bliss EL, Rumel WR, Branch CHH: Psychiatric complications of mitral surgery. Arch Neurol Psychiatry 74:249, 1952
28. Fox HM, Rizzo ND, Gifford S: Psychological observations of patients undergoing mitral surgery. Psychosom Med 16:186, 1954
29. Abram HS: Adaptation to open heart surgery: A psychiatric study of response to the threat of death. Am J Psychiatry 122:659, 1965
30. Blachy PH, Starr A: Post-cardiotomy delirium. Am J Psychiatry 121:371, 1964
31. Merwin SL, Abram HS: Psychologic response to coronary artery bypass. South Med J 70:153, 1977

32. Rabiner CJ, Willner AE, Fishman J: Psychiatric complications following coronary bypass surgery. J Nerv Ment Dis 160:342, 1975

33. Willner AE, Rabiner CJ, Wisoff BG et al: Analogical reasoning and postoperative outcome: prediction for patients scheduled for open heart surgery. Arch Gen Psychiatry 33:255, 1976

34. Layne OL, Yudovsky SC: Postoperative psychosis in cardiotomy patients: the role of organic and psychiatric factors. N Engl J Med 284:518, 1971

35. Lazarus HR, Hagens JH: Prevention of psychosis following open-heart surgery. Am J Psychiatry 124:1190, 1968

36. Surman OS, Hackett TP, Silverberg EL et al: Usefulness of psychiatric intervention in patients undergoing cardiac surgery. Arch Gen Psychiatry 30:830, 1974

37. Schindler BA, Shook J, Schwartz GM: Beneficial effects of psychiatric intervention on recovery after coronary artery bypass graft surgery. Gen Hosp Psychiatry 11:358, 1989

38. American Psychiatric Association: Diagnostic and Statistical Manual of Mental Disorders, 3rd Ed. Rev. American Psychiatric Association, Washington, 1987

39. Breuer AC, Furlan AJ, Hanson MR et al: Central nervous system complications of coronary artery bypass graft surgery: Prospective analysis of 421 patients. Stroke 14:682, 1983

40. Dubin WR, Field HL, Gastfriend DL: Postcardiotomy delirium: A critical review. J Thorac Cardiovasc Surg 77:586, 1979

41. Kornfeld DS, Zimberg S, Malm JR: Psychiatric complications of open-heart surgery. N Engl J Med 273:287, 1965

42. Heller SS, Frank KA, Kornfeld DS et al: Psychological outcome following open-heart surgery. Arch Intern Med 134:908, 1974

43. Aberg T, Kihlgren M: Cerebral protection during open-heart surgery. Thorax 32:525, 1977

44. Bojar RM, Najafi H, DeLaria GA et al: Neurological complications of coronary revascularization. Ann Thorac Surg 36:427, 1983

45. Kolkka R, Hilberman M: Neurologic dysfunction following cardiac operations with low-flow, low-pressure cardiopulmonary bypass. J Thorac Cardiovasc Surg 79:432, 1980

46. Lee WH, Brady MP, Rowe JM et al: Effects of extracorporeal circulation upon behavior, personality, and brain function. Ann Surg 173:1013, 1971

47. Tufo HM, Ostfeld AM, Shekelle R: Central nervous system dysfunction following open-heart surgery. JAMA 212:1333, 1970

48. Tune LE, Holland A, Folstein MF et al: Association of postoperative delirium with raised serum levels of anticholinergic drugs. Lancet ii:651, 1981

49. Sanders KM, Stern TA, O'Gara PT et al: Delirium during intraaortic balloon pump therapy: incidence and management. Abstract NR616. American Psychiatric Association, Annual Meeting, New York, 1990

50. Kornfeld DS, Heller SS, Frank KA et al: Personality and psychological factors in post cardiotomy delirium. Arch Gen Psychiatry 31:249, 1974

51. Henriksen L: Evidence suggestive of diffuse brain damage following cardiac operations. Lancet i:816, 1984

52. Aberg T, Ronquist G, Tyden H et al: Adverse effects on the brain in cardiac operations as assessed by biochemical, psychometric, and radiologic methods. J Thorac Cardiovasc Surg 87:99, 1984

53. Savageau JA, Stanton BA, Jenkins CD et al: Neuropsychological dysfunction following elective cardiac operation. J Thorac Cardiovasc Surg 84:595, 1982

54. Friedman M, Rosenman RH: Association of specific overt behavior pattern with blood and cardiovascular findings. JAMA 169:1286, 1959

55. Friedman M, Ulmer D: Treating Type A Behavior and Your Heart. p. 33. Fawcett/Crest, New York, 1984

56. Matthews KA, Haynes SG: Type A behavior pattern and coronary disease risk: update and critical evaluation. Am J Epidemiol 123:923, 1986

57. Rosenman RH, Brand RJ, Jenkins CD et al: Coronary heart disease in the Western Collaborative Group Study: Final follow-up experience of 8½ years. JAMA 233:872, 1975

58. Blumenthal JA, Williams RB, Kong Y et al: Type A behavior pattern and coronary atherosclerosis. Circulation 58:634, 1978

59. Frank KA, Heller SS, Kornfeld DS et al: Type A behavior pattern and coronary angiographic findings. JAMA 240:761, 1978

60. Zyzanski SJ, Jenkins CD, Ryan TJ et al: Psychological correlates of coronary angiographic findings. Arch Intern Med 136:1234, 1976

61. Dimsdale JE, Hackett TP, Hutter AM et al: Type A personality and extent of coronary atherosclerosis. Am J Cardiol 43:583, 1978

62. The Review Panel on Coronary-Prone Behavior and Coronary Heart Disease: Coronary-prone be-

havior and coronary heart disease: A critical review. Circulation 63:1199, 1981

63. Glass DC, Krakoff LR, Contrada R et al: Effect of harrassment and competition upon cardiovascular and plasma catecholamine responses in type A and type B individuals. Psychophysiology 17:453, 1980

64. Lane JD, White AD, Williams RB: Cardiovascular effects of mental arithmetic in type A and type B females. Psychophysiology 21:39, 1984

65. Williams RB, Lane JD, Kuhn CM et al: Type A behavior and elevated physiological and neuroendocrine responses to cognitive tasks. Science 218:483, 1982

66. Zumoff B, Rosenfeld RS, Friedman M et al: Elevated daytime urinary excretion of testosterone glucuronide in men with type A behavior pattern. Psychosom Med 46:223, 1984

67. Kahn JP, Kornfeld DS, Frank KA et al: Type A behavior and blood pressure during coronary artery bypass surgery. Psychosom Med 42:407, 1980

68. Samuels MA: Electrocardiographic manifestations of neurologic disease. Semin Neurol 4:453, 1984

69. Natelson BH: Neurocardiology: an interdisciplinary area for the 80's. Arch Neurol 42:178, 1985

70. Mikolich JR, Jacobs WC, Fletcher GF: Cardiac arrhythmias in patients with acute cerebrovascular accidents. JAMA 246:1314, 1981

71. Satinsky J, Kosowsky B, Lown B et al: Ventricular fibrillation induced by hypothalamic stimulation during coronary occlusion. Circulation 44 (suppl. II):II-60, 1971

72. Neil-Dwyer G, Walter P, Cruickshank JM et al: Effect of propranolol and phentolamine on myocardial necrosis after subarachnoid hemorrhage. Br Med J 2:990, 1978

73. Eliot RS, Buell JC: The role of the CNS in cardiovascular disorders. Hosp Pract 18:189, 1983

74. Dimsdale JE, Herd JA, Hartley LH: Epinephrine mediated increases in plasma cholesterol. Psychosom Med 45:227, 1983

75. Verrier RL, Lown B: Behavioral stress and cardiac arrhythmias. Annu Rev Physiol 46:155, 1984

76. Friedman M, Byers SO, Rosenman RH: Plasma ACTH and cortisol concentration of coronary-prone subjects. Proc Soc Exp Biol Med 140:681, 1972

77. Hellerstein HK, Friedman EH, Bedar PJ et al: Comparison of personality of males with rheumatic heart disease and with arteriosclerotic heart disease. Circulation 40(suppl. III):III-11, 1969

78. Shekelle RB, Gale M, Norusis M: Type A score (Jenkins Activity Survey) and risk of recurrent coronary heart disease in the Aspirin Myocardial Infarction Study. Am J Cardiol 56:221, 1985

79. Case RB, Heller SS, Case NB et al: Type A behavior and survival after acute myocardial infarction. N Engl J Med 312:737, 1985

80. Shekelle RB, Hulley S, Neaton J et al: The MRFIT behavioral pattern study. II. Type A behavior pattern and incidence of coronary heart disease. Am J Epidemiol 122:559, 1985

81. DeLeo D, Caracciolo S, Berto F et al: Type A behavior pattern and mortality after recurrent myocardial infarction: Preliminary results from a follow-up study of five years. Psychother Psychosom 46:132, 1986

82. Ragland DR, Brand RJ: Type A behavior and mortality from coronary heart disease. N Engl J Med 318:65, 1988

83. Jenkins CD, Rosenman RH, Friedman M: Development of an objective psychological test for the determination of the coronary-prone behavior pattern in employed men. J Chronic Dis 20:371, 1967

84. Dembroski TM, MacDougall JM, Williams RB et al: Components of type A, hostility and anger-in: relationship to angiographic findings. Psychosom Med 47:219, 1985

85. Matthews KA, Glass DC, Rosenman RH et al: Competitive drive, pattern A, and coronary heart disease: a further analysis of some data from the Western Collaborative Group Study. J Chronic Dis 30:489, 1977

86. Cook W, Medley D: Proposed hostility and pharasaic-virtue scales for the MMPI. J Appl Psychol 38:414, 1954

87. Barefoot JC, Dahlstrom WG, Williams RB: Hostility, CHD incidence, and total mortality: A 25-year follow-up study of 255 physicians. Psychosom Med 45:59, 1983

88. Williams RB, Haney T, Lee K et al: Type A behavior, hostility, and coronary heart disease. Psychosom Med 42:539, 1980

89. Dimsdale JE, Hackett TP, Hutter AM et al: Type A behavior and angiographic findings. J Psychosom Res 23:273, 1979

90. MacDougall HM, Dembroski TM, Dimsdale JE et al: Components of type A, hostility and anger-in: Further relationships to angiographic findings. Health Psychol 4:137, 1985

91. Hecker M, Chesney M, Black G et al: Coronary-prone behaviors in the Western Collaborative Group Study. Psychosom Med 50:153, 1985

92. Dembroski TM, MacDougall JM, Costa PT et al: Components of hostility as predictors of sudden death and myocardial infarction in the Multiple Risk Factor Intervention Trial. Psychosom Med 51:514, 1989

93. Siegman AW, Dembroski TM, Ringel MA: Components of hostility and the severity of coronary artery disease. Psychosom Med 49:127, 1987

94. Malzberg B: Mortality among patients with involution melancholia. Am J Psychiatry 93:1231, 1937

95. Murphy JM, Monson RR, Oliver DC et al: Affective disorders and mortality. Arch Gen Psychiatry 44:473, 1987

96. Avery D, Winokur G: Mortality in depressed patients treated with electroconvulsive therapy and antidepressants. Arch Gen Psychiatry 33:1029, 1976

97. Garrity TF, Klein RF: Emotional response and clinical severity as early determinants of six-month mortality after myocardial infarction. Heart Lung 4:730, 1975

98. Carney RM, Rich MW, Freedland KE et al: Major depressive disorder predicts cardiac events in patients with coronary artery disease. Psychosom Med 50:627, 1988

99. Lown B, DeSilva RA, Reich P et al: Psychophysiologic factors in sudden cardiac death. Am J Psychiatry 137:1325, 1980

100. Huang MH, Ebey J, Wolf S: Responses of the QT interval of the electrocardiogram during emotional stress. Psychosom Med 51:419, 1989

101. Tavazzi L, Zotti AM, Rondanelli R: The role of psychologic stress in the genesis of lethal arrhythmias in patients with coronary artery disease. Eur Heart J 7:99, 1986

102. Follick MJ, Gorkin L, Capone RJ et al: Psychological distress as a predictor of ventricular arrhythmias in a post-myocardial infarction population. Am Heart J 116:32, 1988

103. Rainey JM, Pohl RB, Bilolikar SG: The QT interval in drug-free depressed patients. J Clin Psychiatry 43:39, 1982

104. Moss AJ: Prolonged QT-interval syndromes. JAMA 256:2985, 1986

105. Kleiger RE, Miller JP, Bigger JT et al: Multicenter Post-infarction Research Group: decreased heart rate variability and its association with increased mortality after acute myocardial infarction. Am J Cardiol 59:256, 1987

106. Bigger JT, Kleiger RE, Fleiss JL et al: Components of heart rate variability measured during healing of acute myocardial infarction. Am J Cardiol 61:208, 1988

107. Bigger JT, Albrecht P, Steinman RC et al: Comparison of time and frequency domain-based measures of cardiac parasympathetic activity in Holter recordings after myocardial infarction. Am J Cardiol 64:536, 1989

108. Dalack GW, Roose SP: Perspectives on the relationship between cardiovascular disease and affective disorder. J Clin Psychiatry 51:4, 1990

109. Suinn RM, Brock L, Edie CA: Behavior therapy for type A patients. Am J Cardiol 36:269, 1975

110. Suinn RM, Bloom IJ: Anxiety management training for pattern A behavior. J Behav Med 1:125, 1978

111. Roskies E, Spevack M, Surkis A et al: Changing the coronary-prone (type A) behavior pattern in a nonclinical population. J Behav Med 1:201, 1978

112. Roskies E, Kearney H, Spevack M et al: Generalizability and durability of treatment effects in an intervention program for coronary-prone (type A) managers. J Behav Med 2:195, 1979

113. Roskies E, Seraganian P, Oseasohn R et al: The Montreal type A intervention project: Major findings. Health Psychol 5:45, 1986

114. Gill JJ, Price VA, Friedman M et al: Reduction in type A behavior in healthy middle-aged American military officers. Am Heart J 110:503, 1985

115. Jenni MA, Wollersheim JP: Cognitive therapy, stress management training and type A behavior pattern. Cognit Ther Res 3:61, 1979

116. Patel C, Marmot MG, Terry DJ et al: Trial of relaxation in reducing coronary risk: four year follow up. Br Med J 290:1103, 1985

117. Guizzetta CE: Effects of relaxation and music therapy on patients in a coronary care unit with presumptive acute myocardial infarction. Heart Lung 18:609, 1989

118. Thockcloth RM, Ho SC, Wright H, Seldon WA: Is cardiac rehabilitation really necessary? Med J Aust 2:669, 1973

119. Dixhoorn JV, Loos JD, Duivenvoorden HJ: Contribution of relaxation technique training to the rehabilitation of myocardial infarction patients. Psychother Psychosom 40:137, 1983

120. Langosch W, Seer P, Brodner G et al: Behavior therapy with coronary heart disease patients: results of a comparative study. J Psychosom Res 26:475, 1982

121. Thompson DR, Meddis R: A prospective evaluation of in-hospital counselling for first time myocardial infarction men. J Psychosom Res 34:237, 1990

122. Thompson DR, Meddis R: Wives' responses to

counselling early after myocardial infarction. J Psychosom Res 34:249, 1990

123. Naismith LD, Robinson JF, Shaw GB et al: Psychosocial rehabilitation after infarction. Br Med J 1:439, 1979

124. Mayou R, Macmahon D, Sleight P et al: Early rehabilitation after myocardial infarction. Lancet ii:1399, 1981

125. Gruen W: Effects of brief psychotherapy during the hospitalization period on the recovery process in heart attacks. J Consult Clin Psychol 43:223, 1975

126. Dixhoorn JV, Duivenvoorden HJ, Pool J et al: Psychic effects of physical training and relaxation therapy after myocardial infarction. J Psychosom Res 34:327, 1990

127. Oldenburg B, Perkins RJ, Andrews G: Controlled trial of psychological intervention in myocardial infarction. J Consult Clin Psychol 53:852, 1985

128. Frasure-Smith N, Prince R: Long-term follow-up of the Ischemic Heart Disease Life Stress Monitoring Program. Psychosom Med 51:485, 1989

129. Ornish D, Scherwitz LW, Doody RS et al: Effects of stress management training and dietary changes in treating ischemic heart disease. JAMA 249:54, 1983

130. Ornish D, Brown SE, Scherwitz LW et al: Can lifestyle changes reverse coronary heart disease? The lifestyle heart trial. Lancet 336:129, 1990

131. Adsett CA, Bruhn JG: Short-term group psychotherapy for post-myocardial infarction patients and their wives. Can Med Assoc J 99:577, 1968

132. Ibrahim MA, Feldman JG, Sultz HA et al: Management after myocardial infarction: a controlled trial of the effect of group psychotherapy. Int J Psychiatry Med 5:253, 1974

133. Rahe RH, Tuffli CF, Suchor RJ et al: Group therapy in the outpatient management of post-myocardial infarction patients. Int J Psychiatry Med 4:77, 1973

134. Rahe RH, O'Neil T, Hagan A et al: Brief group therapy following myocardial infarction: eighteen-month followup of a controlled trial. Int J Psychiatry Med 6:349, 1975

135. Rahe RH, Ward HW, Hayes V: Brief group therapy in myocardial infarction rehabilitation: three-to-four-year followup of a controlled trial. Psychosom Med 41:229, 1979

136. Stern MJ, Gorman PA, Kaslow L: The group counselling vs. exercise therapy study: a controlled intervention with subjects following myocardial infarction. Arch Intern Med 143:1719, 1983

137. Bilodeau CB, Hackett TP: Issues raised in a group setting by patients recovering from myocardial infarction. Am J Psychiatry 128:73, 1971

138. Horlick L, Cameron R, Firor W et al: The effects of education and group discussion in the post myocardial infarction patient. J Psychosom Res 28:485, 1984

139. Friedman M, Thoresen CE, Gill JJ et al: Feasibility of altering type A behavior pattern after myocardial infarction. Circulation 66:83, 1982

140. Friedman M, Thoresen CE, Gill JJ et al: Alteration of type A behavior and reduction in cardiac recurrences in postmyocardial infarction patients. Am Heart J 108:237, 1984

141. Powell LH, Friedman M, Thoresen CE et al: Can the type A behavior pattern be altered? A second year report from the Recurrent Coronary Prevention Project. Psychosom Med 46:293, 1984

142. Friedman M, Thoresen CE, Gill JJ et al: Alteration of type A behavior and its effect on cardiac recurrences in post myocardial infarction patients: Summary results of the Recurrent Coronary Prevention Project. Am Heart J 112:653, 1986

143. Nunes EV, Frank KA, Kornfeld DS: Psychologic treatment for the type A behavior pattern and for coronary heart disease: A meta-analysis of the literature. Psychosom Med 48:159, 1987

144. Reich P, Gold PW: Interruption of recurrent ventricular fibrillation by psychiatric intervention. Gen Hosp Psychiatry 5:255, 1983

145. Yalom I: The Theory and Practice of Group Psychotherapy. p. 3. 2nd Ed. Basic Books, New York, 1975

146. Mumford E, Schlesinger HJ, Glass GV: The effects of psychological intervention on recovery from surgery and heart attacks: An analysis of the literature. Am J Public Health 72:141, 1982

147. Krantz DS, Durel LA, Davia JE et al: Propranolol medication among coronary patients: Relationship to type A behavior and cardiovascular response. J Hum Stress 8:4, 1982

148. Krantz DS, Contrada RJ, Durel LA et al: Comparative effects of two beta-blockers on cardiovascular reactivity and type A behavior in hypertensives. Psychosom Med 50:615, 1988

149. Krantz DS, Contrada RJ, LaRiccia PJ et al: Effects of beta-adrenergic stimulation and blockade on cardiovascular reactivity, affect, and type A behavior. Psychosom Med 49:146, 1987

150. Stratton JR, Halter JB: Effect of benzodiazepine (alprazolam) on plasma epinephrine and norepinephrine levels during exercise and stress. Am J Cardiol 56:136, 1985

151. Williams RB, Schanberg SM: Influence of alprazolam on neuroendocrine and cardiovascular responses to stress in type A men and patients with panic disorder. Abstract-Protocol 4006. Panic Disorder Biological Workshop, Washington, 1986

152. Roy A, Adinoff B, Linnoila M: Acting out hostility in normal volunteers: Negative correlation with levels of 5HIAA in cerebrospinal fluid. Psychiatry Res 24:187, 1988

153. Sheard MH: Effect of lithium on human aggression. Nature 230:113, 1971

154. Littman AB, Fava M, Lamon-Fava S et al: Treatment of type A behavior in cardiac patients with buspirone. Abstract NR340. American Psychiatric Association, Annual Meeting, New York, 1990

155. Centers for Disease Control: Reducing the Health Consequences of Smoking: 25 Years of Progress. A report of the Surgeon General. Publication CDC 89-8411. US Department of Health and Human Services, Rockville, MD, 1989

156. Vlietstra RE, Kronmal RA, Oberman A et al: Effect of cigarette smoking on survival of patients with angiographically documented coronary artery disease. JAMA 255:1023, 1986

157. Sparrow D, Dawber TR, Colson T: The influence of cigarette smoking on prognosis after a first myocardial infarction. J Chronic Dis 31:425, 1978

158. Blumenthal JA, Levenson RM: Behavioral approaches to secondary prevention of coronary heart disease. Circulation 76(suppl I):I-130, 1987

159. Mann LS, Johnson RW, Levine DJ: Tobacco dependence: Psychology, biology, and treatment strategies. Psychosomatics 27:713, 1986

160. Glassman AH, Jackson WK, Walsh BT et al: Cigarette craving, smoking withdrawal, and clonidine. Science 226:864, 1984

161. Hjalmarson AM: Effect of nicotine chewing gum in smoking cessation: a randomized, placebo-controlled, double-blind study. JAMA 252:2835, 1984

162. Schneider NG, Jarvik ME, Forsyth AB et al: Nicotine gum in smoking cessation: A placebo-controled double-blind trial. Addict Behav 8:253, 1983

163. Fagerstrom KO: A comparison of psychological and pharmacological treatment in smoking cessation. J Behav Med 5:343, 1982

164. Subcommittee of the Research Committee of the British Thoracic Society: Comparison of four methods of smoking withdrawal in patients with smoking-related diseases. Br Med J 286:595, 1983

165. DeWit H, Camic PM: Behavioral and pharmacological treatment of cigarette smoking: End of treatment comparisons. Addict Behav 11:331, 1986

166. Gmur M, Tschopp A: Factors determining the success of nicotine withdrawal: 12-year follow-up of 532 smokers after suggestion therapy (by a faith healer). Int J Addict 22:1189, 1987

167. Hall S, Rugg D, Turnstall C et al: Preventing relapse to cigarette smoking by behavioral skill training. J Consult Clin Psychol 52:372, 1984

168. Tunstall CD, Ginsberg D, Hall SM: Quitting smoking. Int J Addict 20:1089, 1985

169. Cottraux J, Schbath J, Messy P et al: Predictive value of MMPI scales on smoking cessation program outcomes. Acta Psychiatr Belg 86:463, 1986

170. Anda RF, Williamson DF, Escobedo LG et al: Depression and the dynamics of smoking. JAMA 264:1541, 1990

171. Glassman AH, Helzer JE, Covey LS et al: Smoking, smoking cessation, and major depression. JAMA 264:1546, 1990

172. Sirota AD, Curran JP, Habif V: Smoking cessation in chronically ill medical patients. J Clin Psychol 41:575, 1985

173. Burt A, Thornley P, Illingsworth D et al: Stopping smoking after myocardial infarction. Lancet i:304, 1974

174. Burling TA, Singleton EG, Bigelow GE et al: Smoking following myocardial infarction: A critical review of the literature. Health Psychol 3:83, 1984

175. Bass C, Wade C: Chest pain with normal coronary arteries: A comparative study of psychiatric and social morbidity. Psychol Med 14:51, 1984

176. Channer KS, James MA, Papouchado M et al: Anxiety and depression in patients with chest pain referred for exercise testing. Lancet ii:820, 1985

177. McLaurin LP, Raft D, Tate SC: Chest pain with normal coronaries: a psychosomatic illness? Circulation 56(suppl. III):III-174, 1977

178. Ostfeld AM, Lebovits BZ, Shekelle RB et al: A prospective study of the relationship between personality and coronary heart disease. J Chronic Dis 17:265, 1964

179. Wielgosz AT, Fletcher RH, McCants CB et al: Unimproved chest pain in patients with minimal or no coronary disease: A behavioral phenomenon. Am Heart J 108:67, 1984

180. Pasternak RC, Thibault GE, Savoia M et al: Chest pain with angiographically insignificant coronary arterial obstruction. Am J Med 68:813, 1980

181. Weissman MM: The epidemiology of panic dis-

order and agoraphobia. p. 56. In Frances AJ, Hales RE (eds): Review of Psychiatry. Vol. 7. American Psychiatric Press, Washington, 1988

182. Marks L, Lader M: Anxiety states (anxiety neurosis): A review. J Nerv Ment Dis 156:3, 1973

183. Beitman BD, Lamberti JW, Mukerji V et al: Panic disorder in patients with angiographically normal coronary arteries. Psychosomatics 28:480, 1987

184. Rosenbaum, JF: The drug treatment of anxiety. N Engl J Med 306:401, 1982

185. Markowitz JS, Weissman MM, Ouellette R et al: Quality of life in panic disorder. Arch Gen Psychiatry 46:984, 1989

186. Gelenberg AJ: Anxiety. p. 185. In Bassuk EL, Schoonover SC, Gelenberg AJ (eds.): The Practitioner's Guide to Psychoactive Drugs. Plenum, New York, 1983

187. Hyman SE, Arana GW: Handbook of Psychiatric Drug Therapy. Little, Brown, Boston, 1987

188. Schoonover SC: Depression. p. 68. In Bassuk EL, Schoonover SC, Gelenberg AJ (eds.): The Practitioner's Guide to Psychoactive Drugs. Plenum, New York, 1983

189. Keller MB, Klerman GL, Lavori PW et al: Treatment received by depressed patients. JAMA 248:1848, 1982

190. Prien RF, Kupfer DJ: Continuation drug therapy for major depressive episodes: how long should it be maintained? Am J Psychiatry 143:18, 1986

191. Kellner R: Functional somatic symptoms and hypochondriasis. Arch Gen Psychiatry 42:821, 1985

192. Lipowski ZJ: Somatization: the concept and its clinical application. Am J Psychiatry 145:1358, 1988

193. Smith GR, Monson RA, Ray DC: Psychiatric consultation in somatization disorder: a randomized controlled study. N Engl J Med 314:1407, 1986

194. Stern TA: Munchausen's syndrome revisited. Psychosomatics 21:329, 1980

195. Pitt E, Pitt B: Cardiopathica fantastica. Am Heart J 108:137, 1984

196. Stern TA, Murray GB: Complex partial seizures presenting as a psychiatric illness. J Nerv Ment Dis 172:625, 1984

197. Devinsky O, Price BH, Cohen SI: Cardiac manifestations of complex partial seizures. Am J Med 80:195, 1986

198. Kiok MC, Terrence CF, Fromm GH et al: Sinus arrest in epilepsy. Neurology 3:14, 1984

199. Murray, GB: Complex partial seizures. p. 103. In Manschreck, TC (ed.): Psychiatric Medicine Update. Elsevier Science Publishing, New York, 1981

200. Cassem NH: Cardiovascular effects of antidepressants. J Clin Psychiatry 43(11[sect.2]):22, 1982

201. Welch CA, Drop LJ: Cardiovascular effects of ECT. Convulsive Ther 5:35, 1989

202. Greenblatt DJ, Shader RI, Abernathy DR: Current status of benzodiazepines (first of two parts). N Engl J Med 309:354, 1983

203. Stern TA: Psychiatric management of acute myocardial infarction in the coronary care unit. Am J Cardiol 60:59J, 1987

204. Cote P, Gueret P, Bourassa MG: Systemic and coronary hemodynamic effects of diazepam in patients with normal and diseased coronary arteries. Circulation 50:1210, 1974

205. Marty J, Nitenberg A, Blanchet F et al: Effects of midazolam on the coronary circulation in patients with coronary artery disease. Anesthesiology 64:206, 1986

206. Marty J, Gauzit R, Lefevre P et al: Effects of diazepam and midazolam on baroreflex control of heart rate and on sympathetic activity in humans. Anesth Analg 65:113, 1986

207. Goldstein DS: Plasma catecholamines in clinical studies of cardiovascular diseases. Acta Physiol Scand 527:39, 1984

208. Kalsner S, Richards R: Coronary arteries of cardiac patients are hyperreactive and contain stores of amines: a mechanism for coronary spasm. Science 225:1435, 1984

209. Hoar PF, Nelson NT, Mangano DT et al: Adrenergic response to morphine-diazepam anesthesia for myocardial revascularization. Anesth Analg 60:406, 1981

210. Paulson BA, Becker LD, Way WL: The effects of intravenous lorazepam alone and with meperidine on ventilation in man. Acta Anesthesiol Scand 27:400, 1983

211. Adams F: Neuropsychiatric evaluation and treatment of delirium in the critically ill cancer patient. Cancer Bull 36:156, 1984

212. Adams F, Fernandez F, Anderson BS: Emergency pharmacotherapy of delirium in the critically ill cancer patient. Psychosomatics 27(suppl.):33, 1986

213. Kornecki E, Ehrlich YH, Lenox RH: Platelet-activating-factor-induced aggregation of human platelets specifically inhibited by triazolo-benzodiazepines. Science 226:1454, 1984

214. Coull DC, Crooks J, Dingwall-Fordyce I et al: Amitriptyline and cardiac disease: Risk of sudden death identified by monitoring system. Lancet ii:590, 1970

215. Moir DC, Cornwell WB, Dingwall-Fordyce I et al: Cardiotoxicity of amitriptyline. Lancet ii:561, 1972

216. Baldessarini RJ: Chemotherapy in Psychiatry. Harvard University Press, Cambridge, MA, 1985

217. Dec GW, Stern TA: Tricyclic antidepressants in the intensive care unit. J Intensive Care Med 5:69, 1990

218. Glassman AH: Cardiovascular effects of tricyclic antidepressants. Annu Rev Med 35:503, 1984

219. Giardina EGV, Bigger JT, Glassman AH et al: The electrocardiographic and antiarrhythmic effects of imipramine hydrochloride at therapeutic concentrations. Circulation 60:1045, 1979

220. Glassman AH, Bigger JT: Cardiovascular effects of therapeutic doses of tricyclic antidepressants: A review. Arch Gen Psychiatry 38:815, 1981

221. Glassman AH, Johnson LL, Giardina EGV et al: The use of imipramine in depressed patients with congestive heart failure. JAMA 250:1997, 1983

222. Muller OF, Goodman N, Bellet S: The hypotensive effect of imipramine hydrochloride in patients with cardiovascular disease. Clin Pharmacol Ther 2:300, 1961

223. Roose SP, Glassman AH, Giardina EGV et al: Tricycliclic antidepressants in depressed patients with cardiac conduction disease. Arch Gen Psychiatry 44:273, 1987

224. Tesar GE, Rosenbaum JF, Biederman J et al: Orthostatic hypotension and antidepressant pharmacotherapy. Psychopharmacol Bull 23:182, 1987

225. Glassman AH, Bigger JT, Giardina EGV et al: Clinical characteristics of imipramine-induced orthostatic hypotension. Lancet i:468, 1979

226. Freyschuss U, Sjoqvist F, Tuck D et al: Circulatory effects in man of nortriptyline, a tricyclic antidepressant drug. Pharmacol Clin 2:68, 1970

227. Reed K, Smith RC, Schoolar JC et al: Cardiovascular effects of nortriptyline in geriatric patients. Am J Psychiatry 137:986, 1980

228. Roose SP, Glassman AH, Giardina EGV et al: Nortriptyline in depressed patients with left ventricular impairment. JAMA 256:3253, 1986

229. Thayssen P, Bjerre M, Kragh-Sorensen P et al: Cardiovascular effects of imipramine and nortriptyline in elderly patients. Psychopharmacology 74:360, 1981

230. Kragh-Sorensen P, Hansen CE, Baastrup PC et al: Self-inhibiting action of nortriptyline's antidepressive effect at high plasma levels. Psychopharmacology 45:305, 1976

231. Burrows GD, Vohra J, Hunt D et al: Cardiac effects of different tricyclic antidepressant drugs. Br J Psychiatry 129:335, 1976

232. Kantor SJ, Bigger JT, Glassman AH et al: Imipramine-induced heart block: A longitudinal case study. JAMA 231:1364, 1975

233. Vohra J, Burrows G, Hunt D et al: The effect of toxic and therapeutic doses of tricyclic antidepressant drugs on intracardiac conduction. Eur J Cardiol 3:219, 1975

234. Pitts NE: The clinical evaluation of doxepin: A new psychotropic agent. Psychosomatics 10:164, 1969

235. Dumovic P, Burrows JD, Vohra J et al: The effects of cyclic antidepressant drugs on the heart. Arch Toxicol 35:255, 1976

236. Veith RC, Raskind MA, Caldwell JH et al: Cardiovascular effects of tricyclic antidepressants in depressed patients with chronic heart disease. N Engl J Med 306:954, 1982

237. Bigger JT, Spiker DG, Petit JM et al: Tricyclic antidepressant overdose: Incidence of symptoms. JAMA 238:135, 1977

238. Marshall JB, Forker AD: Cardiovascular effects of tricyclic antidepressant drugs: therapeutic usage, overdose, and management of complications. Am Heart J 103:401, 1982

239. Stern TA, O'Gara PT, Mulley AG et al: Complications after overdose with tricyclic antidepressants. Crit Care Med 13:672, 1985

240. Bigger JT, Giardina EGV, Perel JM et al: Cardiac antiarrhythmic effect of imipramine hydrochloride. N Engl J Med 296:206, 1977

241. Connolly SJ, Mitchell LB, Swerdlow CD et al: Clinical efficacy and electrophysiology of imipramine for ventricular tachycardia. Am J Cardiol 53:516, 1984

242. Giardina EGV, Barnard T, Johnson LL et al: The antiarrhythmic effect of nortriptyline in cardiac patients with ventricular premature depolarizations. J Am Coll Cardiol 7:1363, 1986

243. Velebit V, Podrid PJ, Lown B et al: Aggravation and provocation of ventricular arrhythmias by antiarrhythmic drugs. Circulation 65:886, 1982

244. Jefferson JW: A review of the cardiovascular effects and toxicity of tricyclic antidepressants. Psychosom Med 37:160, 1975

245. Thorstrand C: Clinical features in poisonings by tricyclic antidepressants with special reference to the ECG. Acta Med Scand 199:337, 1976

246. Pi EH, Simpson GM: New antidepressants: A review. Hosp Formul 20:580, 1985

247. Hames TK, Burgess CD, George CF: Hemodynamic responses of trazodone and imipramine. Clin Pharmacol Ther 12:497, 1982

248. Byrne JE, Gomoll AW: Differential effects of trazodone and imipramine on intracardiac conduction in the anesthetized dog. Arch Int Pharmacodyn Ther 259:259, 1982

249. Richelson E: Pharmacology of antidepressants in use in the United States. J Clin Psychiatry 43(11[sect.2]):4, 1982

250. Janowsky D, Curtis G, Zisook S et al: Ventricular arrhythmias possibly aggravated by trazodone. Am J Psychiatry 140:796, 1983

251. Pellettier JR, Bartolucci G: Trazodone and cardiovascular side effects. J Clin Psychopharmacol 4:119, 1984

252. Vlay SC, Friedling S: Trazodone exacerbation of VT. Am Heart J 105:604, 1983

253. Ramrize AL: Seizures associated with maprotiline. Am J Psychiatry 140:509, 1983

254. Knudsen K, Heath A: Effects of self-poisoning with maprotiline. Br Med J 1:601, 1984

255. Wenger TL, Cohn JB, Bustrack J: Comparison of the effects of bupropion and amitriptyline on cardiac conduction in depressed patients. J Clin Psychiatry 44:174, 1983

256. Peck AW, Stern WC, Watkinson C: Incidence of seizures during treatment with tricyclic antidepressants and bupropion. J Clin Psychiatry 44:197, 1983

257. Fisch C: Effect of fluoxetine on the electrocardiogram. J Clin Psychiatry 46:42, 1985

258. Cooper GL: The safety of fluoxetine: An update. Br J Psychiatry 153(suppl. 3):77, 1988

259. Teicher MH, Glod C, Cole JO: Emergence of intense suicidal preoccupation during fluoxetine treatment. Am J Psychiatry 147:207, 1990

260. Fava M, Rosenbaum JF: Suicidality and fluoxetine: is there a relationship? Abstract NR 475. American Psychiatric Association, Annual Meeting, New York, 1990

261. Davidson JRT, Miller RD, Turnbull CD et al: Atypical depression. Arch Gen Psychiatry 39:527, 1982

262. Sheehan DV: Delineation of anxiety and phobic disorders responsive to monoamine oxidase inhibitors: Implications for classification. J Clin Psychiatry 457(7[sect. 2]):29, 1984

263. Kronig MH, Roose SP, Walsh BT et al: Blood pressure effects of phenelzine. J Clin Psychopharmacol 3:307, 1983

264. Onrat J, Goldberg MR, Biaggioni I et al: Hemodynamic and humoral effects of caffeine in autonomic failure. N Engl J Med 313:549, 1985

265. Whitworth JA, Saines D, Thatcher R: Differential blood pressure and metabolic effects of 9-alpha

fluorocortisol in man. Clin Exp Pharmacol Physiol 10:351, 1983

266. Sullivan EA, Shulman KI: Diet and monoamine oxidase inhibitors: a reexamination. Can J Psychiatry 29:707, 1984

267. Clark ANG, Mankikar GD: D-Amphetamine in elderly patients refractory to rehabilitation procedures. J Am Geriatr Soc 27:174, 1979

268. Kaplitz SE: Withdrawn, apathetic geriatric patients responsive to methylphenidate. J Am Geriatr Soc 23:271, 1975

269. Katon W, Raskind M: Treatment of depression in the medically ill elderly with methylphenidate. Am J Psychiatry 137:963, 1980

270. Kaufmann MW, Murray GB: The use of d-amphetamine in medically ill depressed patients. J Clin Psychiatry 43:463, 1982

271. Woods SW, Tesar GE, Murray GB et al: Psychostimulant treatment of depressive disorders secondary to medical illness. J Clin Psychiatry 47:12, 1986

272. Kaufmann MW, Cassem NH, Murray GB et al: The use of methylphenidate in depressed patients after cardiac surgery. J Clin Psychiatry 45:82, 1984

273. Askinazi C, Weintraub RJ, Karamouz N: Elderly depressed females as a possible subgroup of patients responsive to methylphenidate. J Clin Psychiatry 47:467, 1986

274. Lydiard RB, Gelenberg AJ: Hazards and adverse effects of lithium. Annu Rev Med 33:327, 1982

275. Roose SP, Nurnberger JI, Dunner DL et al: Cardiac sinus node dysfunction during lithium treatment. Am J Psychiatry 136:804, 1979

276. Schou M: Electrocardiographic changes during treatment with lithium and with drugs of the imipramine-type. Acta Psychiatr Scand 169:258, 1963

277. Jaffe CM: First-degree atrioventricular block during lithium carbonate treatment. Am J Psychiatry 134:88, 1977

278. Worthley LIC: Lithium toxicity and refractory cardiac arrhythmias treated with intravenous magnesium. Anaesth Intensive Care 2:357, 1974

279. Stern TA, Lydiard RB: Lithium therapy revisited. Psychiatr Med 4:39, 1987

280. Jefferson JW, Kalin NH: Serum lithium levels and long-term diuretic use. JAMA 241:1134, 1979

281. Fowler NO, McCall D, Chou T et al: Electrocardiographic changes and cardiac arrhythmias in patients receiving psychotropic drugs. Am J Cardiol 37:223, 1976

282. Bernstein JG: Handbook of Drug Therapy in Psychiatry. p. 201. Wright-PSG, Boston, 1983

283. Branchey MH, Lee JH, Amin R et al: High and low potency neuroleptics in elderly psychiatric patients. JAMA 239:1860, 1978

284. Khan MM, Lopan KR, McComb JM et al: Management of recurrent ventricular tachyarrhythmias associated with Q-T prolongation. Am J Cardiol 47:1301, 1981

285. Settle EC, Ayd FJ: Haloperidol: A quarter century of experience. J Clin Psychiatry 44:440, 1983

286. Shader RI: Extrapyramidal and cardiovascular side-effects of butyrophenones. p. 78. In DiMascio, Shader RI (eds): Butyrophenones in Psychiatry. Raven Press, New York, 1972

287. Sos J, Cassem NH: The intravenous use of haloperidol for acute delirium in intensive care settings. p. 121. In Speidel H, Rodewald G (eds): Psychic and Neurologic Dysfunctions After Open Heart Surgery. Thieme Verlag, Stuttgart, Germany 1980

288. Sos J, Cassem NH: Managing postoperative agitation. Drug Ther 10:103, 1980

289. Stern TA: The management of depression and anxiety following myocardial infarction. Mt Sinai J Med 52:623, 1985

290. Tesar GE, Murray GB, Cassem NH: Use of high-dose intravenous haloperidol in the treatment of agitated cardiac patients. J Clin Psychopharmacol 5/6:344, 1985

291. Sanders KM, Minnema AM, Murray GB: Low incidence of extrapyramidal symptoms in treatment of delirium with intravenous haloperidol and lorazepam in the intensive care unit. J Intensive Care Med 4:201, 1989

292. Alexander HE, McCarty K, Giffen MB: Hypotension and cardiopulmonary arrest associated with concurrent haloperidol and propranolol therapy. JAMA 252:87, 1984

293. Cassem NH: Critical care psychiatry. p. 981. In Shoemaker WC, Thompson WL, Holbrook PR (eds): Textbook of Critical Care. WB Saunders, Philadelphia, 1984

294. Flaherty JA, Lahmeyer HW: Laryngeal-pharyngeal dystonia as a possible cause of asphyxia with haloperidol treatment. Am J Psychiatry 135:1414, 1978

295. McDanal CE: Haloperidol and laryngeal-pharyngeal dystonia (letter). Am J Psychiatry 138:1262, 1981

296. Crowe RR: Electroconvulsive therapy: A current perspective. N Engl J Med 311:163, 1984

297. Brody JI, Bellet S: The use of electric shock therapy in patients with cardiovascular disease. Am J Med Sci 233:40, 1957

298. Lewis WH, Richardson JD, Gahagan LH: Cardiovascular disturbances and their management in modified electrotherapy for psychiatric illness. N Engl J Med 252:1016, 1955

299. Alexander SP, Gahagan LH: Deaths following electrotherapy. JAMA 161:577, 1956

300. Fink M: Efficacy and safety of induced seizures (ECT) in man. Compr Psychiatry 19:1, 1978

301. Hussar AE, Pachter M: Myocardial infarction and fatal coronary insufficiency during electroconvulsive therapy. JAMA 204:146, 1968

302. Sisler GC, Wilt JC: Immediate coronary thrombosis following electroconvulsive therapy. Am J Psychiatry 110:354, 1953

303. McKenna G, Engle R, Brooks H et al: Cardiac arrhythmias during electroshock therapy: significance, prevention, and treatment. Am J Psychiatry 127:530, 1970

304. Deliyiannis S, Eliahim M, Bellet S: The electrocardiogram during convulsive therapy studied by radioelectrocardiography. Am J Cardiol 10:187, 1962

305. Green R, Woods A: Effects of modified ECT on the electrocardiogram. Br Med J 1:1503, 1955

306. Gerring JP, Shields HM: The identification and management of patients with a high risk for cardiac arrhythmias during modified ECT. J Clin Psychiatry 43:140, 1982

307. Dec GW, Stern TA, Welch C: The effects of electroconvulsive therapy on serial electrocardiograms and serum cardiac enzyme values: A prospective study of depressed hospitalized inpatients. JAMA 253:2525, 1985

308. Drop LJ, Welch CA: Anesthesia for electroconvulsive therapy in patients with major cardiovascular risk factors. Convulsive Ther 5:88, 1989

29

Return to Work

Hugh C. Smith, M.D.

Coronary heart disease causes more deaths, disability, and economic loss in industrialized countries than any other disease entity; it is responsible for the single largest health care cost in the United States.[1] Among the many adverse effects of coronary heart disease, the impact of myocardial infarction, coronary artery bypass surgery, and percutaneous transluminal coronary angioplasty (PTCA) upon the work-related activities of individuals and society is particularly profound and widespread. Nearly 1 million patients survive heart attacks in the United States annually; more than 45% of the survivors are younger than 60 years.[1] In 1988, one-half of the 353,000 coronary artery bypass surgical procedures were performed on patients younger than 65 years.[1] In that same year, approximately two-thirds of the 240,000 patients who underwent coronary angioplasty were younger than 65 years.[1] Taken together, more than 750,000 persons under age 65 in the United States currently survive myocardial infarction or undergo coronary artery bypass surgery or PTCA each year.

Return to gainful employment is a major goal in the rehabilitation of patients following myocardial infarction, coronary artery bypass surgery, and PTCA, and return to work is often considered to be an important outcome measurement of the cost effectiveness of rehabilitation programs. Although coronary heart disease remains the leading cause of morbidity and disability, the death rate from myocardial infarction declined by 29.2% from 1978 to 1988.[1] Whether these increased numbers of survivors return to gainful employment or apply for premature (before age 65) disability benefits will have significant national economic impact. Psychological and socioeconomic factors have been shown in many studies to be at least as important as medical or physical factors in determining subsequent employment status. There has been significant progress in the physical rehabilitation of patients with coronary heart disease, but the psychosocial and occupational rehabilitation of these patients has not kept pace.

A review of all factors known to influence work activities in patients after myocardial infarction, coronary bypass surgery, or PTCA is necessary to the process of identifying the major obstacles to resumed employment and developing or focusing rehabilitative efforts to overcome them.

MYOCARDIAL INFARCTION

Reductions in gainful employment following myocardial infarction may occur as a consequence of (1) failure to return to work, (2) prolonged convalescence and delay in returning to work, (3) working diminished hours or at lower intensity than preinfarction levels, or (4) loss of work opportunity as a result of economic factors or employment policies.

Reported rates of return to work are as low as 35%[2] and as high as 95%,[3,4] partly because of significant differences in patient populations (age, socioeconomic class, country), work environment, selection bias (uncomplicated infarctions versus all infarctions), and timing of postinfarction employment assessment. It is estimated that approximately 70 to 75% of all patients in the United States return to work after myocardial infarction. For patients with uncomplicated myocardial infarction, over 85% of those under age 65 who were working before their myocardial infarction resumed employment.[5,6] Most patients return to work within 2 to 3 months of their infarction, but more recent studies document a continued trend toward shorter periods of convalescence and absence from work.[7,8] This trend toward earlier return to work appears to result from several therapeutic advances including reperfusion therapy, better identification of low-risk patients who can participate in accelerated rehabilitation programs, psychosocial rehabilitation, and improved access to coronary rehabilitation programs. However, many patients who initially return to work do not remain employed, and further dropout rates of 20% at 1 year have been reported.[9] This dropout from the work force continues through successive years. Various clinical and psychosocial factors have been identified as predictors of postinfarction employment.

Clinical Factors

Increased severity of myocardial infarction, measured by either Killip class,[8] type of infarction (transmural/nontransmural),[8] or a comprehensive severity profile,[10] was identified by stepwise multivariate analysis as an important predictor of a reduced rate of return to work. This has not been a consistent finding in other studies, in which less comprehensive measures of severity or univariate analyses of different variables were used.[6,11,12] Other clinical predictors of a lower rate of resumed employment include complications of myocardial infarction (arrhythmias, heart failure),[8,13] continued angina, or subsequent hospitalization.[8] Neurologic complications of myocardial infarction, such as moderate to severe memory impairment, are also associated with lower rates of return to work.[14] Conversely, Dennis et al.[7] have noted that although losses in productivity and income may be unavoidable in high-risk patients with severe myocardial infarction or with complications, many of these economic losses are preventable in low-risk patients. In a randomized trial using an occupational work evaluation protocol at 21 days after myocardial infarction, low-risk patients were identified and advised to return to work at 5 weeks after infarction. Patients receiving this intervention returned to work 3 weeks earlier than those randomized to receive usual care.

Psychosocial Factors

Studies employing stepwise multivariate regression analysis have also identified socioeconomic status as reflected by education, physical demands of employment, or type of occupation as an important psychosocial predictor of return to work.[8,12,15] The generally lower rate of return to work associated with lower socioeconomic status is particularly evident among older blue-collar workers.[8,16,17] This finding is consistent with the observations that those who work at jobs with high physical demands are particularly likely not to resume employment.[10] Blue-collar workers also have more apprehension about the physical aspects of their job[6,18] and exhibit more anxiety and depressive symptoms than white-collar workers following myocardial infarction.[9,19] The patients' self-perception of their health status has also been determined by univariate and multivariate analyses to be an important predictor of return to work.[8,10,12,15,20]

Several descriptive studies have also attributed job loss to a number of other psychosocial factors. Although limitations in these studies make identification of the most important factors difficult, the studies provide some understanding of the general nature and extent of the adverse influences upon postinfarction employment.

Most studies have observed lower rates of return to work in older patients, particularly those older than 60 years.[6,8,13,16,20] With advancing years, a psychological "disengagement" from work occurs as part of the mental preparation for eventual retirement,[21] and the occurrence of a life-threatening illness may prompt a reassessment of work in the context of a potentially shorter life span and hence hasten the disengagement process.

Psychological manifestations of distress, particularly anxiety and depression, have also been associated with longer convalescence periods and lower rates of resumed employment.[8,13,22] In an excellent review, Shanfield[23] points out that it is likely that psychiatric affective disorders are better predictors of problems with subsequent work than is the fairly frequent occurrence of anxiety and depression symptoms after myocardial infarction. In contrast, denial and type A behavior patterns are positively associated with higher rates of return to work.[8,9,24] In this regard, failure to return to work should not always be regarded as an adverse outcome. For the older, financially independent "workaholic" reconsidering personal goals after myocardial infarction, the decision to stop or reduce work in order to attain a more "balanced" lifestyle may be a positive adaptive response to a major coronary event.

Most early studies of return to work focused primarily on men. When working women were included, they were found to have longer convalescence periods and lower rates of return to work than men.[2,6,8,13,16,20,25] However, women who sustain myocardial infarction are also generally older and have higher mortality and morbidity rates and more psychosocial problems, particularly depression, than their male cohorts.[9,20,26,27] This increased incidence of depression in women after infarction is consistent with the prevalence of depression in the general population[28,29] (see Ch. 28). Women, particularly married women, may be more often discouraged from returning to work[20] and may have a different attachment to work than men.[20]

The adverse effect of increasing age upon return to work was reported to be greater for women than men in one study,[20] which also found that younger single women with smaller salaries were more likely to return to work. This finding suggests that older married women may have less motivation to return to work after myocardial infarction, possibly because their work provided only supplemental or discretionary family income, and they were previously working both outside the home and as homemaker. Overall, however, the factors that influence work activities in women after myocardial infarction are incompletely understood and merit further study,

particularly because women now constitute an increasing part of the work force[26,30]; also, the incidence of smoking in women has steadily increased over the past two decades, and an increased incidence of myocardial infarction in these working women can be reasonably anticipated (See also Ch. 13).

The presence of moderate family support has also been associated with shorter convalescence and an earlier return to work, but high levels of family support, presumably by fostering the patient's feelings of dependency (or in response to such feelings), was associated with a delayed return to work.[8,15]

The lower rate of return to work for blue-collar workers underscores the concept that the work environment can profoundly influence postinfarction work activities. However, the workplace is a dynamic environment, and there are major trends, favorable and unfavorable, occurring simultaneously, that will significantly modify employment outcome after myocardial infarction. Employer and union regulations and attitudes, through public education about heart disease and advances in therapy, appear to be less restrictive than a decade earlier. There has been a significant increase in automation and mechanization in industry and a progressive shift from a manufacturing to a service economy in Western countries. This has significantly reduced the number of jobs with high physical demands and contributed to a more favorable work environment for the patient with coronary heart disease. However, this automation process and the changing business climates have prompted many employers to reduce their work force by offering favorable early retirement programs or inducements. These may be particularly attractive to employees convalescing from myocardial infarction several years before their planned age-related retirement and may prompt their early departure from the work force. The rising costs of health care have also caused many employers to shift from employee indemnity health insurance to managed health care programs with lower premiums and employer costs. In efforts to contain health care costs, these managed health care programs may have exclusions or increased premiums for workers with certain illnesses such as coronary heart disease, thus creating disincentives to work resumption. The prevalence of these potentially restrictive policies and the magnitude of their impact upon return to work after myocardial infarction are not currently known, but the continued growth of managed care programs makes this an important area for future study. Pell and D'Alonzo,[30] in their comprehensive study of nearly 30 years ago (1964) of the 5-year follow-up of male employees after the first myocardial infarction, first noted the absence of correlation between subsequent work and subsequent survival—the 5-year survival rate was 75 to 80%, but the 5-year employment rate was only 50% for salaried workers and 43% for wage earners. The subsequent studies reviewed in this chapter have all reinforced the early impression that failure to return to work and to remain working after myocardial infarction is a multifaceted problem and that the decline in return to work is more severe than can be explained on clinical grounds alone.

CORONARY ARTERY BYPASS SURGERY

For many patients, the decision to perform coronary artery bypass surgery is made when the level of anginal symptoms has increased to the point of severely limiting daily activities, including the ability to work. Because angina is relieved and functional capacity is improved in the great majority of patients following coronary artery bypass surgery, it was initially believed that this surgery would allow previously disabled persons to return to the active work force. This has not generally been the case. Most studies in the United States,[31–36] although not designed primarily to evaluate return to work, report a net decline in employment after coronary artery bypass surgery that is generally greater than the decline observed following myocardial infarction. The Coronary Artery Surgery Study (CASS) has provided prospective long-term outcome data on patients with coronary heart disease treated medically and surgically. In both the randomized CASS Alabama cohort[31] and the nonrandomized CASS Mayo Clinic cohort,[32] the percentage of

surviving patients under age 65 still working at 2 years was significantly reduced, but was nearly identical for medically and surgically treated patients: 65% in both groups at Alabama, 62% of the medical group and 63% of the surgical group at Mayo Clinic. The similarity of results in these two treatment groups indicates that factors other than mode of treatment and effectiveness exert considerable negative influence on subsequent employment.

Clinical Factors

Smith et al.[32] found that no clinical or angiographic indicators of preoperative severity of coronary heart disease influenced the postoperative employment rate. These data are somewhat in contrast to the myocardial infarction studies cited above, which demonstrated that the severity of infarction and the presence of complications adversely influenced the rate of return to work. The probable explanation for these differences is that in postoperative survivors, unlike myocardial infarction survivors, the preoperative clinical severity factors are no longer operative because the coronary stenoses are bypassed and most patients are relieved of angina. The recurrence of angina after surgery, however, was cited in several studies as the most powerful postoperative determinant for not working.[32,33]

Psychosocial Factors

A review of the studies of work patterns after coronary artery bypass surgery[31–36] underscores the important influence of nonmedical factors upon postoperative employment. In the majority of studies, the most powerful nonmedical predictor of postoperative employment was whether the patients were working before surgery.[32–34] Just as they were important predictors of return to work after myocardial infarction, lower socioeconomic status, as reflected by education or occupation, and increased age were also associated with lower levels of postoperative employment.[32–36]

Patients who fail to return to work by 6 months

after surgery are also less likely ever to do so. There are several possible explanations for the adverse relationship between durations of both preoperative and postoperative unemployment and return to work. The prevailing local levels of unemployment and the patients' attitude to work are continuing influences that are not altered by surgery. Many patients indicate a strong dislike for their work or blame their work for contributing to their coronary condition. A finding similar to that demonstrated after myocardial infarction was that the patients' self-perceptions of their ability to work is important; it was the most powerful predictor of postoperative employment in one study;[37] in another study,[33] 96% of patients not working after coronary artery bypass surgery believed that they were disabled.

Professionals, the self-employed, and those with higher levels of education have the highest rates of working following coronary artery bypass surgery.[32,33,36,38] In earlier reports,[32,34,39,40] physician advice not to work was given by patients as the reason for not resuming work after coronary artery bypass surgery, but this stated reason has not been independently or systematically assessed. It is also not known whether this advice is as prevalent today, or has significant influence; this possible factor merits further study.

In summary, coronary artery bypass surgery in the United States has not achieved its potential to offset its huge national cost (at least $7 billion annually) through an increased productivity by returning workers previously disabled by coronary heart disease to the active work force. A long-term follow-up report of the patients randomized to medical therapy or coronary artery bypass surgery in the CASS cohorts has found no difference in employment status between the two treatment groups at 10 years after randomized therapy.[41] Thus, coronary artery bypass surgery has added to rather than decreased the costs of coronary heart disease to U.S. society.

The demonstrated lack of correlation between levels of postoperative recreational physical activity and postoperative employment[32] further supports the importance of nonclinical factors in determining postoperative employment and reinforces the need for a comprehensive approach to rehabilitation of the patient following coronary artery bypass surgery if its full benefits are to be realized by individual patients and by society.

CORONARY ANGIOPLASTY

The findings regarding return to work after PTCA are similar to those observed for myocardial infarction and coronary artery bypass surgery. There is a lower rate of employment after PTCA than before,[42,43] but the magnitude of the decline is generally less than after myocardial infarction and coronary artery bypass surgery. In two studies, the overall percentage of working patients dropped by 5% following coronary angioplasty: from 68 to 63% in a multicenter U.S. study[42] and from 84 to 79% in a Canadian study.[43] Nonmedical factors also appear to be as important as medical factors in predicting return to work after PTCA, but these have been less extensively studied.[44,45] As expected, convalescence is shorter and return to work occurs earlier after successful percutaneous transluminal coronary angioplasty than for either myocardial infarction or coronary artery bypass surgery.[42–44] In the large National Heart, Lung, and Blood Institute (NHLBI) Percutaneous Transluminal Coronary Angioplasty Registry Study[42] of 2,250 patients, three outcome subsets were examined: (a) successful PTCA, (b) failed PTCA with subsequent surgery, and (c) failed PTCA with subsequent medical therapy. Group (c) had a higher prevalence of prior myocardial infarction and coronary artery bypass surgery and a lower rate of prior employment. Despite differences in both baseline characteristics and therapeutic outcomes, there was a similar decline in work in all three groups at 1.5 years follow-up. The occurrence of chest pain during follow-up was an important predictor of lower rates of return to work, irrespective of the outcome of PTCA. At follow-up, only 77% of patients with chest pain were working compared with 90% of patients without chest pain. This effect is similar to that observed following coronary artery bypass surgery. Generally higher rates of subsequent employment (88 to 98%) have been reported for patients who are under age 60 and working prior to successful PTCA than for similar patients with myocardial infarction or coronary artery bypass surgery,[42–44,46,47] but there is a preponderance of patients with single-vessel disease and no prior myocardial infarction or disability in the PTCA group. Systematic evaluations with longer-term follow-up of the effects of restenosis or medications upon employment rates for patients after PTCA have not been reported. One study[48] comparing the medically treated CASS patients from 1975 to 1979 with the Emory Angioplasty Registry experience from 1981 to 1983 (after statistical correction for 13 known variables) provides some insight into the 3-year effect of PTCA upon employment. After correcting for baseline employment status, age, sex, baseline activity levels, and baseline angina class (excluding baseline retirees and those over 65 years at 3-year follow-up), there was a significantly more favorable work outcome after PTCA than with continued medical therapy. Angina class and activity levels were also better in the angioplasty-treated group. These data, although encouraging, should be interpreted with caution in view of population differences, of time and place, the nonrandomized selection of PTCA patients, and the potential for inadequate or erroneous corrections for known and unknown variables.

REHABILITATION PROGRAMS AND RETURN TO WORK

Only a small percentage (6%) of coronary patients were estimated to have access to rehabilitation programs before 1986, but a recent randomized study of rehabilitation programs reports that approximately one-half the patients in the "usual-care" or control groups received some rehabilitation during their hospitalization.[8] The percentage of these coronary rehabilitation programs that currently include vocational counselors, work evaluation programs (see Ch. 30), and out-of-hospital (home, work site) personnel who can address the socioeconomic obstacles to resumed work activities is not known, but is probably small.

Although return to work and a productive lifestyle are goals of coronary rehabilitation programs,[5,49–51] most research has concentrated on the clinical outcomes of subsequent coronary morbidity and mortality and improvement in exercise capacity. In studies that systematically assessed short-term (6 months to 1 year) return to work after myocardial infarction as an outcome indicator, little or no improvement in rates of return to work have been reported from exercise conditioning programs.[25,52,53] In one long-term study,[54] those receiving rehabilitative care also did not have higher rates of return to work than the control group.

In contrast, Hedback and Perk[55] reported a higher maintained working rate at 2 to 5 years in patients younger than 55 years receiving a comprehensive rehabilitation program in which, in addition to exercise training, risk factor modification was conducted. There was a lower rate of coronary events and use of cardiac and anxiolytic medications in the treated group. Although the benefits of aerobic exercise conditioning programs have been judged inadequate to address short-term problems concerning return to work,[56] their long-term benefits to work maintenance, achieved through successful secondary prevention as shown by Hedback and Perk,[55] should not be overlooked.

Many hospitals have now established coronary rehabilitation programs where none existed before, but the recent dramatic impact of thrombolytic therapy on morbidity and mortality from myocardial infarction and the impact of risk stratification with low-level exercise tests as early as day 5 in hospital has enabled physicians to identify very early those low-risk patients who may not require further extensive (and expensive) evaluation and treatment. These patients may be discharged as early as 6 to 7 days following myocardial infarction. This abbreviated hospitalization may make it impossible for the personnel in rehabilitation programs to address all the patient's and family's needs in the hospital setting, including vocational counseling; continued counseling on an outpatient basis, individually as part of an ambulatory rehabilitation program, or in groups such as "Coronary Clubs" may be necessary.

Just as medical treatment is stratified according to the individual patient's risk or need assessment, increasingly stratified coronary rehabilitation programs should be developed to best meet the vocational needs of the individual patient. It is probable that low-risk patients, with abbreviated hospitalizations and no complications of myocardial infarction, will need less vocational counseling or psychosocial interventions, as they have less perception of physical disability and will have high rates of return to work and earlier resumption of employment. Dennis et al.[7] have demonstrated significantly earlier return to work following myocardial infarction in patients identified to be at low risk who were advised about early return to work than in patients receiving usual care.

In a subsequent study[57] of the cost benefits of this program, Pickard et al. determined that medical costs were lower and occupational income higher in patients who returned to work early as a consequence of this identification and intervention process, and they forecast an annual economic benefit in excess of $800 million when projected to the similar 300,000 low-risk employed patients under 60 years of age who survive myocardial infarction in the United States each year. The increasingly widespread use of thrombolytic therapy to reestablish myocardial perfusion in the early hours of acute myocardial infarction has resulted in a significant increase in acute and long-term survival, and the spectrum of functional impairment and risk in patients following current therapy for myocardial infarction will also be significantly altered. This increased diversity in the spectrum of clinical risk and impairment in patients with myocardial infarction following current therapy further underscores the economic necessity of work risk stratification, so that expensive rehabilitation resources can be directed to high-risk patients, who stand to benefit the most, and less costly care and accelerated rehabilitation programs can be provided to low-risk patients, who have an excellent prognosis and the capability to return to work early without increased clinical risks.

Recognition of the failure of the usual exercise-conditioning and patient-counseling coronary rehabilitation programs to significantly modify the rate of return to work after myocardial infarction has prompted several investigators to develop and evaluate rehabilitation programs with vocational counseling and psychosocial interventions specifically focused upon improving the rates of return to work. The comprehensive approach is similar to that of the American Heart Association–sponsored Work Classification Clinics of the 1950s and 1960s. Various in-hospital, home, and workplace interventions were used for groups and for individual patients. There was evidence of less psychological stress and dependence upon family in the treated groups, and real and perceived barriers to reemployment were removed. Although convalescence was generally shorter with an earlier return to work in the treated groups, there was no significant increase in return to work over the control groups by 6 months to 1 year.[58–60]

In a carefully performed study, Burgess et al.[8] reported that both the vocational and psychosocial treatment groups and the "usual-care" group (over 50% received some rehabilitation) had an identical high rate (88%) of return to work. These results and those of others[58–60] led Burgess et al.[8] to conclude that rehabilitation programs with psychosocial and occupational interventions specifically designed to return patients to work were not wholly justified. However, the high rate of return to work in their control group leaves only a small margin for improvement, and the small numbers of patients in their study ($n = 68$ in each group) and a low predicted difference between groups raises the possibility of a beta error. The rate of return to work of the 32 dropouts (18%) from their rehabilitation programs was not included in their analysis. If these rehabilitation program dropouts are also those with a high dropout rate from the work force (a likely scenario), the high rate of return to work in both treatment and control groups may reflect a selection bias, and vocational rehabilitation efforts may have to be refocused on these program dropouts.

A more realistic assessment of the cost effectiveness of coronary rehabilitation programs with specific vocational rehabilitation goals requires that they be selectively aimed at patients who, on the basis of the research cited earlier in this chapter, can now be identified as being at high risk for not returning to work.

Analysis of determinants of success or failure

in the vocational rehabilitation of the coronary patient would not be complete without an examination of the role of the patient's physician or surgeon. This individual can potentially provide to the patient and family much of the motivation, encouragement, and reassurance that may be necessary on a continuing basis for a patient to return to work, and remain employed, after a major coronary event. There is some evidence that this can be a powerful determinant of subsequent employment. The single notable exception to the postoperative decline in employment noted in other studies of coronary artery bypass surgery in the United States is the report by Liddle et al.[61] Prior to operation, all patients in this Utah community were advised by their surgeons that work rehabilitation was a major purpose and benefit of the coronary artery bypass operation. Only 46% of the 413 men younger than 65 years were working before surgery, but 85% returned to work after surgery. These authors emphasized that the most important factors in rehabilitation and postoperative employment are the psychological preparation of patients and their families regarding recovery and the attitudes of the patients' physicians and employers regarding vocational rehabilitation.

SUMMARY

Coronary rehabilitation has made tremendous strides in improving exercise capacity and reducing the subsequent coronary morbidity and mortality in patients who survive myocardial infarction and in patients who undergo coronary artery bypass surgery or PTCA. The significant decline in employment noted following all three of these major events for patients with coronary heart disease has been much more resistant to change. Current rehabilitation programs that improve cardiac performance have not had a significant impact upon return to work. However, much of the important groundwork has been laid for significant future advances in the vocational rehabilitation of the coronary patient. Many of the clinical and nonclinical predictors for not return-

ing to work have been identified, and programs with specific psychosocial and vocational goals have been developed. The few coronary vocational rehabilitation programs reporting results to date have had, at best, only a modest impact upon return to work, but they have not been selectively applied to patients at high risk for subsequent unemployment.

Surprisingly, more information is still needed on the factors that influence the subsequent employment of working women, the effects of physician and family advice, the patients' attitudes toward their work, and the factors that determine the subsequent losses from the work force of those patients who initially returned to work. The potential unintended adverse impact upon return to work of the various cost containment measures of managed health care programs, the effects of continuing changes in our work environment and society, and whether the early "employment benefits" of PTCA over coronary artery bypass surgery will be reduced or lost long-term because of restenosis are all issues that require further study.

The cost effectiveness of vocational rehabilitation programs for the coronary patient will have to be assessed after their selective application to patients who are identified by vocational risk stratification techniques as being at high risk for subsequent nonemployment. The recent major changes in the management of myocardial infarction, resulting in much shorter hospitalizations, and the major influence of nonclinical factors upon subsequent employment, will require that current and future coronary rehabilitation vocational programs be flexible and respond to the continuously changing medical and work environment. These vocational coronary programs will have to be based much less in the hospital and much more in the home and continuing work environment. Ongoing rehabilitation programs in the work environment may at first glance appear costly, but the economic consequences of premature disability or nonemployment of a large and growing number of coronary patients with little or no coronary disability after myocardial infarction, coronary artery bypass surgery, or PTCA has reached enormous proportions. These comprehensive rehabilitation programs are essential to the optimal vocational outcomes of the more than 6 million U.S. citizens who currently have overt coronary heart disease.

REFERENCES

1. American Heart Association: Heart Facts 1991. American Heart Association, Dallas, TX
2. Vuopala U: Resumption of work after myocardial infarction in Northern Finland. Vol. 7. Department of Medicine, University of Onter, Onter, Finland, 1972
3. Brown LB, Antic R, Hetzel BS: Social effects of myocardial infarction in men under the age of 50 years: A review after one to eight years. Med J Aust 2:125, 1969
4. Mulcahy R, Hickey N, Coughlin N: Rehabilitation of patients with coronary heart disease. Geriatrics 3:120, 1972
5. Wenger NK, Hellerstein HK, Blackburn H et al: Physician practice in the management of patients with uncomplicated myocardial infarction—changes in the past decade. Circulation 65:421, 1982
6. Kjoller E: Resumption of work after acute myocardial infarction. Acta Med Scand 199:379, 1976
7. Dennis C, Houston-Miller N, Schwartz RG et al: Early return to work after uncomplicated myocardial infarction. JAMA 260:214, 1988
8. Burgess AW, Lerner DJ, D'Agostino RB et al: A randomized control trial of cardiac rehabilitation. Soc Sci Med 24:359, 1987
9. Stern MJ, Pascale L, Ackerman A: Life adjustment post-myocardial infarction: determining predictive variables. Arch Intern Med 137:1680, 1977
10. Smith GR, O'Rourke DF: Return to work after a first myocardial infarction. JAMA 259:1673, 1988
11. Lloyd GG, Cawley RH: Psychiatric morbidity after myocardial infarction. Q J Med 201:33, 1982
12. Trelawney RC, Russel O: Social and psychological responses to myocardial infarction: multiple determinants of outcome at six months. J Psychosom Res 31:125, 1987
13. Maeland JG, Havik OE: Return to work after myocardial infarction: The influence of background factors, work characteristics and illness severity. Scand J Soc Med 14:183, 1986
14. Moller M, Holm B, Sindrup E: Electroencephalographic prediction of anoxic brain damage after resuscitation from cardiac arrest in patients with acute myocardial infarction. Acta Med Scand 203:31, 1978
15. Mayou R: Prediction of emotional and social outcome after a heart attack. J Psychosom Res 28:17, 1984
16. Shapiro S, Weinblatt E, Frank CW: Return to work after first myocardial infarction. Arch Environ Health 24:17, 1972
17. Heatley MA, Haney T, Barefoot JC: Medical, psychological and social correlates of work disability among men with coronary artery disease. Am J Cardiol 58:911, 1986
18. Mayou R, Foster A, Williamson B: Psychosocial adjustment in patients one year after myocardial infarction. J Psychosom Res 22:447, 1978
19. Wishnie HA, Hackett TP, Cassem NH: Psychological hazards of convalescence following myocardial infarction. JAMA 215:1292, 1971
20. Chirikos TN, Nickel JL: Work disability from coronary heart disease in women. Women Health 9:55, 1984
21. Super D: A life span, life space approach to career developments. p. 197. In Brown D, Brooks L (eds): Career Choice and Development. 2nd Ed. Jossey Bass Co., San Francisco, 1990
22. Cay EL, Vitter N, Phillip A, Dugard P: Return to work after a heart attack. J Psychosom Res 17:231, 1973
23. Shanfield SB: Return to work after an acute myocardial infarction: A review. Heart Lung 19:109, 1990
24. Degre-Coustry C, Grevisse M: Psychologic problems in rehabilitation after myocardial infarction: Non-institutional approach. Adv Cardiol 29:126, 1982
25. Giese H, Schomer HH: Life style changes and mood profile of cardiac patients after an exercise rehabilitation program. J Cardiopulmonary Rehabil 6:30, 1986
26. Wenger NK: Coronary disease in women. Annu Rev Med 36:285, 1985
27. Walling A, Tremblay GJ, John J et al: Evaluating the rehabilitation potential of a large population of post-myocardial infarction patients: Adverse prognosis for women. J Cardiopulmonary Rehabil 8:99, 1988
28. Stern MJ, Pascale L, McLoone JB: Psychosocial adaptation following acute myocardial infarction. J Chronic Dis 29:513, 1976
29. Boyd JH, Weissman MM, Thompson WD, Myers JK: Screening for depression in a community sample: Understanding the discrepancies between

depression symptoms and diagnostic scales. Arch Gen Psychiatry 39:1195, 1982

30. Pell S, D'Alonzo CA: Immediate mortality and five year survival of employed men with a first myocardial infarction. N Engl J Med 270:915, 1964

31. Oberman A, Wayne JB, Kouchoukos NT: Working status of patients following coronary bypass surgery. Circulation 65(Suppl. II):II-115, 1982

32. Smith HC, Hammes L, Gupta S et al: Employment status after coronary artery bypass surgery. Circulation 65(Suppl. II):II-120, 1982

33. Almeida D, Bradford JM, Wenger NK et al: Return to work after coronary bypass surgery. Circulation 68(Suppl. II):5, 1983

34. Hammermeister KE, de Rouen TA, English MT et al: Effect of surgical versus medical therapy on return to work in patients with coronary artery disease. Am J Cardiol 44:105, 1979

35. Rimm AA, Barboriak JJ, Anderson AJ et al: Changes in occupation after aortocoronary vein bypass operation. JAMA 236:361, 1976

36. Barnes GK, Ray MJ, Oberman A et al: Changes in working status of patients following coronary bypass surgery. JAMA 238:1259, 1977

37. Stanton BA, Jenkins CD, Denlinger P et al: Predictors of employment status after cardiac surgery. JAMA 249:907, 1983

38. Love JW: Employment status after coronary bypass operations and some considerations. J Thorac Cardiovasc Surg 80:68, 1980

39. Kuschner B, Fox KM, Tomlinson IW et al: The effect of a predischarge consultation on the resumption of work, sexual activity, and driving following acute myocardial infarction. Scand J Rehabil Med 8:155, 1976

40. National Institutes of Health Consensus Development Conference Statement: Coronary artery bypass surgery: Scientific and clinical aspects. N Engl J Med 304:680, 1981

41. Rogers WJ, Coggin CJ, Gersh BJ et al: Ten year follow up of quality of life in patients randomized to medical therapy versus coronary artery bypass surgery. The Coronary Artery Surgery Study (CASS). (Abstract.) Circulation 78(Suppl. II):II-258, 1988

42. Holmes DR, VanRaden MJ, Reeder GS et al: Return to work after coronary angioplasty: A report from the National Heart, Lung and Blood Institute Percutaneous Transluminal Coronary Angioplasty Registry. Am J Cardiol 53:48C, 1984

43. Boulay F, David P, Guiteras VP et al: Benefices socio-economiques de la dilatation coronarie. Arch Mal Coeur 77:426, 1984

44. Holmes DR, Vlietstra RE, Mock MB et al: Employment and recreational patterns in patients treated by percutaneous transluminal coronary angioplasty: A multicenter study. Am J Cardiol 52:710, 1983

45. Russell RO, Mansour PA, Wenger NK: Return to work after coronary bypass surgery and percutaneous transluminal angioplasty: Issues and potential solutions. Cardiology 73:306, 1986

46. Meier B, Charves V, Segesser L et al: Vocational rehabilitation after coronary angioplasty and coronary bypass surgery. p. 171. In Walter PJ (ed): Return to Work After Coronary Bypass Surgery. Psychosocial and Economic Aspects. Springer-Verlag, Berlin, 1985

47. Kelly ME, Taylor GJ, Moses HWE et al: Comparative costs of myocardial revascularization, percutaneous transluminal coronary angioplasty and coronary artery bypass surgery. J Am Coll Cardiol 5:16, 1985

48. Ellis SG, Fisher L, Duschman T et al: Comparison of coronary angioplasty with medical treatment for single and double vessel coronary disease with left anterior descending involvement: Long-term outcome based upon an Emory-CASS Registry study. Am Heart J 118:208, 1989

49. Atwood JA, Nielson DH: Scope of cardiac rehabilitation. Phys Ther 65:1812, 1985

50. Wenger NK: Rehabilitation of the coronary patient: Status 1986. Prog Cardiovasc Dis 29:181, 1986

51. Parmley WW: President's page: Position report on cardiac rehabilitation. J Am Coll Cardiol 7:451, 1986

52. Stern MJ, Gorman PA, Kaslow L: The group counseling versus exercise therapy study: A controlled intervention with subjects following myocardial infarction. Arch Intern Med 143:1719, 1983

53. Ott CR, Sivarajan ES, Nuoton KM et al: A controlled randomized study of early cardiac rehabilitation: The Sickness Impact Profile as an assessment tool. Heart Lung 12:162, 1983

54. Erdman RA, Duivenvoonden HJ, Verhage F et al: Predictability of beneficial effects in cardiac rehabilitation: A randomized clinical trial of psychosocial variables. J Cardiopulmonary Rehabil 6:206, 1986

55. Hedback B, Perk J: Five-year results of a comprehensive rehabilitation programme after myocardial infarction. Eur Heart J 8:234, 1987

56. Blodgett C, Pekarik G: Program education in car-

diac rehabilitation. Overview of evaluation issues. J Cardiopulmonary Rehabil 7:316, 1987

57. Pickard MH, Dennis C, Schwartz RG et al: Cost-benefit analysis of early return to work after uncomplicated acute myocardial infarction. Am J Cardiol 63:1308, 1989

58. Groden BM, Cheyne AI: Rehabilitation after cardiac illness. Br Med J 2:700, 1972

59. Bengtsson K: Rehabilitation after myocardial infarction. Scand J Rehabil Med 15:1, 1983

60. Mayou R, MacMahon D, Sleight P, Florencio MJ: Early rehabilitation after myocardial infarction. Lancet ii:1399, 1981

61. Liddle HV, Jensen R, Clayton PD: The rehabilitation of coronary surgical patients. Ann Thorac Surg 34:374, 1982

VOCATIONAL ASPECTS OF REHABILITATION

30

Work Evaluation

Herman K. Hellerstein, M.D.

Rehabilitation of the coronary patient involves the restoration, attainment, and maintenance of an optimal emotional, psychologic, physical, sexual, social, and occupational status. For young and middle-aged patients, the return to full physical and mental functioning is a particularly high priority, for medical, social, and economic reasons. Work is considered psychologically therapeutic for the recovering coronary patient. In addition, the economic survival of the coronary patient and the family generally depends on gainful employment and self-sufficiency.

Interventional techniques such as coronary artery bypass surgery (CABG), percutaneous transluminal coronary angioplasty (PTCA), thrombolysis, and exercise training have prolonged survival but have not been consistently associated with increased productivity and return to work of patients who were previously employed or those who have been disabled or limited in work capacity.[1-3] Unfortunately, although rehabilitation programs have brought about dramatic improvement in the functional capacity and psychologic well-being of the coronary patient, in terms of resumption of gainful employment, they have been less successful[4] (see Chs. 20, 28, 29).

Each year in the United States several million men and women develop clinical coronary heart disease, angina, or acute myocardial infarction, and several hundred thousands undergo such interventional techniques as CABG, PTCA, or thrombolysis. Of the annual 800,000 U.S. survivors of acute myocardial infarction, as many as 200,000 are candidates for occupational work evaluation, appropriate risk stratification, and return to work.[4,5] One study estimated that the medical cost savings for these individuals might approximate $100 million, and the additional earned income $400 million (in 1990 dollars).[4] This would total $500 million in cost savings and additional income alone. Another $300 million would be saved by the employer, including such costs as disability insurance. Similar data are not readily available on patients undergoing PTCA or CABG surgery.

The success of cardiac rehabilitation in returning patients to work is usually evaluated in terms of the percentage of patients who return to work, the time between the acute coronary event and return to work, the number of hours worked per week, and the compensation therein.

Decisions concerning return to work of coronary heart disease (CHD) patients are complex and are affected by many factors. Table 30-1 demonstrates the predominantly nonmedical factors influencing the return to work of these patients.[6,7] Physical job requirements do not pose a major problem for the majority of young and middle-aged coronary patients. They are rarely excessive and unmodifiable.[8-11]

In highly industrialized societies, the physical energy requirements of work have constantly decreased since 1900,[12] and even more remarkably so in the past several decades, with the introduction of mechanization, automation, robotization, and computer technology. Greater emphasis is now placed upon other aspects of performance (particularly psychological), intellectual competence, interpersonal relations, and skills with

523

Table 30-1. Factors Influencing the Return to Work of Coronary Heart Disease Patients after a Coronary Event

Patient Factors	Work Factors
Disease-related	General
Older age at onset of event	Occupational status and category
Medical prognosis	Previous employment
Severity of cardiovascular disease and complications	Patient's concern about work safety
Degree of disability	Physical requirements of work
Other significant diseases	Emotional, cognitive, mental requirements
Socioeconomic	Favorable outlook
Lower educational level	Professionals, managers, executives
Lower social class	Higher skills
Psychoemotional	Unfavorable outlook
Emotional stability	Unemployed prior to the event
Personality	Lower skills
Perception of health	Negative employer attitude
Perception of illness as being job-related	Physician-related
Unresolved concerns	Advice regarding work
Family-related	Lack of encouragement, counseling
Overprotection	Economic
Lack of family support	Benefits, pensions
	Legislation and employment benefits
	Nonwork income

lower energy requirements.[13] Furthermore, heavy work is usually assigned to younger workers.

Coronary patients often come from a stable, middle-aged working population. Over 40% of such subjects have worked 15 years or more in the same occupation. One study demonstrated that 56% of coronary patients had worked more than 5 years at the last place of employment, 39% more than 10 years, and 23% more than 20 years.[10] Furthermore, the occupational categories are usually of a higher skill; in one study 37% were classified as skilled, 43% as semiskilled, and less than 20% as unskilled.[10]

The requirements for employment of cardiovascular patients have been stated succinctly by the World Health Organization (WHO) Expert Committee on Rehabilitation of Patients with Cardiovascular Diseases.[14]

1. The occupation should not increase the gravity of the overall condition of the patient by either excessively high or excessively low physical requirements.
2. It should make the best possible use of the individual's ability.

3. It should provide maximum satisfaction for the individual, adequate remuneration, and, if possible, opportunity for security and promotion.

The return to work requires an evaluation of the individual's capabilities and limitations, and appropriate matching with job(s) whose requirements can be estimated accurately or have been measured in similar patients or age-matched normal subjects.

The evaluation of the patient with coronary heart disease should be comprehensive. It should include not only quantification of functional capacity (see Chs. 7 and 8), but also an overall evaluation of the total health status (presence of significant, potentially limiting, comorbid disease[s], especially peripheral and cerebral vascular disease), prognosis, therapeutic needs, and psychological state.

Psychological dysfunction is common in coronary heart disease patients (see Ch. 28) but is commonly transient and infrequently requires formal psychotherapy.[4,11] However, severe psychological dysfunction often antedates the acute coronary event. In such patients, the psychologic state can influence the adjustment to work, especially if they experience exacerbation of anxiety and depression, not only in the acute event, but also well into convalescence and beyond. This occurs commonly in patients who continue to have unstable angina, uncontrolled arrhythmias, or diabetes mellitus after the acute event.

To patients with CHD, the emotional milieu of the job may be more significant than its energy requirements. The status of the job and the perceived stress imposed by an overly demanding employer, by the pressure of competition in a piecework job, or by the patient's having accepted responsibility for which he or she feels unfit are important facets. Although the influence of the economic and family pressures generated at home may prevail during the working hours, more commonly the opposite pertains; that is, many patients have their attacks of angina only at home. It should be emphasized, however, that in almost all cases, the satisfaction, restoration of self-respect, and relief from financial worry that result from the return to work outweigh most detrimental emotional stresses associated with a job. A suitable job, thus, must provide status, self-esteem, and remuneration and be within the individual patient's present and future capacity.

The identification of specific demands of a large variety of jobs and the quantification of functional capacity of individual coronary patients are essential for appropriate work prescription. Risk stratification provides guidelines not only for medical management, but also for work prescription and vocational rehabilitation.[4,5] It is important to distinguish coronary patients who can be identified as having a poor prognosis for survival and successful reemployment,[10] from those who can be identified as having excellent functional capacity and being able to return to previous work under unmodified conditions.[4] Some patients can be identified as being likely to return normally to work without limitations; another group could work with limitations; and a third group should not or could not work because of marked physical impairments and the low likelihood of finding a position whose demands are low enough.[4] Risk assessment and stratification focus on assigning coronary patients into one of three gross categories, high-, intermediate-, and low-risk, on the basis of left ventricular dysfunction and myocardial ischemia—spontaneous or as elicited by diagnostic techniques such as electrocardiograms (ECGs), hemodynamic changes, and myocardial imaging at rest or with effort.[4] The demonstration of the low energy requirements of many jobs[8–10,15,16] has facilitated the safe and successful return to work of patients classified not only as low-risk, but also of those classified as intermediate-risk and, in

Table 30-2. Relationship of Physiologic Classification to Work Energy Capacity of Cardiacs and Work Classification

Work Classification[a]	Cardiac Functional Classification	Physiologic Symptoms	METs
Heavy to very heavy	Normal	Normal	⩾6
Medium to heavy	I	Cardiac disease with no limitation of physical activity. Ordinary physical activity causes no discomfort.	>5
Light to medium	II	Cardiac disorder with slight to moderate limitation of physical activity causes discomfort.	3–4
Sedentary to light	III	Moderate cardiac disorder with moderate to great limitation of physical activity. Less than ordinary physical activity causes discomfort.	2–3
Sedentary	IV	Cardiac disorder unable to carry on any physical activity without discomfort.	1–2

[a] U.S. Department of Health and Human Services[17]
(Adapted from Ford and Hellerstein,[22] and from Turell and Hellerstein,[50] with permission.)

special instances, of those classified as high-risk (equivalent to the New York Heart Association classes I, II, and III, respectively),[5] to specific jobs whose demands are well within their limited capacities (Table 30-2).

GENERAL RECOMMENDATIONS FOR ACTIVITY LIMITATIONS AND WORKING CONDITIONS

Synthesis of Evaluative Data

A synthesis of the New York Heart Association Functional Classification, risk stratification, exercise test performance, and Social Security Disability Evaluation[4,15,17] follows:

Class I patients are those with cardiac disease (coronary disease) but without resulting limitations of physical activity at 5 or more METs. These are low-risk patients.[4] Ordinary activity does not cause undue fatigue, palpitations, dyspnea, anginal pain or other evidence of myocardial ischemia or arrhythmias. In terms of *activity limitations*, no restrictions should be placed on walking, climbing, crawling, kneeling, standing, stooping, bending, high rate of speed, tension, or reaching arms overhead. Some *limitations* are advised. Patients should avoid running when possible. They may lift 25 to 50 lbs occasionally, while frequent lifting or carrying of objects weighing up to 25 lbs is permissible. Concerning *working conditions*, there are no restrictions outside, nor any involving temperature, humidity or wetness, dusty, mechanical hazard, cramped quarters, high places, electrical hazard, nightshifts or motor vehicle driving. An 8-hour shift with occasional overtime is suggested.

This corresponds to the classification of *medium work*, according to the disability evaluation under the Social Security Administration.[17] Medium work involves lifting no more than 50 lbs at a time, with frequent lifting or carrying of objects weighing up to 25 lbs. If an individual can do medium work, such a person can also do sedentary and light work.

Class II patients have cardiac disease (coronary disease) resulting in slight limitation of physical

activity at 3 to 4 METs. These are intermediate-risk patients.[4] They are comfortable at rest. Ordinary physical activity results in fatigue, palpitations, dyspnea, anginal pain, or mild myocardial ischemia at their peak tolerance. There are no *activity limitations:* on crawling, kneeling, standing, stooping, bending, high rates of speed, tension, or stretching arms overhead. Some *limitations* should be observed. Patients may walk at their own pace, should avoid running, may climb up to two flights of stairs three times an hour, and may lift or carry 20 to 25 lbs, with frequent lifting or carrying of objects weighing up to 10 lbs. In terms of *working conditions*, there are no restrictions in regard to humidity or wetness, dust, motor vehicle driving (private), mechanical hazards or nightshifts. However, some *limitations* apply. Outside activity should not exceed ordinary activity. Exertion or prolonged exposure to extremes of hot and cold temperatures should be avoided, as should cramped quarters, high places, electrical hazards, and driving public conveyance. Working 8 hours a day with no overtime is recommended.

This corresponds to *light work* as defined by the Social Security Administration.[17] Light work involves lifting no more than 20 lbs at a time, with frequent lifting or carrying of objects weighing up to 10 lbs. Although the weight lifted may be very little, a job is in this category when it requires a good deal of walking or standing or when it involves sitting most of the time with some pushing or pulling of arm or leg controls. To be considered capable of performing a wide or full range of light work, the coronary patient must have the ability to do substantial amounts of all of these activities. If the coronary subject can do light work, he or she should also be able to do sedentary work unless there are limiting factors such as loss of fine dexterity or inability to sit for long periods of time.

Class III patients have cardiac disease (coronary disease) resulting in marked limitation of physical activity at 2 to 3 METs. They are high-risk patients.[4] They are comfortable at rest. Less than ordinary physical activity causes fatigue, palpitations, dyspnea, anginal pain, or objective evidence of myocardial ischemia. There are some *activity limitations*. Walking is permissible as limited by symptoms. Patients should avoid running, crawling, and kneeling. They may occasionally climb one or two flights of stairs, may stand up to 10% of time, may carry or lift a maximum of 10 lbs several times an hour, and may push or pull up to 10 to 15 lbs several times an hour. They should avoid stooping and bending, high rates of speed, tension, and reaching arms overhead. In terms of *working conditions*, they should avoid outside exposure to extremes of hot and cold temperatures. They should also avoid mechanical hazards, cramped quarters, high places, electrical hazards, and prolonged motor vehicle driving. Their hours may be part time.

This corresponds to *sedentary work* as defined by the Social Security Administration.[17] Sedentary work involves lifting no more than 10 lbs at a time and occasionally lifting or carrying articles such as files, ledgers, and small tools. Although a sedentary job is defined as one that involves sitting, a certain amount of walking and standing is often necessary in carrying out job duties. Jobs are sedentary if walking or standing are required occasionally and other sedentary criteria are met.

Class better than I refers to coronary patients who have attained a functional aerobic capacity that is equal to or better than that of age-matched normal sedentary or active subjects and who may have a maximal aerobic capacity of 10 to 12 METs, as determined by multistage exercise tests. This corresponds to *heavy work* as defined by the Social Security Administration.[17] Heavy work involves lifting no more than 100 lbs at a time, with frequent lifting or carrying of objects weighing up to 50 lbs. If the coronary patient can do heavy work, he or she can also do medium, light, and sedentary work.

A rare coronary patient is capable of *very heavy work*. This involves lifting objects weighing more than 100 lbs at a time, with frequent lifting or carrying of objects weighing 50 lbs or more. If a coronary patient can do very heavy work, he or she also can do heavy, medium, light, and sedentary work.

Selected Proscriptions

Uncontrolled repeated episodes of cardiac syncope or near loss of consciousness, unrelated to physical exertion (but due to paroxysmal tachy-

arrhythmias, high degrees of atrioventricular block, malfunction of an artificial pacemaker, postural hypotension, transient cerebral ischemic attacks, etc.), would merit the designation of high-risk, until controlled, regardless of a favorable functional classification in event-free periods. Even in patients with an occasional or single episode, special care should be taken in a job in which loss of control could have disastrous effects on the patient, fellow workers, and others. Thus, jobs such as crane operator, public vehicle driver or any involving proximity to moving machines (lathes, etc.) would be contraindicated.

Associated obstructive arterial disease such as claudication with marked impairment of the peripheral arterial circulation (with resting ankle-to-brachial systolic blood pressure ratio of less than 0.50) would preclude work that involves a significant amount of walking.[17] However, such coronary patients could perform sedentary or light work involving the upper extremities and the use of other capabilities for communication and administration.

Options with Work Requirement/ Functional Capacity Mismatch

In addition to performing a comprehensive evaluation of the coronary patient including functional capacity and risk stratification, it is necessary to characterize the demands of prescribed work. In most cases, the patient can return to the previous work. However, when there is a mismatch, that is, when the work requirements exceed the individual's capacity, there are several options:

1. *Job modification* to reduce the work demands by altering the environmental demands, changing the design of work, or changing jobs.
2. *Selective placement* in other jobs with lesser demands, by transferring to a different job, ideally within the same place of employment.
3. *Vocational training* to improve the capacity by vocational counseling, vocational training, or retraining for jobs with higher or different skill requirements and lower energy demands.
4. *Enhancement of the individual's capacity*

through exercise training, psychological and emotional support, and/or other medical therapies, including drugs, surgery, angioplasty, etc.

5. *No employment or retirement* if none of the above are feasible.

Requirements of Work

The requirements of work (demands, stresses, loads) can be divided into two major categories: physical and intellectual-psychological.

Physical Requirements

The energy expenditure of a job can be expressed in terms of external work in kilogram-meters, foot-pounds, oxygen uptake in milliliters of oxygen per minute per kilogram body weight (METs), calories per minute, or levels of energy expenditure peak vs. steady-state. Other features include pace (fast or slow), pauses, remaining stationary versus locomotion, skills, aptitudes, training, and past work experience. Environmental conditions include noises, dusts, fumes, thermal (heat or cold) stress, and illumination.

Intellectual-Psychological Requirements

Intellectual-psychological requirements encompass knowledge, cognition, mental ability, judgment, decision-making, interpersonal relationships, and motivation.

ENERGY EXPENDITURE AT WORK

The energy expenditures and demands of work can be estimated (1) by *indirect* measures of the job, predicating the worker's responses on the basis of an exercise test or past work performance; or (2) by *direct* measurement of the job and the responses of the worker.

Indirect Measurements

From Activities at Work

Indirect evaluation is based on analysis of activities carried out under various conditions and whose caloric values have been measured.

The energy expenditures of a given job can be assessed from a detailed description and analysis of the job, including the type, speed, pace, official rest pauses; the number of cycles carried out per hour or per day of work; the pattern of work; the environment in which it is performed; the skills required; time spent sitting, standing, walking, and stair climbing; any bending, lifting, and stooping that is involved; movement of arms, hands, and whole body; and the transportation necessary to and from work and on the job.[13]

Several methods have been used[13]:

1. The timing of all activities by an observer (time and motion study)
2. The timing and recording of activities by the subject (the diary technique)
3. The recall of activity after the event, either directly by the subject (through questionnaire) or by means of interviews
4. Accelerometry and pedometry
5. Ciné or time-lapse photography

These techniques give a rough indication of work activity. However, simplified version of the diary and recall techniques in a large number of subjects can be used to define groups, but not individuals, who are involved in heavy, moderate, and sedentary work.[13]

From Job Descriptions

An estimate of the average oxygen uptake or calories can be calculated from detailed job descriptions (found in the *Dictionary of Occupational Titles* and other manuals),[18-21] standard tables, and published studies of the energy levels of jobs.[8-10,22-27] Unfortunately, such descriptions of jobs tables of energy levels of jobs, compiled in certain communities and plants rarely apply for a given job in a specific locale, due to changing technology and work practices and variations in the caloric expenditure within the same occupation. The tables cannot take into account the efficiency of a given subject or the possible environmental conditions or psychological factors involved in a specific job. The values in most tables correspond to average energy expenditure for prolonged activity lasting more than several minutes. Most industrial activities, however, are cyclic and have a cycle of less than a minute. The expenditure for peak activities is infrequently specified.[23] The peak activities in coronary (and other cardiac) patients may constitute the main factor limiting muscular activities.

Despite the above limitations, job descriptions, analyses, and classifications are valuable in counseling the coronary patient about work.[22-27] The general characterization of the same or similar jobs, ideally available locally, enable the counselor (physician, vocational consultant, etc.) to identify specific and appropriate jobs whose demands and requirements would fall within the coronary patient's evaluated physical, emotional, and functional capacity, and would be appropriate for the patient's level of education, age, past and present work experience, skills, aptitudes, work attitude, and functional classification and risk stratification.[4,15]

From Daily Dietary Intake and Nonwork Activities

The energy expenditures during the work shift have been roughly approximated by subtracting from the daily dietary energy intake the nonwork energy expenditures, calculated from tables of energy expenditure. This method is not only imprecise, but is also time-consuming. It is difficult to obtain reliable data. Although total and average values are provided, information is not provided about peak levels. Also, this technique suffers from a significant shortcoming; namely, that "a considerable time elapses before changes in activity are accurately reflected by changes in food intake, and dietary studies are unlikely to give a true indication of the level of activity unless they extend over at least five days."[28]

From Physiologic Responses at Work

Physiologic responses are an indirect measure of the responses of the body to "all stimuli, including physical activity, oxygen uptake, mental and intellectual activity, and environmental factors such as temperature and noises."[13] Certain cir-

culatory responses reflect physical activity more reliably than do others.

In exercise tests, the heart rate, blood pressure, and minute ventilation ($\dot{V}E$) increase linearly with effort and oxygen uptake ($\dot{V}O_2$). Because of the simplicity and ease of recording, heart rate has been used as an index of "the difficulty" and energy expenditure of individuals at work. The assumption has been made that the heart rate at work can be equated with the oxygen uptake of an equal heart rate (HR) obtained during a multistage exercise test of the individual subject.[24] This is the *method of HR-O$_2$ intake equivalence.*

Unfortunately, this linear relationship does not prevail in the majority of occupational tasks, in large part because of the combined effects of emotions, heat stress and other environmental factors, especially during periods of low energy expenditure.

The method of HR-O$_2$ intake equivalence has been shown to be invalid in cardiac and normal subjects (Table 30-3) whose peak oxygen uptake at work is below 1 L of oxygen per minute (4 to 5 METs), which is higher than that required by most occupations in Western societies (Table 30-4). Above this level, that is, with high intensity work, better correlations between HR and oxygen uptake can be anticipated.[8-10,28,29]

In job situations with low levels of energy expenditure and variable emotional and psychological stresses (factory, business, radio, television,

Table 30-3. Comparison of Measured and Equivalent Oxygen Uptake of 142 Normal and Coronary Subjects at Work

Occupation	No. Patients	$\dot{V}O_2$ Measured (ml/kg/min)		$\dot{V}O_2$ Equivalent from Exercise Test HR (ml/kg/min)	
		Average	Peak	Average	Peak
Businessmen	15	5.1	5.9	7.2	11.9
Anesthetists	26	5.2	5.5	5.8	10.9
Surgeons	39	5.3	6.0	11.3	16.5
Factory	62	5.3	6.3	13.5	18.6

Abbreviation: HR, heart rate.
(From Hellerstein,[16] with permission.)

Table 30-4. Mean and Peak Energy Expenditure During Typical Working Day by Subjects Without[a] and with Heart Disease

Measured in Cardiac and Control Subjects[a] (METs)	Measured in Normal Subjects[b] (METs)

Mean 1.0–1.2, peak 1.2–2.3
    Attendant; clerical; electrician; foreman; garage attendant; painter; supervisor
	Mean 1.3–1.6
	    Sheet metal; lawyer; radio and television

Mean 1.3–1.6, peak 1.6–3.3
    Anesthetist; assembler; bench work; business, box maker; clerk; control operator, drill press, factory; foreman guard; inspector; machine operator; maintenance; supervisor; surgeon; tool grinder; warehouse
	Mean 1.6–2.0
	    Automobile driving; desk work; clerical; filing; typing; electric calculator computer; light domestic; light machine

Mean 1.6–2.0, peak 1.8–3.4
    Domestic work (light); inspector; machine operator, (e.g., clutch tester, burnisher, drill press, scarfing, stube lathe); maintenance millwright; matron; steel mill; supervisor
	Mean 2.0–2.5
	    Automobile repair; bartending; domestic—window cleaning; radio and television repair; stock picker; walking level, 2 mph

Mean 2.0–2.5, peak 2.5–5.4
    Fireman; foreman; furnace worker; janitor; maintenance; supervisor; welder
	Mean 2.5–3.0
	    Agricultural work, automobile repair; industrial (e.g., loading, unloading, machine assembler); janitor; truck driving; walking level, 2.5 mph; welding

	Mean 3–4 Bed-making; brick laying; heavy manual labor (digging); walking level, 3 mph; light carpentry; machine assembly; paper-hanging; plastering; trailer-truck driving; welding; window-cleaning

[a] References 8–11, 16, 22, 27.
[b] References 4, 7, 14, 23, 24, 31.

law, medicine [especially surgery], and heat-stressful occupations), the relationship between heart rate and oxygen uptake is poor and can be misleading as a measure of the oxygen uptake of the body.

Although the heart rate has limited value in estimating the body's oxygen uptake, especially at low levels of energy, heart rate during the work shift can be used as a measure of myocardial oxygen uptake $(M\dot{V}o_2)^{29}$ (see Ch. 7). There is an excellent correlation between HR and $M\dot{V}o_2$.

The heart rate also provides excellent insight into cumulative fatigue, as indicated by a rise in the resting heart rate, higher heart rates after a given effort in the same environment at work (Fig. 30-1), and higher heart rates after working hours. Increasing fatigue persisting after work hours, increasing cardiac symptoms at work and at home, and the need for more medications may cast doubt on the suitability of a job or indicate a change in the clinical course of the underlying heart disease. Obviously, periodic retesting and vocational reevaluations are recommended.

Direct Measurements

In the early 1950s and 1960s, a large number of normal and only a few cardiac subjects were evaluated for their energy expenditure, with emphasis on special tasks involved in a variety of jobs.[23–25] Only recently has technology developed that can measure oxygen consumption and other parameters during a large part of a work shift without impairing work performance or without evidence of a hampered efficiency or productivity because of the study. In addition to the direct measurement of oxygen uptake, the following responses of workers have been measured:

1. *Cardiovascular responses:* heart rate, blood pressure, and ECG changes.

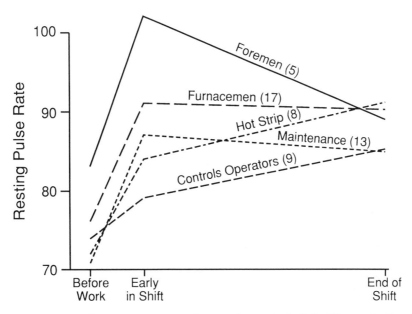

Fig. 30-1. Average resting pulse rate at 3 points during the work shift for 52 men in five job categories in a steel mill (13 class I, 7 class II). Twenty had CHD, 14 were age-matched control subjects, and 18 were normal male subjects holding typical jobs in a steel mill in which no cardiac subjects were engaged at the time of the study. Standard deviations are of the order of 12 pulse beats per minute. The rising resting pulse indicated fatigue. (From Ford et al,[9] with permission.)

2. *Respiratory responses:* ventilation volume per minute and ventilation rate. Minute ventilation increases linearly with oxygen uptake.[30]

3. *Temperature-regulation responses:* body temperature and perspiration rate, especially in heat-stressful occupations such as in steel mill worker and firefighter.

4. *Metabolic responses:* the lactic acid in heavy work, and the catecholamines in mental and emotionally stressful work and in hazardous and physically stressful work such as firefighting.

My associates and I evaluated over 500 workers with various types of heart diseases (the majority of whom had CHD) and matched control subjects (normals) in a great variety of jobs, some with low energy requirements and low or high psychological or emotional stress (factory, business, radio and television, court of law, surgeons and anesthetists in the operating room), and some with higher physical demands, often with high ther-

mal stress as encountered in the steel mill or foundry work and in firefighting.[8,9,16,27]

Clinical, Laboratory, and On-the-Job Studies

All subjects were evaluated by means of a medical history, physical examination, standard twelve-lead ECG, multistage exercise tests, psychological tests such as the Minnesota Multiphasic Personality Inventory (MMPI), and a work history. The subjects were studied at their usual work throughout a typical day's shift by the methods previously reported.[8,9] A detailed log was kept of the exact duration of each activity in which the subject engaged during the day. Five-minute samples of expired air were collected to measure oxygen uptake energy expenditure during each activity. ECGs and respiratory rate were recorded as the samples were taken and blood pressures recorded either during or immediately after the determination. Multiple observations were made on any activity that occupied more than an hour of the subject's time. In no case did a worker fail to meet a quota for the day or show other objective evidence of decreased productivity due to the study. Radiant heat was measured with a black globe thermometer, air speed, and wet and dry bulb temperature. Heat stress was estimated from the charts of Belding and Hatch.[9] Data recorded included age, diagnosis, environmental conditions, time breakdown, heat stress, and physiologic responses. The subjects with coronary disease were also individually matched with control subjects performing the same job. ECGs were recorded throughout the working day, with telemetry, direct writing, or Holter ambulatory apparatus. The firefighters not only were studied at work but also performed a maximal or supramaximal bicycle exercise test at a later time, while clad in their firefighting clothes, which weighed approximately 31 lbs.

The coronary patients (all men) were found working in all areas of the factory and steel mill, even in some of the most strenuous jobs, and performed fully the duties of the other occupations studied. The surgeons and anesthetists were studied while performing 47 operative procedures in the operating room. The procedures included routine and more sophisticated operations including thoracovascular, general, gynecologic, urologic, and orthopedic surgery.

Comparisons were made between average and peak HRs, blood pressure, caloric expenditure, METs, myocardial oxygen uptake ($M\dot{V}O_2$), oxygen uptake ($\dot{V}O_2$), ratio of $M\dot{V}O_2/\dot{V}O_2$ as the relative cost of $M\dot{V}O_2$, and body $\dot{V}O_2$ responses at work and those of exercise tests. The average and peak HR costs of work were also expressed as percentages of age-predicted maximal HR or peak HR attained during exercise testing. The measured energy requirements at work were compared with those estimated from the HR at work on the basis of the demonstrated linear relationship of HR to external work and $\dot{V}O_2$ in exercise tests, (the method of equivalence).

Table 30-5 lists the physical characteristics of 333 subjects studied on the job. The functional aerobic capacities, based on multistage exercise tests, were low in all subjects except the firefighters.

Table 30-6 lists the average and peak HR, blood pressure, and $M\dot{V}O_2$. The mean average and mean peak caloric expenditure ranged between 2.0 and 2.5 calories/min in the factory and in the operating room. The mean expenditure in the steel mill was higher, at 2.5 calories/min, with an average peak expenditure of 4.05 calories/min. The factory workers, health professionals, and businessmen expended between 1.5 and 2.0 METs, and the steelworkers up to 3 METs (Figs. 30-2 and 30-3). These levels of energy expenditure correspond to low levels of exercise testing: less than walking on a treadmill at 2.0 mph on a 3.5% grade, or for one or two minutes at 1.7 mph on a 10% grade, or pedaling on a bicycle ergometer at less than 300 kpm/min.

The mean HRs at work were generally below 100 bpm. The mean peak heart rate value (the highest recorded at any time for each individual) was less than 120 bpm, except for occasional television performers while on the air and firefighters and steelworkers who were exposed to high heat stress and high energy expenditure.

The energy expenditures for the coronary patients and control subjects were not statistically different. The cardiac patients tended to have a slightly higher systolic blood pressure at rest than did the control subjects (136 versus 122 mmHg) and at peak work (153 versus 134 mmHg). This was significant at the 0.02 level.

Different jobs required different patterns of energy expenditure. In each job, the magnitude and duration of energy expenditure and sequence of tasks were consistent and were not modified by the presence of heart disease. Two basic patterns were observed: (1) a low rate of energy expenditure maintained fairly steadily; and (2) high peaks of energy expenditure alternating with inactive periods (Fig. 30-4).

The majority of jobs studied resembled the low energy pattern. The workers took an average of nine to ten breaks during the working shift for an average total of almost 2 hours. This time included rest periods and meals but not time away from work necessitated by the study procedures. Again, no significant difference in the frequency or duration of rest periods was noted between the cardiac workers and the control subjects.

The ECG changes in the coronary patients and in the control groups were similar, except for ventricular premature beats during work, occurring only in the coronary group.

Table 30-5. On-the-Job Study: Physical Features

Occupation	No. of Subjects	N	HD	Height (cm)	Weight (kg)	BSA (m²)	Age (yrs)	$\dot{V}_{O_2}$ max (ml O₂/kg BW)	FAC (%)
Factory worker[a]	62	26	36	177.8	76.0	1.86 (.15)	HD 50.6 (9.4) N 41.5 (12.3)	33.2[b]	90
Steel mill worker[a]	53	33	20	179.1	78.3	1.96 (.13)	HD 50 (9.0) N 37.4 (9.0)		
Surgeon[a]	39	32	7	181.4 (2.8)	80.9 (8.2)	1.995 (.118)	40.7 (10.0)	28.5	72
Anesthetist	26	19	7	174.8 (5.0)	75.7 (9.8)	1.93 (.17)	36.3 (6.7)	26.7	67
Firefighter	105	105	0	180.4 (.55)	87.3 (1.04)	2.05 (.12)	40.3 (.75)	33.7 (0.64)	86
Broadcaster	33	31	2	177.8 (6.6)	77.4 (4.7)	1.94 (.15)	35.0 (9.0)		
Businessperson	15	0	15	179.6 (3.8)	78.7 (2.8)	1.98	53.4 (10.0)	27.5	76
Total	333	246	87						

[a] Oxygen uptake measured on the job.
[b] Assumed.
    Abbreviations: N, normal; HD, heart disease; FAC, functional aerobic capacity; BW, body weight; BSA, body surface area.
    (From Hellerstein,[16] with permission.)

Table 30-6. On-the-Job Study of Hemodynamics and Aerobic Requirements

Occupation	On-the-Job HR Average	Peak	Blood Pressure Average	Peak	cal/min Rest	Average	Peak	L/min Average	Peak	$\dot{V}_{O_2}$ Avg Peak (L/min)	Avg Peak (ml O₂/ kg/min)
Factory worker	102	122	136/81	153/89	HD 1.34 N 1.30	2.03 1.97	2.38 2.29	.406	.476	5.3	6.3
Steel mill worker	87	158[a]			1.34	2.51	4.05	.502	.810	6.4	10.3
Broadcaster	92	116	126/81	136/89							
Businessperson	82	103				2.01	2.32	.401	.464	5.1	5.9
Anesthetist	83	108	121/79	140/86		1.98	2.08	.397	.416	5.2	5.5
Firefighter	89	140	116/80	156/108							
Surgeon	104	118	132/84	147/92	1.42	2.12	2.41	.425	.482	5.3	6.0

[a] Average of 17 patients.
    Abbreviations: HR, heart rate; HD, heart disease; N, normal.
    (From Hellerstein,[16] with permission.)

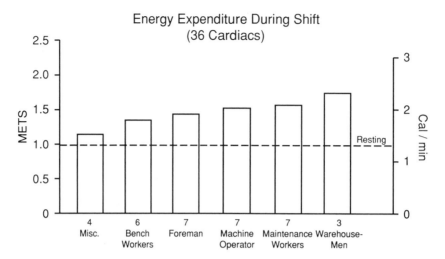

Fig. 30-2. Average energy expenditure of individual jobs performed by 36 workers (2 not shown) with CHD during an 8-hour shift in a factory. Note the increasing energy expenditure as progressively larger muscle groups are used. The same pattern was evident in the control group. (From Ford and Hellerstein,[8] and Ford et al,[9] with permission.

Pulse Rate. In the factory, the average pulse rate increased from 84 bpm at rest to an average of 102 bpm during work. Sinus tachycardia (over 110 bpm) occurred in an equal number of control and cardiac subjects. Tachycardias were disproportionate to the rate of energy expenditure, since tachycardia occurred at energy rates of 1.8 to 4.3 cal/min. In the factory, working pulse rate in excess of 120 bpm suggested sustained anxiety or limited cardiovascular reserve (Fig. 30-5). In contrast, in the steel mill, where the heat stress was considerably higher, there was a rough correlation between the rate of working energy expenditure and pulse rates at low heat stress. At

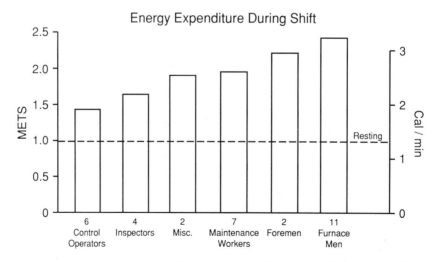

Fig. 30-3. Average energy expenditure of individual jobs performed by 32 workers with coronary heart disease during an 8-hour shift in a steel mill. Note the increasing caloric expenditure in jobs requiring walking, climbing, and lifting.[9] (From Ford et al,[9] with permission.)

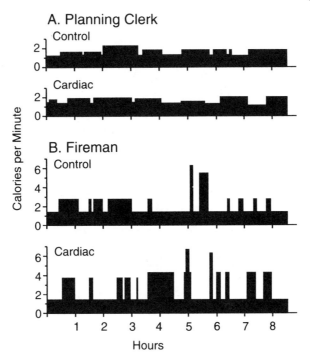

Fig. 30-4. Patterns of energy expenditure during work shifts for two types of jobs performed by workers with CHD and by matched control subjects in a factory. (**A**) Low rate of energy expenditure maintained steadily. (**B**) Intermittent high peaks of energy expenditure alternating with inactive periods. No significant difference is seen in the frequency or duration of rest periods and breaks in a comparison of the coronary workers with control subjects. (From Ford and Hellerstein,[8] with permission.)

high heat stress, the pulse rate tended to be higher for a given rate of energy expenditure, which is consistent with the effects of heat stress.[9,31] Respiratory rates at rest and at peak effort were 17 per minute and 26 per minute, respectively, with no difference between the coronary and control groups in the factory or in the steel mill.

ELEVATED BLOOD PRESSURE RESPONSES AT WORK

In our study, the peak blood pressure responses at work rarely approached or exceeded those obtained at high submaximal or peak exercise testing. In the subjects monitored during work, at the factory, steel mill, radio or television station, or operating room (surgeons and anesthetists), blood pressure responses were more

characteristic of individuals than of the job situation. Blood pressure rose transiently into a hypertension classification (more than 160/95 mmHg) in 22.0% of anesthetists, 25.6% of surgeons, 30.1% of steelworkers, and 69.0% of firefighters.[27]

In our study of 105 firefighters, 10.0% of subjects had values that could be classified as hypertensive while at rest in the firehouse or while in the exercise laboratory. Hypertensive responses occurred in 69.0% of the normotensive subjects during firefighting. The elevation of blood pressure during high physical and emotional stress cannot, thus, be indicative of hypertension per se. The cardiovascular responses of firefighters were considered to be due to a combination of physical effort, external and internal heat load (heat-conserving fire clothes), and exposure to noxious fumes, as well as, in a few instances, some degree of physical fitness. It has been well demonstrated that physically unfit sub-

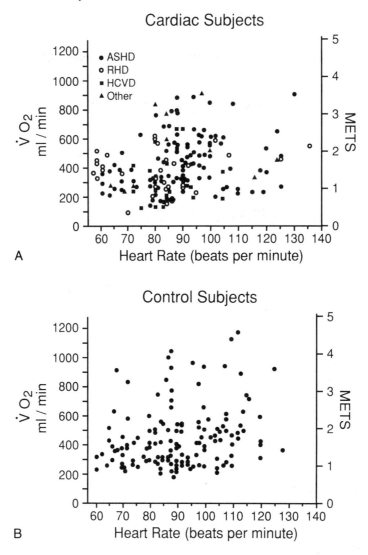

Fig. 30-5. (**A**) Pulse rate and oxygen consumption: 157 observations on 36 subjects with heart disease during a work shift in a factory.[8] (**B**) Pulse rate and oxygen consumption: 144 observations on 26 control subjects during the work shift in the same factory. These figures show a poor correlation between pulse rate and oxygen consumption, both for control and cardiac subjects. At these relatively low levels of exertion other factors such as emotion, temperature, and inter-individual variation influence pulse rate so greatly as to make it useless as a criterion of energy expenditure at work. See text for further discussion. (From Ford and Hellerstein,[8] with permission.)

jects have higher blood pressures relative to the external work performed.

The question may be raised as to what value should be ascribed to the elevation of blood pressure at work. Pickering et al. used the ninetieth percentile as the upper limit when investigating ambulatory blood pressure ranges in normal subjects.[32] With 1.5 standard deviations of the upper limit of normal, the peak blood pressure for many normal subjects reached or exceeded 145/90. This occurred particularly in subjects who were in their 50s, 60s, and 70s.[33] Ambulatory blood pressure monitoring of normal subjects has revealed that a significant percentage of individuals attain blood pressure values at or above 1.5 to 2.0 standard deviations above the so-called upper limits of normal. Thus, an important question as yet unanswered concerns the value that should be considered the maximal allowable value designated as normotensive.

OCCUPATIONAL WORK DEMANDS AND FUNCTIONAL STATUS

Automation and mechanization have markedly reduced energy demands of all occupational work during the past 30 years. Thus, only 5% of patients now perform "heavy" occupational work as compared with 65 percent in the 1950s.[34] Rarely does a contemporary worker have peak caloric expenditure of as much as 4 cal/min. In general, in a great variety of jobs, the peak caloric expenditure is less than 3 cal/min. Müller and Franz have estimated that the endurance limit of regular daily work for normal subjects averaged 5 cal/min.[35] However, the majority of modern industrial work jobs require average energy expenditure at half that rate or less. Patients convalescing from an acute myocardial infarction, who are able to wash, shave, and dress (approximately 3 cal/min, 2 METs), walk around the block at 6.6 cal/min (5 METs) are, in all probability, expending as much energy at home as they would at work. Recognition by the physician of the relatively high energy cost of such simple ordinary activities will enable the physician to advise the patient to resume work, without fear of overtaxing the heart.

The inability to perform 5 METs of exercise without developing either ischemic ST changes on the ECG or arrhythmias has been used as a criterion by the Social Security Administration for disability evaluation.[17] Such subjects would be classified as being in the high-risk category.[4] However, some patients with impaired left ventricular function can have relatively well-preserved exercise capacity and may be capable of gainful employment in occupations that require

energy expenditures consistent with those found in the factory, business or management, and many other professions. Often, a simple adjustment or job modification can be made to eliminate a single peak-energy load that would otherwise make a job impossible. For example, a fellow worker might tighten a lathe chuck or lift heavy parts into place for the worker who could not expend 5 or 6 METs. If indicated, a brief conference with an employer or with a labor representative can allow for a relatively simple change in working conditions that make a job more suitable.

REALISTIC EXERCISE TESTS FOR WORK PRESCRIPTION

On-the-job evaluations, of both normal subjects and coronary and other cardiac patients, have provided valuable insight into the magnitude and types of stresses and the responses to them in a variety of occupations. Exercise tests of coronary patients have been used to evaluate their aerobic capacity and hemodynamic responses to known energy expenditures, and to provide a basis for work recommendations, (Table 30-2) risk stratification[4], and eligibility for Social Security disability benefits when certain abnormalities occur at 5 or less METs.[17] When the functional capacity is related to the energy demands of various jobs, specific work classifications can be made for sedentary, light, medium work. A comparison of these stresses with those imposed during standardized exercise tests reveals such marked differences as to challenge the unreserved use of standard exercise tests in formulating a work prescription.[36]

Occupational physical stresses or energy expenditures are often of low or submaximal muscular effort and of brief duration, and they are rarely sustained at high levels for more than 2 or 3 minutes.[36] That is, they are intermittent rather than continuous (Fig. 30-4). Work is characteristic, with rest or relative rest characterizing 30 to 45% of a work shift.[8,9] The subjects at work perform their muscular effort while fully clad, often after the ingestion of food, coffee, tobacco, and prescribed medications, etc., in contrast to the controlled setting of an exercise laboratory. Major muscles in the upper extremities, rather than in the lower extremities, are called upon more extensively at work than at traditional exercise testing. The physical and emotional environments are rarely as well-controlled at work or during leisure activities as in the exercise laboratory. Extremes of temperature, noises and dust, mental, intellectual, and cognitive demands, interpersonal relationships, deadlines and supervision, monetary and other societal pressures, rather than aerobic work expenditures, constitute the major occupational stresses in most societies.

Contemporary exercise tests thus rarely simulate real-life situations. Standard exercise test conditions of prior sleep, relative fasting, privacy, controlled temperature, graded submaximal or maximal effort primarily of the lower extremities, considerate and trained personnel, safety provisions, etc., have many advantages, especially those of reproducibility and of quantitative assessment of cardiovascular function. However, their extrapolation to real-life settings is limited.

The aerobic stresses of most exercise tests exceed those required by most occupations in Western societies and fail to account for many of the other important determinants of successful performance at work cited above.[36] Few occupations require as much as 50% of a worker's aerobic capacity.[8,9]

Information obtained at exercise testing, however, has some relevance to work performance in gauging realistic ranges of anticipated aerobic activities.[36] In addition, clinical exercise tests have diagnostic and prognostic value in detecting objective evidence of myocardial ischemia and potentially life-endangering ventricular arrhythmia. They can also quantitate aerobic and chronotropic capacities under controlled conditions. For example, the occurrence of complex ventricular arrhythmia and of ECG ST-T displacement during exercise testing is predictive of similar changes at work of similar intensity.[27] Exercise tests are often more sensitive than on-the-job observations because characteristically they exceed the energy demands of most types of work. For example, in our study of firefighters, the physi-

ologic responses during maximal exercise testing in the laboratory exceeded the maximal responses on the job of 80 to 85% of the subjects.[27] However, in the remainder, the heart rate, blood pressure, and double product exceeded those in the exercise laboratory due to the combined effects of extremes of heat, dust, fumes, physical effort, realistic life-threatening hazards, and the heat-retaining effects of the fire clothes and mask in the midst of a working fire.[27]

Modifications of present exercise testing techniques can enhance their value in meaningful vocational counseling.[36] Exercise and other stress testing may be expanded to include (1) standardized effort for diagnostic and quantitative purpose; (2) reality stress testing, with one or more stresses in various combinations, designed to simulate an anticipated work situation[37] (this could include stresses of effort of muscle groups used on the job, cold, heat, noise, food, problem-solving, mental stress tests,[38–47] simulated work tests[48] [see Ch. 28], and decision-making); and (3) situational testing (on-the-job evaluations that can be performed either indirectly with automatic portable equipment to record ECGs and blood pressure or with direct monitoring of these components, as well as by direct measurements of oxygen uptake and job performance, as discussed earlier).

Thus, standard exercise tests must be considered as having limited value in the formulation of work recommendations. Occupational stresses differ in type and magnitude from those imposed at exercise testing. Cardiovascular responses to muscular work differ from those in exercise tests, where heart rate, blood pressure, and minute ventilation increase linearly with increasing effort and oxygen uptake. At work, the combined effects of emotions, heat or other environmental stress, and a generally low caloric expenditure are encountered. Abnormal responses to standard, high-intensity exercise tests rarely preclude working, at most jobs.

The present status of mental stress tests in the laboratory has similarly limited applicability in work prescription or proscription. Currently, popular mental stress tests include mental arithmetic, consisting of 3 to 10 minutes of rapid, urgent, 59-serial subtractions (for example, 17 from 1,013 until 10 is reached and repeated, etc.) and interactive concentration tasks (combination of problem-solving, concentration, and rapid psychomotor performance).[40] These tests reliably induce modest increases in heart rate (10 to 15 bpm),[40,41] and blood pressure (10 to 25 mmHg systolic, and 5 to 15 mmHg diastolic)[40,41] in most coronary patients; and they reliably induce regional wall motion abnormalities and myocardial perfusion deficits and ischemia (often silent), in 15 to 44% of subjects,[42,43] particularly those with *both* resting and exercise-induced ischemia,[42] apparently related to a primary reduction in coronary blood flow.[42] The hemodynamic changes during mental stress tests are relatively trivial compared to those occurring during standard exercise tests, and are generally comparable to walking at a casual pace at work or elsewhere.

The yield of abnormal responses of patients with CHD to mental stress tests varies considerably. In a study of 372 patients,[41] 16% had significant ECG ST segment abnormalities during mental arithmetic and during exercise tests, 57% had them at exercise tests only, and 27 percent had normal ECG ST segment responses to both exercise and mental tests.

Our study of the hemodynamic, metabolic, and ECG responses to a psychologic quiz test[38] showed a consistent increase in diastolic blood pressure and similar increase in heart rate, but with variable ECG responses and, similar to mental stress testing, insensitivity in eliciting evidence of myocardial ischemia in 7 of 42 (17%) men with coronary heart disease. In comparison, 32 of 42 coronary patients (76%) showed ischemic ECG responses to treadmill exercise tests. However, a quiz testing abnormality was highly specific for exercise-induced ST depression; all subjects with quiz-induced ischemic ECG changes showed similar or greater exercise-induced ECG ST depression. The diastolic blood pressure increased 26% at peak quiz but decreased 19% at peak exercise. Although norepinephrine levels increased during both types of tests,[46] the local metabolic changes and vasodilatation in exercising muscles counteracted the vasoconstriction of

the norepinephrine. Although the oxygen uptake at peak exercise increased to 8 METs, the calculated ratio of the myocardial oxygen uptake to the body oxygen uptake ($M\dot{V}O_2/\dot{V}O_2$) decreased from 22.6 at rest to 13.6 at peak effort.[38] In contrast, although the oxygen uptake during the quiz test increased only to 1.2 METs, the $M\dot{V}O_2/\dot{V}O_2$ ratio increased from 22.6 to 40.1 at peak quiz. However, this disproportionate oxygen demand on the myocardium elicited myocardial ischemic ST segment displacement in only a few subjects. Psychologic stress responses differ markedly from those consistently elicited by physical exercise.

Our study of normal and coronary subjects at work with low energy expenditure but with significant cognitive mental and intellectual demands (in the factory, radio and television, business, and the operating room [surgeons, anesthetists], and during marital sexual activity in the privacy of the home[8,9,27]), consistently revealed that the hemodynamic responses were modest and far less than those of standard exercise tests. The peak heart rate in these "stressful" situations rarely exceeded 120 bpm; an exception occurred in several surgeons during trying episodes. An equal percentage of control and coronary subjects developed sinus tachycardia of over 110 bpm (10 of 26 normal and 7 of 36 coronary subjects, considered to be disproportionate to the rate of energy expenditure in the factory). The ECG changes in control and coronary subjects were similar, except that 4 of 36 coronary subjects had rare ventricular premature complexes at work and at submaximal but not maximal exercise tests. Although ventricular arrhythmia was more frequent in the coronary patients at work and in the exercise tests than in the control subjects, in no instance did any subject develop malignant ventricular rhythms similar to those recorded by Lown et al. in their mental and psychological stress study of high-risk coronary patients with a history of previous serious ventricular arrhythmia.[49]

In general, mental and psychological stress responses are consistently of lesser magnitude, more variable and less predictable, and appear to depend in large part upon differences in the symbolic interpretations and attitudes toward the tests. The prognostic significance of such transient myocardial ischemia during mental stress tests in the laboratory is still unclear and remains moot.[45] The validity of mental stress testing to predict work performance or response to therapy remains doubtful at present.[41,44]

In specific cases where there is a question as to whether the mental, cognitive or interpersonal demands are excessive and may provoke significant deleterious ischemia and arrhythmias, ambulatory ECG and blood pressure monitoring at the work site may be indicated. My associates and I observed rare instances in which the rate-pressure product (a measure of myocardial oxygen demand), during emotionally and intellectually stressful situations, approximated that found at peak treadmill exercise of 8 to 9 METs.[27] In such cases, counseling or selective placement was indicated.

The emotional and psychological status (depression, anxiety, fear, and low self-esteem) (see Ch. 28) associated with the advent of clinical CHD may be, in over half of coronary subjects, the primary determinant of return to work (excluding other factors cited previously, such as age, job opportunities, and pension benefits), despite asymptomatic status and adequate aerobic capacity. Precision in recommendations about work and nonwork activities helps dispel myths and unfounded beliefs that even mild exertion is dangerous.[11] The successful performance of a multistage exercise test whose energy demands far exceed those of a specific job may be sufficient to change the patient's perception of personal inadequacy. Further counseling, on-the-job monitoring, and/or psychological therapy (see Ch. 28) may be indicated in relatively few coronary patients.

REFERENCES

1. Barnes GK, Ray MJ, Oberman A et al: Changes in working status of patients following coronary bypass surgery. JAMA 238:1259, 1977
2. Davidson DM: Return to work after cardiac events: A review. J Cardiac Rehabil 3:60, 1983
3. Roskamm H, Golkhe H, Samek L et al: Long-term effect of aortocoronary bypass surgery on exercise tolerance and vocational rehabilitation. p. 10. In Proceedings of II World Congress on Cardiac Rehabilitation: Abstracts of Free Communications. Jerusalem, 1981
4. DeBusk RF: The Stanford University cardiac rehabilitation program. J Myocard Isch 2:28, 1990
5. Dennis C, Houston-Miller N, Schwartz RG et al: Early return to work after uncomplicated myocardial infarction: Results of a randomized trial. JAMA 260:214, 1988
6. Davidson DM, Taylor CB, DeBusk RF: Factors influencing return to work after myocardial infarction or coronary artery bypass surgery. Cardiac Rehabil 10:1, 1979
7. Franklin BA: Getting patients back to work after myocardial infarction or coronary artery bypass surgery. Physician Sports Med 14:183, 1986
8. Ford AB, Hellerstein HK: Work and heart disease I. A physiologic study in the factory. Circulation 18:823, 1958
9. Ford AB, Hellerstein HK, Turell DJ: Work and heart disease II. A physiologic study in a steel mill. Circulation 20:537, 1959
10. Parran TV, Hellerstein HK, Cohen D et al: Results of studies at the Work Classification Clinic of the Cleveland Area Heart Society. p. 330. In Rosenbaum FF, Belknap EL (eds): Work and the Heart. Hoeber, New York, 1959
11. Hellerstein HK, Ford AB: Comprehensive care of the coronary patient. Optimal (intensive) care, recovery, and reconditioning. An opportunity for the physician. Mongraph No. 2, p. 132. In Blumgart H (ed): Symposium on Coronary Heart Disease. 2nd Ed. Vol. 2. American Heart Association, Dallas, 1968.
12. Stamler J: Lectures on Preventive Cardiology. Grune & Stratton, Orlando, FL, 1967, p. 138
13. World Health Organization: Exercise test in relation to cardiovascular function. Report of a WHO meeting. WHO Tech Rep Ser 388, 1968
14. World Health Organization: Expert Committee on Rehabilitation of Cardiovascular Patients. Report. WHO Tech Rep Ser 270, 1964
15. Criteria Committee of the New York Heart Association: Diseases of the Heart and Blood Vessels. Nomenclature and Criteria for Diagnosis. 6th Ed. Little, Brown, Boston, 1964, p. 112
16. Hellerstein HK: Work demands and environmental factors influencing cardiac rehabilitation. Physiologic aspects, physical performance tests, and work responses. In Proceedings of Sixth Interna-

tional Conference on Cardiac Rehabilitation, Cairo, Sept. 18–21, 1977, p. 189, 1980

17. U.S. Department of Health and Human Services, Social Security Administration: Disability Evaluation under Social Security. SSA Publication No. 05-10089, February 1986. Sect. 404.1567, Physical Requirements. 20 CFR, Ch. 111. U.S. Dept. of Health and Human Services, Washington, DC, April 1, 1989

18. U.S. Department of Labor, Employment and Training Administration: Dictionary of Occupational Titles. 4th Ed. U.S. Govt. Printing Office, Washington, DC, 1977

19. Tindall T, Mihayl VP: Directory of Occupational Information. Georgia Southern Press, Athens, GA, 1990

20. University of Wisconsin: Handbook for Analyzing Jobs. Reprint no. 13. Material Development Center, Stout Vocational Rehabilitation Institute, University of Wisconsin—Stout, Menomonie, WI, 1972

21. Field JE, Field TF: Classification of Jobs. Vol. 1. Georgia Southern Press, Athens, GA, 1988

22. Ford AB, Hellerstein HK: Energy cost of the Master two-step test. JAMA 164:1868, 1957

23. Durnin JVG, Passmore R: Energy, work and leisure. Heinemann, London, 1967

24. Poulsen E, Asmussen E: Energy requirements of practical jobs from pulse increase and ergometer test. Ergonomics 5:33, 1962

25. Karpovich PV: Physiology of muscular activity. 4th Ed. WB Saunders, Philadelphia, 1953

26. Fox SM, Naughton JP, Haskell WL: Physical activity and the prevention of coronary heart disease. Ann Clin Res 3:404, 1971

27. Hellerstein HK: Prescription of vocational and leisure activities. Adv Cardiol 24:105, 1978

28. The Rehabilitation of Patients with Cardiovascular Diseases. Report on a Seminar. Noordwijk aan Zee, October 2–7, 1967. Regional Office for Europe. World Health Organization, Copenhagen 1969, EURO 0381

29. Kitamura K, Jorgensen CR, Gobel FL et al: Hemodynamic correlates of myocardial O_2 consumption during upright exercise. J Appl Physiol 32:516, 1972

30. Ford AB, Hellerstein HK: Pulmonary ventilation as an index of energy expenditure. Clin Res Proc 5:227, 1957

31. Christensen EH: Physiological evaluation of work in Nykroppa Iron Works p. 93. In Floyd WF, Welford AT (eds): Symposium on Fatigue. Ergonomics Research Society. HK Lewis, London, 1953

32. Pickering TG, Harshfield GA, Kleinert HD et al: Blood pressure during normal daily activities, sleep, and exercise: Comparison of values in normal and hypertensive subjects. JAMA 247:992, 1982

33. Zachariah PK, Sheps, SG, Bailey KR et al: Age-related characteristics of ambulatory blood pressure load and mean blood pressure in normotensive subjects. JAMA 265:1414, 1991

34. DeBusk RF, Blomqvist CG, Kouchoukos NT et al: Identification and treatment of low-risk patients after acute myocardial infarction and coronary-artery bypass surgery. N Engl J Med 314:161, 1986

35. Müller EA, Franz J: Energieverbrauchsmessungen bei Beruflicher Arbeit mit einer Verbesserten Respirations-gasuhr. Arbeitsphysiologie 14:499, 1952

36. Franklin BA, Hellerstein HK: Realistic stress testing for activity prescription. J Cardiovasc Med 7:570, 1982

37. Hellerstein HK, Franklin BA: Exercise testing and prescription. p. 197. In Wenger NK, Hellerstein HK (eds): Rehabilitation of the Coronary Patient. 2nd Ed. Churchill Livingstone, New York, 1984

38. Franklin BF, Hellerstein HK, Kaimal KO et al: Psychologic vs. exercise stress: comparison of hemodynamic, metabolic and ECG responses. Med Sci Sports Exerc 12:(2)116, 1980

39. Schiffer F, Hartley LH, Schulman CL et al: The Quiz Electrocardiogram: a new diagnostic and research technique for evaluating the relation between emotional stress and ischemic heart disease. Am J Cardiol 37:41, 1976

40. Zotti AM, Bettinardi O, Soffiantino F et al: Psychophysiological stress testing in postinfarction patients. Circ 83 (suppl II):II-25, 1991

41. Specchia G, Falcone C, Traversi E et al: Mental stress as a provocative test in patients with various clinical syndromes of coronary heart disease. Circ 83 (suppl II):II-108, 1991

42. L'Abbate A, Simonetti I, Carpeggiani C et al: Coronary dynamics and mental arithmetic stress in humans. Circ 83 (suppl II):II-94, 1991

43. Giubbini R, Galli M, Campini R et al: Effects of mental stress on myocardial perfusion in patients with ischemic heart disease. Circulation 83 (suppl. II):II-100, 1991

44. Steptoe A, Vogele C: Methodology of mental stress testing in cardiovascular research. Circulation 83 (suppl. II):II-14, 1991

45. Weiner H: Stressful experience and cardiorespiratory disorders. Circulation 83 (suppl. II):II-2, 1991

46. Dimsdale JE, Ziegler MG: What do plasma and urinary measures of catecholamines tell us about human responses to stressors? Circulation 83 (suppl. II):II-36, 1991

47. Gottdiener JS, Krantz DS, Helmers K et al: Silent ischemia induced by mental arousal is not predicted by ambulatory ST segment monitoring. J Am Coll Cardiol 15(2):120A, 1990

48. Sheldahl LM, Wilke NA, Tristani FE et al: Response to repetitive static-dynamic exercise in patients with coronary artery disease. J Cardiopulm Rehabil 5:139, 1985

49. Lown B, Temte JV, Reich P et al: Basis for recurring ventricular fibrillation in the absence of coronary heart disease and its management. N Engl J Med 294:623, 1976

50. Turrell, Hellerstein HK: Evaluation of cardiac function in relation to specific physical activities following recovery from acute myocardial infarction. Postgrad Cardiovasc Dis 1:237, 1958

31

Community Resources for Rehabilitation

Kathy Berra, B.S.N.

Coronary rehabilitation services have become synonymous with an intensive approach to lowering coronary risk factors and enhancing functional capacity in order to decrease morbidity and mortality in persons with known coronary heart disease (CHD). Coronary rehabilitation implies a comprehensive plan of recovery. It includes health education designed to increase knowledge (see Chs. 25, 26, 27); measures to retard or reverse the underlying atherosclerosis (see Chs. 4 and 5); exercise designed to restore and improve functional capacity compatible with a return to usual social, vocational, and occupational interests (see Chs. 20–24, 29, 30); and psychological interventions designed to provide support and encourage "heart-healthy" behaviors (see Ch. 28).[1–10] All of these interventions have the common goal of an improvement in the quality of life of coronary patients.[11–15]

Advances in the medical and surgical management of coronary patients have heralded a new era for coronary rehabilitation. These advances have lengthened the life expectancy of the coronary patient. In addition, they have enhanced the quality of life of the coronary patient through the introduction of new medications, new invasive procedures, and new techniques for the management of angina, arrhythmias, ischemia, and sudden cardiac death.

The purpose of this chapter is to define the role of community resources in providing coronary re-habilitation services. The role of a medical program in a nonmedical facility will be discussed, and appropriate procedures for developing a community-based coronary rehabilitation program will be defined.

HISTORICAL PERSPECTIVES

YMCArdiac Therapy (YCT) was developed in 1970 to address the long-term needs of coronary patients in a cost-effective manner through community-based facilities.[16] YCT was based on the pioneering efforts of successful programs, whose methods and approaches were recognized as safe and effective in this relatively new field of health care. These programs were used as the foundation for the development of a community-based cardiovascular rehabilitation model through the YMCA.*

Why a YMCA, why a Jewish Community Center, why a Junior College for a medical program? The American Heart Association (AHA) estimates

---

* Early leaders in the field, cited alphabetically, included Drs. Joseph Acker, John Boyer, Loring Brock, John Cantwell, Robert DeBusk, Gerald Fletcher, Sam Fox, William Haskell, Herman Hellerstein, Fred Kasch, Albert Kattus, Howard Pyfer, Pate Thomson, Nanette Wenger, and Lenore Zohman.

that 66 million U.S. residents have diseases of the heart and blood vessels.[17] In addition, it was estimated that in 1990 1.5 million would sustain acute myocardial infarction; nearly 300,000 would receive coronary artery bypass graft surgery (CABG)[17]; and well over 150,000 would receive percutaneous transluminal coronary angioplasty (PTCA).[18] There is no lack of potential participants for coronary rehabilitation programs. Why, then, is it estimated that as few as 25% of potential patients actually participate in formal coronary rehabilitation programs?[19] If one considers the enormity of the problem, the numbers of potential participants, the high cost of overhead at most medical facilities, as well as problems of space, location, and the lack of exercise facilities at many medical centers, the need for additional locations for coronary rehabilitation programs seems obvious.

Since 1970 many successful community-based programs have provided coronary rehabilitation services. Their unique contribution to this important field can be seen in their ability to provide long-term, cost-effective approaches to solving the challenge of coronary rehabilitation.

THE CHALLENGE TO THE COMMUNITY

Coronary rehabilitation involves health care professionals from many disciplines.[4] Their professional expertise, their ability to facilitate important coronary risk factor interventions, and their continued surveillance of patients during the rehabilitation process enhance the speed of recovery and the success of long-term lifestyle modifications.[5,7,8,20-33] To most patients, the term "coronary rehabilitation" means exercise. What remains a challenge to persons with coronary disease and to health care professionals is the maintenance of new behaviors, beyond exercise, that will promote heart health over a lifetime. There are many of these new behaviors for some patients and only a few for others. They include

1. Taking medications daily for an indefinite period. (Complex regimens are often required.)

2. Giving up smoking for life.
3. Being aware of the long-term effects of certain foods on cholesterol, triglyceride, and blood sugar levels; on sodium intake; and on weight.
4. Being willing to exchange old, comfortable food habits for new and healthier food habits for life.
5. Learning new ways to respond during times of acute stress, and learning how to manage stressful situations.
6. Becoming a patient in an often confusing and frustrating health care system.
7. Accepting the importance of regular aerobic exercise, and finding exercise routines that are enjoyable as well as safe and effective.
8. Knowing how to evaluate the signals received from the body, especially the heart, and knowing when to ask for help.
9. Managing coexisting health problems.
10. Seeing themselves as an active partner in their health care, together with their physician, family, and friends.

In considering the many demands that face coronary patients, can health care providers expect such important lifestyle changes to occur in the 8 to 12 weeks designated by many third-party payors as adequate for coronary rehabilitation? Community-based programs can offer long-term, cost-effective interventions that are safe and efficacious. They have a unique advantage in being able to provide

1. A healthy atmosphere for persons with chronic illness.
2. A sense of community participation through membership in a community center.
3. The ability to draw from patient populations over a wide geographic area.
4. The ability to provide services to many individuals who would not have been referred had the program been offered by competing hospitals or clinics.
5. A medical advisory committee involving local experts regardless of their specific clinic or hospital affiliation.
6. Facilities such as outdoor exercise areas, pools, large gymnasiums, lockers, showers, and meeting areas.

7. Programs for families and group activities.
8. A not-for-profit corporation that can provide low-cost, high-quality health care services and scholarship subsidies.

The goals and objectives of community programs do not differ significantly from those of hospital- or clinic-based programs. They generally have an open-ended enrollment that allows patients to participate for longer periods. They usually serve larger numbers of patients per session because of their facilities. They provide health education and coronary risk factor intervention programs run by health care professionals from the community, in addition to the program staff. As cardiovascular technology advances, with resultant decreases in the duration of hospitalization and fewer admissions, our ability to "capture" the coronary audience is constantly being challenged.[34-37] The need to provide intensive rehabilitation services, especially risk factor intervention, remains. However, with earlier return to work and to usual lifestyles, the coronary patient needs options including home-based rehabilitation, rehabilitation programs at the work site, and community-based rehabilitation programs for optimal care.[14,38-44]

PROGRAM DESIGN

Administration

In designing a community-based program, it is important to assess the goals and objectives of the organization, as well as the needs of the community, the facility, and other available supportive services.[14]

The goals of the organization should include a commitment to the maintenance of health through lifestyle intervention programs. They should also include an awareness of the importance of interrelationships of the family, the social, and the work environments in the maintenance of health.

An assessment of community needs will provide critical information about the potential success of a rehabilitation program. Important questions to ask are

1. Is there a perceived lack of long-term lifestyle intervention programs for persons with CHD in the community?
2. Does the medical community support such programs?
3. Is your organization acknowledged as a provider of adult health enhancement programs?

The facility itself also contributes to a successful program. Items of concern regarding facilities include

1. Is the location convenient, with easy access? This becomes more critical if the population served includes individuals with physical handicaps.
2. Are the times available for exercise and educational sessions convenient to the population being served? Offering programs early in the morning and later in the evening to span the workday will increase the number of participants who can use rehabilitation services.
3. Is space available for group and individual educational sessions?
4. Are appropriate amenities such as showers and lockers available for use by participants following exercise sessions?

If the community facility can provide the space and the support services, and if the community supports such a program, an important step in the developmental phase is the establishment of a medical advisory committee. The purpose of the medical advisory committee is to provide the following:

1. Support for medical staff in a nonmedical facility.
2. Input regarding policies and procedures.
3. Evaluation of program goals and objectives.
4. Expertise in the multidisciplinary functions of the coronary rehabilitation program.
5. A referral base for patients.

The medical advisory committee is responsible for the control of the quality of medical care. It should include members of the community who have expertise in areas relevant to coronary rehabilitation. These encompass psychologists, exercise physiologists, nutritionists, physicians, nurses, social workers, and others, such as rep-

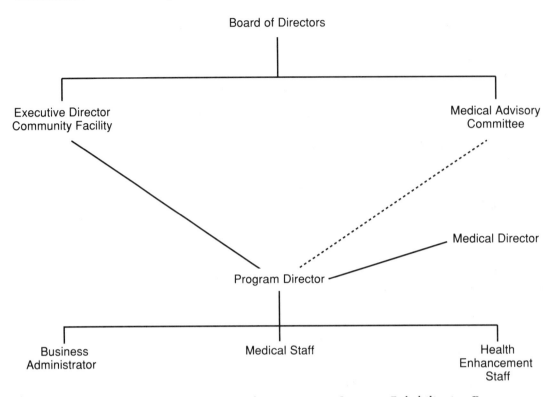

Fig. 31-1. Scheme for Administration of a Community Coronary Rehabilitation Program

resentatives from the AHA. This group acts as a liaison with the medical community to provide credibility for the program. It is advisable that the committee consist of a broad range of physicians, representing community hospitals, clinics, and other medical groups. Figure 31-1 describes an organizational model.

Patient Services and Program Entry

The patient population served by community-based programs will include those with a wide variety of diagnoses. These diagnoses include, but are not limited to, patients who have experienced unstable angina, myocardial infarction, CABG, PTCA, heart transplantation, heart failure, life-threatening arrhythmias, automatic implantable cardioverter defibrillators (ICDs), valvular surgery, and other medical and surgical interventions. The type of patient appropriate for a community facility will be based upon the abil-

ity of the facility to provide close supervision and other supportive services such as advanced cardiac life support (ACLS). The overall risk of participation in coronary rehabilitation programs is very low.[45–50] Procedures designed to evaluate the stability of cardiovascular signs and symptoms and to educate patients prior to entry into a rehabilitation program are the foundations of patient safety. There are several important steps in the maintenance of patient safety in community rehabilitation programs. These are discussed below.

Referral Data and Entry Criteria

Referral data should include information regarding cardiac procedures, hospitalization course, historical summaries of cardiovascular and other medical conditions, and current data on known coronary risk factors (Fig. 31-2). Referral data should also include a recent resting electrocardiogram (ECG) and results of a *current* maximal or high submaximal sign- or symptom-limited ex-

Patient's Name _____

I. Cardiovascular Diagnoses (check if positive):

❐ Myocardial infarction   Date _____   Hospital _____

❐ Transmural   ❐ Subendocardial   ❐ Inferior   ❐ Anterior   ❐ Lateral

Complications _____

❐ Angina pectoris, stable for at least 3 months   ❐ PCTA _____

❐ Unstable angina pectoris. Date _____   ❐ Arrhythmia. Kind _____

❐ Coronary by-pass surgery. Date _____   ❐ Abnormal exercise test

❐ Hospital _____   ❐ Essential hypertension

❐ Other _____   ❐ Arteriosclerosis obliterans

II. Most recent laboratory data: (Please fill in blanks or attach this information)

	Chol.	HDL	LDL	Trigly.	Blood Sugar	K +	Chest X-ray
Result							
Date							

III. Other significant medical diagnoses _____

_____

IV. Current medications, including dose

_____

_____

Please enclose copies of:

1. Hospital discharge summary following MI/unstable AP/CABG/PTCA.
2. Patient's most recent ECG/Treadmill Test.
3. Report of coronary arteriography.
4. Report of coronary artery bypass surgery.
5. Report of long-term arrhythmic monitoring.

I agree to have my patient participate in the YMCArdiac Therapy Program. I have no reason to believe that an exercise stress test nor any individually prescribed therapeutic exercise program based on that test will be harmful to my patient.

I agree to have my patient counseled in measures designed to lower coronary risk factors.

I agree to continue the regular care of my patient throughout the participation in YMCArdiac Therapy.

Signature _____ MD

Date _____

Fig. 31-2. Sample Physician Referral Form (Courtesy of YMCArdiac Therapy.)

ercise test. Also included should be information about current medications, recommended dosages, and schedule of administration. As part of the referral process, the referring physician should be made aware of the circumscribed role of the rehabilitation program in the total care of the patient. The referring physician remains the critical manager of the long-term care of the patient. The program should not be viewed as a threat to the integrity of the referring physician–patient relationship. The program services are defined as therapeutic exercise, health education, and coronary risk factor intervention and education. The quality of communication between the rehabilitation program director and the referring physician is often the key component to a successful rehabilitation program. Referring physicians should be continually informed of the progress of their patients and of problems that occur. In addition, patients must understand that the program does not supplant the usual and continuing care received from their physician. An integral part of the referral data is an acknowledgment on the part of the patients that they intend to participate fully in the rehabilitative process, including coronary risk factor intervention as well as therapeutic exercise (Fig. 31-3).

Intake Evaluation

The intake evaluation includes appropriate testing and evaluation of cardiovascular function, psychosocial function, attitudes about rehabilitative care, and evaluation of coronary risk factors. Cardiovascular tests and laboratory procedures can be performed by the rehabilitation program or can be accepted as part of the data provided by the referring physician. Assessment of noncardiovascular health information is also important. These data include information about the stability of coexisting medical conditions, such as hypothyroidism, diabetes mellitus, or chronic pulmonary disease.

A key component of the intake evaluation is a review of the participant's self-reported medical history (Fig. 31-4). It is through this approach that the patient's knowledge regarding the cardiovascular history can be assessed, information regarding other potential medical or orthopedic complications from the patient's perspective can

be reviewed, and the importance of the patient's perceptions of and attitudes to participation in the rehabilitative process can be ascertained.

The initial medical history need not be complex. It should be used as a tool to elicit discussion with the patient and is valuable in establishing initial communication. At the same time, a physical examination to rule out unstable conditions should also be performed. The medical director provides the important final acknowledgment of patient stability. It is not unusual for coronary patients to have been seen by their regular physician within the weeks immediately preceding their desire to join a rehabilitation program and, in the interim, to develop unstable conditions such as atrial fibrillation, ventricular arrhythmias, or worsened angina. In summary, the intake evaluation should include a review of the self-reported medical history, a comprehensive physical examination to establish cardiovascular stability, performance of exercise testing, and evaluation of coronary risk factors.

Intake Education

The educational process can begin following the intake evaluation. The education of the coronary patient has been covered in depth in Chapters 26 and 27. The emphasis here is the importance of a comprehensive approach to coronary risk factor education, including

1. Acknowledgment of personal risk factors.
2. Identification of appropriate and acceptable interventions for each individual patient.
3. The use of contracts, reward, and relapse prevention techniques as a method of confirming commitment and giving patients tools with which they have a greater chance of succeeding with the necessary interventions.

SELF-MONITORING SKILLS

A unique component of the education of the coronary patient is the development of self-monitoring skills for use during therapeutic exercise and in daily life. These self-monitoring skills include the awareness and assessment of angina,

I hereby agree to participate in YMCArdiac Therapy in an attempt to lessen my coronary risk factors. I understand the program is being undertaken because of evidence that such endeavor lessens the possibility of recurrent heart attacks.

I understand that YMCArdiac Therapy is in no way a substitute for the medical care rendered by my personal physician. I hereby authorize YMCArdiac Therapy to release to my physician information about my progress in the program. I also authorize YMCArdiac Therapy to request information about my health from my personal physician and/or any hospital where I have received care.

I agree to attend the exercise sessions as scheduled. I also agree to attend those Risk Factor Clinics prescribed by the program director, in agreement with my personal physician.

I agree to be responsible for the payment each month of the fees incurred in the program during that month. I understand that my payment of the monthly fees is not dependent upon my reimbursement by my medical health insurance policy, but is solely my responsibility.

Date _____

_____
Signature of Applicant

_____
Print Name of Applicant

_____
Address

_____
City

(   ) _____ (   ) _____
Telephone (Home)   (Work)

_____
Name of Personal Physician

_____
Address

_____
City   State   Zip

(   ) _____
Telephone

Fig. 31-3. Sample Application Form for Participant in a Community Coronary Rehabilitation Program (Courtesy of YMCArdiac Therapy.)

INITIAL MEDICAL HISTORY

CARDIOVASCULAR HISTORY

HAVE YOU HAD: (PLEASE CIRCLE)

1. A HEART ATTACK?
   IF YES, DATE(S): _____   YES   NO

2. UNSTABLE ANGINA PECTORIS?
   IF YES, DATE(S): _____   YES   NO

3. RHEUMATIC HEART DISEASE?
   IF YES, DATE(S): _____   YES   NO

4. CONGENITAL HEART DISEASE?
   IF YES, WHAT?: _____   YES   NO

5. A HEART MURMUR?   YES   NO

6. CORONARY ARTERIOGRAPHY?
   IF YES, DATE(S): _____   YES   NO

7. CARDIAC PACEMAKER?
   IF YES, WHEN?: _____   YES   NO

8. CORONARY ARTERY BYPASS SURGERY?
   IF YES, DATE(S): _____   YES   NO

9. CARDIAC VALVE REPLACEMENT?
   IF YES, DATE(S): _____   YES   NO

10. ANGIOPLASTY (PTCA)?
    IF YES, DATE(S): _____   YES   NO

11. ATHERECTOMY?
    IF YES, DATE(S): _____   YES   NO

12. SURGERY ON ARTERIES OTHER THAN YOUR HEART?
    IF YES, DATE(S): _____   YES   NO

13. OTHER CARDIOVASCULAR PROCEDURES?
    IF YES, PLEASE DESCRIBE: YES   NO

    _____

    _____

Fig. 31-4. Sample Form for Patient's Report of Medical History

14. HAVE YOU EVER HAD PAIN, PRESSURE, TIGHTNESS, BURNING, ACHING, OR OTHER TYPE OF DISCOMFORT IN YOUR CHEST, NECK, JAW, SHOULDERS, BACK, OR ARMS?

                                                                   YES   NO

(IF NO, PLEASE GO TO QUESTION NUMBER 27)

15. WHEN DID YOU FIRST EXPERIENCE THIS DISCOMFORT?
DATE:

16. HAVE YOU HAD THIS DISCOMFORT IN THE PAST THREE MONTHS?

                                                                   YES   NO

17. IS YOUR DOCTOR AWARE THAT YOU HAVE THIS DISCOMFORT?

                                                                   YES   NO

18. IS THERE *MORE* OR *LESS* DISCOMFORT IF YOU PRESS ON YOUR CHEST, ARMS, NECK, OR BACK WHEN YOU HAVE THE DISCOMFORT?

                                                           MORE   LESS

19. DOES THE DISCOMFORT WORSEN WITH A DEEP BREATH?

                                                                   YES   NO

20. DOES THE DISCOMFORT WORSEN WITH, OR CHANGE WITH, CERTAIN BODY POSITIONS?

                                                                   YES   NO

21. DURING THE PAST THREE MONTHS, HAS THIS DISCOMFORT OCCURRED

	YES	NO
WITH PHYSICAL EFFORT	____	____
WITH EMOTIONAL UPSET	____	____
WITH EXPOSURE TO COLD	____	____
WITH OR JUST AFTER MEALS	____	____
SPONTANEOUSLY	____	____

22. THIS DISCOMFORT IS RELIEVED BY

	YES	NO
REST	____	____
NITROGLYCERINE	____	____
OTHER MEDICATION	____	____

23. THIS DISCOMFORT OCCURS
____ TIMES PER DAY
____ TIMES PER WEEK
____ TIMES PER MONTH

24. PLEASE GRADE THE USUAL INTENSITY OF YOUR DISCOMFORT ON THIS SCALE OF 1–4.
GRADE 1 = ONSET OF THE DISCOMFORT
GRADE 2 = MORE INTENSE
GRADE 3 = INCREASING INTENSITY
GRADE 4 = WORST DISCOMFORT YOU HAVE EVER EXPERIENCED
THE USUAL GRADE OF MY DISCOMFORT IS _____.

Fig. 31-4 *(continued)*

25. PLEASE INDICATE ON THIS DIAGRAM WHERE YOUR DISCOMFORT IS LOCATED

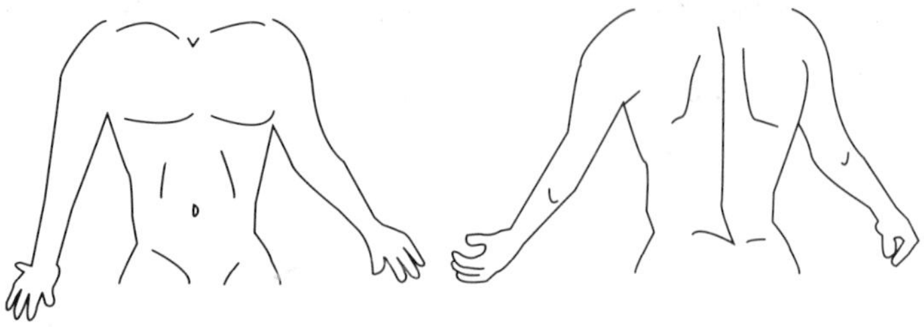

26. PLEASE DESCRIBE YOUR DISCOMFORT IN YOUR OWN WORDS:

_____

_____

SCORE _____

ABNORMAL HEART RHYTHMS

27. DURING THE PAST YEAR, HAVE YOU HAD ANY ABNORMAL HEART RHYTHMS?
(SKIPS OR RAPID HEART RATES)   YES   NO

(IF NO, GO TO QUESTION NUMBER 29.)
IF YES, WHAT WAS YOUR DOCTOR'S DIAGNOSIS?

_____

IF YES, WERE YOU GIVEN ANY MEDICATIONS TO TREAT THIS ABNORMAL HEART
RHYTHM?   YES   NO

IF YES, PLEASE NAME THEM:

_____

28. THIS ABNORMAL RHYTHM OCCURS   YES   NO

	YES	NO
DURING EXERCISE	___	___
AFTER EXERCISE	___	___
UNRELATED TO EXERCISE	___	___
DURING SLEEP AND AWAKENS YOU	___	___
AND MAKES YOU DIZZY OR LIGHTHEADED	___	___
WITH ALCOHOL	___	___
WITH EMOTIONAL UPSET	___	___
WITH COFFEE, TEA, OR CAFFEINATED FOOD	___	___
OR DRINKS	___	___
WITH FATIGUE	___	___
OTHER	___	___

SCORE ____

Fig. 31-4 *(continued)*

CONGESTIVE HEART FAILURE

29. HAVE YOU EVER HAD ANY OF THE FOLLOWING SYMPTOMS?

	AT ANY TIME		IN THE LAST THREE MONTHS	
	YES	NO	YES	NO
SHORTNESS OF BREATH THAT HAS AWAKENED YOU FROM SLEEP	____	____	____	____
UNDUE OR UNEXPECTED BREATHLESSNESS OR FATIGUE DURING EXERTION	____	____	____	____
SWELLING OF BOTH ANKLES THAT WAS PRESENT ON MORNING WAKENING	____	____	____	____
SUDDEN UNEXPLAINED WEIGHT GAIN	____	____	____	____

STROKE OR IMPENDING STROKE

30. HAVE YOU EVER HAD DIFFICULTY SPEAKING COMBINED WITH WEAKNESS OF AN ARM OR LEG?   YES   NO
(IF NO, GO TO QUESTION NUMBER 34)
IF YES, WHEN: _____

31. HAVE YOU EVER HAD THESE SYMPTOMS OCCUR ABRUPTLY, THEN CLEAR COM-PLETELY: DIFFICULTY SPEAKING OR SEEING, WEAKNESS OR CLUMSINESS OF AN ARM OR LEG?   YES   NO
IF YES, WHEN? _____
IF YES, HAVE ANY OF THESE SYMPTOMS OCCURRED WITH EXERCISE?
          YES   NO

32. HAVE YOU EVER BEEN TOLD THAT YOU HAVE HAD A STROKE?
          YES   NO

33. HAVE YOU EVER BEEN TOLD THAT YOU HAVE HAD A TRANSIENT ISCHEMIC ATTACK?   YES   NO

INTERMITTENT CLAUDICATION

34. HAVE YOU EVER HAD MUSCLE ACHING IN EITHER YOUR BUTTOCK OR LEGS THAT OCCURS WITH WALKING AND IS RELIEVED WITH LESS THAN TEN MINUTES OF REST? (IF NO, GO TO QUESTION NUMBER 36)   YES   NO
IF YES, WHERE DOES THIS DISCOMFORT OCCUR?

	BUTTOCK	THIGH	CALF
RIGHT	_____	_____	____
LEFT	_____	_____	____

35. IF YES, HOW MANY BLOCKS CAN YOU WALK AT A *NORMAL* PACE BEFORE THIS DISCOMFORT STOPS YOU FROM WALKING?   # OF BLOCKS: _____
IF YES, HOW MANY BLOCKS CAN YOU WALK AT A FAST PACE BEFORE THIS DISCOMFORT STOPS YOU FROM WALKING?   # OF BLOCKS: _____

Fig. 31-4 *(continued)*

553

MUSCULOSKELETAL HISTORY

36. HAVE YOU EVER HAD ANY SEVERE JOINT, BACK MUSCLE, OR TENDON PAIN?

     YES   NO

     IF YES, PLEASE DESCRIBE:

     _____

37. HAVE YOU EVER HAD ANY SURGERY ON YOUR MUSCLES, JOINTS, OR BONES?

     YES   NO

     IF YES, PLEASE DESCRIBE:

     _____

CORONARY RISK FACTORS

38. *SMOKING:* WHAT IS YOUR CURRENT SMOKING STATUS?

     NONSMOKER

     EX-SMOKER – PLEASE NOTE QUIT DATE: _____

     YEARS SMOKED: _____   PACKS PER DAY SMOKED: _____

     CURRENT SMOKER: PACKS PER DAY SMOKING: _____

     YEARS YOU HAVE SMOKED: _____

39. *HIGH BLOOD PRESSURE:* HAVE YOU EVER BEEN TOLD THAT YOUR BLOOD PRES-
     SURE WAS TOO HIGH?   YES   NO

     IF YES, WHEN? _____

40. *HIGH BLOOD LIPIDS:* HAVE YOU EVER BEEN TOLD THAT YOU HAVE HIGH BLOOD
     CHOLESTEROL?   YES   NO

     HIGH BLOOD TRIGYLCERIDES?

     DO YOU HAVE A FAMILY HISTORY OF HIGH BLOOD LIPIDS?

                                                           YES   NO

41. *BODY WEIGHT:* WHAT IS YOUR CURRENT WEIGHT? _____LBS

     WHAT DO YOU CONSIDER TO BE YOUR IDEAL WEIGHT? _____LBS

42. *DIABETES:* HAVE YOU EVER BEEN TOLD THAT YOU HAVE "SUGAR" DIABETES?

                                                           YES   NO

43. *FAMILY HISTORY*: PLEASE ANSWER THE FOLLOWING:

	AGE IF LIVING	AGE AT DEATH	MAJOR DISEASES	CAUSE OF DEATH*
FATHER				
MOTHER				
AUNT(S)				
UNCLE(S)				

Fig. 31-4 *(continued)*

	AGE IF LIVING	AGE AT DEATH	MAJOR DISEASES	CAUSE OF DEATH*
GRANDFATHER(S)				
GRANDMOTHER(S)				
BROTHER(S)				
SISTER(S)				
SON(S)				
DAUGHTER(S)				

*MAJOR DISEASES AND CAUSES OF DEATH:
1. CORONARY HEART DISEASE
2. STROKE
3. HIGH BLOOD PRESSURE

4. CANCER
5. ACCIDENT
6. HEART FAILURE

7. OTHER

PHYSICAL ACTIVITY

44. *OCCUPATION:* DURING AN AVERAGE WEEK, DO YOU

	ALL	HALF	LESS THAN HALF	NEARLY NONE
SIT ON THE JOB	___	___		
WALK ON THE JOB	___	___		
LIFT OR CARRY HEAVY OBJECTS (GREATER THAN 30 LBS)	___	___		

45. PLEASE DESCRIBE YOUR USUAL LEISURE TIME PHYSICAL ACTIVITY:

WORK SITUATION

46. WHAT IS YOUR OCCUPATION? _____

47. DO YOU HOLD MORE THAN ONE JOB?   YES   NO

48. HOW MANY HOURS PER WEEK DO YOU WORK? _____

49. HOW MANY WEEKS VACATION DO YOU TAKE PER YEAR? _____

50. HOW MANY WEEKS PER YEAR DO YOU SPEND OUT OF TOWN ON BUSINESS?
_____

51. ARE YOU
VERY SATISFIED   _____
SATISFIED   _____
DISSATISFIED   _____
    (WITH YOUR WORK)

Fig. 31-4 *(continued)*

52. DOES YOUR JOB ENTAIL EXTREMES OF ENVIRONMENTAL TEMPERATURE?

	YES	NO
BIG, QUICK, IMPORTANT DECISIONS?	YES	NO
COMPETITION?	YES	NO
SIGNIFICANT NERVOUS TENSION OR STRESS?	YES	NO

53. DO YOU HAVE ANY SERIOUS FAMILY PROBLEMS?   YES   NO

OTHER MEDICAL PROBLEMS

54. PLEASE DESCRIBE ANY OTHER SIGNIFICANT MEDICAL PROBLEMS YOU HAVE THAT HAVE NOT BEEN INCLUDED IN THIS QUESTIONNAIRE.

_____

_____

MEDICATIONS

55. PLEASE LIST ALL MEDICATIONS THAT YOU CURRENTLY TAKE, THE TIMES THAT YOU TAKE THEM, THE DOSAGE AND REASON THAT YOU ARE TAKING THEM.

MEDICATION	DOSAGE	FREQUENCY PER DAY	REASON FOR TAKING	DATE AND TIME LAST TAKEN

PREPARATION FOR YOUR EXERCISE TEST

1. IF YOU SMOKE, AT WHAT TIME TODAY DID YOU LAST SMOKE? _____
2. WHEN WAS YOUR LAST LARGE MEAL? _____
3. HAVE YOU EXERCISED VIGOROUSLY TODAY?   YES   NO
4. DID YOU SLEEP WELL LAST NIGHT?   YES   NO
5. ARE YOU FEELING WELL TODAY?   YES   NO
6. HAVE YOU DEVELOPED ANY NEW OR DIFFERENT SYMPTOMS OR PROBLEMS SINCE YOU LAST SAW YOUR DOCTOR?   YES   NO
   IF YES, WHAT?

_____

BRIEFLY DESCRIBE THE GOALS YOU WISH TO ACHIEVE BY JOINING THIS PROGRAM.

_____

_____

_____

Fig. 31-4 *(continued)* (Courtesy of YMCArdiac Therapy.)

arrhythmias, medications, and responses to therapeutic exercise. There has been repeated affirmation that participants in coronary rehabilitation programs *can* learn techniques of self-monitoring. Through these self-monitoring techniques, patients know when to contact the health care system. Self-efficacy, or the ability of an individual to believe that he or she can master an agreed-upon or identified behavior, is important in coronary rehabilitation.[51-54] A patient's ability to self-monitor and appropriately intervene will be influenced by personal experiences in the rehabilitation program, by verbal persuasion by the rehabilitation staff, and by knowledge of his or her physiologic data. "Self-monitoring skills" are a fundamental component to enhance the self-efficacy of coronary patients.

Self-monitoring skills for therapeutic exercise can be divided into two categories: those for anginal symptoms and those for arrhythmias and heart rate assessment. Self-monitoring skills for angina include the ability of patients to answer the following questions:

1. What does my usual angina feel like? (tightness, heaviness, fullness, banding)
2. Where is it located? (in the chest, neck, jaw, arm, back)
3. How often do I usually experience angina? (once a week, twice a day)
4. What are my usual triggers or causes? (eating, severe emotional upset, exposure to cold or exertion)
5. How severe is my usual angina? (grade 1 through 4, with 4 the most severe)
6. What usually relieves my angina? (rest, nitroglycerin)
7. Does my angina ever wake me from my sleep? Does it occur at rest or without provocation?
8. Am I taking any medications preventively, before known provocations, and/or to control my anginal symptoms? If yes, what are they?

Self-monitoring skills for heart rate assessment and arrhythmias include the ability of patients to answer the following questions:

1. What is my usual resting heart rate?
2. Do I usually have irregular heartbeats? If so, what is the frequency in a 3-minute period?

3. What heart rate guidelines has my doctor given me for my exercise program?
4. Do I have trouble achieving this heart rate, or do I exceed my heart rate easily while exercising?
5. Do I have increased numbers of irregular heartbeats during or after exercising?
6. Am I taking any medications that may alter my usual heart rate response to exercise? If so, should I take these medicines before exercising?
7. If I have irregular heartbeats, do I ever feel dizzy or faint?
8. Does my doctor want me to call if I develop frequent irregular heartbeats?

If patients are given the information and directions for self-assessment, they are more likely to make appropriate choices about seeking medical care when necessary. Simple daily logs for monitoring angina and arrhythmias can be used by patients until they become confident of their assessment skills (Fig. 31-5). Self-monitoring skills during exercise therapy consist of a series of self-assessments and documentation of cardiovascular responses. The self-assessments include

1. Confirmation of prescribed heart rate guidelines.
2. Documentation of achieved heart rates with therapeutic exercise.
3. Measurement of exercise performance.
4. Recording of other physiologic data such as weight and perceived exertion.
5. Documentation of signs or symptoms.
6. Documentation of orthopedic difficulties.
7. Assessment of other physiologic parameters of concern.
8. Documentation of stability of medications.
9. Other data to support attendance and/or other communications with the program staff.

Periodic follow-up evaluations should be scheduled between the program staff and patient:

1. To reassess stability of coronary signs and symptoms.
2. To review progress of identified coronary risk factor interventions.
3. To reestablish goals and commitments.

DAILY LOG FOR ARRHYTHMIAS						
# OF EPISODES						
TRIGGER (IF KNOWN)						
# PER MINUTE						
MANAGEMENT						
REST						
MEDICATION						
OTHER						

DAILY LOG FOR ANGINA							
# OF EPISODES							
TRIGGERED							
SPONTANEOUS							
GRADE (1-4)*							
DURATION							
MANAGEMENT							
REST							
NTG							
OTHER							

* Grade one is the onset of angina.
Grade four is the worst angina you have experienced.

Fig. 31-5. Sample Daily Log for Arrhythmias and Angina (Courtesy of YMCArdiac Therapy.)

4. To evaluate the efficacy of the therapeutic exercise.
5. To redesign appropriate interventions as indicated.
6. To address new issues as appropriate.

It is also important that follow-up evaluations include physiologic testing, laboratory analysis, or psychosocial measurements to determine changes and improvements in functional capacity and psychological status. Favorable changes are important in achieving self-confidence and a sense of accomplishment, and they are a significant reward for hard work. The timing of follow-up evaluations should be individually scheduled for each patient. The frequency will depend on the seriousness of the coronary disease and the complexity of recommended lifestyle interventions. Further evaluations should be based on individual patient needs, with all patients being evaluated at least annually.

PROGRAM SAFETY

Prescriptive exercise for persons with known CHD entails some risk.[45–50] This risk is generally related to many factors, including

1. Age.
2. Severity of disease.
3. Symptoms of angina.
4. History of prior cardiac arrest.
5. Left ventricular dysfunction.
6. Compromised exercise capacity.
7. Coexisting medical problems such as chronic obstructive pulmonary disease, chronic renal failure, and diabetes mellitus.
8. Severe orthopedic problems.
9. Psychological instability.

What is known about the safety of coronary rehabilitation programs, and how do these safety data further identify patients at higher risk for complications?

In a recent study by Van Camp and Peterson,[45] historical, clinical, and cardiac catheterization findings were identified in the population of patients who had sustained cardiac arrest and/or myocardial infarction while participating in rehabilitation exercise programs.

Historical features of importance were

1. A history of congestive heart failure.
2. Prior cardiac arrest.
3. A history of ventricular tachycardia by exercise ECG or Holter (ambulatory ECG) monitor recording.

Clinical features of importance were

1. Poor exercise capacity (less than 4.5 minutes of Bruce protocol, 6 METs).
2. ST segment depression with exercise, beginning at a heart rate of less than 120 beats/min.

3. Peak systolic blood pressure of less than 120 mmHg.
4. Exertional hypotension of at least a 10-mmHg drop in systolic blood pressure.
5. Ventricular tachycardia.

Cardiac catheterization findings of importance were

1. Left ventricular ejection fraction (EF) of less than 40%.
2. Left main and/or three-vessel coronary disease.

In an earlier article, these authors assessed total cardiovascular complications in exercise rehabilitation programs. The conditions and results of the study were as follows[46]:

1. One hundred sixty-seven randomly chosen exercise rehabilitation programs, representing 51,303 participating patients from January 1980 to December 1984, were evaluated for cardiac arrest.
2. The 51,303 patients in these programs during this 48-month period exercised for 3,251,916 hours.
3. Twenty-one cardiac arrests (8.9 per one million exercise hours), three fatalities (1.3 per one million exercise hours), and 8 myocardial infarctions (3.4 per one million exercise hours) occurred.

This study indicates a very low rate of complications in a population of known coronary patients, and a very high rate of successful resuscitation. These results are most encouraging. The study is comparable to an earlier one reported by Haskell.[50] We can learn two important concepts from this study:

1. Serious cardiovascular events are rare for all patients in a supervised setting.
2. High-risk patients are most likely to derive greater benefit from monitored and supervised exercise rehabilitation programs than are moderate- and low-risk patients. The expected mortality of 35 to 40% in the high-risk patient may be favorably altered by the increased supervision of exercise rehabilitation programs.[55,56]

The study also found that 86% of the 167 programs represented reported no major cardiovascular complication (either cardiac arrest or myocardial infarction) during this 4-year period.

Community-based programs provide safety through procedures designed to

1. Evaluate clinical status.
2. Educate patients regarding warning and premonitory signs and symptoms.
3. Ascertain stability of exercise-related cardiovascular responses.
4. Ascertain influences of coexisting illnesses as they relate to exercise safety.
5. Ascertain intercurrent events.
6. Provide heart rate guidelines consistent with cardiovascular status based on dynamic exercise evaluation.
7. Regularly reevaluate patients' clinical status and alter exercise guidelines if necessary.
8. Provide ACLS by licensed and certified medical supervisory personnel.
9. Coordinate ACLS with local hospitals and paramedic units for transport of emergency cases for further care.
10. Communicate regularly with referring physicians to enhance patient supervision.
11. Educate the coronary rehabilitation staff in new techniques for the management of patients.
12. Direct patients to become their own best "care givers." As patients become active participants in their care through information and education, they will be able to make informed decisions about their health status. This education and information encourages patients to heed the signs and symptoms and have the knowledge and confidence to act appropriately as change occurs.

Risk stratification of coronary patients has been addressed in a previous chapter (see Ch. 11). The knowledge of a patient's level of risk is the critical component to long-term patient safety in community-based programs.[57] All patients should be given specific heart rate guidelines, symptom-limiting guidelines, perceived exertion guidelines,[58] and guidelines for medication management to ensure the safety of exercise (Table 31-1).

High-risk patients pose a unique challenge to community-based programs. Many patients will remain "high risk" for the remainder of their lives. Given the medical and surgical interventions available to patients today, high-risk patients no longer face a life of certain invalidism. Through adequate supervision, comprehensive evaluation, and appropriate goals for exercise, these patients can safely participate in exercise rehabilitation. What do we know about high-risk coronary patients? A review of the literature of exercise therapy for carefully screened patients with severe left ventricular dysfunction showed beneficial responses to exercise training without apparent increased risk. A study by Cody et al. in Australia reported an annual mortality of 9% in an exercise training group versus an expected mortality of 35 to 40% in a similar matched patient population with ventricular dysfunction who were not exercising.[55] Mayo Clinic data are similar for patients with severe left ventricular dysfunction who exercise.[56] Patients with left ventricular dysfunction and arrhythmia who qualify for therapeutic exercise can expect a greater increase in their quality of life compared with relatively uncomplicated coronary patients. The complicated patient who can increase his or her functional capacity to 4 to 6 METs can expect to experience a change from being relatively homebound to living a significantly more active and normal life.

OTHER COMMUNITY RESOURCES AND PROGRAM MODELS

In addition to the formal rehabilitation model, other services and programs are available in communities to provide additional resources for coronary rehabilitation. Such resources include the AHA, Mended Hearts Inc., State Vocational Rehabilitation (VR) Services, and services provided by the U.S. federal government. In addition, programs developed in other countries offer important models to consider when developing community-based programs.

Table 31-1. Exercise Therapy Guidelines Using Risk Stratification Definitions

Low Risk[a]

Asymptomatic Patients (functional capacity of 8 METs; uncomplicated coronary history)

1. Heart rate guidelines based on treadmill exercise test.
2. Perceived exertion consistent with moderate exercise.
3. Symptom guidelines based on self-reported history and cardiovascular exam.
4. Continuous self-monitoring.
5. ECG monitoring only as indicated.
6. Exercise guidelines consistent with functional capacity.
7. Recreational guidelines consistent with functional capacity and appropriate goals.

Intermediate Risk[b]

Patients at risk for a recurrent coronary event; functional capacity is <8 METs; patients who have experienced shock, congestive heart failure, or abnormal exercise ECG or who are unable to self-monitor

1. Heart rate guidelines based on treadmill exercise test.
2. Perceived exertion consistent with moderately low-level exercise.
3. Symptom guidelines based on self-reported history and cardiovascular exam.
4. Continuous self-monitoring.
5. Intermittent ECG monitoring to establish cardiovascular response to therapeutic exercise.
6. Moderate exercise guidelines consistent with functional capacity and symptoms. More frequent exercise sessions with a slower progression of exercise intensity.
7. Recreational guidelines consistent with functional capacity and the estimated energy cost and other variables, such as weather and competition.

High Risk[c]

Patients with severely depressed left ventricular function (ejection fraction [EF] less than 30%); resting complex arrhythmias; arrhythmias that increase with exercise; a demonstrable drop in systolic blood pressure with exercise; marked exercise-induced ischemia (greater than 2 mm ST depression); or survivors of sudden cardiac death

1. Heart rate guidelines based on treadmill exercise test.
2. Perceived exertion consistent with low level exercise.
3. Symptom guidelines based on self-reported history and cardiovascular exam.
4. Continuous self-monitoring.
5. Continuous or intermittent ECG monitoring as indicated by cardiovascular signs, symptoms and history; graduating to intermittent monitoring as soon as usual cardiovascular responses are documented.
6. Low-level exercise guidelines consistent with functional capacity and symptoms. Modification of exercise type, intensity, frequency and duration to provide low level stimulus.
7. Temporary postponement of resumption of recreational activities until cardiovascular responses to exercise are established and functional capacity is consistent with desired activity.

[a] For definitions, the source is the American College of Physicians.[58a] For recommendations, the source is the author.[4,16]

The American Heart Association

The AHA,[59] through its national center, has developed an impressive array of educational materials for both primary and secondary prevention of CHD. The materials are available in written and video format and can be used for individual and/or group programs. The AHA has recently developed an educational video series designed especially for the hospitalized coronary patient, *Active Partnership in the Health of Your Heart.* This is a series of six videos designed to be viewed in the hospital and during the early phases of recovery following hospital discharge. The videos review important topics including the interpretation of tests and procedures, coronary risk factor assessment, smoking cessation, healthy eating habits, exercise programs, and stress reduction. The series is accompanied by a workbook that is designed to enhance the effectiveness of the videos by stressing goals for behavioral change, formal contracting, relapse prevention, and regular self-evaluations.

The AHA also has special coronary risk factor reduction materials packaged for the physician's office (Heart RX), the work place (Heart at Work), and the school (Heart Treasure Chest, Getting to Know Your Heart, Heart Decisions). These informational programs and written materials have been developed by national experts, will be reviewed and updated frequently, and can provide important educational materials for community-based coronary rehabilitation programs.

Mended Hearts, Inc.

Mended Hearts, Inc.,[60] is a national, nonprofit U.S. service organization providing support for persons who have undergone CABG and other surgery. Mended Hearts, Inc., provides both educational materials and group or individual support through regular meetings at local hospitals and rehabilitation centers. During hospitalization, trained Mended Hearts volunteers are available to visit patients who have just undergone open-heart surgery. The purpose of the visit is to provide visible evidence of a successful recovery and to provide additional support to families as necessary.

Mended Hearts, Inc., assists in research programs designed to benefit coronary surgery patients. The organization is also actively working to remove unnecessary and unwarranted barriers to return to full and gainful employment following recovery from heart surgery. Its membership includes individuals who have had heart surgery, their spouses, families, friends, and all others who are interested and committed to these goals. It serves a complementary function to community-based rehabilitation programs.

State Vocational Rehabilitation Services

Individual states vary widely in the provision of VR services, enabled by federal legislation, designed specifically for cardiac patients. The state of Arizona,[61] for example, has an excellent model developed specifically to provide cardiac rehabilitation services. Through the coordinator for cardiac rehabilitation, referral services are available, as well as financial support, for participation in rehabilitation programs. Although economic handicaps are generally a prerequisite for eligibility, the rehabilitative services can be an adjunct to other insurance programs. Some areas that can be positively addressed by the use of state VR services include

1. Work area modification to facilitate return to usual employment if physical limitations are a result of the cardiovascular problem (e.g., a chain hoist to assist with heavy lifting, as in mechanical work).
2. Job retraining if resumption of the former occupation is not possible as a result of the cardiovascular condition.
3. Participation in a coronary rehabilitation exercise program to restore normal functional capacity necessary for return to work.
4. Assistance to homemakers limited by their coronary disease to regain ability to perform household activities and achieve self-sufficiency.[62]

The VR counselor also works directly with employers to facilitate participation in coronary rehabilitation programs as a means of enhancing earlier return to work and employability.

The National Heart, Lung, and Blood Institute

The National Heart, Lung, and Blood Institute (NHLBI) produces excellent materials for medical professionals for use in health education of patients. An excellent example of such service is the National Cholesterol Education Program.[63] This educational program is based on the 1987 report of the National Cholesterol Education Program Expert Panel on Detection, Evaluation, and Treatment of High Blood Cholesterol in Adults (Adult Treatment Panel). It provides a classification of various hyperlipidemic patterns and recommended dietary and drug interventions for the various forms of hyperlipidemia. To supplement this program, the National Cholesterol Education Program for Physicians (NCEP) and the Cholesterol Education Program for Nurses (CEPN)[59] was developed by the NHLBI in cooperation with the AHA and other agencies. Both the NCEP and CEPN focus on

1. The pathophysiology of hyperlipidemia.
2. Screening and identification of high-risk individuals.
3. Dietary interventions through education and counseling.
4. Pharmacologic interventions.

These resources and programs, plus many others, are available through the NHLBI and can provide nationally endorsed guidelines and program implementation for coronary risk factor intervention.

International Models

Models for cardiac rehabilitation outside the United States have been developed that use both full care (residential format) and the integration of a centralized outpatient rehabilitation program with other services available in the community.[1] A model for the centralized administration plus community volunteer organization programs is the North Karelia Project in rural Finland.[65] This model has not been adopted in the United States but warrants careful consideration. Significant success has been reported in reduction of recurrent myocardial infarction and decreased costs to the state for disability due to CHD.

SUMMARY

Coronary rehabilitation programs have successfully been offered in community facilities for over 30 years. Community facilities are eager to encompass health-related programs. Such programs expand their ability to provide comprehensive service to their membership and to the community. Health-related services such as blood pressure screening; weight loss, physical fitness, stress reduction, and smoking cessation

programs; heart-healthy cooking; and cholesterol screening are examples of services provided by coronary rehabilitation programs in community facilities, which have a wide applicability to the community at large.

The ability to meet the needs of large numbers of patients; to provide cost-effective interventions; to involve the medical community in a cooperative venture; and to positively influence families and social groups is found over recent decades and predicts a bright future for community-based coronary rehabilitation programs.

REFERENCES

1. Wenger NK, Hellerstein HK: Rehabilitation of the Coronary Patient. 2nd Ed. Churchill Livingstone, New York, 1984
2. Pollock ML, Schmidt DH: Heart Disease and Rehabilitation. Houghton Mifflin, Boston, 1980
3. McHenry PL, Ellestad MH, Fletcher GF et al: A position statement for health professionals by the Committee on Exercise and Cardiac Rehabilitation of the Council on Clinical Cardiology, American Heart Association. Circulation 81:396, 1990
4. American Association of Cardiovascular and Pulmonary Rehabilitation: Guidelines for Cardiac Rehabilitation. Human Kinetics Publishers, Champaign, Ill., 1990
5. Leon AS, Certo C, Comoss P et al: Position Paper of the American Association of Cardiovascular and Pulmonary Rehabilitation: Scientific evidence of the value of cardiac rehabilitation services with emphasis on patients following myocardial infarction. Section 1. Exercise conditioning component. J Cardiopulmonary Rehabil 10:79, 1990
6. Miller NH, Taylor CB, Davidson DM et al: Position Paper of the American Association of Cardiovascular and Pulmonary Rehabilitation: Scientific evidence of the value of cardiac rehabilitation services with emphasis on patients following acute myocardial infarction. Section 2. The psychosocial component. J Cardiopulmonary Rehabil 10:198, 1990
7. Kallio V, Hamalainen H, Hakkila J, Luurila OJ: Reducation of sudden deaths by a multifactorial intervention program after acute myocardial infarction. Lancet ii:1091, 1979
8. Hamalainen H, Luurila OJ, Kallio V et al: Long-

term reduction in sudden deaths after a multifactorial intervention programme in patients with myocardial infarction: 10-year results of a controlled investigation. Eur Heart J 10:55, 1989

9. Oldridge N, Guyatt G, Fischer M, Rimm A: Cardiac rehabilitation after myocardial infarction: combined experience of randomized clinical trials. JAMA 260:945, 1988

10. The Multiple Risk Factor Intervention Trial Research Group: Mortality rates after 10.5 years for participants in the Multiple Risk Factor Intervention Trial. JAMA 263:1795, 1990

11. Wenger NK, Mattson ME, Furberg CD, Elinson J: Assessment of quality of life in clinical trials of cardiovascular therapies. Am J Cardiol 54:908, 1984

12. Siegrist J: Impaired quality of life as a risk factor in cardiovascular disease. J Chronic Dis 40:571, 1987

13. Applegate W, Schron E, Pequegnat W: Quality of life assessment in clinical trials with symptomatic populations. Task Force Report, in press. J Prev Med

14. Wenger NK: The concept of quality of life: an appropriate consideration in clinical decision making affecting patients with cardiovascular disease. Qual Life Cardiovasc Care 8:42, 1984

15. Croog SH, Levine S, Testa MA et al: The effects of antihypertensive therapy on the quality of life. N Engl J Med 314:1657, 1986

16. Fry G, Berra K: YMCArdiac Therapy: Community Based Cardiac Rehabilitation. Carolyn Bean Associates, San Francisco, 1981

16a. Hellerstein HK, Hirsch HZ, Cumler W, et al: Reconditioning of the coronary patient. A preliminary report. In Likoff W and Moyer JH (eds): Coronary Heart Disease. Grune & Stratton, New York, 1963

17. American Heart Association: 1990 Heart and Stroke Facts: American Heart Association, 7320 Greenville Avenue, Dallas, TX 75231, 1990

18. Holmes DR, Vliestra RE, Reiter SJ, Bresnahan DR: Advances in interventional cardiology. Mayo Clin Proc 65:565, 1990

19. DeBusk RF: Stanford University cardiac rehabilitation program. J Myocardial Ischemia 2:28, 1990

20. Ben-Ari E, Rothbaum DR, Linnemeier TJ, et al: Benefits of a monitored rehabilitation program versus physician care after emergency percutaneous transluminal coronary angioplasty: follow-up of risk factors and rate of restenosis. J Cardiopulmonary Rehabil 7:281, 1989

21. Position Paper of the American Association of Cardiovascular and Pulmonary Rehabilitation: Scientific evidence of the value of cardiac rehabilitation services with emphasis on patients following myocardial infarction. J Cardiopulmonary Rehabil 10:79, 1990

22. Southard DR, Broyden R: Psychosocial services in cardiac rehabilitation: a status report. J Cardiopulmonary Rehabil 10:255, 1990

23. Blumenthal J, Levenson RM: Behavioral approaches to the secondary prevention of coronary heart disease. Circulation 76(suppl. I):I-30, 1987

24. The 1988 Report of the Joint National Committee on Detection, Evaluation, and Treatment of High Blood Pressure. Arch Intern Med 148:1034, 1988

25. Blankenhorn DH, Nessim SA, Johnson RL et al: Beneficial effects of combined colestipol-niacin therapy on coronary atherosclerosis and coronary venous bypass grafts. JAMA 257:3233, 1987

26. Superko HR, Haskell WL: Cardiac rehabilitation: time for a more intensive approach to lipid-lowering therapy. J Cardiopulmonary Rehabil 7:220, 1987

27. Tyroler HA: Review of lipid-lowering clinical trials in relation to observational epidemiological studies. Circulation 76:512, 1987

28. Wilhelmsen L: Cessation of smoking after myocardial infarction: effects on mortality after ten years. Br Heart J 49:416, 1983

29. Higgins C, Schweiger MJ: Smoking termination patterns in a cardiac rehabilitation population. J Cardiac Rehabil 3:55, 1983

30. Mulcahy R: Influence of cigarette smoking on morbidity and mortality after myocardial infarction. Br Heart J 49:410, 1983

31. Miller NH: Smoking cessation strategies in prevention of coronary heart disease. Cardiovasc Nursing 24:45, 1988

32. Wenger N, Cleeman JI, Herd JA, McIntosh HD: Education of the patient with cardiac disease in the twenty-first century: an overview. Am J Cardiol 57:1187, 1986

33. Haskell WL: Mechanisms by which physical activity may enhance the clinical status of cardiac patients. p. 276. In Pollock M and Schmidt D (eds): Heart Disease and Rehabilitation. Houghton Mifflin, Boston, 1979

34. Karliner, JS: When do you discharge patients? Cardiovasc Med 61, 1985

35. Topol EJ, Burek K, O'Neill WW et al: A randomized controlled trial of hospital discharge three days after myocardial infarction in the era of reperfusion. N Engl J Med 318:1083, 1988

36. Dennis C, Houston-Miller N, Schwartz RG: Early

return to work after uncomplicated myocardial infarction: Results of a randomized trial. JAMA 260:214, 1988

37. Burek KA, Kirscht J, Topol EJ: Exercise capacity in patients 3 days after acute, uncomplicated myocardial infarction. Heart Lung 18:575, 1989

38. Miller N, Haskell W, Berra K, DeBusk R: Home versus group training for increasing functional capacity after myocardial infarction. Circulation 70:645, 1984

39. DeBusk RF, Haskell WL, Miller NH et al: Medically directed at-home rehabilitation soon after clinically uncomplicated acute myocardial infarction: A new model for patient care. Am J Cardiol 5:251, 1985

40. Kinsey MG, Fletcher BJ, Rice CR et al: Coronary risk factor modification followed by home-monitored exercise in coronary bypass surgery patients: a four-year follow-up study. J Cardiopulmonary Rehabil 9:207, 1989

41. Greenland P, Chu JS: Efficacy of cardiac rehabilitation services. Ann Intern Med 109:650, 1988

42. DeBusk RF, Houston N, Haskell W et al: Exercise training soon after myocardial infarction. Am J Cardiol 44:1223, 1979

43. Stevens R, Hansen P: Comparison of supervised and unsupervised exercise training after coronary bypass surgery. Am J Cardiol 53:1524, 1984

44. Williams S, Miller H, Krisch P et al: Guidelines for unsupervised exercise in patients with ischemic heart disease. J Cardiac Rehabil 1:213, 1981

45. Van Camp SP, Peterson RA: Identification of the high risk cardiac rehabilitation patient. J Cardiopulmonary Rehabil 9:103, 1989

46. Van Camp SP, Peterson RA: Cardiovascular complications of outpatient cardiac rehabilitation programs. JAMA 256:1160, 1986

47. Koplan JP, Siscovick DS, Goldbaum GM: The risks of exercise: a public view of injuries and hazards. Public Health Rep 100:189, 1985

48. Hossack KF, Hartwig R: Cardiac arrest associated with supervised cardiac rehabilitation. J Cardiac Rehabil 2:402, 1982

49. Fardy PS, Doll N, Taylor J, Williams M: Monitoring cardiac patients: how much is enough? Physician Sportsmed 10:146, 1982

50. Haskell WL: Cardiovascular complications during exercise training of cardiac patients. Circulation 57:920, 1978

51. Bandura A, Watters RH: Social Learning and Personality Development. Rinehart and Winston, New York, 1963

52. Bandura A: Self-efficacy: toward a unifying theory of behavioral change. Psychol Rev 84:191, 1977

53. Jenkins LS: Self-efficacy: new perspectives in caring for patients recovering from myocardial infarction. Prog Cardiovasc Nursing 2:32, 1987

54. Ewart CK, Taylor CB, Reese LB, Debusk RF: Effects of early post-myocardial testing on self perception and subsequent physical activity. Am J Cardiol 51:1076, 1983

55. Cody DV, Dennis AR, Ross DA et al: Early exercise testing, physical training and mortality in patients with severe left ventricular dysfunction. J Am Coll Cardiol 2(suppl. 1):718, 1983

56. Squires RW, Lavie CJ, Branat TR et al: Cardiac rehabilitation in patients with severe ischemic left ventricular dysfunction. Mayo Clin Proc 62:997, 1987

57. The Multicenter Postinfarction Research Group: Risk stratification and survival after myocardial infarction. NEJM 309:331, 1983

58. Borg GAV, Noble BJ: Perceived exertion. p. 131. In Wilmore JH (ed): Exercise and Sports Science Review. Academic Press, New York, 1974

58a. Cardiac Rehabilitation Services: Position Paper, Health and Policy Committee, American College of Physicians. Ann Intern Med 109:671, 1988

59. The American Heart Association, National Center, 7320 Greenville Avenue, Dallas, TX 75231

60. Mended Hearts, Inc., 7320 Greenville Avenue, Dallas, TX 75231

61. Arizona Department of Economic Security. Vocational Rehabilitation, 3033 North Central, Suite 600 140D, Phoenix, AZ 85012

62. Kolnick V: Vocational Rehabilitation: returning the cardiopulmonary patient to work and recreation. American Association of Cardiovascular and Pulmonary Rehabilitation (AACVPR) Fourth Annual National Convention Syllabus. Available through AACVPR, 7611 Elmwood Avenue, Suite 201, Middleton, WI 53562.

63. National Cholesterol Education Program. Coordinated by the National Heart, Lung and Blood Institute. U.S. Department of Health and Human Services, C-200, Bethesda, MD 20892

64. Salonen JT, Puska P: A community programme for rehabilitation and secondary prevention for patients with acute myocardial infarction as part of a comprehensive community programme for control of cardiovascular diseases (North Karelia Project). Scand J Rehabil Med 12:33, 1980

32

Medicolegal Aspects of Rehabilitation of the Coronary Patient

David L. Herbert, J.D.
William G. Herbert, Ph.D.

The development of rehabilitation services for the coronary patient is of relatively recent origin. While such health-provider activities were undergoing development and implementation, the medical profession was also undergoing change and turmoil. Some providers and lawyers alike contend that a litigation explosion, as well as a medical malpractice crisis, has engulfed the United States in the past three decades. Regardless of the debate surrounding such statements, the law has necessarily and dramatically had an impressive impact on the practice of medicine during this period.

Health professionals who practice coronary rehabilitation should consider many potential problems when planning and delivering services to their patient population. These include the development of policies and procedures of the program; the purchase, maintenance, and use of equipment; the hiring and training of personnel; the implementation of the principles and practices of informed consent; and the use of exercise testing and prescription, programming, monitoring, and leadership. Other considerations also pertain to recommendations for off-site exercise and monitoring techniques, emergency response protocols, risk management, insurance, the use of waivers or prospective releases, and a host of other matters. Although a detailed examination of all these areas would be an ambitious undertaking,[1] an ongoing examination of developing practices and their medicolegal aspects may be necessary, given the rapid developments in medical practice and standards, and the so-called litigation explosion.[2] A review of basic and important medicolegal information should serve as a foundation and background for rehabilitation professionals to apply to program practices.

THE REHABILITATION MODEL

The provision of coronary rehabilitation services must be reviewed within a medical model. The medicolegal aspects of such services must also be examined from such a perspective. Even though a number of licensed and nonlicensed professionals practice within the field, certain basic principles pertain regardless of the professional perspective. Although not all members of the rehabilitation team may perform the same services within a particular program, in the event of an injury or death, the conduct of all will be judged from a negligence and malpractice perspective. An examination of the tort system within which such conduct would be judged should help those attempting to define and manage their own conduct or prospectively to evaluate it.

THE TORT SYSTEM AND THE STANDARD OF CARE

The tort system is confined to the resolution of noncontractual civil wrongs. The word *tort* means to twist or wrong, and the tort system exists to resolve these wrongs. The tort system generally examines conduct that is either intentional or negligent and involves harm to another, proximately caused by an act or an omission that deviates from accepted norms or standards of conduct. In medical cases, the applicable standard of conduct is generally peer set, but judicially is recognized as the so-called "standard of care." Questionable conduct is examined within this tort system by reference to what various witnesses testify is the standard of care owed by given professionals to specific patient populations.

In the past, many standards were set on a case-by-case basis, through individual opinions of expert witnesses, who, at the time of trial, would give their opinions about what standard of care was owed to particular patients. Some have contended that this system allowed for an overreliance on "good" witnesses, rather than on what most practitioners would define as the established standard of care in the community of the case being considered. Moreover, some contend that these developments contributed to the malpractice and litigation crisis by allowing individualized standards to be established in particular cases, sometimes resulting in inconsistent verdicts and uncertainty about the appropriate delivery of patient care and practice.

In the 1980s, the medical profession began to combat this problem by recommending the adoption of widely endorsed and authoritatively written standards of care to provide an appropriate reference source for the examination of provider practices. The movement toward adoption of such standards was called the top medical story of the year by the American Medical Association (AMA) in late 1988.[3]

The effort to develop such standards has affected those engaged in the provision of rehabilitative services for coronary patients. Several authoritative and respected national organizations have already participated in these efforts, including the American Heart Association (AHA),[4,4a] the American College of Sports Medicine (ACSM),[5] the American College of Cardiology (ACC),[6,6a,6b,6c] and the American Association of Cardiovascular and Pulmonary Rehabilitation (AACVPR).[7] Publication of standards of practice by these and other groups has had and will continue to have a dramatic impact on the so-called standard of care owed to patients within this population.[8]

NEGLIGENCE AND MALPRACTICE

Although probably incapable of precise definition, negligence amounts to a failure to conform one's conduct to a generally accepted standard or duty. Malpractice is a form of negligence, but generally is limited to negligence committed by a variety of professionals, including physicians and other health care providers. A cause of action for negligence is established by proof of a breach of conduct owed by one person to another, proximately resulting in harm or damage to the injured party. A cause of action for malpractice is essentially the same, except that proof of breach of duty is provided by reference to the applicable standard of professional care as set by the profession under examination. Proof of that standard and its breach is generally established through expert witnesses at time of trial. Such testimony, although sometimes subject to individualized opinions, is often based on professional group guidelines, standards, recommendations, consensus statements, position papers, or similar written documents.

STANDARDS OF PRACTICE

Existing standards of practice are the reference points likely to be used by those examining provider conduct in a judicial arena to determine whether the professional under examination adhered to the appropriate standard of care in service provision to the patient. An examination of applicable standards from a legal perspective is helpful to those considering the variety of medicolegal concerns affecting their practices toward patients. A number of professional "standards" developed by the above professional organizations deserve brief examination. One or more of these standards could be (and have been) used as reference points for determination of the appropriate standard of care in a judicial setting.

The American Heart Association

The AHA was the first to develop written standards related to the coronary rehabilitation model. A position paper in 1972 was comprehensively updated in 1979 with the publication of *The Exercise Standards Book*.[4a] These standards were further refined and upgraded in late 1990.[4] These standards are physician-oriented and deal with rehabilitative care in regard to evaluation of the patient, exercise testing and prescription, and monitoring and supervision of exercise.

The American College of Cardiology

In 1986 the ACC adopted standards of practice dealing with cardiovascular rehabilitation services.[6] Although somewhat broad and generalized in certain respects, these standards deal with formal and informal, as well as supervised and unsupervised, rehabilitative exercise programs. Despite adoption of these written statements, much is left to "individual determination and discretion".[1] Two subsequent Task Force Reports expanded the original recommendations.[6b,6c]

The American College of Sports Medicine

The ACSM has developed a comprehensive set of written guidelines dealing with preventive and rehabilitative cardiac exercise programs. The publication delineates the standard of care related to screening, exercise testing and prescription, and similar topics. It was first published in 1975 and subsequently revised in 1980, 1986, and 1991.[5]

These guidelines emphasize a team approach to the provision of services and do not necessarily or explicitly require direct involvement of a physician for some program activities. In certain respects, these guidelines may be in conflict with those of the AHA, for example. Such conflict may create additional legal concerns for those practicing independent of a physician; the guidelines of another association could be used in litigation to establish a failure to conform with that other association's statement on the standard of care.

American Association of Cardiovascular and Pulmonary Rehabilitation

In 1986, the AACVPR paper[7] dealing with the provision of rehabilitative services presented the association's view of the need, effectiveness, and clinical value of cardiac rehabilitation, but did not provide a comprehensive standard of reference for cardiac rehabilitation programs. A set of program standards for cardiac rehabilitation activities and means of assessing outcomes is currently available.[8]

Other Groups

A variety of other groups including the Young Men's Christian Association (YMCA), the International Dance Exercise Association (IDEA), now known as the American Council on Exercise (ACE), and the Aerobic Fitness Association of American (AFAA) have published statements that may have an impact on certain aspects of the standard of care related to coronary rehabilitation programs.[9] While not as specifically applicable to coronary rehabilitation as standards promulgated by the previously mentioned organizations, these statements may have implication for certain activities carried on within the coronary rehabilitation setting.

INFORMED CONSENT

Since coronary rehabilitation programs must be viewed and examined within the medical model, the provision of service must be preceded by the steps necessarily required of medical personnel providing similar procedures within other settings of the model. Informed consent, when viewed through the medical model, is a process by which a patient agrees and consents to a procedure, with a full understanding and appreciation of the facts and circumstances of treatment. Without a valid informed consent, a "normal" treatment scenario by a medical practitioner would be impossible and would make the practitioner liable for civil battery, as well as for any untoward event that occurred to the patient due to the treatment or procedure.

For an informed consent process to be valid, the patient must be provided with specific information about the procedure, its risks and benefits, and a review of applicable alternatives. On the basis of these factors, the patient must voluntarily and knowingly agree to undergo the procedure. The patient must be given the opportunity to ask questions and to receive an explanation of all material factors associated with the event.

Failures in the informed-consent process can result in litigation in the event of harm to the patient, which can concomitantly result in judgment against the rehabilitation professional. For example, in the case of *Hedgecorth v. United States*, 618 F. Supp. 627 (Dist. Ct., E.D. Mo. 1985),[10] an elderly plaintiff underwent a graded exercise test at a Veterans Administration (VA) facility. He had performed another test shortly before, but the results of that test were not obtained by the VA facility or its practitioners. The plaintiff complained of a loss of vision and chest pain during the procedure. It was subsequently learned that he sustained a stroke and blindness due to the stroke that occurred during the test. Although the plaintiff signed an informed-consent document prior to the procedure, it did not contain a risk disclosure provision as to the possibility of stroke occurring during the test. The court determined that:

> "The credible medical evidence presented at trial demonstrates that giving the [VA-conducted] stress test to the plaintiff . . . was a deviation from the appropriate standard of care. The purpose of a stress test is, as the name implies, to place a stress on the heart through physical exercise and thereby derive information concerning the heart's condition. Because of the nature of the test certain dangers accompany its administration. These dangers include the possibility that the patient will suffer a stroke. The patient should be warned that a stroke could result from the administration of the test, and plaintiff Lowell Hedgecourth was not warned of this danger. Thus, plaintiff . . . did *not* take the test with informed consent of its dangers," *Hedgecorth v. United States*, 618 F. Supp. 627 (1985) at pages 631–632.

As a result of this finding, the court held:

> "As a direct result of the negligent acts and omissions of the defendants, the plaintiff . . . suffered an infarct in the right occipital lobe of his brain. This stroke directly caused plaintiff'(s) . . . total and permanent disability," at page 632.

The plaintiff and his wife were awarded almost one million dollars as a result of these negligent acts.[10]

Even though the traditional view of the informed-consent disclosure process would mandate that only material risks be disclosed during the process, the law is moving toward requiring ever-broadening disclosure of risks to the patient. Some jurisdictions have adopted the rule that patients must be supplied with information on the basis of their need for it.[11]

Although it is not possible to disclose all possible and rare risks, the trend is to require the provision of more information to the patient. In light of this trend, practitioners are advised to seek counsel to review their informed-consent practices, as failures in this regard can result in the practitioner's being liable for all subsequent untoward events. Sample informed-consent forms for exercise rehabilitation and exercise testing are reproduced in Appendices 32-1 and 32-2.

EXERCISE TESTING, EXERCISE PRESCRIPTION, AND MONITORING OF EXERCISE TRAINING

Exercise testing, exercise prescription, and monitoring of exercise activities raise significant legal concerns related to the provision of rehabilitative care to coronary patients. Within the medical model applicable to rehabilitative care, exercise testing and prescription must be viewed as medical; as a consequence, physician involvement with exercise testing and prescription is probably mandated at some level. However, whether this requires the actual presence of the physician for each exercise test and training activity is a matter of debate and uncertainty when applicable standards are compared with state statutory or administrative declarations.[12] Provision should be made for the management of complications, especially the presence of qualified personnel certified in the conduct of exercise tests, in monitoring and detection of signs suggestive of impending serious complications, and in the immediate management of complications. Documentation of protocols and scheduled rehearsals of the management of complications, including detection, institution of therapy, and transportation to nearby tertiary-care facilities and professionals, is necessary.

Assuming that testing and prescription are medical in nature, the same principles that apply within the general medical model apply to coronary rehabilitation activities. That is, only properly licensed and authorized care givers may be responsible for these procedures when carried out for medical purposes. Should individuals proceed to test or prescribe within the rehabilitation-medical model without the involvement of a properly licensed and authorized practitioner, these individuals would be exposed to at least two potential adverse consequences.

Virtually all states have enacted statutes making the unauthorized provision of health care a criminal offense, usually a misdemeanor, punishable by fine and/or imprisonment for up to 1 year. Such statutes typically provide that the practice of medicine is "generally regarded as the diagnosis of an individual's symptoms to determine with what disease or illness he is afflicted, and then to determine on the basis of that diagnosis what remedy or treatment should be given or prescribed to treat that disease and/or relieve the symptoms."[13]

Aside from this potential consequence, a nonphysician who is found to be engaged in the unauthorized practice of medicine is also subject to being held to a higher standard of care in the event of an untoward incident and injury to a patient. In such an event, the practitioner's conduct would be compared with the presumed conduct of a physician acting under the same or similar circumstances, a standard of care which cannot be met by nonphysicians. As a consequence, a finding of negligence is almost assured in such circumstances.

Exercise testing can result in significant claim and litigation. For example, in the recent case of *Tart v. McGann*, 697 F.2d.75 (2d. Cir. 1982), an airline pilot who was undergoing an annual physical examination was required to undergo a graded exercise test. During the final stage of the test he apparently began to experience "difficulty," but did not overtly express this. Following the test, he sustained a myocardial infarction and subsequently brought suit contending that the physicians who performed the test did so negligently and under circumstances where the test should have been stopped early. Although the jury returned a defense verdict, the case was settled for a substantial sum.[14] A principal focus of the case, as well as the deliberations of the jury that followed the presentation of evidence, centered on the issue of whether this plaintiff's facial expressions of fatigue during the final stages of the test should have been sufficient to mandate termination of the test.

A number of other cases, filed and decided or pending, with respect to exercise testing will ultimately add to the judicial examination of this procedure.[15–17] The existence and frequency of these lawsuits will probably increase in the years to come to coincide with the dramatic increase in the use of such tests for diagnostic purposes.[18]

Monitoring of coronary rehabilitation exercise activities will also become the subject of more frequent claims and litigation in years to come, as patients are discharged earlier from hospitals and from supervised coronary rehabilitation programs as a result of reimbursement regulations. The medical profession has necessarily moved toward development of unsupervised, self-monitored exercise programs for coronary patients so that exercise may be undertaken off site by the patient. Some of these activities necessarily carry a higher significance of claim and suit.[19]

POLICIES AND PROCEDURES, COMMUNICATION AND RECORD-KEEPING, AND LIABILITY INSURANCE

On the basis of promulgated standards of care by professional associations, coronary rehabilitation programs should develop individualized policies and procedures for their activities and programs. Such documents should be developed in conjunction with legal and medical consultation and should also cite the standards upon which such policies are based.

Establishment of policies and procedures of the program will serve as the initial line of defense for the program's activity in the event of claim and suit. However, if those policies and procedures are not followed by the program personnel, proof of negligence may come from within the documents themselves. Under these circumstances, negligence and/or malpractice may be established simply by reference to and proof of program policies and breach thereof by program personnel, sometimes even without the requirement of expert testimony.[20] Policies and procedures must be followed, or proof of negligence may come from the documents themselves when compared with the actions or omissions of the personnel in question.

Although policies and procedures may be the first line of defense from claim and suit, thorough and comprehensive communication and record-keeping are close behind. Comprehensive, readable, well-written, and well-documented records are necessary to provide not only acceptable patient care, but also defensible program activity. Many lawyers who represent injured parties say that if a particular notation about a particular procedure is not written and contained within a patient record, such an event did not happen. Those deciding these issues in malpractice cases sometimes agree. As consequence, it is imperative for records of both negative and positive findings to be recorded and for a proper chronological sequence of documentation to be established in patient records. Although the length of time for record retention may vary from state to state, such records should probably be retained for as long as possible owing to the ever-changing rules regarding so-called statutes of limitation. These enactments normally limit the time within which lawsuits may be filed; however, because of rapidly changing court rulings and new legislative enactments, the law in some jurisdictions on this subject may be somewhat confusing.

A last, but necessary, line of defense, is provided to coronary rehabilitation professionals through liability insurance. Practitioners in this health care field must secure and maintain such coverage or face exposure of their personal assets to claim and suit.

RISK MANAGEMENT

Risk management is a series of proactive, ongoing activities designed to prevent untoward events and subsequent claims and suits. Such activities can minimize exposure to claim and suit and may result in reduced liability insurance premiums. These activities can also provide independent, objective evaluation of coronary rehabilitation programs and their compliance with standards and requirements of the industry. Risk management recommendations should also result in better patient care and practice. As a consequence, risk management procedures should be adopted by all coronary rehabilitation programs.

MINIMIZATION OF RISKS

On the basis of the foregoing, recognized medicolegal risks associated with service provision to the coronary patient should be apparent. These risks can be minimized by

1. Development of program protocols and procedures in accordance with nationally recognized practice parameters
2. Proper utilization of personnel for such programs in accordance with the requirements of state licensing laws
3. Appropriate use of program service providers in accordance with established and recognized standards of care
4. Adherence to applicable informed consent requirements as established within the facilities' jurisdiction;
5. Effective and ongoing communication with patients and referring providers
6. Implementation of systematic risk management procedures designed to uncover deficiencies in program policies while adapting as necessary to professional developments and the ever-changing standard of care
7. Purchase of sufficient professional liability insurance for the program and its personnel

SUMMARY

A variety of complex legal questions arise for professional consideration in coronary rehabilitation activity. The nature and diversity of the services rendered necessitate legal counsel assistance. Although a general review of the legal concerns related to coronary rehabilitation activities should benefit practitioners, there must also be a thorough and ongoing examination of all factors related to the professional care owed to the coronary patient undergoing rehabilitative care in order for the practitioner to meet the ex-

pected standard of care and to minimize personal exposure to claim and suit. A number of references are provided for further reading.[21-38]

REFERENCES

1. Herbert DL, Herbert WG: Legal Aspects of Preventive and Rehabilitative Exercise Programs. 2nd Ed. Professional Reports Corp, Canton, OH, 1989
2. The Exercise Standards and Malpractice Reporter. Professional Reports Corp, Canton, OH
3. Year End Review, Medicine by the Book. p. 1. AMA News, January 6, 1989
4. American Heart Association: Special report: Exercise standards, a statement for health professionals. Circulation 82:2286, 1990
4a. American Heart Association: The Exercise Standards Book. American Heart Association, Dallas, TX, 1980
5. American College of Sports Medicine: Guidelines for Graded Exercise Testing and Exercise Prescription. 4th Ed. Lea & Febiger, Philadelphia, 1991
6. American College of Cardiology: Position report on cardiac rehabilitation: Recommendations of the American College of Cardiology on cardiovascular rehabilitation. J Am Coll Cardiol 7:451, 1986
6a. Herbert, DL: An examination of the recommendations for cardiovascular services adopted by the American College of Cardiology. The Exercise Standards and Malpractice Reporter 1:69, 1987
6b. Wenger NK, Balady GJ, Cohn LH et al: Ad Hoc Task Force on Cardiac Rehabilitation: Cardiac rehabilitation services following PTCA and valvular surgery: Guidelines for use. Cardiology 19:4, 1990
6c. Wenger NK, Haskell WL, Kanter K et al: Ad Hoc Task Force on Cardiac Rehabilitation: Cardiac rehabilitation services after cardiac transplantation: Guidelines for use. Cardiology 20:4, 1991
7. American Association of Cardiovascular and Pulmonary Rehabilitation: Cardiac Rehabilitation Services: A Scientific Evaluation. American Association of Cardiovascular and Pulmonary Rehabilitation, Middleton, WI, 1986
8. American Association of Cardiovascular and Pulmonary Rehabilitation: Guidelines for Cardiac Rehabilitation Programs. Human Kinetics Books, Champaign, IL, 1991
9. Herbert, Herbert, Berger: A trial lawyer's guide to the legal implications of recreational, preventive

and rehabilitative exercise program standards of care. Am J Trial Advocacy 11:433, 1988

10. Herbert: Informed consent and new disclosure responsibility for exercise stress testing: The case of *Hedgecorth v. United States*. Exercise Stand Malpract Rep 1:30, 1987

11. Risk disclosure in the informed consent process; Judging the adequacy of disclosure in light of the patients' need for information, an emerging trend. Exercise Stand Malpract Rep 2:56, 1988

12. Is physician supervision of exercise stress testing required?, Exercise Stand Malpract Rep 2:6, 1988

13. ibid 1, p. 113

14. Edelman, The case of *Tart v. McGann:* Legal implications associated with exercise stress testing. Exercise Stand Malpract Rep 1:21, 1987

15. Treadmill fall results in defense verdict. Exercise Stand Malpract Rep 2:30, 1988

16. Are GXTs required for screening of all men over 40? Exercise Stand Malpract Rep 2:30, 1988

17. Herbert: Exercise stress testing lawsuit results in defense verdict. Exercise Stand Malpract Rep 4:23, 1990

18. Dramatic increase in diagnostic testing for MI patients reported. Exercise Stand Malpract Rep 2:28, 1988

19. Herbert: Selected liability considerations of prescribed but unsupervised cardiac rehabilitation activities. Exercise Stand Malpract Rep 2:89, 1988

20. Standard of care and deviation therefrom can be established without expert testimony. Exercise Stand Malpract Rep 3:12, 1989

21. Bacorn R: Legal aspects of exercise stress testing and exercise prescription. p. 156. In Zohman L, Phillips R (eds): Progress in Cardiac Rehabilitation: Medical Aspects of Exercise Testing and Training. Intercontinental Book Corp, New York, 1973

22. Falvo D: Informed consent. p. 193. In Effective Patient Education: A Guide to Increased Compliance. Aspen Systems, Rockville, MD, 1985

23. Haskell W, Stoedefalke K, Seigel G, Wenger N: Law and cardiac rehabilitation. p. 387. In Naughton J, Hellerstein HK (eds): Exercise Testing and Exercise Training in Coronary Heart Disease. Academic Press, New York, 1973

24. Herbert: Selected liability considerations of prescribed but unsupervised cardiac rehabilitation activities. Exercise Stand Malpract Rep 2:33, 1988

25. Herbert: Cardiac rehabilitation services and cost containment measures: Questions of patient safety and provider liability. Exercise Stand Malpract Rep 2:1, 1988

26. Herbert: Informed consent documents for stress testing to comport with *Hedgecorth v. United States*. Exercise Stand Malpract Rep 1:81, 1987

27. Herbert: The use of prospective releases containing exculpatory language in exercise and fitness programs. Exercise Stand Malpract Rep 1:75, 1987

28. Herbert: The application of informed consent principles to exercise stress testing procedures. Exercise Stand Malpract Rep: Lawyers Ed 1:43, 1987

29. Herbert: New perspectives on professional practices in cardiopulmonary rehabilitation: The AACVPR evaluation statement. Exercise Stand Malprac Rep 1:28, 1987

30. Herbert: Standards of practice: The report on cardiac rehabilitation services from the AACVPR. Exercise Stand Malpract Rep 1:9, 1987

31. Herbert W, Herbert D: Legal considerations. In Blair S, Painter P, Pate R et al (eds): Resource Manual for Guidelines for Exercise Testing and Prescription. Lea & Febiger, Philadelphia, 1988

32. Herbert, Herbert: Legal considerations of exercise testing and prescription. In: ACSM Resource Manual for Guidelines for Exercise Testing and Training. Lea & Febiger, Philadelphia, 1988

33. Herbert, Herbert: Legal aspects of cardiac rehabilitation exercise programs, Physician Sportsmed 16:105, 1988

34. Herbert, Herbert: Exercise testing in adults: Legal and procedural considerations for the physical educator and exercise specialist. JOPHER 17–19, 1975

35. Parr, R, Kerr J: Liability and Insurance in Adult Fitness and Cardiac Rehabilitation. University Park Press, Baltimore, 1975

36. Sagall E, Gumatay R: Exercise testing, exercise training programs, and the law, p. 233. In N. K. Wenger (ed): Exercise and the heart. FA Davis, Philadelphia, 1978

37. Sagall E: Legal implications of cardiac rehabilitation programs. p. 640. In Pollock M, Schmidt D (eds): Heart Disease and Rehabilitation. Houghton-Mifflin, Boston, 1979

38. Siegel G: The law and cardiac rehabilitation. p. 387. In Naughton J, Hellerstein H, Mohler I (eds), Exercise Testing and Exercise Training in Coronary Heart Disease. Academic Press, New York, 1973

Appendix 32-1
Informed Consent for Exercise Rehabilitation of Patients with Known or Suspected Heart Disease

Name _____

1. Purpose and Explanation of Procedure

In order to improve my physical exercise capacity and generally aid in my medical treatment for heart disease, I hereby consent to be placed in a rehabilitation program that will include cardiovascular monitoring, physical exercises, dietary counseling, stress reduction, and health education activities. The levels of exercise which I will perform will be based upon the condition of my heart and circulation as determined through a laboratory graded exercise evaluation given at the beginning of the program. I will be given exact instructions regarding the amount and kind of exercise I should do. I agree to participate three times per week in the rehabilitation program. A physician will be present at each session[a] and professionally trained clinical personnel will provide leadership to direct my activities and monitor my electrocardiogram and blood pressure to be certain that I am exercising at the prescribed level. I understand that I am expected to attend every session and to follow physician and staff instructions with regard to any medications which may have been prescribed, exercise, diet, stress management, and smoking cessation. If I am taking prescribed medications, I have already so informed the program staff and further agree to so inform them promptly of any changes which my doctor or I have made with regard to use of these. I will be given the opportunity for periodic re-evaluation with laboratory evaluations at 3 and 6 months after the start of my rehabilitation program. Should I remain in the program beyond 6 months, less frequent evaluations will also be provided. The program physicians may change the foregoing schedule of evaluations for individuals if it is considered necessary for medical management.

I have been informed that in the course of my participation in exercise, I will be asked to complete the activities unless such symptoms as fatigue, shortness of breath, chest discomfort or similar occurrences appear. At that point, I have been advised it is my complete right to stop exercise and that it is my obligation to inform the program personnel of my symptoms. I recognize and hereby state that I have been advised that I should immediately upon experiencing any such symptoms or if I so choose, reduce or stop exercise and inform the program personnel of my symptoms.

---

[a] or will be readily available, as appropriate for the program

NOTE: The law varies from state to state and no form should be adopted or used by any program without individualized legal advice. Reprinted with permission from Herbert & Herbert, Legal Aspects of Preventive and Rehabilitative Exercise Programs: Second Edition. © 1989 by Professional Reports Corporation, Canton, Ohio. All other rights reserved.

(Continues)

I understand that during the performance of exercise, a trained observer will periodically monitor my performance and perhaps take my electrocardiogram, pulse, blood pressure or make the observations for the purpose of monitoring my progress and/or condition. I also understand that the observer may reduce or stop my exercise program, when findings indicate that this should be done for my safety and benefit.

2. Risks

It is my understanding and I have been informed that there exists the possibility during exercise of adverse changes including abnormal blood pressure, fainting, disorders of heart rhythm, and very rare instances of heart attack, stroke, or even death. Every effort I have been told, will be made to minimize these occurrences by proper staff assessment of my condition before each exercise session, staff supervision during exercise and my own careful control of exercise effort. I have also been informed that emergency equipment and personnel are readily available to deal with unusual situations should these occur. I understand that there is a risk of injury, heart attack, stroke, or even death as a result of my exercise, but knowing those risks, it is my desire to participate as herein indicated.

3. Benefits to be Expected and Alternatives Available to Exercise

I understand that this medical treatment may or may not benefit my health status or physical fitness. Generally, participation will help determine what recreational and occupational activities I can safely and comfortably perform. Many individuals in such programs also show improvements in their capacity for physical work. For those who are overweight and able to follow the physician's and dietitian's recommended dietary plan, this program may also aid in achieving appropriate weight reduction and control.

4. Confidentiality and Use of Information

I have been informed that the information which is obtained in this rehabilitation program will be treated as privileged and confidential and will consequently not be released or revealed to any person without my express written consent. I do however agree to the use of any information which is not personally identifiable with me for research and statistical purposes so long as same does not identify my person or provide facts which could lead to my identification. Any other information obtained however, will be used only by the program staff in the course of prescribing exercise for me, planning my rehabilitation program, or advising my personal physician of my progress.

5. Inquiries and Freedom of Consent

I have been given an opportunity to ask certain questions as to the procedures of this program. Generally these requests which have been noted by the interviewing staff member and his/her responses are as follows.

_____

_____

_____

_____

_____

NOTE: The law varies from state to state and no form should be adopted or used by any program without individualized legal advice. Reprinted with permission from Herbert & Herbert, Legal Aspects of Preventive and Rehabilitative Exercise Programs: Second Edition. © 1989 by Professional Reports Corporation, Canton, Ohio. All other rights reserved.

(Continues)

I further understand that there are also other remote risks that may be associated with this program, which have been reviewed with me. Despite a generalized review of these risks, it is still my desire to participate.

I acknowledge that I have read this document in its entirety or that it has been read to me if I have been unable to read same.

I consent to the rendition of all services and procedures as explained herein by all program personnel.

Date _____   _____

                                    Participant's Signature

_____

Witness' Signature

_____

Program Supervisor's Signature

NOTE: The law varies from state to state and no form should be adopted or used by any program without individualized legal advice. Reprinted with permission from Herbert & Herbert, Legal Aspects of Preventive and Rehabilitative Exercise Programs: Second Edition. © 1989 by Professional Reports Corporation, Canton, Ohio. All other rights reserved.

Appendix 32-2
Informed Consent for Exercise Testing of Patients with Known or Suspected Heart Disease

Name _____

1. Purpose and Explanation of Test

I hereby consent to voluntarily engage in an exercise test to determine my exercise capacity and state of cardiovascular health. I also consent to the taking of samples of my exhaled air during exercise to properly measure my oxygen consumption. I also consent, if necessary, to have a small blood sample drawn by needle from my arm for blood chemistry analysis, to the performance of lung function, body fat (skin fold pinch) and standard psychological tests. It is my understanding that the information obtained will help me evaluate future physical activities in which I may engage and aid my doctor in his determination of an appropriate medical treatment for me.

Before I undergo the test, I certify to the program that I am in good health and have had a physical examination conducted by a licensed medical physician within the last _____months, and that my physician has recommended the exercise test and referred me to this particular center for performance of the test. Further, I hereby represent and inform the program that I have completed the pre-test history interview presented to me by the program staff and have provided correct responses to the questions as indicated on the history form or as supplied to the interviewer. It is my understanding that I will be interviewed by a physician and perhaps another person prior to my undergoing the test. In the course of these interviews, it will be determined if there are any reasons which would make it undesirable for me to take the test. Consequently, I understand that it is important that I provide complete and accurate responses to the interviewer and recognize that my failure to do so could lead to possible unnecessary injury to myself during the test.

The test which I will undergo will be performed on a motor driven treadmill or bicycle ergometer with the amount of effort gradually increasing. As I understand it, this increase in effort will continue until I feel and verbally report to the operator any symptoms such as fatigue, shortness of breath or chest discomfort which may appear. It is my understanding and I have been clearly advised that it is my right to request that a test be stopped at any point if I feel unusual discomfort or fatigue. I have been advised that I should immediately upon experiencing any such symptoms or if I so choose, inform the operator that I wish to stop the test at that or any other point. My wishes in this regard shall be absolutely carried out.

NOTE: The law varies from state to state and no form should be adopted or used by any program without individualized legal advice. Reprinted with permission from Herbert & Herbert, Legal Aspects of Preventive and Rehabilitative Exercise Programs: Second Edition. © 1989 by Professional Reports Corporation, Canton, Ohio. All other rights reserved.

(Continues)

It is further my understanding that prior to beginning the test, I will be connected by electrodes and cables to an electrocardiographic recorder which will enable the program personnel to monitor my cardiac (heart) activity. During the test itself, it is my understanding that a physician or (if the physician is in a room nearby) his trained observer will monitor my responses continuously and take frequent readings of blood pressure, the electrocardiogram, and my expressed feelings of discomfort or effort.

Once the test has been completed, but before I am released from the test area, I will be given special instructions about showering and recognition of certain symptoms which may appear within the first 24 hours after the test. I agree to follow these instructions and promptly contact the program personnel or medical providers if such symptoms develop.

2. Risks

It is my understanding and I have been informed that there exists the possibility of adverse changes during the actual test. I have been informed that these changes could include abnormal blood pressure, fainting, disorders of heart rhythm, stroke, and very rare instances of heart attack or even death. Every effort I have been told, will be made to minimize these occurrences by preliminary examination and by precautions and observations taken during the test. I have also been informed that emergency equipment and personnel are readily available to deal with these unusual situations should they occur. I understand that there is a risk of injury, heart attack, stroke, or even death as a result of my performance of this test but knowing those risks, it is my desire to proceed to take the test as herein indicated.

3. Benefits to be Expected and Alternatives Available to the Exercise Testing Procedure

I understand that the possible beneficial results of this test depend upon my doctor's medical reasons for requesting it. It may be helpful in determining my chances of having heart disease that should be treated medically.[a] If my doctor suspects or knows already that I have heart disease, this test may help to evaluate how this disease affects my ability to safety do certain types of physical work or exercises and how to best treat the disease. Other tests for determining the presence or severity of heart disease may be available as alternatives to this exercise test, as are alternative ways to assess my physical fitness. I have had an opportunity to ask about these and have been given answers regarding advantages/disadvantages as noted below:

_____

4. Confidentiality and Use of Information

I have been informed that the information which is obtained in this exercise test will be treated as privileged and confidential and will consequently not be released or revealed to any person without my express written consent. I do, however, agree to the use of any information for research or statistical purposes so long as same does not provide facts which could lead to the identification of my person. Any other information obtained, however, will be used only by the program staff to evaluate my exercise status or needs.

_____

[a] Concept includes both medical and surgical therapies.

(Continues)

5. Inquiries and Freedom of Consent

I have been given an opportunity to ask questions as to the procedure. Generally these requests which have been noted by the testing staff and their responses are as follows:

_____

_____

I further understand that there are also other remote risks that may be associated with this procedure, which have been reviewed with me. Despite a generalized review of these risks, it is still my desire to proceed with the test.

I acknowledge that I have read this document in its entirety or that it has been read to me if I have been unable to read same.

I consent to the rendition of all services and procedures as explained herein by all program personnel.

Date _____   _____
                     Patient's Signature

_____
Witness' Signature

_____
Test Supervisor's Signature

NOTE: The law varies from state to state and no form should be adopted or used by any program without individualized legal advice. Reprinted with permission from Herbert & Herbert, Legal Aspects of Preventive and Rehabilitative Exercise Programs: Second Edition. © 1989 by Professional Reports Corporation, Canton, Ohio. All other rights reserved.

THE FUTURE OF CORONARY REHABILITATION

33

Rehabilitation of the Coronary Patient in the 21st Century: Challenges and Opportunities*

Nanette K. Wenger, M.D.

The enormous advances in the care of the patient with coronary heart disease during the past half century will doubtless substantially influence the scope of and approaches to coronary rehabilitation in the century to come. A position paper of the American College of Cardiology defines cardiovascular rehabilitation as "those exercise and counselling services which will reduce symptoms or improve cardiac function."[1] This preview of tomorrow highlights several of the diverse contributors to changes in coronary rehabilitative care: the changed spectrum and time course of therapy for acute coronary events; the increased scope of patients eligible for exercise rehabilitation; the increased incorporation of a behavioral approach to risk reduction in education and counseling of coronary patients; the relevance of psychosocial factors, including return to work, in comprehensive coronary care; the emergence of quality of life as a health care issue; and the evolving trend toward individualization of coronary rehabilitation services.

---

* Adapted in part from an invited Plenary Lecture at the XI World Congress of Cardiology, Manila, Philippines, February 11–16, 1990, and an invited paper in the Ten Year Anniversary issue of Journal of Cardiopulmonary Rehabilitation, March/April 1991 (with permission).

CHANGED SPECTRUM AND TIME COURSE OF THERAPY FOR ACUTE CORONARY EVENTS

Bed rest was the predominant treatment for acute myocardial infarction in the first part of the 20th century; most hospitalized patients remained virtually immobile for at least 4 to 6 weeks after even an uncomplicated myocardial infarction. Restriction of physical activity during convalescence lasted at least several months, and return to work, if it occurred, was much delayed; many such individuals were retired from their jobs or at best returned to lower levels of activity and responsibility. Coronary care units and electrocardiographic (ECG) monitoring techniques had not yet been developed; and most antianginal preparations in current use were not therapeutic considerations at that time. Even the use of sublingual nitroglycerin during acute myocardial infarction was challenged. Cardiac catheterization and coronary angiography, coronary bypass surgery (CABG), cardiac pacemakers, and coronary angioplasty (PTCA) were advances for the future.

The most dramatic changes in the clinical outcome of myocardial infarction during the past decade have been the lessened pathophysiologic consequences and improved survival from the acute illness; these relate predominantly to earlier and more intensive diagnostic and therapeutic interventions during the acute phase of myocardial infarction. The result of coronary thrombolysis, using a variety of pharmacologic preparations, with and without subsequent myocardial revascularization procedures (CABG or PTCA) when appropriate, has been a decrease in the pathophysiologic severity of the residual disease among patients so treated during the course of acute infarction. At discharge from the hospital, coronary patients have less myocardial necrosis, less residual myocardial ischemia, and less resultant myocardial dysfunction than previously. Therefore, survivors of acute myocardial infarction have less physical disability, a greater likelihood of both early and late survival, and a lower risk of proximate recurrent coronary events. Exercise rehabilitation can be initiated earlier and often at higher intensity than previously; and return to work or to usual pre-illness activities often can be undertaken promptly.

Even among patients not suitable for the dramatic myocardial revascularization interventions just described, a substantial decrease has occurred in the time course of their coronary care, such that the period of restriction and disability has been compressed. This has resulted in a shortened hospitalization and more prompt institution of multifaceted medical management.

This changing spectrum of coronary care has engendered both opportunities and challenges in that the shortened period of illness, often termed a "compression of morbidity," is characterized both by advantages and by disadvantages. For example, a patient with an initial episode of angina pectoris may be hospitalized to exclude myocardial infarction, undergo coronary angiography and PTCA if appropriate on the next day, and return home the following morning with a remedied coronary artery morphology, not having sustained myocardial damage and thus having a more favorable prognosis, requiring no restriction of activity, and able to promptly resume his or her prior lifestyle; unquestionably, this is an advantageous outcome. The challenge is that these patients, as a consequence of the brief illness and hospitalization, often fail to understand that they have a significant underlying illness;

this results in a decreased perception of the need for or interest in preventive care and less adherence to the recommendations for risk reduction.[2] These patients must adopt lifestyles designed to limit the progression of their atherosclerosis, i.e., conventional coronary risk reduction, if the favorable outcome of the myocardial revascularization procedure is to be maintained. Further, these patients must appreciate their requirement for serial medical surveillance, despite the brief episode of acute illness, because this brief episode represented a potentially life-threatening event. Even for patients who have undergone myocardial revascularization procedures following myocardial infarction or for the low-risk postinfarction patients, the challenge in their rehabilitative care, because they are likely to do well at least for the short term, is to meet their continuing need for preventive coronary care. The occurrence of myocardial infarction and the consequent requirement for the acute interventions cited indicate that this subset of patients has accelerated atherosclerosis; progression of the atherosclerosis must be prevented and efforts at inducing regression attempted[3] if subsequent recurrent acute coronary events are to be averted or delayed.

At the other extreme of the spectrum is the seriously chronically ill and often elderly coronary patient. Contemporary coronary care has offered the advantage of enabling many patients in this category to survive two or three decades of recurrent coronary events, including episodes of unstable angina pectoris, recurrent myocardial infarction, congestive heart failure, and a variety of arrhythmias, often punctuated by intercurrent PTCA or CABG surgery. Despite the 10- or 20-year survival with accelerated coronary atherosclerosis, the typical outcome is end-stage ischemic cardiomyopathy, for which cardiac transplantation is the only current therapeutic option and is not available to aged coronary patients. Even for these transplant candidates, interim rehabilitative care[4] must overcome the systemic physical deconditioning that has resulted from prolonged and disabling symptoms of decreased cardiac output and often from the inactivity related to the protracted hospitalizations for ischemic cardiomyopathy. These patients' emotional problems relate to both the anxiety and depression attendant on the symptomatic and disabling illness and the anxiety about incipient cardiac transplantation; both must be addressed. Further, candidates for cardiac transplantation must learn the alterations in lifestyle needed to decrease conventional coronary risk attributes since, in part owing to the immunosuppressant therapies, coronary atherosclerosis is accelerated in the transplanted heart. Although most patients following cardiac transplantation, after a regimen of exercise training, have an adequate physical work capacity, detailed attention to their rehabilitative care may be required to address relatively complex issues of psychosocial adjustment, as well as the needs for coronary risk modification.[4]

These extremes in the diversity of the clinical profile of coronary patients have necessitated diversity in all therapeutic approaches to coronary heart disease, including rehabilitative care. Nowhere is this more evident than in the changing characteristics of exercise rehabilitation. Today there is uniform early initiation of physical activity after a coronary event, with ambulatory exercise rehabilitation often commencing shortly after discharge from the hospital. Newer data have documented a satisfactory training effect from an exercise regimen of lesser intensity than that previously undertaken,[5] with the decrease in exercise intensity compensated for by a somewhat longer duration of exercise. Exercise training at a target heart rate range of 60 to 75% of the highest heart rate safely achieved at exercise testing, as compared with the prior 70 to 85% target heart rate range, appears associated with better adherence because of greater comfort during exercise and more enjoyment of the exercise. The lower exercise intensity is further characterized by greater safety in that coronary patients exercise further from their ischemic threshold; therefore, a decreased amount and duration of professional supervision of exercise is entailed, with a resultant decrease in cost. Finally, this approach fosters a progressive transition to independence in exercising, which is likely to encourage lifelong exercise habits.

The conduct of exercise training for coronary patients has also changed substantially from the early years, when professional supervision was ubiquitous because little was known about the safety of exercise for coronary patients; however, supervision during the initial years did not entail continuous ECG monitoring, because ECG telemetry was not available. Contemporary experience has confirmed the safety of non-ECG-monitored exercise regimens for low-risk coronary patients.[6] Patients hospitalized for an acute coronary event now characteristically undergo risk stratification procedures to determine the need for invasive interventions or more intensive therapies. These data characterizing risk status, available at the time of discharge from the hospital, can enable decisions about the need for supervision of exercise rehabilitation. High-risk coronary patients are referred for myocardial revascularization procedures; those not suitable for this intervention require at least initial supervision of their exercise training, often with ECG monitoring. Generally accepted high-risk characteristics include a significantly reduced functional capacity (less than 6 METs); depressed ventricular function (manifested by a decreased ejection fraction, cardiac enlargement, or a third heart sound); development of angina pectoris or ECG evidence of myocardial ischemia at low intensities of exercise (a heart rate below 120 beats/min or an exercise work load of less than 6 METs); or an abnormal hemodynamic response to exercise, typically exercise-related hypotension, that reflects exercise-induced ischemic ventricular dysfunction with a resultant decrease in cardiac output. Often, several of these features are present simultaneously in high-risk coronary patients. Other attributes associated with increased risk include complex or sustained ventricular arrhythmias, a prolonged QT interval on the ECG, and survival after ventricular fibrillation not associated with myocardial infarction. Patient characteristics, rather than disease status, also define another high-risk patient subset, which includes patients unable to monitor their exercise heart rate or perceived level of exertion[7] and those who habitually exceed their recommended intensity for exercise training.

About half of all survivors of myocardial infarction are characterized as at low risk, and unsupervised exercise or home exercise training regimens for these patients are feasible and safe.[8]

The improvement in functional capacity appears comparable with supervised and unsupervised exercise. Although there is consensus in the literature that more rapid improvement in functional capacity occurs in a supervised exercise setting, much of this advantage appears related to the higher intensity of exercise training for patients enrolled in supervised exercise programs.

Information about adherence to unsupervised exercise regimens is available to supplement these data about the efficacy of unsupervised exercise training. Different reports in the literature describe better adherence, worse adherence, and comparable adherence to unsupervised as compared with supervised exercise modalities.[9–14] Most of the differences appear dependent on patient and family characteristics, such that patients with prior exercise experience are more likely to adhere to the regimen, as are patients with family and social support.[15] Cigarette smokers and overweight persons are less likely to adhere to an exercise regimen, as are patients who perceive their health status as poor. These features can help physicians identify subsets of coronary patients likely to do well with unsupervised exercise as compared with other subsets for whom supervision appears preferable.[10]

The advantages of unsupervised exercise are that coronary patients with this option have a greater availability of exercise rehabilitation, particularly patients who live far from a medical center. Other advantages include lower cost and increased patient satisfaction. The convenience is great in that patients do not have to adhere to a program schedule or commute to a program site; the time that would have been spent commuting is recommended to be translated into engaging in a longer duration of exercise to compensate for the lower intensity of exercise rehabilitation that is characteristic of unsupervised regimens. However, the long-term adherence to unsupervised exercise has not yet been ascertained.

The disadvantages of unsupervised exercise offer challenges for the future. Absence of supervision limits or obviates the opportunity to teach middle-aged or older adults, many of whom have had no exercise experience since childhood, the signs and symptoms of exercise excess or exercise intolerance. Complications may occur because patients have not adequately learned how to self-monitor their intensity of exercise; how to limit musculoskeletal problems and other orthopedic injuries; how to select appropriate clothing, footwear, and equipment for exercise; and how to modify their intensity of exercise on the basis of environmental considerations, particularly extremes of temperature and humidity. A further disadvantage is the lack of opportunity to teach patients about coronary risk reduction. The relative roles of peer support and professional support in the total rehabilitative process remain uncertain, but neither is available in an unsupervised exercise setting.

The challenge is to extend the benefits of supervised exercise training to coronary patients for whom unsupervised exercise otherwise appears appropriate. Short-term exercise supervision offers patients the opportunity to practice newly acquired exercise skills and to receive the support needed by some for maintenance of an exercise regimen. But, for example, how can exercise adherence be improved? Is there a role for heart rate recorders or similar equipment to document exercise adherence, intensity, and duration at home? What about resuscitation from the rare cardiac event? Resuscitation is characteristically successful in a supervised exercise setting; can a non-health care professional, i.e., a friend or an exercising companion, provide comparable safety? Is there a role for telephone contact with health professionals? Will these factors enable an improved response to patient concerns and questions in the early weeks following a hospitalization? Such questions are typically rapidly and effectively addressed during a supervised exercise regimen. Most important, in regard to educational aspects, how can technology help? As will be discussed below, educational and exercise videocassettes are available for use at home. Is this or other technology of value in encouraging exercise adherence and providing satisfactory nonexercise education and counseling?

INCREASED SCOPE OF PATIENTS ELIGIBLE FOR EXERCISE REHABILITATION

In the early years of exercise rehabilitation, this modality was considered suitable predominantly for patients recovered from uncomplicated myocardial infarction. Many categories of patients who, in prior years, were arbitrarily excluded from exercise rehabilitation, now constitute a large percentage of the enrollees in structured exercise rehabilitation programs. These include elderly coronary patients; high-risk or symptomatic coronary patients with combinations of myocardial ischemia, arrhythmia, or compensated congestive heart failure; and a variety of other medically complex patients.

Exercise regimens for these patients are characterized by lower intensity, longer duration, and often an initial requirement for supervision and ECG monitoring.[1,16] The goal of exercise for these categories of patients is often an improvement in functional status so as to enable maintenance of independent living[17]; this contrasts with the goal of improvement of functional capacity to permit a return to remunerative work, which is a frequently desired outcome for younger and less impaired patients.

Major demographic changes in the population, not only in the United States but worldwide, have been characterized by a progressive increase in the population older than 65 years. In both industrialized and developing nations, the population older than 80 years is the subset whose numbers are increasing most rapidly. A large proportion of elderly persons in the United States live independently and are reasonably well, alert, and active; many of the "oldest old" are likely to be encountered among coronary patients.[18]

This contemporary population explosion among the alert and functional elderly, for whom coronary heart disease is a frequent health problem, has resulted in their increased use of the expensive high technology involved in cardiovascular diagnostic and therapeutic procedures. More than one-third of all coronary angiography, PTCA, CABG, and pacemaker implantation procedures currently performed in the United States are undertaken in patients older than 65 years; the 12% of the U.S. population in this age group now uses one-third of all health care resources.

Physicians increasingly recommend graduated exercise programs for their elderly coronary patients, both those with an uncomplicated clinical course and those with medically complex situations. Walking programs are considered optimal for elderly patients in that they require no special exercise skills, facilities, or equipment. Walking provides an adequate training stimulus for most elderly coronary patients as it constitutes a substantial percentage of the lesser total aerobic capacity characteristic of aging. The age-dependent relative aerobic costs of walking at a constant pace have been emphasized by Bruce et al., who noted that, whereas walking may not provide a reasonable training stimulus for individuals between ages 30 and 60, populations in their 80s and 90s obtained an excellent training effect from walking at the same pace.[19] In addition to improving the physical work capacity of many elderly coronary patients, walking and other forms of exercise help to decrease anxiety and depression and to aid in weight control. A modest improvement in physical work capacity, coupled with the teaching of techniques of work simplification, may enable the protracted maintenance of independent living, an outcome valued by most elderly coronary patients and a cost-saving feature of rehabilitative care as well; in most societies, one of the most costly components of health care for the elderly is custodial care.

Much has also been learned about the exercise training of symptomatic coronary patients. Only in recent decades have patients with angina pectoris, as well as those with symptomless myocardial ischemia (evident at exercise testing), been enrolled in exercise rehabilitation programs. Patients with angina pectoris typically have more physiologic impairment both before and after myocardial infarction than do many patients without residual myocardial ischemia or those recovered from successful myocardial revascularization procedures. Patients with angina pectoris, both with and without myocardial infarction, were previously often underserved in regard to their need for rehabilitative services, particularly exercise rehabilitation. A further major recent advance has been the documentation that patients receiving multiple categories of anti-ischemic (antianginal) drugs can benefit from exercise training and can achieve a training effect; this includes nitrate drugs, calcium-blocking drugs, beta-blocking drugs, and combinations of these. The predominant effect of these drugs, a reduction in myocardial oxygen demand, lessens symptoms and allows training to proceed, with resultant improvement in the patient's functional capacity. It has also been learned that exercise testing for exercise prescription should be undertaken with patients on the drug regimen to be used during exercise training. An additional advance of recent years has been the delineation that the degree of ventricular dysfunction correlates poorly with the patient's exercise capacity. Many patients with ventricular dysfunction and compensated congestive cardiac failure have successfully and safely undergone exercise training, with a resultant improvement in their functional capacity, without undue risk, and typically without deterioration of ventricular function. The training effect is predominantly or exclusively peripheral, involving intact skeletal muscle, such that trained skeletal muscle increases its oxygen extraction from the perfusing blood, with a resultant decrease in myocardial oxygen demand at submaximal levels of exercise. The lessened myocardial oxygen demand in the trained individual is further determined by a redistribution of the exercise cardiac output, a decrease in systemic vascular resistance, and a variety of autonomic adaptations; the lower heart rate response to exercise is a major result of these peripheral adaptations resulting from exercise training. The low- to moderate-intensity exercise training characteristic for patients with residual ischemia or ventricular dysfunction, or other medically complex coronary patients, results either predominantly or exclusively in peripheral adaptations to training; cardiac adaptations are described only with high-intensity and long-duration exercise training of selected coronary patients. Nevertheless, the optimal mode(s), duration, and surveillance needs for the exercise training of these patients have yet to be determined.

Even among elderly, impaired, and otherwise high-risk coronary patients, exercise training affords additional benefits including favorable metabolic changes such as lowered triglyceride levels, increased sensitivity to insulin, improved high-density lipoprotein (HDL) to low-density lipoprotein (LDL) or total cholesterol ratios, greater ease of weight control, and important psychological adaptations, particularly the renouncing of sick role behaviors. Musculoskeletal benefits involve, in addition to the improved work capacity, an increase in joint mobility and stability and improved neuromuscular coordination.

Also new to this decade has been the demonstration that mild to moderate resistance exercise training can safely and effectively improve both strength and cardiovascular endurance,[20,21] enabling the performance of a variety of tasks of daily living that require both physical strength and muscular exertion. This can improve performance both in the workplace and at leisure activities. Resistance training also provides diversity in the exercise regimen, which may increase patient interest and adherence.

INCORPORATION OF A BEHAVIORAL APPROACH TO RISK REDUCTION IN THE EDUCATION AND COUNSELING OF CORONARY PATIENTS

Coronary patients in the 21st century will require an elaborate spectrum of education and counseling that encompasses coronary preventive aspects (particularly coronary risk reduction) and therapeutic aspects including diet, activity, and medications and addresses individual expectations of outcome, including return to work. Return to work is likely to become an economic imperative for many patients in the 21st century. Based on a recent Harris poll, 60% of U.S. coronary patients aged 35 and older have a high school education or less, so that physicians treating these patients must work harder to improve the efficacy of communication with them. Weed observed that "the most important member of the health-care team is the patient, highly motivated, not costing anything, even willing to pay—and there is one for every member of the population."[22] Stated another way, we must accept the challenge to inform, educate, and counsel the coronary patient, the most important member of our health care team.

There is also accumulating evidence that conventional coronary risk reduction results in both survival and morbidity benefits in elderly patients,[23] so that the education and training for coronary risk reduction should be incorporated in their rehabilitative care.

Secondary prevention is an integral part of rehabilitation. Those experienced in adult education are well aware that the isolated provision of cognitive information is inadequate in attempting to change lifestyle characteristics. Education and counseling must include training in the skills needed for the adoption of health-related behaviors, provision of an opportunity to practice these skills in coronary risk reduction, and subsequent serial measurement of benefit and periodic reinforcement of successful coronary risk reduction.[24] Opportunities to initially institute coronary risk reduction are often limited by the short hospitalization; also, patients not enrolled in supervised exercise regimens have less access to education and counseling. Are educational telephone conference calls of value? Can home videocassettes provide nonexercise education and counseling?

The diverse populations of coronary patients, however, are likely to have diverse educational preferences. Some may elect the traditional didactic presentation of information, with lectures and group discussions, that were characteristic of most patient education programs during the recent decades. Other patients may prefer teaching tapes, films, or pamphlets that may be reviewed either individually at home or together with family members. Yet others may learn better by participatory activities such as workshops that teach cooking, purchase and preparation of food designed for weight reduction, sodium restriction, or cholesterol lowering; or other participatory demonstrations such as techniques for handling stressful situations or other concerns. Combinations of these techniques are likely to be valuable.

Can technology help? Can technologic advances aid primary care physicians to deliver more effective, predictable, and high-quality teaching that will enable better learning? Can technology help provide appropriate and timely reinforcement and extend the influence and services of a variety of health care professionals?[25]

A number of new technology-based educational approaches are currently available, and more are likely to appear in routine use. Integra-

tion of currently available technology into techniques for patient education and behavior modification has gained increasing acceptance. Educational interactive microcomputer programs and a variety of audiovisual aids are now available, including videocassettes designed for use at home with workbooks for record keeping; interactive home computer software; and a variety of other equipment-based educational approaches. The challenge will be to select the best among them to meet the learning needs of an individual patient or of groups of patients. Appropriately used, technology may extend the influence of health care professionals and provide effective teaching and reminders; inappropriately used, technology may detract from the educational message and squander valuable resources that could better be used to improve the information and skills of the coronary patient.

PSYCHOSOCIAL FACTORS, INCLUDING RETURN TO WORK, IN COMPREHENSIVE CORONARY CARE

Although White stated, a number of years ago, that "it is of importance to realize that the heart may recover more rapidly than the depressed mental state which is so often a complication,"[26] a current unmet need is effective psychosocial assessment and interventional counseling for coronary patients.

An initial need, yet in the research setting, is to explore the most appropriate techniques for formal assessment of psychosocial complications of coronary illness. Will it be possible to identify the patient at high risk of adverse psychosocial outcomes, as is currently possible for medical complications of the coronary illness? Will this identification enable the categorization of psychosocial impairment and the targeting of early interventions; and can these components of care improve the return to employment, to sexual function, and to family and community roles? Are there psychosocial problems unique to elderly or severely impaired coronary patients?

Women with coronary disease have less favorable psychosocial outcomes than do men, but it remains uncertain whether this reflects gender, age, comorbidity, severity of illness, and/or a less effective social support system for women in coronary rehabilitation programs and in the community. More information is needed to enable appropriate targeted intervention strategies.

Much has been learned about the characteristics of coronary patients at high risk for failing to return to work, both after myocardial infarction and after myocardial revascularization procedures: older age, adequate nonwork income, anxiety or depression, occurrence of symptoms with effort, lower social class, less education, higher physical activity level of the work, perception of the coronary illness as job-related, more than 6 months of unemployment following a coronary event, and lack of physician advice to resume work.[27,28] Successful return to work is one measure of satisfactory rehabilitation and social integration. Obviously, each adverse aspect just cited offers opportunities for amelioration; different patient subsets present different problems. Return to work is less common among women and occurs earlier after PTCA than after CABG surgery.

A number of pilot studies have shown improvement in the perception of health status when coronary patients are informed of the implications of the physiologic results obtained at exercise testing as they relate to the performance of daily living and occupational and recreational activities.[29] Other studies have shown an improved perception of health status based on review of the benefits that can be expected to occur from effective coronary risk reduction.

QUALITY OF LIFE AS A HEALTH CARE ISSUE

The increased prevalence of chronic illness in recent decades has contributed importantly to the emergence of quality of life as a health care issue. Chronic illness, by definition, is one for which therapies are not curative, but are rather designed to limit the disabling consequences of the illness. Thus, in a medical care context, quality of life encompasses the ways in which a patient's life is affected both by the illness and by the components of its care; this has been described by Spitzer as "clinically relevant human attributes."[30]

Clinicians are becoming more aware of the dimensions of quality of life, the components to be examined if quality of life is to be used as an outcome measure for the assessment of health care. As a response to treatment, health-related quality of life encompasses the patient's resultant comfort, sense of well-being, and life satisfaction; the ability to maintain physical, sexual, emotional, and intellective function; and the ability to participate in valued activities in the home, the workplace, and the community. This is a uniquely subjective evaluation, in that it addresses the values and expectations of individual patients. For example, what do patients desire as an outcome of the care for coronary heart disease? Do they want only to survive and recover? Do they want to feel better, or do they want to feel completely well? Do they want to resume an independent and active lifestyle, or is a return to work an option? As patient satisfaction with outcomes of medical care is examined, a major determinant appears to relate to the quality of life attributes just cited.

Mosteller et al. summarized the challenge of ascertaining life quality, applicable as an outcome of rehabilitative care, in observing that "public impression to the contrary, the bulk of medical and surgical treatment is not life-saving, but is aimed at improving the state or quality of life. Most diseases are not dramatically fatal, but chip away at comfort and happiness. At the same time, treatments for life-threatening diseases often have different impacts on patient comfort. To the extent that we are unable to measure and compare the effects of treatments on the quality of the patient's life, we are unable to document advantages of treatments as well as their defects."[31] Whereas much of the detailed ascertainment of quality of life is conducted in research settings, there is increasing emphasis on the development of very brief instruments that can be used by the clinician in office practice to help guide rehabilitative and other care.

As outcomes of exercise training are examined,

particularly in very low-risk coronary patients, who are likely to be more common in the future, these patients with less severe disease are unlikely to demonstrate an improvement in survival or a lessening of reinfarction as an outcome of rehabilitative care or most other interventions. Despite the demonstration by meta-analysis that exercising patients in exercise trials of prior years had a 25% survival advantage and a lessening of reinfarction, the contemporary application of coronary thrombolysis, myocardial revascularization when appropriate, and improved pharmacotherapy have so lowered the postinfarction mortality and recurrence of proximate reinfarction that there is little likelihood that exercise rehabilitation or other interventions will provide further benefit in short-term survival or reduced reinfarction in a statistically demonstrable fashion. Morbidity and mortality outcomes must, then, be considered insensitive measures of the efficacy of an intervention in this very low-risk population; hence, quality-of-life attributes are likely to receive greater consideration as outcome measures for coronary rehabilitative care.

Quality-of-life issues are particularly relevant to rehabilitative care in that the goals of rehabilitation for coronary patients address precisely the quality-of-life domains just outlined. Rehabilitative care is designed to alleviate or lessen activity-related symptoms, to improve functional capacity, to limit the adverse psychological consequences that may lead to unwarranted invalidism, to retard the progression of the underlying coronary atherosclerosis, and to enable the patient to return to a productive and personally satisfying role in society. Quality of life is a relevant outcome variable for coronary rehabilitative care because it also reflects the patient's personal value system, life satisfaction, and judgments about perceived health status. Perceived health status, in turn, has been demonstrated to correlate better with mortality risk than did many more objective measures of disease[32-34] and to correlate better with work performance than did objectively measured functional capacity. Of added interest, perceived health status may be favorably altered by education and counseling in a setting of coronary rehabilitative care.

INDIVIDUALIZATION OF CORONARY REHABILITATION

In the early years of coronary rehabilitation, the programs available were highly structured, relatively inflexible, and constituted as rather impersonal regimens to which most or all patients were required to conform. These programs were often elaborate and entailed what many perceived to be an excess of time and costs. During the past decade, a major change has occurred that is characterized by a trend toward the delivery of the specific rehabilitative services that are appropriate for an individual patient's characteristics, requirements, and preferences. This approach may prove the most cost-effective concept in coronary rehabilitative care in that highly individualized care is ideal to address the diverse populations of coronary patients with respect to age, severity of illness, comorbidity, and expectations of outcome. Even within these diverse populations, integrated multidisciplinary rehabilitative care must be tailored to an individual patient's needs, as is routinely done with other aspects of coronary care.[35]

Several selected examples can illustrate the concept of individualization in coronary rehabilitation. The first involves a patient recovered from a recent myocardial infarction, who has been determined to be at low risk for a proximate recurrent coronary event by appropriate risk stratification procedures. This patient can therefore exercise independently (with this optimally undertaken after a brief orientation to exercise) and does not require ECG-monitored or even supervised exercise training. The major rehabilitative needs of this category of patients are the education and skill-building required to undertake and maintain effective coronary risk reduction and a healthy lifestyle. Subsequent periodic surveillance can ascertain the improvement in physical work capacity as a result of home exercise. By contrast, a second coronary patient is at high risk for a recurrent coronary event because of residual myocardial ischemia, but has been determined to be unsuitable for myocardial revascularization procedures; this patient, at least initially, requires close observation of exercise training, probably including real-time ECG monitoring. Even after functional restoration is achieved, this patient may also require work assessment and vocational counseling, because the high-risk status may limit certain occupations and moderate or high intensities of physical activity. There may be complicating psychosocial problems.

These, again, illustrate the extremes, but it is likely that with the current greater emphasis on comprehensive coronary risk reduction, psychosocial assessment, and vocational assessment, including vocational counseling, a variety of differing specific educational and counseling components will be selected for specific patients.

The challenge in the 21st century will be to select, from among the rehabilitative services available, those appropriate for an individual coronary patient and to tailor the method of delivery of those services. These selections will be based both on medical recommendations and on patient preferences, but should always be designed to encourage progressive independence in coronary rehabilitation and long-term comprehensive care. This concept is attractive to patients, to their physicians, and to those responsible for the costs of care.

To ascertain the cost effectiveness of these rehabilitative interventions, we should define, in the initial plan of care, both quantitatively and on a temporal basis, the desired and anticipated goals of each of the rehabilitative therapies recommended. As an example, one patient should increase his or her exercise capacity as a result of exercise training, with a specified improvement in the MET level anticipated to occur within 3 months; at the same time a specified amount of weight reduction or cholesterol lowering should be anticipated within a set number of months, as response to either dietary counseling or pharmacologic therapy, or both. Analysis of outcomes in this manner will identify the components of rehabilitative care with successful outcomes for an individual patient and those that should be replaced by other approaches to improve the effectiveness of the therapy. For structured rehabilitation programs, the sum of outcomes in each category across patients will determine whether a particular component of rehabilitative care is successful in obtaining the desired outcome or whether that component warrants reformatting or other alteration in the plan of care.

Cost effectiveness assessment of coronary rehabilitation services must also consider quality-of-life attributes, particularly in the polar situations (very high-risk and very low-risk groups), in which morbidity and mortality are insensitive and inadequate measures of the efficacy of an intervention. Favorable outcome features likely to derive from coronary rehabilitation programs are those that enable patients to cope with the problems of a chronic illness such that a personally satisfactory lifestyle is attained.

Over time, and probably with the aid of newer technology, even more varied patterns of delivery of rehabilitative services are likely to develop. These different approaches to coronary rehabilitative care may increase their applicability to a variety to settings, enabling not only hospital-based but also community-based care in a variety of settings—home, workplace, community clinic, or senior adult center, to name a few. This should also foster rehabilitative care that is applicable to a wide spectrum of severities of coronary illness. The major challenge is to encourage informed, motivated, and innovative health professionals to develop and provide the multifaceted components of the coronary rehabilitative care needed for the patient of the 21st century.

REFERENCES

1. American College of Cardiology: Position report on cardiac rehabilitation: Recommendations of the American College of Cardiology on cardiovascular rehabilitation. J Am Coll Cardiol 7:451, 1986
2. Kinsey MG, Fletcher BJ, Rice CR et al: In-hospital coronary risk factor education in patients after coronary bypass surgery followed by home monitored exercise: A four-year follow-up. J Cardiopulmonary Rehabil (abstract). 7:501, 1987
3. Ornish D, Brown SE, Scherwitz LW et al: Can lifestyle changes reverse coronary heart disease? The Lifestyle Heart Trial. Lancet 336:129, 1990
4. American College of Cardiology Ad Hoc Task

Force: Cardiac rehabilitation services after cardiac transplantation: Guidelines for use. Cardiology 20:4, 1991

5. Blumenthal JA, Rejeski WJ, Walsh-Riddle M et al: Comparison of high- and low-intensity exercise training early after acute myocardial infarction. Am J Cardiol 61:26, 1988

6. VanCamp SP, Peterson RA: Cardiovascular complications of outpatient cardiac rehabilitation programs. JAMA 256:1160, 1986

7. Borg G: Psychophysical bases of perceived exertion. Med Sci Sports Exercise 14:377, 1982

8. Wenger, NK: Home versus supervised exercise training after myocardial infarction and myocardial revascularization procedures. Pract Cardiol 15:47, 1989

9. DeBusk RF, Haskell WL, Miller NH et al: Medically directed at-home rehabilitation soon after clinically uncomplicated acute myocardial infarction: A new model for patient care. Am J Cardiol 55:251, 1985

10. Erdman RAM, Duivenvoorden HV, Verhage F et al: Predictability of beneficial effects in cardiac rehabilitation: A randomized clinical trial of psychosocial variables. J Cardiopulmonary Rehabil 6:206, 1986

11. Hands ME, Briffa T, Henderson K et al: Functional capacity and left ventricular function: The effect of supervised and unsupervised exercise rehabilitation soon after coronary artery bypass graft surgery. J Cardiopulmonary Rehabil 7:578, 1987

12. Miller NH, Haskell WL, Berra K, DeBusk RF: Home versus group exercise training for increasing functional capacity after myocardial infarction. Circulation 70:645, 1984

13. Stevens R, Hanson P: Comparison of supervised and unsupervised exercise training after coronary bypass surgery. Am J Cardiol 53:1524, 1984

14. Heath GW, Maloney PM, Fure CW: Group exercise versus home exercise in coronary artery bypass graft patients: Effects on physical activity habits. J Cardiopulmonary Rehabil 7:190, 1987

15. Friis R, Taff GA: Social support and social networks, and coronary heart disease and rehabilitation. J Cardiopulmonary Rehabil 6:132, 1986

16. Williams RS, Miller H, Koisch FB, Jr, et al: Guidelines for unsupervised exercise in patients with ischemic heart disease. J Cardiopulmonary Rehabil 3:213, 1981

17. Squires RW, Lavie CJ, Brandt TR et al: Cardiac rehabilitation in patients with severe ischemic left ventricular dysfunction. Mayo Clin Proc 62:997, 1987

18. Wenger NK, Marcus FI, O'Rourke RA (eds): 18th Bethesda Conference. Cardiovascular disease in the elderly. J Am Coll Cardiol, 10(Suppl. A), 1987

19. Bruce RA, Larson EB, Stratton J: Physical fitness, functional aerobic capacity, and responses to physical training or bypass surgery in coronary patients. J Cardiopulmonary Rehabil 9:24, 1989

20. Kelemen MH, Stewart KJ, Gillilan RE et al: Circuit weight training in cardiac patients. J Am Coll Cardiol 7:38, 1986

21. Franklin BA, Bonzheim K, Gordon S, Timmis GC: Resistance training in cardiac rehabilitation. J Cardiopulmonary Rehabil 11:99, 1991

22. Weed LL: A touchstone for medical education. p. 13. In: Harvard Medical Alumni Bulletin. Harvard University Press, 1974

23. Hermanson B, Omenn GS, Kronmal RA et al: Beneficial six-year outcome of smoking cessation in older men and women with coronary artery disease: Results from the CASS Registry. N Engl J Med 319:1365, 1988

24. Blumenthal JA, Califf R, Williams S, Hindman M: Cardiac rehabilitation: A new frontier for behavioral medicine. J Cardiac Rehabil 3:637, 1983

25. Wenger NK (ed): The Education of the Patient with Cardiac Disease in the Twenty-first Century. LeJacq Publishing Inc, New York, 1986

26. White PD (ed): Heart Disease, MacMillian, New York, 1951

27. Almeida D, Bradford JM, Wenger NK et al: Return to work after coronary bypass surgery. Circulation 68(Suppl. II):II-205, 1983

28. Walter PJ (ed): Return to Work After Coronary Artery Bypass Surgery: Psychosocial and Economic Aspects. Springer-Verlag, New York, 1985

29. Taylor CB, Bandura A, Ewart CK et al: Exercise testing to enhance wives' confidence in their husbands' cardiac capability soon after clinically uncomplicated acute myocardial infarction. Am J Cardiol 55:635, 1985

30. Spitzer WO: Keynote address. State of science 1986: Quality of life and functional status as target variables for research. J Chronic Dis 40:465, 1987

31. Mosteller F, Gilbert JP, McPeek B: Reporting standards and research strategies for controlled trials. Controlled Clin Trials 1:37, 1980

32. LaRue A, Bank L, Jarvik L, Hetland M: Health in old age: How do physicians' rating and self-ratings compare? J Gerontol 34:687, 1979

33. Kaplan GA, Camacho TC: Perceived health and mortality: A nine year follow-up of the human population laboratory cohort. Am J Epidemiol 117:292, 1983

34. Mossey JM, Shapiro E: Self-rated health: A pre-dictor of mortality among the elderly. Am J Public Health 72:800, 1982

35. Berra K, Franklin BA, Hall LK et al: Guidelines for Cardiac Rehabilitation Programs. AACVPR. Human Kinetics Books, Champaign, IL, 1991

Index